Textbook of Anaesthesia

Textbook of Anaesthesia

Edited by

G. Smith BSc, MD, FFARCS
Professor of Anaesthesia,
University of Leicester School of Medicine, Leicester, UK

A. R. Aitkenhead BSc, MB, ChB, FFARCS
Senior Lecturer in Anaesthesia,
University of Leicester School of Medicine, Leicester, UK

CHURCHILL LIVINGSTONE
EDINBURGH LONDON MELBOURNE AND NEW YORK 1985

CHURCHILL LIVINGSTONE
Medical Division of Longman Group Limited

Distributed in the United States of America by Churchill
Livingstone Inc., 1560 Broadway, New York, N.Y.
10036, and by associated companies, branches and
representatives throughout the world.

First published 1985

ISBN 0 443 02825 7

British Library Cataloguing in Publication Data
A Textbook of anaesthesia.
  1. Anesthesia
  I. Smith, G. (Graham) II. Aitkenhead, A.R.
  617′.96   RD81

Library of Congress Cataloging in Publication Data
Main entry under title:
Textbook of anaesthesia.
  1. Anesthesiology. I. Smith, G. (Graham)
II. Aitkenhead, A. R. (Alan R.) [DNLM: 1. Anesthesia.
WO 200 T355]
RD81.T44 1984   617′.96   84–4223

Printed in Hong Kong by Sing Cheong Printing Co Ltd

Preface

For several years we have felt the necessity for a concise, readable but comprehensive text to bridge the gap between those volumes which are appropriate for the undergraduate and those intended for use by anaesthetists in the latter part of training. Such a book should be easy to read, provide sound practical advice in the administration of anaesthetics but, above all, be presented as an integrated development from the basic sciences. It should satisfy the needs of the new recruit into anaesthesia (and perhaps be appropriate for the undergraduate undertaking an elective period of study) during the first 1–2 years in the specialty. The trainee should be encouraged to use the text both as a practical guide in the operating theatre and also as the foundation of his theoretical learning before moving on to the larger textbooks, monographs and journals, in order to increase his breadth and depth of knowledge.

This textbook is our modest attempt to achieve these aims and we are grateful to all who have helped in this endeavour. Clearly a single author approach would have been preferable in many respects by producing uniformity of style. However, all our contributors have been generous in permitting the editors to undertake widespread revision of manuscripts in an attempt to achieve conformity. Hence any errors are entirely the fault of the editors. Since it is intended that some chapters may be read in isolation, for example, in preparation for undertaking specific anaesthetic operating theatre lists, a small element of repetition has been deemed necessary. In addition, it is hoped that this book is sufficiently portable to accompany the trainee during his practical duties, and so a substantial appendix has been incorporated to provide rapid access to commonly used reference material.

Applied physiology and pharmacology are the key stones of sound anaesthetic practice. Although a comprehensive discussion is clearly impractical in a text of this size, we have included a synopsis of the relevant basic sciences in order to emphasise those areas of greatest importance and stimulate application in the clinical arena.

We are also indebted to the publishers, Messrs Churchill Livingstone, who have embraced the concept of this book with enthusiasm and who have been instrumental in producing a text as modestly priced as possible. In addition, all the figures and diagrams have been prepared or redrawn from original articles by Angela Chorley, Margaret Gold and Julia Polanski of the Audio Visual Services Department, University of Leicester, and we are particularly grateful for the high quality of artwork which has been attained. Our gratitude must also be recorded to Jan Wapples, AIMBI of the Medical Illustration Department, Leicester Royal Infirmary for the majority of the photography in the text, Kim Moulding BA(Hons), Principal Secretary in the University Department of Anaesthesia for substantial secretarial work, and Drs D. R. Derbyshire and C.A. Pinnock for their invaluable assistance.

This textbook was planned and commenced before the Faculty of Anaesthetists announced changes for the FFARCS examination. It is fortuitous therefore that this book should be suited ideally to those anaesthetic trainees preparing for the new Primary FFARCS examination and DA(U.K.) diploma. In addition this text should serve as a primer for the new European Diploma of Anaesthesiology.

Leicester, 1985   G.S.
A.R.A.

Contributors

Alan R. Aitkenhead BSc MB ChB FFARCS
Senior Lecturer, University Department of Anaesthesia,
Leicester Royal Infirmary, Leicester, UK

Douglas S. Arthur MB ChB FFARCS
Consultant, Department of Anaesthesia, Royal Infirmary,
Glasgow, UK

David B. Barnett MD MB ChB FRCP
Professor of Applied Pharmacology and Therapeutics,
University of Leicester School of Medicine, Leicester Royal
Infirmary, Leicester, UK

Paul S. Cossham MB ChB FFARCS
Consultant, Department of Anaesthesia, Leicester Royal
Infirmary, Leicester, UK

Brian R. Cotton BSc MB BS FFARCS
Consultant, Department of Anaesthesia, Leicester Royal
Infirmary, Leicester, UK

David R. Derbyshire MB ChB FFARCS
Lecturer, University Department of Anaesthesia, Leicester Royal
Infirmary, Leicester, UK

Robert Ellis MB ChB FFARCS
Assistant Professor of Anesthesia, Department of Anesthesia,
Medical College of Virginia, Richmond, Virginia, USA

David Fell MB ChB FFARCS
Senior Registrar, Department of Anaesthesia, Leicester Royal
Infirmary, Leicester, UK

Valerie A. Goat MB ChB FFARCS
Consultant, Nuffield Department of Anaesthetics, John Radcliffe
Hospital, Oxford, UK

Ian S. Grant MB ChB MRCP FFARCS
Consultant, Department of Anaesthesia, Ninewells Hospital,
Dundee, UK

Ronald Greenbaum MB ChB, FFARCS DObst RCOG
Consultant, Department of Anaesthesia, University College
Hospital, London, UK

J. Martin Hampson MB BS FFARCS
Consultant, Department of Anaesthesia, Leicester Royal
Infirmary, Leicester, UK

Christopher D. Hanning BSc MB BS FFARCS
Senior Lecturer, University Department of Anaesthesia,
Leicester Royal Infirmary, Leicester, UK

Stephen A. Hudson M.Pharm MPS
Principal Pharmacist and Clinical Tutor, Eastern General
Hospital and Heriot-Watt University, Edinburgh, UK

Philip C. W. Hunt MB BS FFARCS
Senior Registrar, Department of Anaesthesia, Leicester Royal
Infirmary, Leicester, UK

R. Hugh James MB BS FFARCS DTM&H
DObst RCOG DA
Consultant, Department of Anaesthesia, Leicester Royal
Infirmary, Leicester, UK

John H. Kerr DM BM BCh FFARCS
Consultant, Nuffield Department of Anaesthetics, John Radcliffe
Hospital, Oxford, UK

Richard L. J. Kohn MB ChB FFARCS
Consultant, Department of Anaesthesia, Leicester Royal
Infirmary, Leicester, UK

Ing-Marie Larsson MD
Department of Anaesthesia, Centrallasarettet, Västerås, Sweden

D. Geoffrey Lewis, BA MA MD MB BChir FFARCS
Consultant, Department of Anaesthesia, Leicester Royal
Infirmary, Leicester, UK

Una M. MacFadyen BSc MB ChB MRCP DCH
Lecturer, University Department of Child Health, Leicester
Royal Infirmary, Leicester, UK

Peter J. McKenzie MB ChB FFARCS
Consultant, Nuffield Department of Anaesthetics, John Radcliffe
Hospital, Oxford, UK

Christopher J. D. Maile MA MB BChir FFARCS
Senior Registrar, Department of Anaesthesia, Leicester Royal
Infirmary, Leicester, UK

Anne E. May MB BS FFARCS
Consultant, Department of Anaesthesia, Leicester Royal
Infirmary, Leicester, UK

Walter S. Nimmo BSc MB ChB FFARCS MRCP MD
Professor of Anaesthesia, University of Sheffield Medical School,
Sheffield, UK

John Norman PhD MB ChB FFARCS
Professor of Anaesthesia, University Department of Anaesthesia,
Southampton General Hospital, Southampton, UK

Timothy M. O'Carroll MB BS FFARCS DObst RCOG
Consultant, Department of Anaesthesia, Leicester Royal
Infirmary, Leicester, UK

Colin A. Pinnock MB BS FFARCS
Lecturer, University Department of Anaesthesia, Leicester Royal
Infirmary, Leicester, UK

David G. Raitt MB ChB FFARCS DA
Consultant, Department of Anaesthesia, Leicester Royal
Infirmary, Leicester, UK

Graham Smith BSc MB BS MD FFARCS
Professor of Anaesthesia, University of Leicester School of
Medicine, Leicester, UK

Colin M. Stray MB BS FFARCS
Consultant, Department of Anaesthesia, Leicester Royal
Infirmary, Leicester, UK

Susan Taylor MB BS FFARCS DA
Senior Registrar, Department of Anaesthesia, Leicester Royal
Infirmary, Leicester, UK

John Thorburn MB ChB FFARCS DA DObst RCOG
Consultant, Department of Anaesthesia, Western Infirmary,
Glasgow, UK

Gerald C. Tresidder MB BS FRCS
Lecturer, Department of Anatomy, University of Leicester
Medical School, Leicester, UK

Douglas A. B. Turner MB ChB FFARCS
Senior Registrar, Department of Anaesthesia, Leicester Royal
Infirmary, Leicester, UK

Mairlys Vater MB BCh FFARCS DA
Senior Registrar, Department of Anaesthesia, Leicester Royal
Infirmary, Leicester, UK

Peter G. Wallace MB ChB FFARCS DObst RCOG
Consultant, Department of Anaesthesia, Western Infirmary,
Glasgow, UK

John Walls MB ChB FRCP
Consultant, Renal Unit, Leicester General Hospital, Leicester,
UK

Malcolm J. H. Wellstood-Eason MB ChB FFARCS
Consultant, Department of Anaesthesia, Leicester Royal
Infirmary, Leicester, UK

John A. W. Wildsmith MB ChB FFARCS MD
Consultant, Department of Anaesthesia, Edinburgh Royal
Infirmary, Edinburgh, UK

Sheila M. Willatts MB BS MRCP FFARCS DObst
RCOG DA
Consultant, Department of Anaesthesia, Frenchay Hospital,
Bristol, UK

J. Keith Wood MB ChB FRCP MRCPath
Consultant, Department of Haematology, Leicester Royal
Infirmary, Leicester, UK

Contents

1

Anatomy

A knowledge of anatomy is very important to the anaesthetist. In the conduct of anaesthesia it is required to enable him to cannulate veins and arteries, to undertake laryngoscopy for endotracheal intubation, to undertake bronchoscopy which he may be required to perform in the absence of surgical assistance for urgent removal of aspirated material, and to undertake a variety of local anaesthetic blocks. In addition, a sound knowledge of anatomy is necessary in cardiopulmonary medicine and to understand the surgeon's techniques and requirements.

Clearly, this short chapter cannot cover all the anatomical knowledge required of the anaesthetist. Its purpose is to describe in detail only those aspects relevant to the conduct of general anaesthesia and spinal/extradural anaesthesia and to indicate areas for further study in the standard textbooks of anatomy.

VENEPUNCTURE

Upper limb

The superficial veins form varying patterns, but the common arrangements are shown in Figures 1.1 and 1.2.

The arrangement of the arteries is less varied than that of the veins. However, developmental anomalies do occur and it is wise to inspect and palpate for arterial pulsation before undertaking venepuncture. An 'ulnar' artery may leave the brachial artery in the arm and, passing superficial to the common attachment of the superficial flexor muscles of the forearm, lie immediately deep to the median cubital vein — without the intervention of the bicipital aponeurosis. Similarly a 'radial' artery may arise proximally and be situated superficially in the forearm.

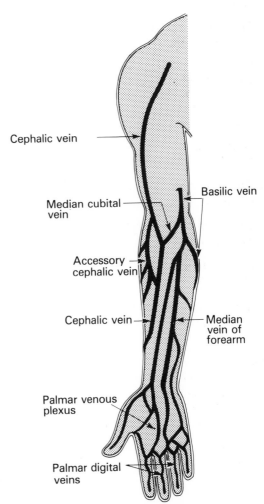

Fig. 1.1 Superficial veins of right upper limb.

Metacarpal veins, lying superficially on the back of the hand, drain blood from the digits and hand (Fig. 1.2). These veins join together to form the dorsal venous arch. From the lateral and medial ends of the

1

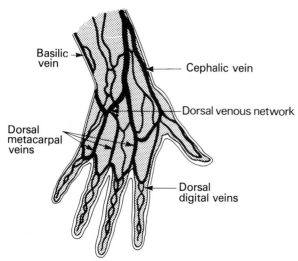

Fig. 1.2 Dorsal metacarpal veins of right hand.

dorsal venous arch, the blood is carried centripetally by the cephalic and basilic veins respectively. These veins also receive tributaries from the skin and superficial tissues of the forearm thus draining, respectively, the pre- and postaxial borders of the upper limb. The basilic vein, having received the brachial veins, continues as the axillary vein. The cephalic vein, after passing through the deltopectoral groove, drains into the axillary vein.

Venepuncture may be performed at the following sites:

1. On the back of the hand and lateral aspect of the wrist in one of the dorsal metacarpal veins (Fig. 1.2).

2. On the anterior aspect of the forearm in the cephalic or median veins (Fig. 1.1), or one of their tributaries. Usually there are useful veins also on the posterior aspect.

It is preferable to cannulate veins on the back of the hand and on the forearm rather than those at the elbow because the cannula may be secured more easily in situ.

When a venepuncture is to be made at or below the elbow greater venous distension can be obtained in an obstructed vein if the front of the forearm is massaged by firm pressure from the wrist upwards. This delivers blood from the superficial veins and from the deep (communicating) vein (Fig. 1.3) which drains the deeper structures of the forearm. A conscious patient should be asked to flex and extend the digits forcibly several times and then to clench the fist firmly. Subsequently the forearm should be massaged from the wrist upwards.

3. At the elbow in either the cephalic or median cubital vein (Fig. 1.3). Usually the median cubital vein is the larger and more mobile of the two, but, if

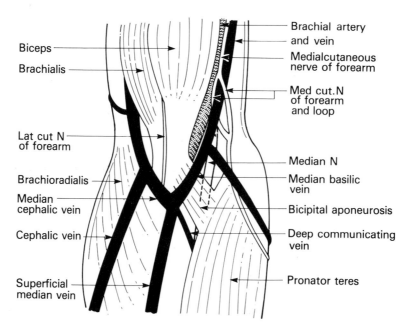

Fig. 1.3 Veins at the right elbow.

used inexpertly, there may be complications. If the needle is inserted too deeply, it may pass through the bicipital aponeurosis and penetrate the brachial artery. The pulsation of this artery can be felt immediately medial to the tendon of the biceps. Medial to the brachial artery lies the median nerve. An anomalous ulnar artery may lie just deep to the median cubital vein and be at risk if the vein is penetrated too deeply (Fig. 1.3). Withdrawal of arterial blood in a pulsatile stream indicates that this has happened.

The medial cutaneous nerve of the forearm divides into its anterior and posterior branches at the elbow (Fig. 1.3) and sometimes these form a loop around the median cubital vein. Thus perivenous piercing with the needle, extravasation of fluid, or the occurrence of a haematoma at this site may damage nerve fibres and in the conscious patient cause acute pain along the inner border of the forearm.

4. Below the clavicle in the subclavian vein (Fig. 1.4). Use of the right subclavian rather than the left provides easier access to the superior vena cava and right atrium. The subclavian vein — the continuation of the axillary — runs from a point just below and medial to the midclavicular point. From here it arches upwards, then, passing downwards and forwards

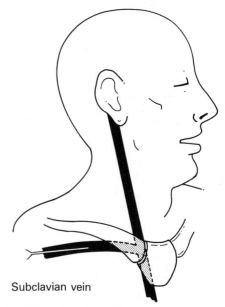

Subclavian vein

Fig. 1.4   Right subclavian and jugular veins.

(Fig. 1.5) it joins the internal jugular to form the brachiocephalic vein posterior to the sternoclavicular joint. The subclavian vein lies in a groove on the superior surface of the first rib. The subclavian artery lies above and behind the vein with the scalenus

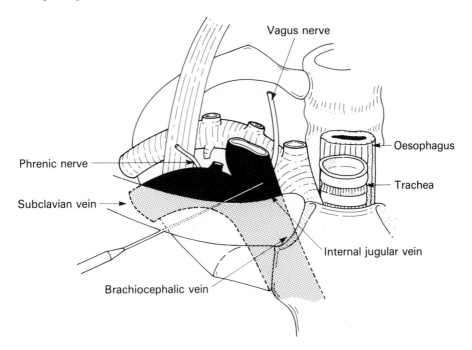

Fig. 1.5   Right subclavian vein.

anterior tendon intervening. The phrenic nerve lies deep to the prevertebral layer of the cervical fascia covering the scalenus anterior. By puncturing the skin below the clavicle — at the junction of its middle and medial thirds — the needle is passed upwards and medially in the direction of the sternoclavicular joint. The vein should be entered at its confluence with the internal jugular vein.

Neck and head

Venepuncture may be performed above the clavicle in the external and internal jugular veins. For puncture of the external and internal jugular veins the patient should be lying in a slight Trendelenburg position with the head turned away from the side of puncture. This position provides easy access to and distension of the veins and minimises the risk of air embolism. Finger pressure just above the middle of the clavicle also produces distension of the external jugular vein.

The external jugular vein, receiving blood from the scalp and face, is formed by the union of the posterior auricular vein and the posterior division of the retromandibular vein (Fig. 1.6). It runs vertically downwards from just behind the angle of the mandible to pass posterior to the clavicle lateral to the sternocleidomastoid tendon, where it terminates in the subclavian vein. In its course it lies deep to the skin and the platysma muscle, and superficial to the investing layer of the deep cervical fascia and sternocleidomastoid muscle. Puncture of the vein should be made one finger's breadth above the clavicle.

The internal jugular vein (Fig. 1.6) is the continuation of the sigmoid sinus. It runs from its superior bulb (dilation) just below the base of the skull to terminate posterior to the sternoclavicular joint, where its inferior bulb is joined by the subclavian vein to form the brachiocephalic vein. The internal jugular lies deep to the sternocleidomastoid muscle on the lateral side of the internal and common carotid arteries (Fig. 1.7).

It is safest to puncture the internal jugular vein using a 'high approach'. A common technique is to approach the vein at the apex of the triangle formed by the sternal and clavicular heads of sternocleidomastoid muscle (Fig. 1.8). This is usually found at the level of the cricoid cartilage where it may be crossed by the external jugular vein. At this point a needle is directed downwards at an angle of 30° to the skin in the direction of the ipsilateral nipple. If the internal jugular vein is not encountered, the needle is redirected medially. Complications include entry of the common carotid artery, branches of the costocervical trunk, the thoracic duct (on the left side) and damage to the sympathetic trunk. The 'high approach' reduces the chance of injury to the pleura and lung.

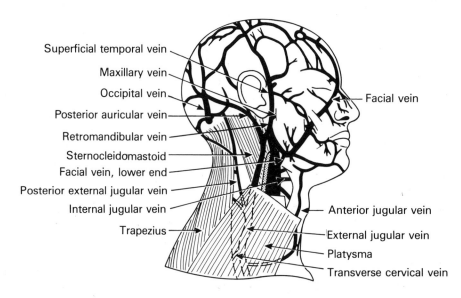

Fig. 1.6 Veins of right side of the head and neck.

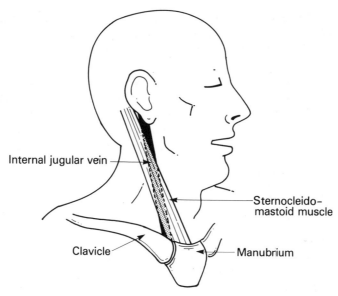

Fig. 1.7 Right internal jugular vein.

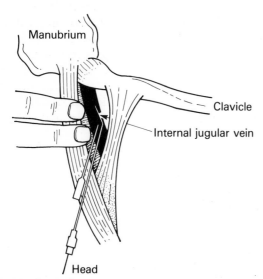

Fig. 1.8 Approach to right jugular vein. Catheter inserted through cannula.

On the right side, cannulation of the right atrium is easy since the right internal jugular vein, brachiocephalic vein, superior vena cava and right atrium lie almost in a straight line.

Lower limb

There are several different patterns of the superficial saphenous system. Various direct and indirect communications exist between the long (great) and short (small) saphenous veins (Fig. 1.9). Throughout their courses these veins both receive tributaries from the skin and subcutaneous tissues and also give off perforating branches which join the deep veins. The perforating veins normally convey blood from the superficial to the deep system. All the veins of the lower limb have bicuspid valves which are arranged so that blood is directed towards the heart. The flow of blood may be reversed when varicosity of the veins is present.

Dorsal metatarsal veins, which receive blood from the toes, run together to form a dorsal venous arch which lies across the foot over the heads of the metarsal bones. This dorsal network of veins also receives blood from the sole and sides of the foot. The medial end of the dorsal venous arch is continued as the long saphenous vein, the lateral end continues as the short saphenous. These veins respectively mark the pre- and postaxial borders of the lower limb.

The long saphenous vein lies, with the saphenous nerve, immediately anterior to the medial malleolus at the ankle (Fig. 1.9). As the vein ascends (still accompanied by the saphenous nerve) along the medial side of the leg, it passes obliquely across the lower part of the tibia to become posteromedial at the medial condyles of the tibia and femur. From here, often accompanied by branches of the medial femoral cutaneous nerve, the vein passes upwards and obliquely forwards to pass through the saphenous opening of the deep fascia which lies two finger breadths below and lateral to the pubic tubercle to enter the femoral vein, which lies medial to the femoral artery. When puncturing the long saphenous vein, any perivenous probing with the needle or spread of injection fluid, or the occurrence of a haematoma, may damage the accompanying nerve and cause acute pain in the conscious patient.

Venepuncture may be performed:

1. On the dorsum of the foot in the dorsal venous arch or one of its tributaries (Fig. 1.9). This provides the best site in the lower limb for i.v. infusions in the operating theatre.

2. On the anteromedial aspect of the leg using either the long saphenous vein or one of its tributaries (Fig. 1.9). The saphenous vein has a thick wall and therefore a sharp needle is required. The lowest part of the vein, in its own fascial sheath, lies in direct contact with the periosteum over the tibia and care should be taken to avoid injuring these structures.

UPPER RESPIRATORY AIRWAY

The upper airway consists of passages extending from the anterior nares down to and including the larynx. The nasal cavity extends from the nostrils (anterior nares) to the posterior nares or choanae where it opens into the nasopharynx or postnasal space. The cavity is divided by the nasal septum into right and left halves. Each half consists of three regions.

The nose

The nasal vestibule lies just inside the nostril. It is the widest part (up to 1 cm) of the cavity. The vestibule is

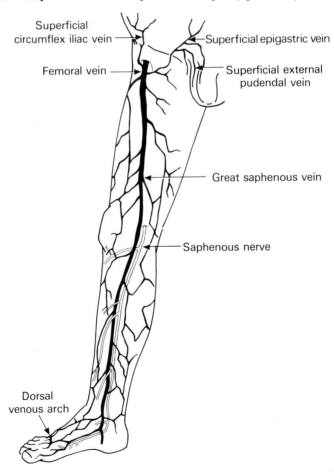

Fig. 1.9 Superficial veins of the right lower limb.

lined by skin which bears coarse hairs (the vibrissae) and sebaceous and sweat glands. At approximately 2 cm distance from the nostrils, the skin becomes continuous with the mucous membrane of the *respiratory region of the nasal cavity*. This membrane consists of columnar or pseudostratified ciliated epithelium with occasional goblet cells. Beneath the basal lamina lie mucous and serous glands with a vascular cavernous tissue containing arteriovenous communications.

The olfactory region is situated in the roof of the nasal cavity. This region is covered with olfactory epithelium extending over the superior part of the septum medially and the superior concha laterally.

The floor of the cavity is formed, from before backwards, by the hard palate comprising the palatal processes of the maxillae and in its posterior quarter the horizontal plates of the palatine bones. The soft palate is attached to the posterior margin of the hard palate. The floor is almost horizontal as it passes posteriorly; it is gently concave from side to side. These bones are covered by periosteum to which the thin overlying mucous membrane is intimately adherent.

The medial wall of the cavity is formed by the nasal septum. After the age of seven years, the septum is often deviated from the median plane. This diminishes the size of one half of the cavity and increases that of the other. The septum is comprised of the vomer bone and the perpendicular plate of the ethmoid bone. Anteriorly lies the septal cartilage. These structures are covered respectively by periosteum and perichondrium over which lies a thick layer of mucous membrane (Fig. 1.10).

The lateral wall of the nose is constituted on the outside by cartilage and bone. In front and below lie three nasal cartilages. The lower cartilages meet in the midline forming the point of the nose. Above and posteriorly, the nasal bone and the frontal process of the maxilla form the remainder of the side wall. On the inside of the nose, the lateral wall of the nasal cavity (Fig. 1.11) is formed by the nasal surfaces of the maxilla anteriorly and inferiorly, posteriorly by the perpendicular plate of the palatine bone and superiorly by the ethmoid. From the latter the superior and middle conchae form projections into the cavity. The inferior concha is a separate bone articulating with the maxilla and palate. The lateral wall, formed mainly by the three projecting conchae, is covered by a thick and very vascular mucous membrane. Below each concha is a passage or meatus. The paranasal sinuses open into the meatuses — the posterior ethmoidal sinus opens into the superior meatus; the remainder open into the middle meatus.

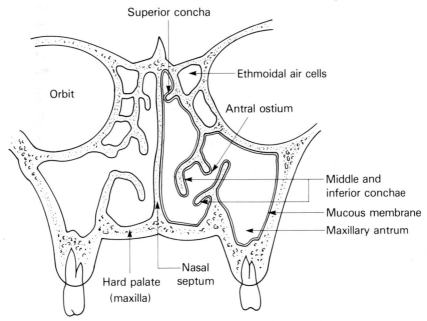

Fig. 1.10 Coronal section of nasal cavities and sinuses.

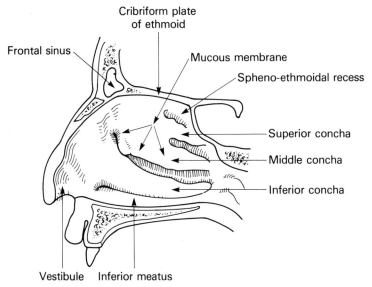

Fig. 1.11   Right nasal cavity: lateral wall.

The nasolacrimal duct opens into the anterior part of the inferior meatus. Just beyond the posterior end of the inferior meatus above the level of the soft palate, in the nasopharynx, lies the opening of the pharyngotympanic (Eustachian) tube with the tubal tonsil attached to its posterior lip.

The nasopharynx or post-nasal space, in its upper part, is the direct posterior continuation of the nasal cavity. The nasopharynx lies just above and behind the soft palate which forms the anterior boundary in its lower part.

The rigid roof and posterior wall of the nasopharynx are formed by bones covered with periosteum and mucous membrane. Passing from above downwards are the body of the sphenoid, the basilar part of the occipital bone and the anterior arch of the atlas (Fig. 1.12). The lateral walls are composed of muscle (mainly the superior constrictor) and the thick pharyngobasilar membrane which is inelastic. Thus the airway through the nasopharynx is always kept patent for breathing. The cavity is lined by respiratory epithelium.

The nerve supply of the mucous membane lining the nose and nasopharynx is derived mainly from cranial nerve V (trigeminal) and both sympathetic and parasympathetic parts of the autonomic nervous system.

Cranial nerve I (olfactory) carries the special sensation of smell from the roof and adjoining walls of the nose to the brain. The anterior ethmoidal branch of the ophthalmic division of the trigeminal nerve conveys afferent somaesthetic impulses from the anterosuperior quadrant of the lateral wall of the nasal cavity and the corresponding part of the septum. The remainder of the lateral wall and most of the medial (septal) wall receives its sensory supply from branches of the pterygopalatine ganglion. This ganglion, lying in the pterygopalatine fossa, is suspended by two branches from the maxillary nerve, which is the second division of the trigeminal nerve. Additional nerves, branches of the maxillary and its anterior superior alveolar branch, supply the lateral wall and floor respectively.

The parasympathetic nerves conduct secretor impulses from the superior salivatory nucleus (in the pons) to the mucous and serous secreting cells in the mucous membrane of the nose and nasopharynx. These impulses pass via the nervus intermedius, along its continuing fibres forming the greater petrosal nerve, which is joined by sympathetic fibres. This nerve synapses in the pterygopalatine ganglion whence the postganglionic fibres pass, with the sensory branches of the ganglion, to the mucous membrane. Stimulation produces mucous and serous secretions.

Some afferent nerve fibres conveying the special sense of taste from the oral surface of the soft palate travel through the pterygopalatine ganglion into the

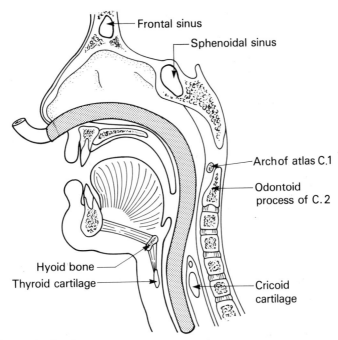

Fig. 1.12 Right side of pharynx: intubated.

greater petrosal nerve. These fibres are the peripheral processes of unipolar cells in the geniculate ganglion of the facial nerve. The central processes travel in the nervus intermedius to join the fasciculus solitarius and then end in its nucleus in the medulla oblongata.

The sympathetic nervous supply for the head has its cells of origin at the level of the first thoracic segment of the spinal cord. From here fibres pass upwards to synapse in the superior cervical sympathetic ganglion. The second neurone fibres pass along the wall of the internal carotid artery. Some of the sympathetic fibres, named the deep petrosal nerve, branch off to join with fibres of the greater petrosal nerve in the formation of the nerve of the pterygoid canal. The sympathetic fibres pass through the pterygopalatine ganglion without synapsing. They are distributed with the other branches of the ganglion to supply constrictor impulses to the smooth muscle in the walls of blood vessels.

The main arterial supply of the inside of the nose comes from the maxillary artery. The maxillary artery, a terminal branch of the external carotid artery, continues through the infratemporal fossa and eventually through the pterygopalatine fossa to give branches to the lateral and medial walls of the nasal and nasopharyngeal cavities. These arterial branches accompany branches of the pterygopalatine ganglion. Anterior and posterior ethmoidal arteries, branches of the ophthalmic artery, supply the upper part of the nasal cavity. The ascending pharyngeal artery (a vertically ascending branch arising from the commencement of the external carotid artery) and the ascending palatine branch of the facial artery, supply the nasopharynx and soft palate.

The veins draining the nose and nasopharynx correspond to the arteries. These veins, passing through the pterygopalatine fossa drain into the pterygoid plexus. This plexus of veins, which has valves, lies within and around the lateral pterygoid muscle. Two large vessels, the maxillary veins, pass backwards from the plexus to join the superficial temporal veins to form the retromandibular vein. Other venous communications are made with the facial and ethmoidal veins.

Most of the lymphatic vessels draining the nasal and nasopharyngeal cavities pass either directly to the upper deep cervical lymph nodes or indirectly via the retropharyngeal and parotid nodes. Beneath the mucous membrane there is a collection of lymphoid tissue, the (naso) pharyngeal tonsil or 'adenoids'. This lies on the upper part of the posterior wall of the nasopharynx. The pharyngeal tonsil is prolonged laterally to join the tubal tonsil. In children hypertrophy of the pharyngeal tonsil may obstruct the airway and, if the tubal tonsil enlarges, the pharyngotympanic tube may be obstructed.

Deviation of the nasal septum is a common occurrence. It usually results from direct trauma to the nose. Rarely it may occur before the age of seven years. There may be overgrowth of the cartilage alone, or excessive growth of the vomer and perpendicular plate of the ethmoid may lead to 'buckling' of the cartilage. Deviation of the septum can lead to occlusion of the nasal cavity into which it projects.

Deflections of the septum, and hypertrophic rhinitis and vascular engorgement affecting the middle and inferior conchae may reduce the size of one or other nasal cavity. Nasal polyps, growing from the mucosa overlying the conchae may also protrude into the upper and middle meatuses. Usually it is easy to pass a lubricated tube through a nostril and along the inferior meatus to enter the nasopharynx although any of these defects may make this difficult.

The mouth

The mouth is bounded externally in front and at the sides by the lips and cheeks; the vestibule of the mouth is the space between its external boundaries and the internal boundary provided by the teeth and gums. The remainder of the mouth constitutes the oral cavity which is separated from the nasal cavities above by the palate. The floor of the mouth is occupied mainly by the muscular tongue. Posteriorly, at the sides, the palatoglossal folds arch upwards and with the upper surface of the tongue form the oropharyngeal isthmus between the mouth and oropharynx.

The mouth is lined by mucous membrane covered with stratified squamous epithelium which continues on to the anteroinferior surface of the soft palate and over the whole tongue. Beneath the mucous membrane lie mucous glands.

The prehensile anterior part of the tongue is covered by filiform papillae. These provide a certain roughness (under the moist surface) and so facilitate the tongue being firmly gripped between finger and thumb. At the sides and tip of the tongue there are fungiform papillae which bear taste buds. Taste buds are found also in all vallate papillae. These lie dorsally at the V-shaped site of fusion of the derivatives of the embryological first and third branchial arches from which the definitive tongue is derived.

The muscles of the tongue are striated. Except for the palatoglossus muscles, supplied from the pharyngeal plexus, all the muscles of the tongue are supplied by cranial nerve XII (hypoglossal).

Most of the lining mucous membrane of the mouth including that over the anterior two-thirds of the tongue is supplied by the lingual nerve — a branch of the 3rd (mandibular) division of the trigeminal nerve. Afferent impulses from the taste buds in the anterior two thirds of the tongue and floor of mouth pass along the chorda tympani nerve. The central processes of its cells, lying in the geniculate ganglion of the facial nerve, pass in the nervus intermedius to terminate in the nucleus of the fasciculus solitarius.

The efferent parasympathetic supply to the salivary glands in the tongue and floor of the mouth takes origin from the superior salivatory nucleus in the pons. The nerves travel in the nervus intermedius, initially in company with the facial nerve, to continue in the chorda tympani nerve. These nerve fibres synapse in the submandibular ganglion whence the postganglionic fibres pass with the branches of the lingual nerve to convey secretor impulses to the salivary glands.

The oropharynx communicates anteriorly through the oropharyngeal isthmus with the upper part of the oral cavity. Superiorly, through the pharyngeal isthmus, it communicates with the nasopharynx. The former is closed by contraction of the palatoglossal muscles and by drawing the tongue backwards and upwards to press against the tensed soft palate. The pharyngeal isthmus is closed by contraction of the levator palati muscles; these raise the soft palate upwards and backwards against the forward movement caused by contractions of the upper part of the superior constrictor muscles and of the highest fibres of the palatopharyngeal muscles. When the fibres of the latter contract they produce the horseshoe-shaped ridge of Passavant within the surrounding superior constrictor muscle.

Anteroinferiorly the oropharynx is bounded by the back of the tongue. This has a smooth moist surface which facilitates the onward movement of a bolus.

Beneath the mucous membrane are scattered nodules of lymphoid tissue, the lingual tonsils, which are prolonged laterally to join the palatine tonsil. The posterior third of the tongue extends from the vallate papillae to the two valleculae.

The (palatine) tonsil, lying between the palato-glossal arch (anteriorly) and palatopharyngeal arch (posteriorly), and the pharyngeal constrictor muscles form the lateral wall of the oropharynx. The constrictor muscles meet in a midline raphe posteriorly. At the level of the oropharynx the constrictors lie in front of the 2nd and 3rd cervical vertebrae. At the level of the upper free border of the epiglottis the oropharynx becomes continuous with the laryngopharynx.

The pharyngeal plexus of nerves and the pharyngeal plexus of veins lie on the outer surface of the middle constrictor muscle about the level of the hyoid bone. The former supplies sensory and motor nerves to the oropharynx. Cranial nerves IX (glossopharyngeal), X (vagus) and XI (accessory) and sympathetic fibres mingle to form the pharyngeal plexus. The somaesthetic impulses leave the plexus to travel via the glossopharyngeal and vagal nerves. The unipolar cells of these nerves may be in either their inferior or superior ganglions. In the medulla the central processes from the inferior ganglions terminate in the nucleus of the fasciculus solitarius and those of the superior ganglions in the nucleus of the spinal fasciculus of the trigeminal nerve. The 'gag' reflex in the unanaesthetised state is induced by touching the mucous membrane covering the posterior third of the tongue, soft palate or lateral and posterior walls of the oropharynx. Pathways from the nuclei in the medulla convey impulses to the nearby nucleus ambiguus and hypoglossal nucleus, leading to efferent, motor, impulses. These travel via cranial nerves IX, X, XI, and XII causing contraction of palatal, pharyngeal and lingual muscles, the effect of which is to close the pharynx completely.

Impulses of the special sense of taste also travel in cranial nerves IX and X; their unipolar cells are in their inferior ganglions and their central processes terminate in the nucleus of fasciculus solitarius. Efferent parasympathetic fibres travel from the inferior salivatory nucleus (in the upper medulla) via the glossopharyngeal nerve. After synapsing in small ganglia in the mucous membrane of the oropharynx they convey secretor impulses to its mucous and serous glands.

The vascular supply of both the oro- and laryngopharynx is as follows:

The arterial supply comes from the ascending pharyngeal, ascending palatine and tonsillar branches of the facial artery and branches of the lingual, superior and inferior laryngeal arteries. The venous drainage is into the pharyngeal plexus of veins which drains upwards to the pterygoid plexus and downwards into the internal jugular vein. Lymphatic drainage is to the deep cervical lymph nodes.

The laryngopharynx is the continuation of the oropharynx. In the upper part of the laryngopharynx, the paths for food and air cross. A bolus of food or fluid is projected downwards and backwards from the oral cavity through the oro- and laryngopharynx and into the oesophagus. In so doing it inevitably crosses the airway which is passing from the nasopharynx, downwards through the oropharynx and across the upper part of the laryngopharynx to pass forwards to the larynx.

As a result of this chiasma it is possible for fluid, food or foreign bodies taken into the mouth to pass down forwards into the larynx to reach the bronchi. In the conscious state this is prevented by the mechanism of deglutition. In this act respiration is momentarily suspended. The bolus is pushed onwards by successive contractions of the pharyngeal constrictor muscles (assisted by gravity). At the same time the larynx is elevated by contraction of the stylo-, salpingo- and palatopharyngeus muscles. This elevation assists in closing the laryngeal inlet. Further elevation of the larynx is achieved by raising the hyoid bone from which the larynx is suspended. Entrance through the inlet into the vestibule of the larynx is also restricted by being covered by the tilting of the epiglottis backwards and downwards.

In vomiting, particularly in the unconscious state when the reflex pathways are out of action, it is possible for the regurgitated gastric contents to be expelled up the oesophagus, through the crico-pharyngeal 'ring' of muscle, into the laryngopharynx and then forwards across to the vestibule and so downwards through the larynx and trachea to the lungs.

It is also possible for air and material expectorated from the lungs and lower respiratory airways to enter the oesophagus and stomach. This is prevented normally by the sphincter-like contraction of the cricopharyngeal part of the inferior constrictor muscles.

Anteriorly, the upper limit of the laryngopharynx is marked by the upper free edge of the epiglottis. Bounding the sides of the inlet to the larynx are the aryepiglottic folds passing posteriorly to the arytenoid cartilages, which articulate inferiorly with the cricoid cartilage. At the sides the salpingo-, stylo- and palatopharyngeus muscles are passing downwards (within the inferior constrictor) to gain attachment to the posterior (vertical) border of the thyroid cartilage and to the fibrous layer of the wall of the pharynx. The overlapping inferior constrictor and the middle and superior constrictor muscles form the rest of the lateral and entire posterior wall of the laryngopharynx. Posteriorly the constrictors are in relation to the anterior longitudinal ligament which is adherent to the periosteum over the lower part of the 3rd cervical vertebra and the succeeding 4th, 5th and 6th vertebrae.

The lining mucous membrane extends laterally as folds from the sides of the epiglottis. Above, it covers the deep aspect of the thyrohyoid membrane, and below, the thyroid cartilage. Spreading backwards it lines the muscles forming the lateral and posterior walls of this part of the pharynx. A longitudinal furrow is formed on each side between the bulge of the larynx, covered by its posterolateral muscles and the overlying mucous membrane, and the concavity of the thyroid cartilage which contains it. These are the right and left piriform fossae (Fig. 1.13).

THE LARYNX

The larynx is the continuation of the airway from the laryngopharynx to the trachea. The cavity of the larynx extends from its inlet to the lower border of the cricoid cartilage. In men its length is approx. 45 mm and its anteroposterior diameter 35 mm; in women, these measurements are approx. 35 mm and 25 mm respectively.

The framework of the larynx comprises cartilages, ligaments and membranes. The outer wall is made up in part by the following cartilages: thyroid; cricoid; paired arytenoids lying on the vertical lamina of the cricoid; the small paired corniculate and cuneiform cartilages; and the cartilage of the epiglottis (Fig. 1.14).

Extrinsic ligaments — thyrohyoid and cricotracheal — join the larynx to the hyoid bone above and to the trachea below. Intrinsic membranes form the inner tube of the 'skeleton' of the larynx. There are two of these bilateral fibroelastic membranes: the upper one — the vestibular or quadrate membrane — extends between the arytenoid and thyroid cartilages and the epiglottis; its free lower border forms the vestibular fold. The fissure between the right and left folds is termed the rima vestibuli. The free upper border forms the aryepiglottic fold which encircles the almost vertical laryngeal inlet or aditus.

The lower membrane — the cricovocal or cricothyroid membrane — connects the cricoid and arytenoid cartilages to the thyroid cartilage. It is attached anteriorly in the notch of the thyroid cartilage and posteriorly to the tip of the anterior angle (the vocal process) of the arytenoid cartilage. Its free upper border forms the vocal fold. The slit, which becomes a space when the vocal folds are separated, is known as the rima glottidis. This is the narrowest part of the airway in the adult; in the infant, the trachea just below the level of the cricoid is the narrowest part. The lower thin part of the cricovocal membrane is attached to the superior border of the cricoid cartilage.

The vestibule of the larynx lies between the inlet and the rima vestibuli. The intrinsic muscles of the larynx run between attachments to the laryngeal cartilages and membranes. The two aryepiglottic muscles encircling the laryngeal inlet act as a sphincter. The two posterior crico-arytenoid muscles rotate the arytenoid cartilages around a vertical axis and draw them downwards and outwards. The effect of these movements is to separate the vocal folds and thereby widen the rima glottidis. The two actions of the posterior crico-arytenoids are antagonised by the lateral crico-arytenoid and transverse arytenoid muscles respectively: their contractions close the glottis.

There is a mucous membrane lining the larynx. Above, it is continuous with that of the laryngopharynx; it is attached loosely and has a stratified squamous surface. Over the vocal folds the mucous membrane is thin and intimately adherent. Below the folds, the mucous membrane has a ciliated columnar epithelium. Except over the vocal folds the mucous membrane contains many mucous glands.

Laryngeal branches of the superior and inferior thyroid arteries supply the larynx. The veins draining the larynx pass to the internal jugular and

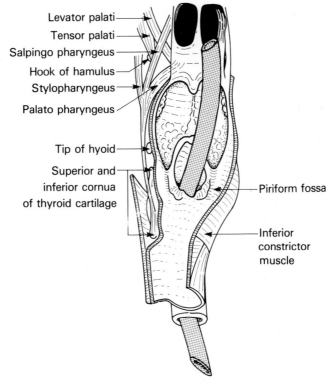

Levator palati
Tensor palati
Salpingo pharyngeus
Hook of hamulus
Stylopharyngeus
Palato pharyngeus

Tip of hyoid

Superior and
inferior cornua
of thyroid cartilage

Piriform fossa

Inferior
constrictor
muscle

Fig. 1.13 The pharynx seen from behind: intubated.

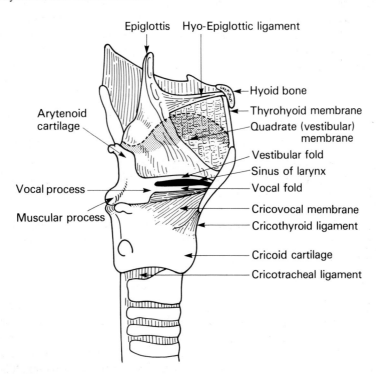

Epiglottis   Hyo-Epiglottic ligament

Arytenoid
cartilage

Hyoid bone
Thyrohyoid membrane
Quadrate (vestibular)
membrane
Vestibular fold
Sinus of larynx
Vocal fold
Cricovocal membrane
Cricothyroid ligament
Cricoid cartilage
Cricotracheal ligament

Vocal process

Muscular process

Fig. 1.14 Cartilages and ligaments of the larynx — from the right side.

brachiocephalic veins. The vocal folds form a watershed for lymphatic drainage. Vessels pass upwards and downwards to join the deep cervical lymph nodes.

The cranial part of the accessory nerve travels with the fibres of the vagus nerve and is distributed with its superior and recurrent laryngeal branches. These supply all the intrinsic muscles of the larynx with efferent motor impulses from the nucleus ambiguus. If one recurrent laryngeal nerve is partially damaged the vocal fold on the same side moves towards the midline because the paralysis affects mainly the posterior cricothyroid muscle. If the recurrent nerve paralysis is complete the affected vocal fold lies in the neutral (cadaveric) position and there is hoarseness of the voice. With increased adduction of the unaffected vocal fold the rima glottidis again approaches its normal shape and size and so the voice is restored. In bilateral partial paralysis the vocal folds are apposed (due to unopposed action by the adductors) thereby obstructing the airway and causing respiratory stridor or total airway obstruction. Bilateral complete paralysis leads to a valve-like obstruction as a result of the slack vocal folds flapping together. This is accompanied by respiratory stridor and there is also loss of voice because the vocal folds cannot be approximated.

All the sensory impulses from the mucosa of the larynx are also conveyed, as afferents, in the two laryngeal nerves. With their unipolar cells in the inferior ganglion of the vagus the fibres pass to end probably in the nucleus of the fasciculus solitarius.

The parasympathetic (visceral) efferent fibres of the vagus arise from the dorsal nucleus of the vagus. Travelling in the superior and recurrent laryngeal nerves they convey secretor impulses to the glands in the mucous membrane of the larynx. The sympathetic nerves travel along the arteries supplying the larynx. These postganglionic fibres pass to the arteries from the middle cervical ganglion.

The larynx and the succeeding trachea form midline structures in the neck. The vocal folds lie just below the notch of the thyroid cartilage behind the laryngeal prominence (Adam's apple). The upper poles of the thyroid gland are at the sides of the larynx. Posterolateral to the thyroid gland lie the great vessels of the neck. The gland and the vessels are covered by the infrahyoid muscles and the sternocleidomastoid muscle, the deep cervical fascia, the platysma muscle and skin.

LOWER RESPIRATORY AIRWAY

The lower airway consists of the trachea and bronchi. The trachea is suspended from the cricoid by the cricotracheal ligament. This passes from the lower border of the cricoid to the first ring of the trachea and is continuous below with the fibrous membrane investing the tracheal rings. When the larynx is elevated in deglutition the upper part of the trachea also rises, its fibroelastic wall being stretched. Below, the trachea bifurcates about the level of the sternal angle — the joint between the manubrium and body of the sternum (level with the disc between the 4th and 5th thoracic vertebrae).

The trachea is freely moveable. It is a midline structure except above its bifurcation where it deviates slightly to the right side. It is 10–12 cm long. In deep inspiration, the trachea is lengthened (by 3–5 cm) by the drawing downwards of its bifurcation and the two principal bronchi. In the adult the diameter of the lumen is about 2.5 cm; in the infant the diameter is less than 3 mm.

A number (16–20) of C-shaped rings of hyaline cartilage maintain the patency of the fibroelastic membrane. Posteriorly, the circumference is flattened slightly by the presence of the unstriped trachealis muscle stretching between the ends of each cartilaginous ring. Contraction of this unstriped muscle narrows the lumen of the trachea and prevents its overdistension when the intraluminal pressure is raised, e.g. during abdominal straining. The trachea is lined by respiratory type mucous membrane. There is a plentiful supply of mucous and serous glands.

Vagal (recurrent laryngeal branches) and sympathetic nerve fibres supply the trachea. The general visceral afferent impulses are conducted to the nucleus of the fasciculus solitarius; the cell bodies of these neurones are in the inferior ganglion of the vagus. Efferent parasympathetic fibres arise from the dorsal nucleus of the vagus to pass in its recurrent laryngeal branch to supply motor impulses to the unstriped trachealis muscle. Other efferent fibres convey secretor impulses to the glands in the lining of the trachea. Vasoconstrictor sympathetic fibres, with their cell bodies in the middle cervical ganglion, pass with the inferior thyroid artery and its branches to reach the trachea.

The inferior thyroid artery is the main arterial supply, although the bronchial arteries also contribute. The trachea is drained by veins emptying either directly into the brachiocephalic veins or indirectly via the inferior thyroid venous plexus. The lymph is drained to the lower deep cervical lymph nodes and to the pre- and paratracheal nodes.

In the neck the trachea lies immediately in front of the oesophagus. The recurrent laryngeal nerve lies in the groove between the two. Posterolateral to the trachea lies the carotid sheath with the thyroid gland intervening. The isthmus of the thyroid gland is anterior and adherent to the 2nd, 3rd and 4th tracheal rings.

In the superior mediastinum, the trachea continues to lie anterior to the oesophagus. In front, the brachiocephalic artery passes obliquely to the right and the left brachiocephalic vein crosses at or above the upper border of the manubrium. The pleural sacs overlap these vessels. On the left of the trachea, lower down, lies the arch of the aorta with the common carotid and subclavian arteries arising from it; on bronchoscopy the pulsation of the aorta is visible. The superior vena cava lies to the right of the trachea. On each side the nearby lung, covered by pleura, envelops the trachea and the structures surrounding it.

The bronchi (Fig. 1.15)

The trachea bifurcates behind the beginning of the arch of the aorta. The deep part of the cardiac plexus of autonomic nerves lies anterior to the bifurcation; below and on each side of the trachea lie tracheobronchial lymph nodes.

At the bifurcation arise the right and left primary (principal, main) bronchi. The right main bronchus continues more nearly in the vertical line of the trachea than does the left; its calibre is larger and its length (2.5 cm) shorter than that of the left (5 cm). The azygos vein arches over the upper aspect of the right bronchus; below initially and then crossing anterior to it is the right pulmonary artery. After the superior lobe (secondary) bronchus branches off, the main bronchus continues downwards, crossing posterior to the pulmonary vessels, to enter the hilum of the lung. There it divides into middle and inferior lobe (secondary) bronchi. The left main bronchus crosses almost transversely beneath the arch of the aorta to lie anterior to the oesophagus and descending aorta. The bronchus at first passes behind and then below the left pulmonary artery to enter the hilum of the left lung where it divides into superior and inferior lobe (secondary) bronchi.

The tertiary segmental bronchi from each lobar bronchus are given off to supply segments of the lobes. These structural units are known as bronchopulmonary segments; they are numbered and are named in accordance with the part of the lung in which each lies. Each bronchopulmonary segment has its own bronchovascular supply. Surgically it is possible to develop planes of separation between segments. Thus segmental resections in addition to lobectomy or pneumonectomy may be carried out at operation.

On bronchoscopy the lining of the trachea and bronchi may be seen and the openings of the secondary lobar bronchi can be identified. The trachea appears as a glistening pinkish-red tube with spaced white rings (the underlying cartilages). Above its bifurcation, aortic arch pulsation can be seen anteriorly and on the left. At its bifurcation the carina appears as a sharp sagittal ridge. The right main bronchus separates off from the vertical at about 25° and the left at 45°. By inspection through a bronchoscope and using the figures on the face of a clock the following orifices can be identified at measured distances from the carina.

Right side:
   Upper lobe bronchus: 3 o'clock at 2.5 cm
   Middle lobe bronchus: 12 o'clock at 4.0 cm
   Lower lobe bronchus: 6 o'clock at 4.5 cm

Left side:
   Lower lobe bronchus: 3 o'clock at 5.0 cm
   Upper lobe bronchus: 9 o'clock at 5.5 cm
   (Lingular bronchus: central at 5.5 cm)

The basic structure of the bronchi is similar to that of the trachea. The bronchi are supplied by bronchial arteries, usually branches from the descending aorta. The veins from the right bronchi drain into the azygos and those on the left enter the left superior hemiazygos vein. The lymphatic vessels of the bronchi drain to nodes at the hilum of the lung and then to the tracheobronchial group.

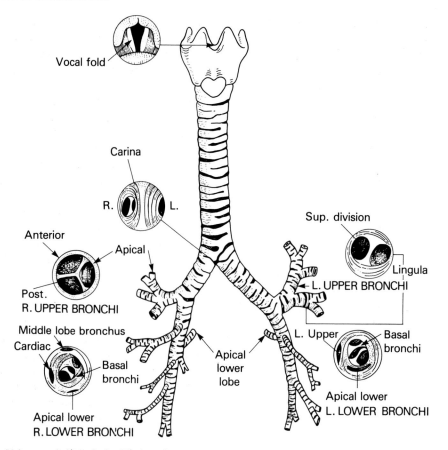

Fig. 1.15   Bronchial tree and views obtained by bronchoscopy.

The pulmonary plexus of nerves supplies the bronchi. This plexus is formed from parasympathetic (vagal) and sympathetic contributions. The pulmonary plexus lies in front of and behind the root of the lung. Networks of nerves pass from the plexus to surround and supply the bronchi. The general visceral afferent fibres of the vagus have their cell bodies in its inferior ganglion and pass (visceral) sensory impulses to the nucleus of the fasciculus solitarius. The efferent vagal fibres conveying motor impulses to the unstriped bronchial muscle arise from the dorsal motor nucleus of the vagus. This nucleus also supplies secretor efferent impulses to the glands in the bronchi. The parasympathetic preganglionic branches of the vagus synapse in ganglia on the walls of the bronchi. The sympathetic supply originates from the 2nd to the 5th thoracic segments of the spinal cord. The postganglionic fibres take origin from synapses in the upper four thoracic ganglia.

SPINAL PUNCTURE

The vertebral canal in the vertebral column is triangular in cross-section. There are openings placed symmetrically at the sides through which the spinal nerves emerge. Anteriorly the wall of the canal is formed by the posterior surfaces of the bodies of the vertebrae (covered by periosteum) and of the intervertebral discs. Both these are covered (posteriorly) by the tough posterior longitudinal ligament. This ligament has serrated margins and narrows gradually as it descends. The serrations are widest where they are attached very firmly to the intervertebral discs. In the intervening narrow sections the ligament is attached to the periosteum over the upper and lower parts of the backs of the vertebral bodies. The posterior wall of the vertebral canal is formed by the anterior surfaces of the laminae (lined by periosteum) of the vertebrae and by the intervening ligamenta flava (Fig. 1.16). The latter, consisting mainly of yellow elastic tissue, extend medially from the capsules of the joints between the superior and inferior articular processes. The right and left ligaments meet each other medially, leaving small intervals in the midline for the passage of veins joining the internal and external vertebral venous plexuses. Each ligamentum flavum passes in an almost vertical plane from a ridge on the lower part of the anterior surface of a lamina above to the upper margin and adjoining posterior surface of the lamina below.

The deepest part of the thin interspinous ligament merges with the posterior aspect of the midline meeting of the ligamenta flava. Superficially the interspinous ligaments are continuous with the deep anterior borders of the supraspinous ligaments, which join the tips of the spinous processes. The ligamenta flava and the interspinous ligaments are thickest between the lumbar vertebrae. When opened up by flexion of the spine the space between successive spinous processes and laminae is greatest in the lumbar region.

The wall of the vertebral canal is incomplete at the sides. From the lateral borders of each vertebral body a pedicle projects posteriorly. The pedicles are shorter (in the vertical plane) than the height of the corresponding vertebra, thus an intervertebral foramen is produced between successive pedicles. In the intervertebral foramen lie the spinal nerve and dorsal root ganglion, covered by sleeves of all three meninges, which merge with the epineurium of the spinal nerve immediately lateral to the foramen. Spinal arteries, veins, lymphatics and fat also pass through the intervertebral foramen. Lining the spinal canal is a layer of extradural fat in which lies the internal vertebral venous plexus.

Within the vertebral canal lies the dura mater, which is formed of dense fibrous tissue. The ensheathing sac of dura contains the spinal cord and nerve roots covered by the leptomeninges. As already indicated the dura mater and leptomeninges extend laterally as sheaths for the dorsal and ventral roots of each spinal nerve. Superiorly the spinal dura mater is a prolongation of the inner, investing layer of the cranial dura. It is attached around the circumference of the foramen magnum. The spinal dura is also attached to the posterior longitudinal ligament and periosteum overlying the backs of the bodies of the second and third cervical vertebrae. This attachment to the posterior longitudinal ligament continues down the length of the dura. By this means, the dural sac is held forwards against the backs of the vertebral bodies and intervertebral discs. Inferiorly the spinal dura mater extends down to the level of the lower border of the second piece of the sacrum where it is closely apposed to and merges with the arachnoid mater. From here it continues, with the arachnoid, as a cover of the filum terminale, which is the connective tissue projection of the pia mater from the apex of the conus medullaris. The filum terminale (after lying centrally in the cauda equina) emerges below the sacral hiatus

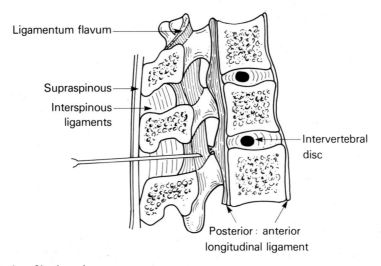

Fig. 1.16 Sagittal section of lumbar spine.

Ligamentum flavum

Supraspinous

Interspinous
ligaments

Intervertebral
disc

Posterior : anterior
longitudinal ligament

to pass posterior to the sacrococcygeal joint to be attached to the dorsal aspect of the coccyx.

The arachnoid mater is a thin tubular membrane lining the dural sac. It envelops the spinal cord and nerve roots, which are covered by pia mater. Where it is in close relation to the spinal cord, the arachnoid is joined to the pia mater by delicate strands of connective tissue, the web-like appearance of which gives its name to the membrane. The cerebrospinal fluid is found between the arachnoid and pia mater. The spinal arachnoid and pia maters are continuations at their upper ends of the cranial leptomeninges.

The pia mater forms a very thin, intimate membranous cover to the spinal cord and nerve roots. Blood vessels run on the surface of the pia and pierce it to supply the cord. From right and left sides of the entire length of the spinal cord — from the foramen magnum to the second lumbar vertebra — the covering pia mater forms a fibrous flange midway between the ventral and dorsal nerve roots. This is termed the ligamentum denticulatum. Laterally the border projects with tooth-like processes which pierce the arachnoid to merge with the dura mater. By this attachment of the ligamentum denticulatum the spinal cord is fixed securely to the dura mater.

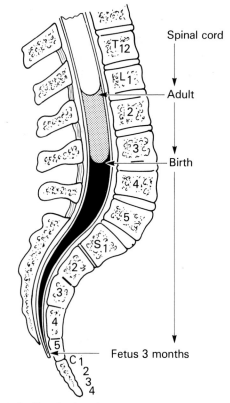

Fig. 1.17 Termination of spinal cord.

The spinal cord and nerves

The spinal cord continues from the medulla oblongata at the level of the foramen magnum. Inferiorly it terminates in a conically-shaped apex called the conus medullaris (Fig. 1.17). In adults the termination of the cord varies, lying higher in women than men, commensurate with the shorter length of the trunk. Thus the cord ends, usually, at a level between the upper and lower borders of the second lumbar vertebra. In the neonate the apex of the conus medullaris lies between the 3rd and 4th vertebrae.

In the early embryo, the spinal nerves pass transversely through the intervertebral foramina at the same level as their segmental origin from the spinal cord. Because of disproportionate growth, most dorsal and ventral nerve roots pass obliquely downwards from their spinal segment to emerge as spinal nerves through their original, but now lower situated, intervertebral foramina. The obliquity is most marked for the lumbar and sacral nerve roots which are known collectively as the cauda equina. These, with the filum terminale, lie within the subarachnoid space.

The spinal cord is made up of centrally placed grey matter, which consists of nerve cells usually arranged in groups, and of white matter consisting of nerve fibres which, except for those ascending fibres conveying impulses of pain, are myelinated. The fibres are arranged in tracts and convey afferent nervous impulses upwards to the brain (ascending) and efferent impulses downwards from the brain (descending). The cauda equina consists of the centrally placed connective tissue filament called the filum terminale, most of the lumbar and all the sacral dorsal and ventral nerve roots. These roots convey respectively afferent and efferent nervous impulses. The dorsal and ventral roots are myelinated. The nerve cells of the spinal cord do not regenerate if traumatised. The axons of the ascending and descending nerve fibres are covered by a myelin sheath. This, however, is produced by oligodendrocytes and not by Schwann cells so no regeneration occurs if the fibres are traumatised.

Thus, the spinal cord is held at its sides by its spinal nerves and is also attached laterally throughout its length to the dura mater by the ligamenta denticulata. The dura is attached anteriorly to the posterior longitudinal ligament and to the periosteum covering the backs of the bodies of the vertebrae and of the intervertebral discs, particularly the upper cervical ones.

Forward bending of the head and trunk with flexion at the occipito-atlantal joint and at the joints between all the vertebrae draws the spinal cord slightly upwards and forwards in the vertebral canal. This movement ensures that the conus medullaris lies as high as possible in the lumbar part of the dural sac. If lumbar puncture is carried out below the level of the 3rd lumbar spinous process in the adult (or the 4th in the infant and young child) the spinal cord cannot be injured by the needle. Besides ensuring the safety of the cord, full forward flexion stretches the supra- and interspinous ligaments and ligamenta flava and so opens up the spaces between successive spinous processes and laminae of the lumbar and 1st sacral vertebra; this effect is greatest between the 3rd and 4th lumbar spines. This allows the anaesthetist more room for manipulation of the needle at lumbar puncture.

The meningeal spaces

A number of spaces, actual or potential, exist within the vertebral canal. From without inwards they are:

1. *The extradural, epidural or peridural space* which extends for the whole length of the spinal dura mater. It is closed superiorly at the foramen magnum. Inferiorly it opens into the cavity of the sacral part of the vertebral canal (Fig. 1.18). This cavity has a fluid capacity of approx. 25 ml. The extradural space lies between the inner surface of the vertebral canal and the outer surface of the dural sac. It is deepest posteriorly where the laminae and ligamenta flava meet in the midline; this feature is most marked in the lumbosacral part of the spine.

The extradural space contains loose fat and a plexus of veins. The fatty areolar tissue extends laterally for a short distance through the intervertebral foramen, surrounding the spinal nerve in its covering. The veins, which are valveless, form the internal vertebral venous plexus. Basivertebral veins, emerging from foramina in the middle of the backs of the vertebral bodies, join this plexus which is formed of two anterior and two posterior longitudinally-running

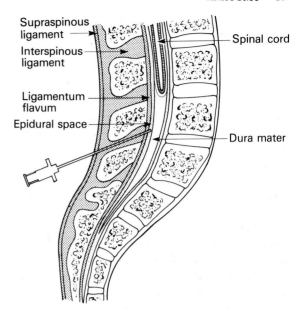

Fig. 1.18   Lower part of spinal cord and meninges.

veins. These are joined, opposite each vertebra, by a series of venous rings encircling the dural sac. It is the transversely-running veins passing posterior to the dura that can be entered by a needle during lumbar puncture. The plexus receives tributaries from the spinal cord and surrounding bones. It communicates, through the intervertebral foramina, with veins running the length of the vertebral column. Fluid injected into the sacral (Figs 1.19 and 1.20) or lumbar parts of the extradural space may spread superiorly to the foramen magnum and laterally through the intervertebral foramina.

In the thoracic part of the spine the extension of the extradural space, through the intervertebral foramina, subjects it to pressures present in the thorax (Fig. 1.21). Any sustained or sudden increase of intrathoracic pressure produces a positive pressure within the extradural space. Deep inspiration lowers, still further, the negative, subatmospheric, intrathoracic pressure which is transmitted to the extradural space. Pressure changes are most marked in the thoracic part of the extradural space, but extend down to the lumbar region.

2. *The subdural space* is a potential space lying between the dura and arachnoid maters. Between the surfaces of these membranes there are capillary and lymphatic vessels for the supply and drainage of the dura mater and extradural fat. Above, the space is in

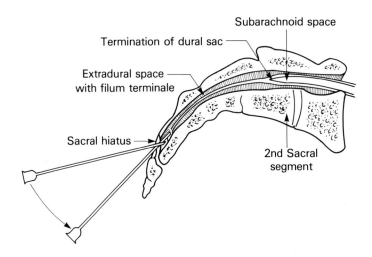

Fig. 1.19   Sacral part of extradural space.

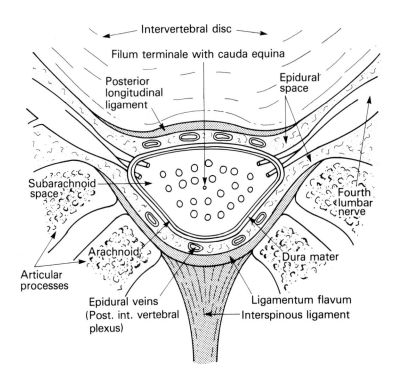

Fig. 1.20   Cross-section of vertebral canal.

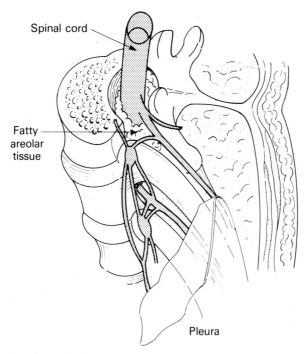

Spinal cord

Fatty
areolar
tissue

Pleura

Fig. 1.21   Extrapleural extension of extradural space.

continuity with that between the cranial dura and arachnoid. At the sides, between these meninges, it extends to the intervertebral foramina., Below, it terminates where the dura and arachnoid fuse at the level of the 2nd sacral vertebra.

3. *The subarachnoid space* lies between the arachnoid mater, lining the dural sac, and the pia mater covering the spinal cord. It contains the cerebrospinal fluid. Superiorly the space is directly continuous with that around the brain. Laterally the

fluid in the space extends to the intervertebral foramina surrounding the dorsal and ventral nerve roots of each spinal nerve (Fig. 1.20). Inferiorly the spinal subarachnoid space is larger than elsewhere. Here it contains the spinal cord, as the latter narrows towards its terminal conus medullaris, and the cauda equina. The space terminates below at the level of the second sacral vertebra, where the tube of arachnoid mater fuses with the inner surface of the lower limit of the dural sac (Fig. 1.19).

FURTHER READING

Brock R C 1952 Lung abscess, 2nd edn. Blackwell Scientific Publications, Oxford
Ellis H, Feldman S 1977 Anatomy for anaesthetists, 3rd edn. Blackwell Scientific Publications, Oxford

Last R J 1978 Anatomy — regional and applied, 6th edn. Churchill Livingstone, Edinburgh
Lee J A, Atkinson R C 1978 Lumbar puncture and spinal anaesthesia. Churchill Livingstone, Edinburgh
Warwick R, Williams P L 1980 Gray's anatomy, 36th edn. Longman, Edinburgh

2

Respiratory physiology

CONTROL OF VENTILATION

The function of respiration is to convey oxygen to the cells and to remove the metabolic product, carbon dioxide. The principal control of ventilation resides in centres in the brain stem, and the activity of the respiratory centre is modified by central and peripheral receptors to permit adequate pulmonary gas exchange. Other reflexes arising from receptors in the lung and respiratory tract modify the pattern of ventilation.

Central control of ventilation

It is known that the essential areas involved in the control of respiration lie in the brain stem, since transection above this level leaves the respiratory rhythm intact. Microelectrode recordings suggest that the main respiratory nuclei lie bilaterally in the medulla. Three main groups have been identified:

1. Located in close proximity to the nucleus retroambigualis in the ventro-lateral medulla are neurones which discharge during inspiration, expiration, and early in the inspiratory phase. These are upper motor neurones supplying the contralateral intercostal muscles. The inspiratory neurones inhibit those of expiration but a reverse inhibition has not been shown.

2. A second group lies bilaterally in the dorsal medulla close to the nucleus of the tractus solitarius. Two types of inspiratory activity have been noted, one of which parallels phrenic nerve discharge, and the other, lung inflation.

3. The third group is the nucleus ambiguus which contains the upper motor neurone cells of the glossopharyngeal and vagus nerves.

Experimental transection of the midpons produces deep breathing with a short expiratory phase; if, in addition, the vagi are cut, breathing is held in inspiration. This sustained gasp is termed apneusis. It is clear therefore that rhythmic ventilation is dependent on the upper pons. This rhythmicity is located in nucleus parabrachialis medialis (NPBM) which was previously known as the pneumotactic centre. Stimulation of dorsal NPBM shortens the phase (inspiration or expiration) during which it is applied; stimulation of the ventral portion shortens inspiration.

Although the evidence suggests that NPBM is essential for rhythmic ventilation, it appears that respiratory rhythm is not generated here. Indeed it has not been possible to locate a 'pacemaker cell', i.e. a rhythmically discharging neurone in phase with respiration but with no synaptic input. Recent hypotheses have suggested that the interconnections of the respiratory neurones may produce an unstable circuit which causes respiratory oscillations.

The effect of ventilation is to modify the O_2 and CO_2 tensions of arterial blood. Alterations in the levels of these variables stimulate chemoreceptors which, in turn, relay the information centrally and thereby modify ventilation. The preservation of normal Pa_{O_2} depends on peripheral chemoreceptors which respond to hypoxia whereas hypercapnia primarily stimulates a brain stem receptor.

Peripheral chemoreceptors

The carotid bodies lie close to the carotid sinus, and the aortic bodies are grouped around the aortic arch. They consist of two types of specialised cell in extremely vascular tissue. The glomus cells (type 1 cells) are innervated by afferent fibres which convey, centrally, information on variations in blood gas tensions. A linear relationship has been noted between peripheral chemoreceptor discharge and CO_2 tension in arterial blood, but it is uncertain if the response is caused by a direct action of CO_2 or hydrogen ion (H^+) concentration. Receptor response has a hyperbolic relationship with Pa_{O_2}. The chemoreceptor response to both hypoxaemia and hypercapnia is not additive but multiplicative. Type 2 cells and their processes surround the type 1 cells but have no known function.

Central receptors

Areas sensitive to changes in P_{CO_2} are located on the ventrolateral surface of the medulla, close to the site of emergence of cranial nerves VII–X. These areas are bathed in cerebrospinal fluid. A further area lateral to cranial nerve XII has a pH-dependent frequency of discharge. The final stimulus may be the extracellular H^+ concentration close to the receptor but, since its level varies with P_{CO_2} in both blood and c.s.f., P_{CO_2} is usually considered to be the stimulus.

Chemoreceptor effects

As the oxygen tension decreases, ventilation shows little change until a level below 8 kPa is reached. The relationship between Pa_{O_2} and ventilation is exponential. Above a Pa_{O_2} of 8 kPa there is little response to steady state changes but increased ventilation has been noted with transient changes in oxygen tension.

Ventilation increases linearly as Pa_{CO_2} increases above 5 kPa; the slope is increased by hypoxia.

In summary, P_{CO_2} (or H^+ concentration) stimulates peripheral and central receptors; hypoxia stimulates the peripheral chemoreceptors but depresses the central receptors as a result of central hypoxia. The resultant effect of chemoreceptor activity is an increase in both the rate and depth of ventilation.

Modified chemoreceptive response

In certain conditions, including chronic lung disease and exposure to high altitudes, abnormal responses are obtained from the chemoreceptors.

1. High altitudes. At high altitude, the reduced atmospheric pressure results in a reduction in inspired, and thus arterial, oxygen tension. Unacclimatised subjects respond to hypoxaemia by hyperventilation, thus reducing Pa_{CO_2}. Acclimatisation results in a decrease in c.s.f. $[HCO_3^-]$ which lowers c.s.f. pH at a given carbon dioxide tension, thereby increasing sensitivity to P_{CO_2}. However, this explanation is probably too simplistic since the increase in ventilation is retained despite a progressive diminution in the response to hypoxaemia in subjects living at high altitudes for many years.

2. Chronic lung disease. In chronic obstructive lung disease there is a reduced response to hypercapnia in 'blue bloater' patients in addition to that caused by mechanical factors. By contrast 'pink puffers' retain their ability to respond to hypercapnia and hypoxaemia in the face of distressing effort.

Other lung receptors

1. Airway stretch receptors at the dorsal ends of the tracheal and bronchial rings are responsible for the Hering-Breuer reflex which, when elicited, terminates inspiration and prolongs expiration. The reflex is excited by inflation of the lungs. It is present in man but appears to vary in intensity from subject to subject. In anaesthetised man it is difficult to detect.

2. Epithelial receptors in the larynx and trachea when stimulated cause coughing, laryngospasm and bronchospasm; stimulation of those in the bronchi causes hyperventilation in addition and may be partially responsible for asthma.

3. J receptors in the alveolar wall close to the pulmonary capillary appear to respond to the presence of alveolar interstitial fluid. In pulmonary congestion and oedema, rapid shallow breathing occurs with laryngeal constriction.

MECHANICS OF VENTILATION

The respiratory muscles perform the work of respiration. The most important muscle is the diaphragm which is assisted by the intercostal and abdominal muscles. The work of ventilation overcomes:

a. the elastic resistance of the tissues; work is proportional to the tidal volume;

b. the frictional resistance of the airways and viscous resistance of the tissues; work varies with gas flow;

c. the inertial resistance of the airways and tissues; work is related to the acceleration of the inflowing gas.

An indication of the amount of work required to overcome the elastic forces is given by the compliance. This is defined as the change in the volume of air in the chest for each kPa change of transthoracic pressure:

i.e. $\Delta V/\Delta P$, where ΔV is the change in volume of the thorax and ΔP is the change in transthoracic pressure.

The dynamic resistance to ventilation is produced by (b) and (c) above; however, the increased work required to overcome inertial resistance is generally ignored as being too small. The contribution of viscous resistance of the tissues is relatively small (20–30%) and relatively constant. The frictional resistance of the airways is more important and more variable and is generally regarded as representing non-elastic resistance (P/rate of volume change [litre/s] where P is the transthoracic pressure).

Compliance

The compliance of the respiratory system comprises that of the conducting airways and that of the lungs and thorax.

1. *The compliance of the respiratory airways.* Any increase in tidal volume contributes to an increase in the inefficiency of respiratory exchange (respiratory deadspace). A figure of 0.02–0.04 litre/kPa has been suggested for airway compliance, most of which resides in the intrathoracic portion of the airways.

2. *Compliance of the thorax.* Both chest wall and lungs have elastic properties which interact to provide an overall value for total thoracic compliance. When a subject is relaxed at the end of a normal expiration, the retractive forces of the lung and the chest wall are in equilibrium. If both were allowed to find their own equilibrium in isolation the lung would contract and the chest expand, as occurs when the chest is opened. At the end of normal expiration in a relaxed subject, the volume of air in the lung is called the functional

residual capacity (FRC). The values for FRC in the average man are 3000 ml when seated and 2200 ml when supine. Variables which alter lung compliance also alter FRC.

Lung compliance (C_L)

This can be estimated by measuring the change in lung volume which occurs with a unit change of pressure across the lung wall (transmural pressure), i.e. the pressure difference between the alveolar space and the intrapleural space. This is performed when a steady state exists and is called the *'static lung compliance'*. In Figure 2.1 the relationship can be seen to be curvilinear, the radii of curvature being greater at lung volume below FRC and close to total lung capacity; however, in the midrange, a constant value can be used as an approximation for lung compliance.

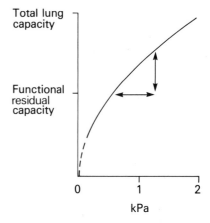

Fig. 2.1 Change in lung volume with change in transmural pressure.

Technically it is difficult to measure intrapleural pressure since the pleural space is only a potential space. It is customary to measure this pressure in the oesophagus using a balloon. In the erect subject the 10 cm balloon is passed into the middle third of the oesophagus. In the supine position the weight of the mediastinal contents may cause the pressure recorded to be erroneously high and adjustment of the site of the balloon may be necessary.

The elastic retractive forces of the lung are caused by the elastic fibres of the lung parenchyma and the surface tension of the liquid/air interface in the alveoli. Indeed, about 50% of the elastic recoil is attributable to the elasticity of the parenchyma and about 50% to the surface tension forces. This knowledge, however, is difficult to reconcile with the increase in surface tension which might be expected in alveoli which are diminishing in size during expiration if, as is generally assumed, alveoli mimic bubbles in their physical properties.

By Laplace's equation, the pressure P within a bubble (pascals) varies directly with surface tension T (mN/m) and indirectly with the radius of curvature r (mm) in the following manner:

$$P = \frac{2T}{r} \qquad (1)$$

As the radius of curvature of the alveolus falls, the pressure inside the alveolus rises; the small alveoli, having higher pressures, would empty into the larger alveoli, rendering the forces within the lung unstable. This does not occur in the lung because in the fluid lining of the alveoli there are surface-active substances called surfactant. These substances consist of phospholipids which are secreted by cuboidal cells with large nuclei at the junctions of septa (type II alveolar cells). As the alveolus decreases in size, the surface film becomes concentrated and the surface tension decreases to approx. 10 mN/m; as the alveolus increases in size, the surface tension rises to approx. 30–40 mN/m.

Lung compliance in the conscious erect average man is approx. 2 litre/kPa decreasing to 1.5 litre/kPa in the supine position.

The compliance of the chest wall (C_{CW}) is difficult to assess because of the activity of the respiratory muscles. It may be calculated theoretically by noting the change in lung volume which occurs during a unit change in the atmospheric-to-intrapleural pressure difference. This is complicated by the inevitable participation of the respiratory muscles in the conscious subject; if the measurement is conducted under anaesthesia, that in itself may bias the calculation. A value of 2 litre/kPa is usually suggested in the supine position but this may increase by 30% in the seated subject.

Total thoracic compliance (C_T) is measured by the change in lung volume which occurs with a unit change in the alveolar/ambient pressure gradient. An approximate value for an average man is 0.85

litre/kPa. Total thoracic compliance can only be measured in conscious subjects if they are trained to relax; therefore it is usually measured in paralysed anaesthetised subjects. (This is also true of chest wall compliance.)

The total compliance of the thorax is related to the other compliances as below:

$$\frac{1}{C_T} = \frac{1}{C_L} + \frac{1}{C_{CW}} \qquad (2)$$

Hysteresis. Elastic bodies exhibit a phenomenon termed hysteresis. This can be demonstrated in the lung. If lung volume above FRC is plotted during inflation against transmural pressure under static conditions, a curve is obtained. The relationship approximates to that of a straight line. However, if the process is repeated during deflation, the inflated lung shows a reluctance to deflate, i.e. the elastic retraction is smaller than expected, and the compliance is greater than expected (Fig. 2.2). This is caused mainly by changes in the surface tension forces and is more marked at the extremes of lung volume.

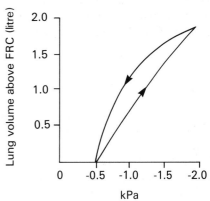

Fig. 2.2. Hysteresis in the lung demonstrated by a comparison of static compliances during inflation and deflation.

Static and dynamic compliance. The above discussion has been confined to static compliance which is an entity of importance in a basic scientific discipline such as physiology because it is an estimate of the elastic retractive forces of the lung. The inflow of air is sufficiently slow to allow the redistribution of gas to be complete.

In a practical discipline such as anaesthesia, a different concept is more relevant. This is dynamic compliance which measures compliance when redistribution of gases within the lung is still taking place although the exchange of flow with the environment is zero. This is the situation which occurs at the end of inspiration and expiration in spontaneously breathing man.

The distribution of air within the lung is dependent only on the compliance of the alveoli when static compliance is measured, whereas the resistance to gas flow within regional airways influences dynamic compliance.

In Figure 2.3 the part of the lung with a low resistance to air flow and a low compliance fills rapidly and is termed a 'fast' alveolus; the part of the lung with a high resistance and a high compliance fills much more slowly and is termed a 'slow' alveolus. In this situation dynamic compliance is smaller than static compliance since, in the time available for the measurement of dynamic compliance, the highly compliant alveolus does not fill completely because of airway resistance. If a patient with chronic obstructive lung disease is anaesthetised, it might be observed that the lungs are 'uncompliant' on controlling ventilation. The dynamic compliance is reduced because of severe airways resistance but, owing to destruction of the lung septa, static compliance may be raised.

Factors which influence compliance

1. Body size. Lung compliance varies with body surface area, height, weight, vital capacity, functional residual capacity and residual volume — all of which are related to body size. In order to make experimental data more widely applicable, specific compliance (lung compliance/FRC) is often calculated.

2. Posture. When the erect patient lies down, compliance decreases but specific compliance is unaltered.

3. The volume history of the lungs. Progressive decrease in lung compliance (of between 23% and 33%) has been recorded during quiet breathing. Deep breaths restore compliance to normal levels. This decrease has been attributed to changes in alveolar configuration.

4. Pulmonary blood volume. A reduction in pulmonary blood volume, as may occur during CPPV (constant positive pressure ventilation) increases compliance.

5. 100% oxygen at low tidal volume. Lung compliance diminishes after breathing 100% oxygen for 2 min. This is not observed when air is breathed.

6. Severe pulmonary disease. Decreases in dynamic lung compliance have been recorded in chronic obstructive lung disease.

7. Age. There is little evidence that compliance varies with age. Changes in functional residual capacity are accompanied by changes in lung compliance.

The effect of anaesthesia on compliance

1. Premedicant drugs. Morphine has little effect on compliance. Anticholinergic drugs increase the compliance of the airways but little is known of their effect on lung parenchyma.

2. General anaesthesia. Dynamic lung compliance is reduced markedly after induction of anaesthesia and the institution of artificial ventilation. It is uncertain if this change is caused by anaesthesia alone or by anaesthesia and artificial ventilation because it is difficult to determine compliance in the

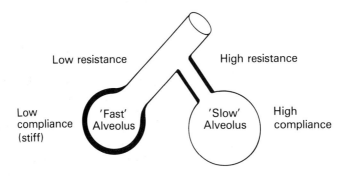

Fig. 2.3   Illustration of differential filling of alveoli in respiratory disease.

spontaneously ventilating subject. A marked reduction in FRC has been recorded during anaesthesia (approx. 20%); a decrease in lung compliance seems the most likely explanation. There is little evidence that compliance falls progressively with time so the greater part of the decrease must occur in the first few minutes of anaesthesia. Hyperinflation or a 'sigh' during ventilation raises compliance briefly, probably by temporarily reducing pulmonary blood volume.

Closing capacity

The lung volume present after a maximum expiration is called residual volume (RV). At this minimum lung volume, there is a reduction in size of the airways and some airways in the lower lung regions close off. The closing capacity (CC) is the lung volume when this closure is first recorded using a marker gas expirogram. A bolus of marker gas such as helium or argon is inspired at residual volume and the subject continues to inspire until the maximum lung volume (total lung capacity, TLC) is reached. The marker bolus is distributed mainly to the upper lung regions because many of the airways in lower lung regions are closed at lung volumes approximating to residual volume and the marker gas does not enter. The trace shown in Figure 2.4 may be divided into four phases: phase I has no marker gas as it consists of expired deadspace; phase II exhibits an increase in marker gas to a plateau; phase III is a plateau; phase IV shows a discrete increase close to residual volume. It is argued that phase III represents a mixture of gas from the upper lung areas (containing marker gas) and of gas from the lower lung areas (free of marker gas). When the airways of the lower lung areas close as residual volume is approached, expired gas empties predominantly from the upper lung areas and the concentration of marker gas rises. Closing capacity is the lung volume at the commencement of phase IV.

Closing capacity increases with age but is apparently independent of body position. Its relationship to FRC is of great importance since if it exceeds FRC there will be some lower airway closure during tidal respiration. Under these circumstances, hypoxaemia results in the part of the lung where airway closure has occurred. Closing capacity in the supine position reaches FRC soon after 40 yr of age; in the erect position it reaches FRC at approx. 60 yr of age. Since a considerable reduction in FRC has been recorded during anaesthesia, it is likely that the closing capacity exceeds FRC and impairs oxygenation during anaesthesia even in younger subjects.

Airway resistance

During inspiration in the spontaneously breathing subject, the chest wall and the lung expand. This causes a reduction in transthoracic pressure (P) which enables the inspired air to overcome the elastic and resistive forces. It can be stated in the following simplified equation that:

$$\Delta P = \underset{\text{(elastic)}}{\frac{V_T}{C}} + \underset{\text{(resistive)}}{R.\dot{V}} \qquad (3)$$

where P is the applied pressure: C is the compliance, V_T is tidal volume, $\dot{V}$ is flow and R is resistance.

The resistance to airflow in the spontaneously breathing normal adult man is approx. 0.05–0.2 kPa/litre/s, the value varying with the tracheobronchial anatomy and the type of gas flow.

The precise relationship between pressure and flow, i.e. the resistance to flow, is dependent on the type of flow — laminar, transitional or turbulent. Calculations of resistance assume that the flow is occurring in straight, smooth, cylindrical tubes which is patently not true when considering the tracheobronchial tree.

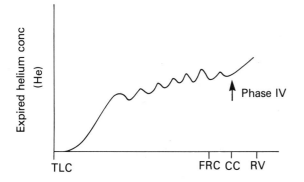

Fig. 2.4 Estimation of closing volume. A slow expiration has taken place after inhalation of a bolus of helium at residual volume. The arrow marks the start of phase IV.

Flow characteristics

Laminar flow describes the movement of gas down straight tubes with a parabolic profile and is the most efficient system of moving gas. The relationship of the pressure decrease (ΔP) across the tube is expressed by the Hagen-Poiseuille Law.

$$\Delta P = \frac{8\eta l \dot{V}}{\pi r^4} \qquad (4)$$

where r is the radius of the tube; l, the length of the tube; $\dot{V}$ the flow rate and η the viscosity of the gas.

Since resistance is equal to $\Delta P/\dot{V}$, it also equals $8\eta l/\pi r^4$. If flow is turbulent, a much greater applied pressure is required, i.e. the resistance is greater. The possibility of turbulent flow occurring may be estimated by calculating Reynolds' number (Re).

$$Re = \frac{v\varrho r}{\eta} \qquad (5)$$

where v is the linear velocity; r is the tube diameter and ϱ is the gas density. If the tube diameter is large and the linear velocity high — as might be expected in the trachea — turbulent flow is more likely to occur. In turbulent flow the resistance to flow is greater than that with laminar flow and is increased more rapidly with increase of flow.

Cooper has suggested that if Reynolds' number is less than 1000, laminar flow is present in the tracheobronchial tree; if Reynolds' number is above 1500, flow is entirely turbulent.

In the lung, Reynolds' number is only likely to exceed its critical value in the trachea and larynx during rapid ventilation; nonetheless the assumption that laminar flow is present is invalid because of the vortices which occur in the inspired air at each division of the bronchial tree.

Since resistance to flow varies with both the flow rate and the flow characteristics, citing a value for airway resistance at one flow rate is of little value. A German physiologist Röhrer suggested an equation for use during transitional flow

$$\Delta P = \underset{\substack{\text{laminar} \\ \text{component}}}{k_1 \dot{V}} + \underset{\substack{\text{turbulent} \\ \text{component}}}{k_2 (\dot{V})^2} \qquad (6)$$

where ΔP is the pressure decrease, $\dot{V}$ is the flow rate, k_1 is the constant for laminar flow and k_2 the constant for turbulent flow.

A more recent modification by Cooper enables a good approximation to be made in an expression of one term

$$\Delta P = 2.4(\dot{V})^{1.3} \qquad (7)$$

which differs by less than 10% from equation (6) over the range 0.2–3.0 litre/s.

Theoretical calculations of the site of the major part of the resistance suggest that it resides in the larger airways and diminishes dramatically in the small airways (less than 2 mm internal diameter, i.e. generations 12–25 in the Weibel classification) to virtually zero in generations 18–25 in the Weibel nomenclature. Thus, severe damage may occur in small airways which will be barely reflected in tests of airway resistance.

Factors which influence airway resistance

The resistance of the upper airways makes the greater contribution to airway resistance. Therefore obstruction of the upper air passages by inhalation of foreign bodies, swelling and oedema of the mucosa caused by inflammation or neoplasm or external pressure on the trachea will increase airway resistance.

The lower airways (those less than 2 mm internal diameter) are the cause of increased resistance in chronic obstructive lung disease, e.g. chronic bronchitis and emphysema and in acute disease, e.g. bronchial asthma. During spontaneous breathing in the normal subject, the pressure within the airways is greater than the intrapleural pressure throughout expiration. During active expiration, the intrapleural pressure may increase sufficiently to overcome the elastic recoil of the airway and result in airway collapse with air trapped distal to the closure. In chronic bronchitis and emphysema the loss of lung tissue reduces the elastic recoil and increases the likelihood of air trapping.

Airway closure may occur also in acute asthma since increased muscular activity and mucosal oedema may narrow the lumina of the bronchioles and predispose to airway closure during active expiration.

Moving from the erect to the supine position causes the functional residual capacity to diminish by almost 1 litre. This results in a decrease in lung volume and airway diameter which increases airway resistance.

THE EFFECT OF ANAESTHESIA ON AIRWAY RESISTANCE

Premedicant drugs. Morphine may cause bronchial constriction by release of histamine. Anticholinergic drugs, e.g. atropine, increase anatomical deadspace by bronchodilation and decrease airway resistance.

General anaesthesia. During anaesthesia airway resistance is markedly increased. Much of this is produced by the tracheal tube and its connections which have a resistance of 0.4–0.6 kPa/litre/s.

A more recently recognised factor is the decrease in functional residual capacity of approx. 20% after induction of anaesthesia. This, it is suggested, reduces the diameter of airways in the lung and thereby increases airway resistance. Healthy anaesthetised patients have an airway resistance of 0.3–0.6 kPa/litre/s. When the trachea is intubated, the resistance increases to 1 kPa/litre/s.

Some anaesthetic induction agents, including Althesin and thiopentone, may cause broncho-constriction, though the belief that d-tubocurarine, the nondepolarising muscle relaxant, causes broncho-constriction has not been substantiated.

THE INEFFICIENCY OF RESPIRATORY GAS EXCHANGE

Under normal circumstances the respiratory muscles ensure that adequate air reaches the lungs so that sufficient oxygen is supplied and carbon dioxide removed from the pulmonary capillary circulation which is in turn maintained by the pumping action of the heart. An increase in metabolic rate is met by increased work of the respiratory muscles and heart.

Factors which increase inefficiency include:

1. Respiratory dead space. The respiratory system is inherently inefficient because the respiratory gases enter and leave the lungs via a common pathway, i.e. anatomical deadspace. Some of the tidal volume enters the alveoli and takes part in respiratory exchange. If some of these alveoli are no longer perfused — after, for example, a pulmonary embolus — an increased portion of the tidal volume is wasted. This will result in hypercapnia unless the central drive increases ventilation. The magnitude of the compensatory increase reflects the extent of the inefficiency.

2. Shunt. If a portion of the cardiac output passing from the right ventricle to the systemic circulation does not come into contact with alveolar gas, it is said to be shunted (the anatomical shunt). Shunt results from Thebesian and bronchial venous blood flow in the normal subject but may also be seen in pathological conditions including lung collapse and cardiac conditions with right-to-left shunting. It amounts to approx. 5% of cardiac output in normal awake man.

3. Ventilation/perfusion ratio inequality $(\dot{V}_A/\dot{Q}_c)$. The greater part of the lungs is both ventilated and perfused. Nonetheless certain factors, e.g. gravity, affect the distribution of both ventilation and perfusion causing some areas to be underventilated (low $\dot{V}_A/\dot{Q}_c$) and other areas to be overventilated (high $\dot{V}_A/\dot{Q}_c$). The overall effect is to increase hypoxaemia and hypercapnia.

4. Diffusion. If molecules of respiratory gases are impeded whilst diffusing from the alveoli across the alveolar capillary membrane to the capillary blood, the efficiency of respiratory gas exchange decreases.

5. Hypoventilation. Hypoventilation results from an inadequate response of the respiratory muscles to metabolic demands causing hypercapnia and hypoxaemia. It may result from muscular weakness or inadequate respiratory drive.

Some of these factors are considered in greater detail below.

Respiratory deadspace

A major concern in the care of anaesthetised patients and of patients in intensive care units is to ensure that both ventilatory exchange in the lungs and the transport of respiratory gases by the circulation is sufficient for the needs of the patient. As some overall index of the efficiency of respiratory gas exchange is necessary, Enghoff modified Bohr's deadspace equation so that the portion of ventilation not taking part in cardiorespiratory gas exchange, i.e. wasted ventilation, can be calculated. This is termed physiological deadspace $(V_{D,PHYS})$.

Bohr-Enghoff equation

$$V_{D,PHYS} = V_T \ \frac{(Pa_{CO_2} - P\bar{E}_{CO_2})}{(Pa_{CO_2} - PI_{CO_2})} \qquad (8)$$

where V_T is tidal volume; Pa_{CO_2} is arterial CO_2 tension; $P\bar{E}_{CO_2}$ is mean expired CO_2 tension and PI_{CO_2} is inspired CO_2 tension.

If the inspired CO_2 concentration is negligible and $V_{D,PHYS}$ is expressed as a proportion of tidal volume,

$$\frac{V_{D,PHYS}}{V_T} = 1 - \frac{P\bar{E}_{CO_2}}{Pa_{CO_2}} \qquad (9)$$

Physiological deadspace is increased in respiratory disease and during anaesthesia. It may be subdivided into anatomical and alveolar deadspace.

Anatomical deadspace $(V_{D,ANAT})$ is customarily used to describe the conducting airways of the respiratory tract which do not take part in respiratory gas exchange. In normal subjects, where alveolar deadspace is very small, anatomical deadspace and physiological deadspace approach the same value. It can be measured planimetrically using Fowler's method of plotting nitrogen concentration against expired volume after inhaling a breath of pure oxygen.

Alveolar deadspace $(V_{D,ALV})$, which cannot be measured directly, results from ventilated but unperfused areas of lung and from an inhomogeneity of ventilation/perfusion ratios within the lung; it varies approximately with the arterial to end-tidal CO_2 tension difference; however, during exercise the end-tidal CO_2 partial pressure (PE'_{CO_2}) may exceed the arterial tension owing to an increased CO_2 output.

Factors which influence deadspace in conscious man

1. *Anatomical deadspace:*

 a. is increased with increase in size of the subject;
 b. is greatest on standing, less when seated and least when supine;
 c. is larger when the neck is extended and the jaw protruded: conversely it is less when the neck is flexed and the chin depressed;
 d. varies directly with tidal volume (about 2–4 ml/100 ml tidal volume);
 e. is increased by catecholamines, e.g. adrenaline and isoprenaline and decreased by histamine and 5-hydroxytryptamine.

2. *Alveolar deadspace* usually has a volume which is close to zero in normal awake, spontaneously breathing man; it is increased if there are areas of lung in which ventilation exceeds perfusion.

Alveolar deadspace:

 a. is increased in subjects who stand motionless for some minutes because perfusion of the lung apices diminishes;
 b. is increased after haemorrhage and fat embolism;
 c. is increased in pulmonary disease, e.g. emphysema.

Effect of anaesthesia on deadspace

1. *Anatomical deadspace.* Antisialagogue drugs increase anatomical deadspace. Hyoscine 0.4 mg i.m. results in a 33% increase in deadspace which may last in excess of two hours.

There is little evidence that anatomical deadspace is increased as a result of induction of anaesthesia (unless an induction agent possessing anticholinergic properties is used).

The effect of muscular paralysis and IPPV on the conducting airways is poorly documented. Indirect evidence suggests that increases in deadspace occur.

2. *Alveolar deadspace.* Anticholinergic premedication reduces pulmonary artery pressure and increases alveolar deadspace by reducing perfusion of the apices of the lung.

There is little evidence that general anaesthesia results in an increase in alveolar deadspace. In addition there is no evidence for any progressive increase in deadspace with duration of anaesthesia. However, it is generally agreed that alveolar deadspace is greater in anaesthetised, artificially ventilated patients compared with unpremedicated, unanaesthetised controls.

Physiological deadspace also increases with decreasing inspiratory/expiratory (I/E) ratio although the greater part of this change is probably attributable to an increase in anatomical deadspace.

Ventilation/perfusion ratio inequality

Distribution of inspired gas in the lung. Inspired gas is distributed unevenly in the lung. A progressive increase in ventilation occurs from the apex to the base of the lung in the erect subject. Ventilation per unit volume of lung is 50% greater at the base than at the apex. This discrepancy is caused by gravity which distorts the shape of the lung causing relative compression at the base and increased transpulmonary pressure at the apex. On inspiration from FRC to TLC the lower resting volume of the basal areas permits greater expansion.

It should be realised that an analogous situation exists in the supine subject. That part of the lung which lies superiorly is less well ventilated; however, since the anteroposterior diameter is much less than the distance from the root of the neck to the diaphragm, the differences in ventilation are less marked. In the lateral position, the dependent lung is better ventilated although this is not the case in the artificially ventilated subject (see p. 370).

Distribution of perfusion. Blood flow also increases from apex to base under the influence of gravity. If the lung is partitioned into three zones, the flow of pulmonary blood is dependent upon the relationship between alveolar pressure (P_A) the arterial pressure (Pa) and the venous pressure (Pv). This is explained most easily if we consider a special type of flow resistor named after Starling (Fig. 2.5). It comprises a length of flexible collapsible rubber tubing which passes through a rigid box. The upstream pressure (Pa) may be overcome by the pressure in the box (P_A) which collapses the tubing and prevents flow, whatever the level of the downstream pressure (Pv). This situation occurs in the upper parts of the lungs (Fig. 2.5).

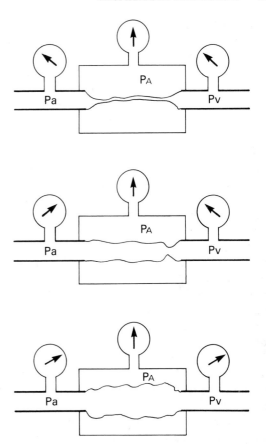

Fig. 2.5 Hydrostatic effects in the lung illustrated by the Starling resistor.

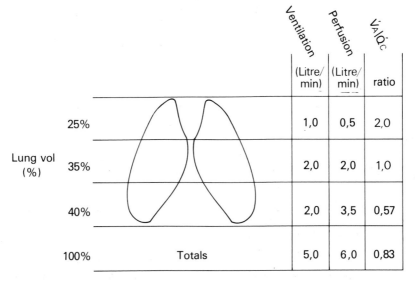

Lung vol (%)		Ventilation (Litre/min)	Perfusion (Litre/min)	$\dot{V}_A/\dot{Q}_C$ ratio
25%		1,0	0,5	2,0
35%		2,0	2,0	1,0
40%		2,0	3,5	0,57
100%	Totals	5,0	6,0	0,83

Fig. 2.6 Ventilation/perfusion ratios in an erect subject.

In the middle section, the arterial pressure exceeds the alveolar pressure; perfusion is dependent on the pressure difference ($Pa–P_A$) and is independent of the venous pressure. This is known as the 'vascular waterfall' because, like a waterfall, the flow is independent of the downstream pressure ($Pa > P_A > Pv$).

In the lower zone, Pv exceeds P_A and perfusion depends entirely on the pressure difference on either side of the box ($Pa–Pv$).

A fourth zone at the base of the lung has been postulated, where perfusion is reduced because of increased pulmonary interstitial pressure affecting the larger vessels.

The gradient in pulmonary perfusion from the apex to the base is similar in direction to the distribution of ventilation but is greater in magnitude.

Similar changes in ventilation and perfusion exist in the supine subject but are less marked because the anteroposterior axis of the thorax is small compared with the distance from the apex to the base of the lung.

Ventilation/perfusion ratios ($\dot{V}_A/\dot{Q}_C$). Radio-isotope techniques allow the inequality of ventilation and perfusion to be measured; results attained in an erect subject could be represented by those shown in Figure 2.6. A wide range of $\dot{V}_A/\dot{Q}_C$ values are obtained which would be greater if the lung were further subdivided. It should be appreciated that the average values of the $\dot{V}_A/\dot{Q}_C$ ratios belie the true effects of $\dot{V}_A/\dot{Q}_C$ ratios on respiratory efficiency.

Assessment of $\dot{V}_A/\dot{Q}_C$ ratios is difficult and requires elaborate equipment. In order to assess the effects of ventilation/perfusion inequalities, Riley and his colleagues proposed a mathematical simplification which assumes that inequalities of $\dot{V}_A/\dot{Q}_C$ ratios do not exist. A three-compartment model of the lung was constructed which assumes that the arterial–alveolar CO_2 difference is negligible and unaffected by inhomogeneity of ventilation and perfusion. The alveoli can then be categorised into three groups:

a. those ventilated but not perfused (alveolar deadspace);
b. those ideally ventilated and perfused ('normality');
c. those perfused but unventilated (venous admixture).

Using the Enghoff modification of Bohr's equation (equation 9) it is possible to calculate physiological deadspace. Since physiological deadspace = anatomical deadspace + alveolar deadspace, alveolar deadspace can be estimated. This will include not only true alveolar deadspace (unperfused alveoli) but an additional deadspace equivalent to the inefficiency caused by alveoli with high $\dot{V}_A/\dot{Q}_C$ ratios.

Shunt

An analogous assessment of alveoli with predominantly low $\dot{V}_A/\dot{Q}_C$ ratios can be calculated as shunt and added to true anatomical shunt. The sum is usually called *venous admixture*.

Venous admixture = anatomical shunt + 'shuntlike' (or frank) effect (from areas of low $\dot{V}_A/\dot{Q}_C$)

Venous admixture is calculated from the 'shunt equation'

$$\frac{\dot{Q}_s}{\dot{Q}_t} = \frac{C_c'O_2 - C_aO_2}{C_c'O_2 - C_{\bar{v}}O_2} \qquad (10)$$

where $\dot{Q}_s$ is venous admixture (litre/min), $\dot{Q}_t$ is cardiac output (litre/min), $C_c'O_2$ is the end-capillary oxygen content (ml), C_aO_2 is the arterial oxygen content and $C_{\bar{v}}O_2$ is the mixed venous oxygen content.

The end-capillary oxygen content is calculated from the alveolar air equation (Table 2.1); a value for the alveolar oxygen tension is obtained; this is in equilibrium with the end-capillary oxygen tension from which the corresponding content can be derived.

Clinically, the alveolar/arterial oxygen partial pressure difference (A−a) Po_2 is often used as an approximation for venous admixture; however a reduction in cardiac output causes a reduction in the mixed venous oxygen tension (if oxygen consumption remains constant) and by lowering arterial oxygen tension leads to an increase in this estimate of venous admixture.

If the Riley method of analysis is used, it would be convenient to differentiate shunt from low $\dot{V}_A/\dot{Q}_C$ ratio inequality. Theoretically if the inspired oxygen tension is raised, venous admixture should be reduced if it is caused chiefly by a scatter of $\dot{V}_A/\dot{Q}_C$ ratios; it should have no effect on true shunt. However, if a high concentration of oxygen is inspired it may cause absorption collapse of the lung, increasing true shunt.

Table 2.1 Alveolar air equations

Ideal alveolar air	$P_{A}O_2 = P_{I}O_2 - \dfrac{P_{a_{CO_2}}}{R}$	where R = respiratory exchange ratio
Riley's equation	$P_{A}O_2 = P_{I}O_2 - \dfrac{P_{a_{CO_2}}}{R}[1 - F_{I}O_2(1-R)]$	
Filley's equation	$P_{A}O_2 = P_{I}O_2 - P_{a_{CO_2}}\left[\dfrac{P_{I}O_2 - P_{\bar{E}}O_2}{P_{\bar{E}}_{CO_2}}\right]$	

Note: 1. Riley's equation assumes that inert gases are in equilibrium and the inspired oxygen concentration constant. Filley's equation permits lack of equilibrium for inert gases.

2. $P_{I}O_2 = F_{I}O_2 \times (P_B - PH_2O)$,

where $F_{I}O_2$ = fractional inspired oxygen concentration
                P_B = barometric pressure
                PH_2O = saturated vapour pressure of water at body temperature.

Effect of anaesthesia on venous admixture

Venous admixture, as measured by the $(A-a)P_{O_2}$ increases after induction of anaesthesia whether ventilation is controlled or not. As yet it is uncertain if this increase in venous admixture is caused by an increase in true shunt or in $\dot{V}_A/\dot{Q}_c$ scatter. Isotope studies in the supine position fail to demonstrate sufficient $\dot{V}_A/\dot{Q}_c$ ratio inequality to account for the increase in venous admixture; thus by default it is assumed to be shunt. 'Microatelectasis', i.e. collapse in the absence of radiological evidence, was suggested to occur with anaesthesia. Early evidence that this change could be reversed by 'sighing' was unsubstantiated.

The spatial inhomogeneity of ventilation and perfusion has been considered in detail because it has proved the most popular explanation for impairment of gas exchange. It is doubtful if this abnormality is of significance in anaesthetised supine subjects unless closing volume approaches functional residual capacity.

It is also possible that failure of the respiratory gases to mix completely during a respiratory cycle might increase the inefficiency of respiratory gas exchange. This is termed 'stratified inhomogeneity of ventilation and perfusion'. Its significance in the anaesthetised subject is uncertain but theoretically concentration gradients would be decreased by a low respiratory frequency and the introduction of a post-inspiratory pause.

A third possibility is that respiratory efficiency might diminish because of cyclical changes in alveolar CO_2 and O_2 partial pressures during the respiratory cycle, i.e. temporal inhomogeneity of ventilation and perfusion. This is negligible in conscious man but is increased during anaesthesia with spontaneous respiration because expiratory flow is exponential. When ventilation is controlled, greater inefficiency might be anticipated because lung volume is greater during the inspiratory phase and perfusion is reduced; perfusion is greatest in the expiratory phase when lung volume is small.

Alveolar–capillary diffusion

The limitation imposed on respiratory efficiency by the diffusion of CO_2 and O_2 across the alveolar–capillary membrane is believed to be small. Since CO_2 has a much higher water solubility than oxygen and can penetrate an aqueous medium 20 times as rapidly as oxygen under normal circumstances (i.e. in the absence of a carbonic anhydrase inhibitor), impaired diffusion tends to cause hypoxaemia rather than hypercapnia.

The oxygen molecules follow a diffusion path from the alveoli across the membrane to the pulmonary capillaries because they diffuse from a high to a low partial pressure. Theoretically hypoxaemia cannot occur in a normal subject at rest provided that the alveolar oxygen tension is normal. It was believed that respiratory exchange was limited by impaired diffusion in the alveolar-capillary block syndrome, e.g. fibrosing alveolitis and interstitial pulmonary oedema; however it seems likely that this inefficiency in gas exchange results from spatial inhomogeneity of ventilation and perfusion because of distortion of tissues. A diffusion defect can be expected (theoretically) if the cardiac output is raised, e.g. during exercise, because equilibrium may not be attained between gas in the alveoli and gas in the capillaries.

The measurement of transfer factor of carbon monoxide was believed to estimate diffusion defects. It now seems more likely that a reduction in transfer factor is caused by a decrease in pulmonary surface area (e.g. lung resection or emphysema), pulmonary arteriovenous shunting or spatial inhomogeneity of ventilation and perfusion.

Anaesthesia and controlled ventilation have little effect on transfer factor.

Summary

The chief factors responsible for inefficiency in respiratory gas exchange are hypoventilation, shunt and spatial inhomogeneity of ventilation and perfusion. The latter two factors are believed to be increased after induction of anaesthesia and control of ventilation; the contribution of stratified and temporal inhomogeneities is uncertain.

CONTROLLED MECHANICAL VENTILATION

The development of intensive therapy since the mid-sixties has resulted in increasing sophistication of methods of ventilatory support often directed to re-establishing spontaneous respiration in patients with poor lung function.

Conventional artificial ventilation of the lungs, also termed IPPV (intermittent positive pressure ventilation) is usually achieved using a tidal volume of 10–15 ml/kg at a rate, in adults, of 10–12 breath/min. Early experiments suggested that IPPV resulted in pulmonary collapse, and 'artificial sighs' were incorporated into most ventilators allowing the tidal volume to double or triple in size once in 30–100 breaths. Later experimental evidence suggests that such a manoeuvre is unnecessary.

In 1948 Cournand suggested that if the intrathoracic pressure increased, this would reduce pulmonary capillary flow and therefore cardiac output. Experimental evidence in dogs has shown that cardiac output does not decrease until the transpulmonary pressure exceeds 1 kPa, but that vena cava flow ceases at peak inspiration (3 kPa).

Efforts were directed to reducing the mean transpulmonary pressure by limiting the duration of inspiration and introducing a postexpiratory pause. There was little improvement because cardiac output diminished significantly with IPPV only in patients with autonomic blockade or decreased circulating volume. If the inspiratory period is reduced to less than 1 s, the efficiency of respiratory gas exchange decreases.

A subatmospheric pressure (NEEP — negative end-expiratory pressure) was used also to reduce the effects of IPPV on mean intrathoracic pressure. It reduces mean intrathoracic pressure but increases the risk of 'air trapping' in the lungs especially in patients with diseased terminal airways, e.g. emphysema. In addition both deadspace and venous admixture increase.

The introduction of an expiratory airway resistance proved of great benefit. The main advantage of PEEP (positive end-expiratory pressure), is that it increases FRC, allowing tidal volume to be raised above closing capacity. This improves gas distribution within the lungs. It also decreases lung water in patients with incipient or frank pulmonary oedema, thereby reducing left ventricular filling pressure and improving cardiac output. Theoretically the increased intrathoracic pressure would be expected to reduce cardiac output but in practice this does not always occur.

In the absence of vasomotor instability and decreased circulatory volume, PEEP often increases arterial oxygenation with reduction of venous admixture. It is recommended when the lungs are 'poorly compliant', e.g. adult respiratory distress syndrome (ARDS) or mitral regurgitation. Nonetheless, the response to PEEP is unpredictable and each patient should be assessed individually to determine the net effect of increased FRC and potential decrease in cardiac output.

The application of an expiratory resistance during spontaneous respiration is termed CPAP (continuous positive airway pressure). This also appears most beneficial in patients with pulmonary disease and is used frequently in children with respiratory distress syndrome (RDS). If PEEP has proved successful in improving oxygenation during artificial ventilation, it is often advisable to use CPAP for a period following the resumption of spontaneous ventilation.

Weaning from controlled mechanical ventilation

Triggering

Triggering enables a patient to initiate a mechanical inflation by lowering the airway pressure, i.e. an attempted spontaneous ventilation. As weaning progresses, the subatmospheric pressure required to initiate a passive inflation is increased. By triggering ventilation in this way, there is less risk that the patient will 'fight' the ventilator whilst being weaned from controlled ventilation.

SIMV (synchronised intermittent mandatory ventilation)

When the patient has started to breathe spontaneously, the frequency of the mandatory breath delivered by the ventilator is gradually reduced. A double circuit is designed so that a patient can breathe spontaneously from one circuit whilst a second circuit conveys mandatory breaths from the ventilator. This is called intermittent mandatory ventilation (IMV). This method has the disadvantage that a mandatory breath might be superimposed upon a spontaneous breath. A recent improvement has allowed IMV to be synchronised with spontaneous respiration (SIMV). If a spontaneous breath occurs within a triggering period, i.e. just before the next mandatory breath is due, it triggers the preset mandatory breath. At other times the patient breathes spontaneously. Sophisticated ventilators enable the spontaneous minute volume to be compared with the total expired volume.

Extended mandatory minute volume (EMMV)

This recent development, also termed mandatory minute ventilation (MMV), allows the ventilator to adjust mandatory ventilation with reference to the patient's spontaneous respiration, whilst the patient is being weaned from the ventilator. Acceptable values for tidal volume and respiratory rate are preset on the ventilator. In the absence of spontaneous respiration they are delivered in the usual way (IPPV); if, however, the patient takes a spontaneous breath, the ventilator delays delivering the preset tidal volume. If sufficient spontaneous breaths are taken the ventilator does not ventilate the patient but, if the patient's respiratory efforts decline, mandatory breaths are again delivered by the ventilator.

Inspiratory assist

Some ventilators can supplement spontaneous breaths mechanically, preventing shallow ventilation. This triggering device is used with SIMV and EMMV.

High frequency ventilation (HFV)

In recent years HFV has excited interest because it can produce good gas exchange by methods not previously explored. Sjöstrand classified HFV into three distinct groups (see also Table 2.2):

1. High frequency jet ventilation (HFJV)
2. High frequency positive pressure ventilation (HFPPV)
3. High frequency forced diffusion ventilation (HFDV), or high frequency oscillatory ventilation (HFOV)

1. High frequency jet ventilation (HFJV). High velocity gas is delivered through a small cannula inserted through the cricothyroid membrane or placed within an endotracheal tube. Air is entrained around the orifice by the Bernoulli Principle. The respiratory frequency is 150—500 breath/min and the tidal volume is generally less than the anatomical deadspace. It usually generates a pressure above atmospheric which is equivalent to a PEEP value of 0.5 kPa. It is currently of interest in the U.K. because a commercially produced ventilator is available (Acutronic Medical Systems AG). It has been used during endoscopy in patients with bronchopleural fistulae and for weaning patients from ventilators.

Both HFJV and HFDV need careful adjustment to ensure adequate CO_2 elimination.

2. High frequency positive pressure ventilation (HFPPV). This technique uses conventional ventilators and the customary technique of endotracheal intubation. It uses lower respiratory frequencies than HFJV (60–150 breath/min) and tidal volumes of 100–300 ml. It differs from HFJV by not entraining air.

3. High frequency forced diffusion ventilation (HFDV), or *high frequency oscillatory ventilation (HFOV).* Sine wave oscillations of frequencies of 500 to 3000 breath/min are used in conjunction with tidal volumes of a few millilitres. There is no bulk flow, so intrapulmonary pressure is low. Although oxygen

Table 2.2   High frequency ventilation

	Frequency (cycles or breath/min)	Air entrainment	V_T (ml)	P_A
High frequency positive pressure ventilation (HFPPV)	60–150	NO	100–300	Higher
High frequency jet ventilation (HFJV)	150–300	YES	< 150	Medium
High frequency forced diffusion (oscillatory) ventilation HFDV/HFOV	500–3000	NO	***	Lower

V_T = tidal volume set at ventilator.
P_A = alveolar pressure.
*** = immeasurable by conventional means.

need only be supplied to satisfy metabolic needs, CO_2 is usually removed by absorption.

The chief advantages of HFV are improved respiratory gas exchange and better patient acceptance of controlled ventilation. Circulatory depression in patients with cardiovascular instability might be expected to be reduced. The reduction of pulmonary barotrauma reported for this technique might prove useful if recent reports of bronchiolectasis, as a result of artificial ventilation with PEEP, are confirmed.

BLOOD GASES

Oxygen transport

During spontaneous respiration in an atmosphere of PO_2 = 21 kPa, a normal individual exhibits an arterial PO_2 of approx. 13.3 kPa (Fig. 2.7). With a normal cardiac output, this results in an *oxygen flux* (arterial oxygen content × cardiac output) of 1 litre/min at rest, which can be raised to 15 litre/min on exercise. Most of this oxygen is carried in blood in chemical combination with haemoglobin. At normal arterial oxygen tension, haemoglobin is almost fully saturated (97.5%); thus increasing the oxygen tension has little effect on haemoglobin saturation.

A small proportion of oxygen is carried in solution (Table 2.3). In arterial blood at 37°C it is 0.0225ml/100 ml/kPa which is approx. 0.3 ml/100 ml blood at normal arterial tension. In mixed venous blood, the oxygen tension is normally 5 kPa, and the dissolved oxygen approx. 0.1 ml/100 ml. Thus only

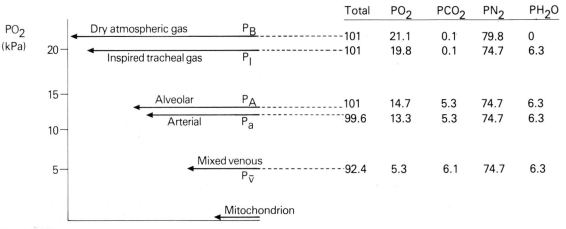

Fig. 2.7   The oxygen cascade.

Table 2.3 Arterial and mixed venous composition

	Arterial	Mixed venous
Oxygen tension ($P\text{O}_2$) (kPa)	13.3	5.3
Oxygen content (ml/100ml)		
Total	20	15
Attached to Hb	19.7	14.9
Dissolved	0.3	0.1
Carbon dioxide tension ($P\text{CO}_2$) (kPa)	5.3	6.0
Carbon dioxide content (ml/100ml)		
Total	50	54
Dissolved	2.5	2.9
Carbamino	2.5	4.9
HCO_3^-	45	46.2

0.2 ml/100 ml blood is available to the tissues from oxygen dissolved in blood when breathing air. The importance of dissolved oxygen is that if the inhaled oxygen concentration is raised to 100% it increases the dissolved arterial oxygen to 2 ml/100 ml blood, although there will be little effect on oxygen carriage by haemoglobin.

Haemoglobin is a complex compound with a molecular weight of 64 500. It contains ferrous iron which forms reversible compounds with oxygen. The theoretical oxygen-carrying capacity of haemoglobin (Hüfner's constant) is 1.39 ml per gram. Experimentally the value is 1.34.

The oxyhaemoglobin dissociation curve (ODC) in Figure 2.8 shows oxygen saturation of haemoglobin on the ordinate and oxygen tension on the abscissa. The position of the curve is defined by the oxygen tension when the haemoglobin saturation is 50% (P_{50}) under standard conditions. P_{50} varies between 3.5 and 3.9 kPa in normal subjects.

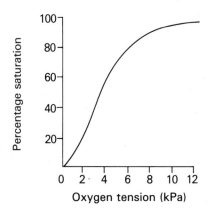

Fig. 2.8 The oxyhaemoglobin dissociation curve.

In venous blood the oxygen tension is normally 5kPa and the haemoglobin saturation is 75%. In the tissues the P_{50} increases, i.e. ODC moves to the right, and more oxygen is released from the haemoglobin at a given tension. If the P_{50} decreases i.e. the ODC moves to the left, less oxygen is available. The affinity of oxygen for haemoglobin is influenced by the following factors:

1. Bohr effect. The Bohr effect is a shift to the right of the ODC, i.e. an increase in P_{50} with increasing hydrogen ion concentration. The classical Bohr effect refers to changes in H^+ concentration resulting from alterations in $P\text{CO}_2$. However, a similar shift of the curve takes place with an increase in H^+ concentration from other causes, e.g. metabolic acidosis. A decrease in H^+ concentration moves the curve to the left.

2. 2,3DPG and CO_2 tension. 2,3 Diphosphoglycerate (2,3DPG) is produced by glycolysis and influences ion changes in the red cell. At constant H^+ concentration the interaction of 2,3 DPG and CO_2 tension reduce the affinity of haemoglobin for oxygen.

3. Temperature. Hypothermia shifts the ODC to the left whereas pyrexia shifts it to the right.

CO₂ carriage

Carbon dioxide is produced by tissue metabolism and conveyed by the venous circulation to the lungs. CO_2 is transported as:

1. Dissolved CO_2. Since the solubility of CO_2 in plasma is 0.5 ml/100 ml/kPa, the dissolved CO_2 in arterial blood amounts to 2.65 ml/100 ml if the arterial tension is 5.3 kPa. The mixed venous tension is 6.0 kPa and this represents an increase in dissolved CO_2 of approx. 0.4 ml/100 ml blood.

2. Bicarbonate. Much of the gaseous CO_2 diffusing from the cells into the venous blood is rapidly hydrolysed to H_2CO_3 (carbonic acid) in the red cells. It then dissociates into H^+ and HCO_3^- ions. The bicarbonate diffuses into the plasma, and chloride diffuses into the red cells to maintain electrical neutrality according to the Gibbs-Donnan equilibrium, since potassium ions cannot leave the red cell. The hydrogen ion is buffered by the reduction of haemoglobin, which normally takes place simultaneously, thereby producing basic forms of histidine on the haemoglobin molecule.

The hydrolysis of CO_2 to carbonic acid can be achieved in the required time only if it is catalysed. Carbonic anhydrase acts as catalyst for this reaction and allows the hydration of one million moles of CO_2/mol of enzyme/min.

The movement of chloride into the red cells is known as the Hamburger shift (or 'chloride' shift) which obscures the important fact that bicarbonate efflux from the red cells is the prime effect and the 'chloride shift' merely a compensatory phenomenon.

3. Carbamino-compounds. CO_2 also combines with the aminoresidues of haemoglobin.

$$HbNH_3 \rightleftharpoons HbNH_2 + H^+$$
$$CO_2 + HbNH_2 \rightleftharpoons HbNHCOOH$$
$$HbNHCOOH \rightleftharpoons HbNHCOO^- + H^+$$

CO_2 carriage is increased because partially-reduced haemoglobin carries more carbamino-compounds than oxyhaemoglobin; this portion is evolved in the lungs. It contributes about 10% to the CO_2 evolved.

CDH effect

The Christiansen-Douglas-Haldane effect relates to the diminished carriage of CO_2 when partially-reduced haemoglobin, a weak acid and buffer, is converted to the stronger acid, oxyhaemoglobin. The CO_2 tension increases with oxygenation although the CO_2 content remains constant.

The decrease in CO_2 content in arterial blood is caused by the loss of the oxylabile carbamino-carriage (10%) and the reduction in bicarbonate ion because of the diminished buffering of H^+ by haemoglobin.

LUNG FUNCTION TESTS (see Appendix XI page 562)

Defects of the mechanical properties of the lung can be easily assessed from simple tests. The readily available portable dry spirometers (e.g. Vitalograph) enable expiratory spirograms to be used in assessing disease. After a maximum inspiration, the expired air is exhaled as rapidly as possible. The total volume expired is the forced vital capacity (FVC) and that portion which is expired in the first second is the forced expired volume at one second ($FEV_{1.0}$). Both values have to be compared with standard values

adjusted for age, height and sex. The ratio $FEV_{1.0}$/FVC compensates for these variations. If a ratio of less than 70% is present, some obstruction of the larger intrathoracic airways is present.

The Wright peak flowmeter measures the peak expiratory flow rate (PEFR) which is sustained for 10 ms. The measurement of lung volumes in conjunction with the above measurement allows the differentiation of the major patterns of defects of lung mechanics. It is desirable to measure total lung capacity (TLC), functional residual capacity (FRC) and residual volume (RV); if one of these variables is measured the others can be computed easily. FRC, for example, may be assessed by the inhalation of a tracer gas (e.g. helium) and the result calculated from its subsequent dilution.

An obstructive pattern present in chronic obstructive lung disease shows a low $FEV_{1.0}$/FVC ratio low PEFR, low VC and high RV.

A restrictive pattern is seen after resection of the lung or certain skeletal defects, e.g. kyphoscoliosis, and is revealed by a normal $FEV_{1.0}$/FVC ratio, low PEFR, low RV and low TLC.

More elaborate tests of mechanical function can be made using a body plethysmograph with an oesophageal balloon to measure intrapleural pressure. Measurements of pressure and volume may be plotted on an X/Y recorder or an oscilloscope. 'Dynamic compliance' can be calculated at the 'no flow' points. The area of the loop is an indication of airway resistance since it represents the work performed by the respiratory muscles (Fig. 2.9).

Gas exchange can be assessed noninvasively by measurement of the transfer factor for carbon

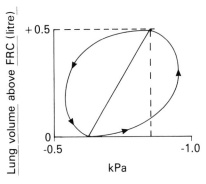

Fig. 2.9 Dynamic pressure/volume loops. Area indicates work performed against resistance. Compliance is $0.5/0.25 = 2$ litre/kPa.

monoxide by the single breath or the steady state method. If the transfer factor is reduced, it suggests the presence of venous admixture or destruction of the lung tissue. This is found in diffuse pulmonary fibrosis, emphysema and pulmonary oedema. It seems unlikely that a defect of diffusion exists and the hypoxaemia results from spatial maldistribution of ventilation and perfusion.

Where severe respiratory disease is present (e.g. causing dyspnoea at rest) arterial blood gas analysis is required.

The assessment of acid base balance — pH and base deficit — in conjunction with the respiratory gases, allows an estimation of the compensatory changes of acidosis and alkalosis which may serve as an index of the severity of respiratory inefficiency.

FURTHER READING

Cotes J E 1979 Lung function — assessment and application in medicine, 4th edn. Blackwell Scientific Publications, London
Nunn J F 1977 Applied respiratory physiology, 2nd edn. Butterworths, London

West J B 1977 Pulmonary pathophysiology — the essentials. Blackwell Scientific Publications, London
West J B 1977 Ventilation/blood flow and gas exchange, 3rd edn. Blackwell Scientific Publications, London
West J B 1979 Respiratory physiology — the essentials, 2nd edn. Blackwell Scientific Publications, London

3

Cardiovascular physiology

The cardiovascular system may be considered under two major headings: the peripheral circulation, which adjusts blood flow to individual tissues, and the heart which generates the sum of the individual flows.

PERIPHERAL CIRCULATION

Under normal physiological conditions, blood flow through an organ is determined by its metabolic requirements. Blood flow per unit mass of tissue varies widely from organ to organ both in the basal resting state and at maximum flow (Fig. 3.1). Disease states, such as hypovolaemia and sepsis, and drug therapy, including anaesthesia, may interfere with autoregulatory mechanisms resulting in excessive or inadequate perfusion.

Blood flow rate is determined by the driving pressure (the difference between mean arterial pressure, MAP, and mean venous pressure, MVP), and the resistance to that flow.

$$\text{Flow} = \frac{\text{MAP} - \text{MVP}}{\text{Resistance}}$$

Resistance to blood flow is determined by three factors: calibre and length of the vessels, viscosity of blood and nature of the flow (turbulent or laminar).

Flow profile

In the absence of irregularities of the vessel wall (e.g. resulting from atheroma), flow in blood vessels is laminar. The relationship between driving pressure

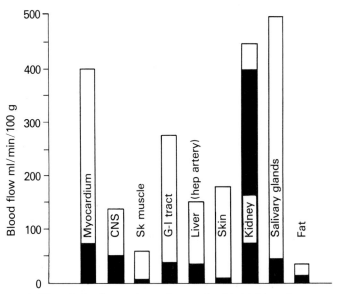

Fig. 3.1 Blood flow at rest (solid portion) and at maximum flow rate (total height) in various organs.

and flow under such conditions is expressed by the Hagen-Poisseuille formula:

$$Q = \frac{\pi r^4 \Delta P}{8 l \eta}$$

where Q is the flow rate, r the radius of the vessel and l its length. ΔP is the driving pressure and η the blood viscosity. This relationship holds true only for steady flow of Newtonian fluids, i.e. those whose viscosity is independent of flow rate. These conditions do not apply to the cardiovascular system, where flow is pulsatile and blood viscosity is determined by flow rate. It is thus an oversimplification, but illustrates the critical role of the vessel radius in determining flow rate, since the relationship is to the *fourth* power of the radius.

Viscosity

Blood is a mixture of solutes (e.g. electrolytes and proteins) and particles (e.g. cells and chylomicrons). At low flow rates, the cells tend to aggregate, thus increasing viscosity. The subject is further complicated by the tendency of cells to concentrate in the centre of the blood vessel where the velocity is greatest. The haematocrit is therefore lowest at the periphery of the lumen where the velocity is lowest. Thus, in vivo, blood tends to act much more as a Newtonian fluid than in vitro. The tendency of erythrocytes to concentrate in the centre of a vessel results in a lower haematocrit in blood which enters side branches. This process is known as plasma skimming, and has obvious implications on flow rate and oxygen delivery.

Anaemia reduces oxygen carrying capacity, leading to an increase in blood flow to maintain oxygen delivery. The increased flow rate is facilitated by reduced viscosity secondary to the reduced erythrocyte count. Clinically, there is little effect on cardiac index until the haemoglobin decreases below 10 g/dl (Fig. 3.2), the usually accepted lower limit for routine anaesthesia.

Volatile anaesthetic agents increase blood viscosity by increasing the rigidity of the erythrocyte membrane. However, the effect is slight in comparison with the effect of anaemia and has no significant effect on tissue blood flow rates.

Blood viscosity is a complex subject and the reader is referred to Stuart and Kenny (1980) for a recent review.

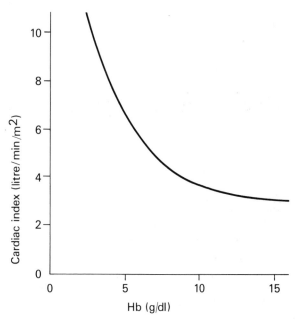

Fig. 3.2   Relationship between haemoglobin and cardiac index in chronic anaemia.

Control of the peripheral circulation

Blood flow through the capillary beds is controlled by local mechanisms and, under normal circumstances, cardiac output adjusts to meet the total flow required. Regulatory mechanisms ensure that the perfusion pressure (arterial pressure) is maintained irrespective of changes in total flow and posture. During periods of stress, e.g. hypovolaemia, the regulatory mechanisms override local control to maintain the blood supply of essential organs including the brain, heart and kidney. These organs also possess autoregulation, i.e. a constant blood flow despite changes in perfusion pressure.

The capillary bed (Fig. 3.3). Capillaries are composed of a single layer of endothelial cells which permit free exchange of nutrients and metabolites between tissues and blood. Not all capillaries are open at any one time and there are generally preferred routes through which blood predominantly flows.

In many tissues, there are also direct arteriovenous anastomoses. In the skin, these facilitate heat loss by increasing tissue flow rate without affecting capillary perfusion.

Control of flow through capillaries is effected by contraction and relaxation of the smooth muscle of the metarterioles and the precapillary sphincters. A

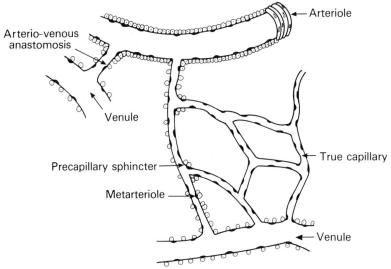

Fig. 3.3 Diagrammatic representation of the microcirculation.

number of metabolic factors including oxygen, ATP and hydrogen ions have been shown to affect capillary flow but the exact mechanism has not been elucidated.

Local regulation of flow by metabolites controls the distribution of blood flow within an organ, in addition to total flow.

Control of the systemic circulation

This section is concerned with the overall control of the circulation and the distribution of blood flow according to priority rather than local needs. It is also concerned with the maintenance of an adequate perfusion pressure and the adjustment of cardiac output by variations in the capacity of the circulation.

The calibre of the arterioles and precapillary sphincters determines blood flow to the peripheral circulation. The calibre depends upon the inherent tone of the smooth muscle, the activity of the autonomic nervous system, circulating hormones, and the local concentration of metabolites (Fig. 3.4).

Inherent tone

Smooth muscle generally exhibits spontaneous contraction in the absence of other stimuli and this is the likely source of inherent tone. Mechanical stretching of the muscle by pulsatile internal pressure may also initiate contractions. In general, those tissues with the poorest sympathetic innervation have the greatest inherent tone. For example vessels in skeletal muscle, brain and myocardium have a high tone whereas those in skin have a low inherent tone.

Autonomic nervous system (Chapters 5 and 12)

Sympathetic adrenergic (Fig. 3.5). The adrenergic sympathetic fibres are the predominant pathway whereby the systemic circulation is controlled. The vasomotor areas in the medulla send descending fibres to the preganglionic cells in the thoracolumbar segment of the spinal cord. The preganglionic fibres synapse with postganglionic fibres in the ganglia of the sympathetic chain from which postganglionic fibres travel to vascular smooth muscle. The activity of the vasomotor centres is influenced by afferent impulses from many sensory areas including baroreceptors, chemoreceptors and skin, and from higher centres in the cortex and hypothalamus. The preganglionic cells in the spinal cord may also be influenced directly by higher centres and by reflex activity at spinal level.

The vasomotor centre is continuously active, resulting in a resting tone in vascular smooth muscle. Increased sympathetic activity does not affect all tissues equally. Those tissues with the highest intrinsic vascular tone respond less well than those with a lower tone (Fig. 3.6). Thus with increased

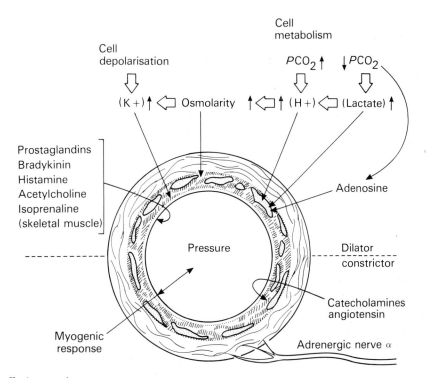

Fig. 3.4 Factors affecting vascular tone.

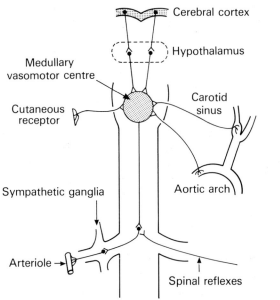

Fig. 3.5 The vasomotor centre.

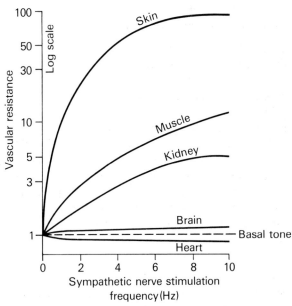

Fig. 3.6 The effect of sympathetic nervous stimulation on vascular resistance in various organs.

adrenergic sympathetic activity there is redistribution of blood from skin, muscle and gut to brain, heart and kidney.

Sympathetic cholinergic. Activation of sympathetic cholinergic fibres results in vasodilatation in skeletal muscle. These fibres are represented centrally in the cerebral cortex and are involved in the anticipatory response to exercise, the 'fight or flight' reaction. Stimulation of the appropriate area of the brain results in redistribution of blood flow from skin and viscera to skeletal muscle.

Dopaminergic receptors. Dopamine is a precursor of noradrenaline and has been shown to have a vasodilator effect on splanchnic and renal vessels mediated through specific receptors. This response is useful pharmacologically but the physiological role of such receptors is unclear.

Humoral control. Adrenaline and noradrenaline are released by the adrenal medulla and from adrenergic nerve endings. Their concentrations may increase dramatically during stress but they probably contribute little to cardiovascular control. Their prime role may be in the metabolic response to stress.

Angiotensin II is a potent vasopressor produced by the conversion of angiotensinogen by renin. Renin is released from the juxtaglomerular apparatus of the kidney in response to a reduction in systemic arterial pressure. Angiotensin II probably plays little part in acute regulation of the circulation but, by increasing the secretion of aldosterone, leads to retention of sodium and hence an increase in circulating volume.

Metabolic control

A number of metabolites influence the calibre of blood vessels, including CO_2, K^+ and H^+. Adenosine, bradykinin and prostaglandins are among the chemicals known to cause vasodilatation. It is likely that different tissues respond more readily to some compounds than others.

Induced hypocapnia resulting from hyperventilation results in generalised vasoconstriction and reduction in tissue blood flow which may be deleterious.

Hypoxia results in vasodilatation in all parts of the circulation except the pulmonary vessels, where vasoconstriction occurs. The vasodilatation is countered by reflex vasoconstriction mediated by the sympathetic nervous system resulting from stimulation of the chemoreceptors. This acts as a protective mechanism to increase blood flow to the brain.

Autoregulation

Blood flow through many organs remains almost constant over a wide range of perfusion pressure. In man, this phenomenon is most marked in the renal and cerebral circulations. The mechanism is unclear, although accumulation or washout of vasodilator metabolites seems a likely explanation. Alterations in the intrinsic tone of vascular smooth muscle have also been proposed.

Measurement of blood flow

The measurement of blood flow in absolute terms through tissues is technically difficult. However, of more importance is the relationship between flow and oxygen consumption. If the imbalance is severe, organ failure occurs and this may be manifest by oliguria, clouding of consciousness, etc. Clinically, it is useful to assess flow in the organ which is most accessible, viz. the skin. Clinical assessment of skin flow by capillary refill may be supplemented by the measurement of the gradient between core temperature and skin temperature, which is normally less than 5°C. Mixed venous oxygen tension may provide a global assessment of the adequacy of tissue perfusion. Normal mixed venous oxygen tension is 6 kPa, and values below 3.7 kPa are associated with a poor prognosis. The value must be interpreted with care particularly in the presence of arteriovenous shunting of blood, when the value may be elevated despite tissue hypoxia.

Capacitance vessels

The veins contain approx. 80% of the blood volume (Fig. 3.7). Venoconstriction and dilatation adjust the capacity of the circulation to maintain a balance with the blood volume, for example during hypovolaemia (vide infra) and with changes in posture. Impairment of venoconstriction by disease or drugs, e.g. anti-hypertensive agents, leads to a reduction in cardiac output and hypotension on standing (postural hypotension).

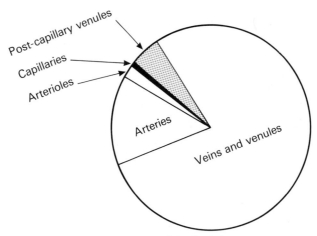

Fig. 3.7   Distribution of blood volume between different parts of the circulation.

The calibre of the veins is adjusted by changes in sympathetic activity, mediated both by nervous and humoral stimulation. The postcapillary venules are also sensitive to local concentrations of metabolites in the same manner as the precapillary sphincters.

Control of arterial pressure

Systemic arterial pressure is controlled closely in order to maintain the driving pressure necessary for tissue perfusion. The normal values vary with age and sex (Table 3.1) in addition to physiological changes including sleep. It must be stressed that although systemic arterial pressure may be measured readily the readings obtained should be interpreted with care. A normal or even elevated arterial pressure is no guarantee of adequate tissue perfusion. Mean arterial pressure (MAP) may be calculated from the formula:

$$MAP = \text{diastolic arterial pressure} + \frac{\text{(pulse pressure)}}{3}$$

Its value is determined by the product of cardiac output (CO) and total systemic peripheral resistance (TPR).

$$MAP = CO \times TPR$$

The units for expressing TPR are confusing. Traditionally, it has been expressed as dyne s/cm^5 and more recently as Newton s/m^5 (1 dyne s/cm^5 = 100 Newton s/m^5).

$$TPR \text{ (dyne s/cm}^5) = \frac{MAP \text{ (mmHg)}}{CO \text{ (litre/min)}} \times 80$$

Thus, if MAP = 100 mmHg and CO = 5 litre/min, TPR = 1600 dyne s/cm^5.

Mean arterial pressure is thus a balance between cardiac output and resistance to flow posed by the vascular beds.

Neurones in the medulla receive and integrate afferent impulses from the baroreceptors, chemo-

Table 3.1   Changes in arterial pressure, cardiac output and peripheral vascular resistance with age.

Age (years)	Arterial pressure (mmHg) Systolic/ diastolic	Mean	Blood flow Cardiac index* (litre/min/m²)	Cardiac output (litre/min)	Peripheral vascular resistance** (mmHg/ litre/min)	(dyne s/cm⁵)
10	100/65	75	4.0	4.8	15	1150
20	110/70	85	3.7	6.7	12	950
30	115/75	90	3.4	6.1	14	1100
40	120/80	92	3.2	5.8	15	1200
50	125/82	95	3.0	5.4	17	1300
60	130/85	98	2.8	5.0	19	1500
70	135/88	102	2.6	4.7	21	1650
80	140/90	105	2.5	4.5	22	1800

*Assuming a body surface area of 1.2m² at age 10 and 1.8m² thereafter
**Assuming a CVP of 5 mmHg

receptors, skin, muscle and viscera, and from higher centres, the hypothalamus and cortex. Classically these neurones have been described as a discrete vasomotor centre but it is now thought that they are distributed in several regions of the medulla. Activity in these neurones leads to increased vasoconstrictor tone and thus an increased arterial pressure, provided that cardiac output does not decrease.

Baroreceptors

Arterial baroreceptors are located in the carotid sinus and the wall of the aortic arch. The nerve endings are not sensitive to pressure but to deformation of the arterial wall (stretch receptors). Stimulation of the baroreceptors leads to reflex reduction in vasoconstrictor and venoconstrictor tone, and to bradycardia. Arterial pressure is thus reduced by diminution of both total peripheral resistance and cardiac output. Conversely a reduction in baroreceptor activity leads to vaso- and venoconstriction and increased heart rate.

Other cardiovascular reflexes

The chemoreceptors located in the carotid and aortic bodies respond to hypoxia and to a lesser extent hypoperfusion. Chemoreceptor stimulation results in a general increase in cardiovascular sympathetic activity, increasing systemic arterial pressure.

A large number of stretch receptors have been described in the heart and great vessels but their role is unclear. Stimulation of receptors in the atria increases sympathetic activity thus aiding the increase in cardiac output which follows increased atrial pressure. Other atrial receptors appear to be responsible for regulation of blood volume by influencing ADH release and thus water balance.

Assessment of baroreceptor responses

The response to change in posture is a useful guide to the ability of a patient to respond to cardiovascular stress. This is of importance in patients with autonomic neuropathy (e.g. diabetics) and those receiving vasodilator drugs.

The Valsalva manoeuvre, a forced expiration against a closed glottis resulting in increased intrathoracic pressure and decreased venous return, is a convenient bedside assessment. In the normal individual, arterial pressure is maintained by a combination of tachycardia and vasoconstriction during the period of increased intrathoracic pressure (Fig. 3.8). On release of the raised intrathoracic pressure there is transient hypertension and bradycardia until the vasoconstriction is reversed. The heart rate response is easiest to detect and may be measured at the bedside.

The baroreceptors may also be tested by external stimulation or by inducing a transient increase in arterial pressure by administration of a short acting vasopressor, e.g. noradrenaline. These tests are more suitable for research than for clinical evaluation.

THE HEART

Anatomy

The heart comprises four chambers; the right and left ventricles, which generate the energy to propel the blood around the pulmonary and systemic circulations respectively, and the atria which serve as reservoirs for blood and as accessory pumps to augment ventricular filling. Uncompensated loss of atrial activity, e.g. atrial fibrillation, reduces cardiac output by approx. 25%.

Cardiac muscle has properties intermediate between those of skeletal and smooth muscle. It has cross-striations similar to those of skeletal muscle and in common with smooth muscle, exhibits spontaneous rhythmic contractions acting as a single unit or syncitium. The muscle fibres are arranged in an interdigitating spiral fashion to form the two ventricles. The left ventricle, which performs approx. six times as much work as the right, has a much thicker wall and is conical in shape. The right ventricular wall is thinner, and applied to the left ventricular wall (Fig. 3.9). The ventricular and atrial muscle fibres are inserted into a fibrous framework at the atrioventricular junction which also provides an attachment for the cardiac valves.

The cardiac valves ensure that blood flows only from atria to ventricles to arterial systems. The aortic and pulmonary valves act passively, opening in response to a pressure gradient between ventricle and artery and closing when the gradient reverses. The tricuspid and mitral valves are prevented from bulging back into the atria during ventricular systole by the papillary muscles and their chordae tendineae.

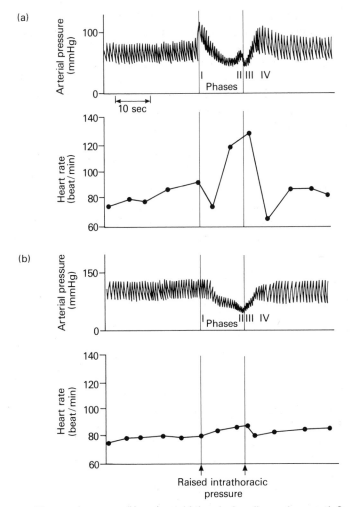

Fig. 3.8 Valsalva manoeuvre. (a): normal response. (b): patient with impaired cardiovascular control. See text for details.

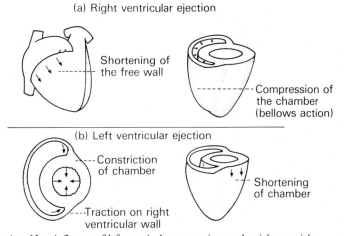

Fig. 3.9 Ventricular contraction. Note influence of left ventricular contraction on the right ventricle.

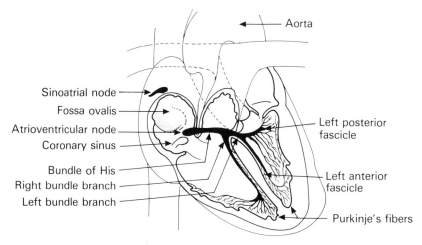

Fig. 3.10 The cardiac conducting system.

The conducting system (Fig. 3.10) comprises fibres of specialised muscle cells and it is responsible for the initiation and spread of cardiac contraction. The sino-atrial (SA) node lies in the wall of the right atrium close to the superior vena cava. An impulse originating here sweeps through the atria, leading to atrial systole and activates the atrioventricular (AV) node. The AV node is continuous with the AV bundle (bundle of His) which pierces the fibrous septum separating atria and ventricles. The AV bundle runs through the ventricular septum and divides into right and left bundles which supply their respective ventricles.

Electrophysiology of the heart

A normal heart beat is initiated by cells of the SA node. The wave of contraction passes around the atria through the AV node and bundle to the ventricles. Cells of the conducting system (pacemaker cells) exhibit spontaneous depolarisation resulting from a relative permeability to sodium ions (Fig. 3.11). At a threshold of -50 mV a sudden sharp depolarisation occurs which is propagated to other cells, initiating a heart beat. The rate of spontaneous depolarisation is fastest in the SA node which thus has the fastest intrinsic rate and this normally determines heart rate. Inhibition of higher parts of the system may result in other cells, for example in the AV node or ventricles, acting as pacemaker at their own slower intrinsic rates. The heart rate is determined by the rate of spontaneous depolarisation which is increased by

sympathetic activity and decreased by vagal activity. Extreme vagal activity may halt spontaneous depolarisation, resulting in asystole until an impulse is generated by a pacemaker cell further down the system (vagal escape).

The action potential of cardiac muscle differs markedly from skeletal muscle. The duration of depolarisation is approx. 200 ms in contrast to the 1–2 ms of skeletal muscle. Cardiac muscle is inexcitable during this period.

The electrocardiogram (e.c.g.)

Electrical currents generated by cardiac muscle during depolarisation and repolarisation are reflected in changes of electrical potential at the skin. The magnitude and polarity of the potential at a particular point depends upon the mass of muscle contracting, and upon its orientation. The P wave reflects atrial depolarisation, the QRS complex ventricular depolarisation and the T wave ventricular repolarisation.

The e.c.g. reflects the *electrical* activity of the heart and it may indicate rate and rhythm in addition to some indication of myocardial damage. It does not reflect the adequacy of mechanical contraction. Normal complexes may be observed in the absence of mechanical activity. For further information on the measurement and interpretation of the e.c.g. the reader is referred to one of the standard texts, e.g. Rollason 1975.

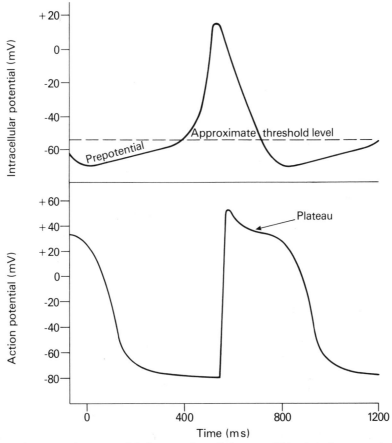

Fig. 3.11 Upper panel: transmembrane potential of a pacemaker cell; heart rate 75 beat/min. Lower panel: cardiac muscle action potential.

The cardiac cycle (Fig. 3.12)

A heartbeat is initiated by spontaneous depolarisation of an SA node pacemaker cell. A wave of depolarisation spreads over the atria, which contract. At this point, the atrioventricular valves are open and the ventricles are filling under the pressure of the venous return — the pulmonary and aortic valves being held closed by the pressure gradient between pulmonary artery and aorta and their respective ventricles. Atrial contraction augments ventricular filling as diastole nears its end. The wave of depolarisation passes through the AV node, along the AV bundle and spreads over the ventricles. Ventricular contraction (systole) follows. As ventricular pressure increases, the AV valves close and a phase of isometric contraction (i.e. increasing tension without shortening) begins. The aortic and pulmonary valves open as ventricular pressures

exceed aortic and pulmonary arterial pressures and the ejection phase commences. Atrial repolarisation occurs during early systole and the atria refill with blood as they relax. Spontaneous depolarisation begins in the SA node.

Towards the end of systole, ventricular repolarisation occurs and the ventricles relax. The pulmonary and aortic valves close as pulmonary arterial and aortic pressures exceed the respective ventricular pressures, marking the end of systole. The closure of the AV valves and aortic and pulmonary valves is audible as the first and second heart sound respectively. The aortic valve normally closes before the pulmonary, splitting the second sound. Aortic valve closure is seen as the dicrotic notch on the aortic pressure waveform.

Relaxation is isometric until ventricular pressure is less than atrial pressure, when the AV valves open

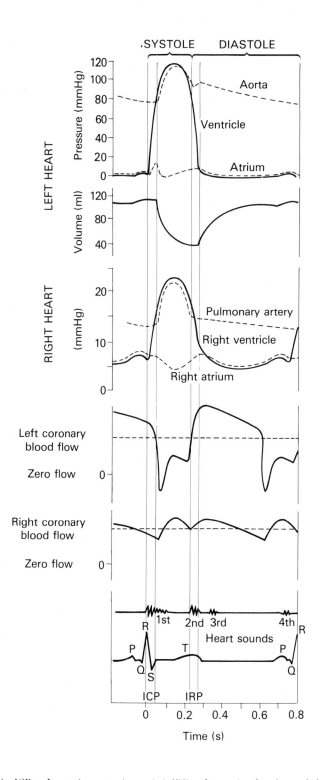

Fig. 3.12   The cardiac cycle. ICP = Isometric contraction period; IRP = Isometric relaxation period.

and ventricular filling begins. Filling continues passively until the SA node initiates a further cardiac cycle. At a normal heart rate of 70 beat/min, a cardiac cycle occupies about 850 ms, of which approx. 220 ms is systole. Increased heart rates are accomplished almost entirely by a reduction in the duration of diastole (and ventricular filling). Thus, the atrial contribution to ventricular filling becomes proportionately more important as heart rate increases.

The passage of cardiac catheters and the interpretation of the waveforms seen is only possible if the cycle of events and their temporal relationship is clearly understood. Figure 3.12 summarises these events. Normal intracardiac pressures and oxygen tensions are shown in Figure 3.13.

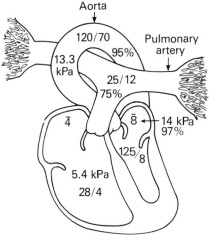

Fig. 3.13 Cardiovascular pressures, oxygen tensions and saturations.

Coronary circulation

The myocardium is supplied by two coronary arteries, the right and left, which supply their respective ventricles. There is often a degree of overlap in the areas supplied but there is little communication between the two vessels. The arteries run over the surface of the heart giving off branches which penetrate the myocardium to supply the capillary beds. Venous drainage from the left ventricle passes via the coronary sinus into the right atrium, that from the right passes via the anterior cardiac vein also into the right atrium. In addition a small proportion of the coronary flow (3–5%) drains directly into the ventricles through the Thebesian veins.

The normal coronary blood flow at rest is approx. 250 ml/min (80 ml/min per 100 g of tissue) and this may increase five-fold during maximal exercise (Fig. 3.1). Myocardial oxygen consumption is approx. 11 ml/100 g/min compared with skeletal muscle at 8 ml/100 g/min. Coronary venous P_{O_2} is very low (approx. 4 kPa [30 mmHg]). Thus increased oxygen consumption by the heart cannot be met by an increased extraction but must be accommodated by increased flow or increase in myocardial efficiency. If increased flow cannot be achieved, increased extraction may result in tissue hypoxia. This feature of the coronary circulation is illustrated by the response to anaemia; if the oxygen carrying capacity of blood is halved (Hb 7 g/dl) and cardiac output is

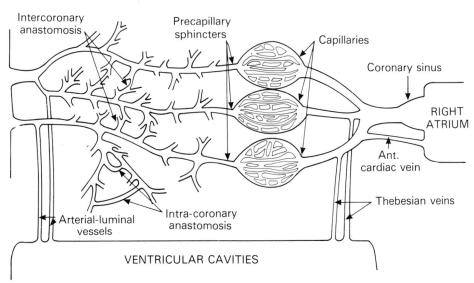

Fig. 3.14 Diagrammatic representation of the coronary circulation.

doubled then myocardial blood flow should *quadruple* if myocardial hypoxia is to be avoided.

The coronary circulation is unique in that blood flows principally during diastole since the intramyocardial vessels are compressed during systole (Fig. 3.12). Increased heart rate shortens diastole and may thus impair myocardial blood supply if flow rate cannot increase during diastole. The intramyocardial pressure is highest in the subendocardial region and lowest at the epicardium. An increased intra-ventricular pressure during diastole, as may occur during sudden hypertension, has a greater effect on flow through the subendocardial vessels and may result in subendocardial ischaemia.

Coronary blood flow is determined predominantly by myocardial metabolic activity. Although there are sympathetic fibres to the heart, changes in myocardial oxygen demand induced by sympathetic stimulation have a predominant effect on coronary vascular resistance in comparison with local vascular effects of the catecholamine transmitters. Although auto-regulation occurs in the coronary circulation, this phenomenon may be difficult to demonstrate in vivo because of changes in myocardial oxygen demand accompanying changes in perfusion pressure.

Cardiac output

Cardiac output ($\dot{Q}$) is the product of stroke volume (SV) and heart rate (HR).

$$\dot{Q} = SV \times HR$$

In a normal 70 kg man at rest, SV = 70 ml, HR = 70 beat/min and $\dot{Q}$ = 5 litre/min. In order to compare the cardiac output of patients of different size, the cardiac output per square metre of body surface area is often calculated. This is termed cardiac index (CI). For example: surface area = 1.7 m^2 in a 70 kg man.

$$CI = \frac{5}{1.7} = 3 \text{ litre/min/m}^2$$

Control of cardiac output

The cardiac output is determined by the metabolic requirements of the body, and over a period of time it equals the venous return (Fig. 3.15). Similarly the output of the two ventricles must also be identical. A consistent difference of 1 ml between the right and left ventricular stroke volumes at a heart rate of 70 beat/min would lead to an imbalance of 1 litre in 14 min. The balancing of venous return and cardiac output, and right and left ventricular outputs is an intrinsic property of the myocardium, and occurs even in a denervated heart with a fixed rate. If this were not so, cardiac transplantation would be impossible and patients with cardiac pacemakers could not exercise.

In 1915 Starling stated the relationship between the force of cardiac contraction and muscle fibre length thus: 'The law of the heart is thus the same as the law of muscular tissue generally, that the energy of

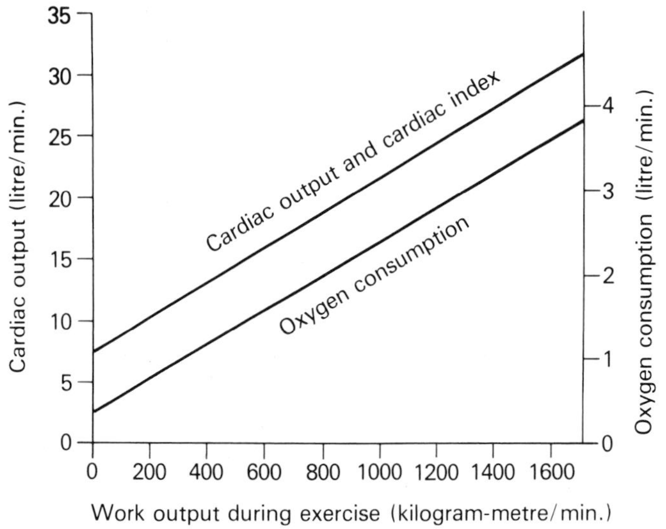

Fig. 3.15 Relationship between exercise, cardiac output and oxygen consumption.

contraction, however measured, is a function of the length of the muscle fibre'. This intrinsic property of cardiac muscle enables the heart to balance venous return and cardiac output and the outputs of right and left ventricles. This mechanism alone compensates for increases in venous return of 2–300% above resting values. Further increases in venous return are met by increases in contractility of the muscle fibres and heart rate. These changes are mediated by the autonomic nervous system.

The mechanism is best understood if the effect of an increase in activity in a muscle group is considered. Increased metabolism in muscle leads to locally-induced vasodilatation and increased blood flow. The increased flow rate increases venous return, which distends the right atrium and ventricle. The resulting increased force of contraction increases right ventricular stroke volume which leads to left ventricular distension. This in turn causes increased left ventricular stroke volume and an increase in cardiac output if heart rate remains constant. The increased cardiac output is maintained until reduced muscle metabolism leads to vasoconstriction, reversing the process. If the vasodilatation is sufficient to reduce peripheral vascular resistance, arterial pressure decreases transiently. Baroreceptor activity diminishes and vasoconstriction and increases in heart rate and contractility occur as a result of increased sympathetic activity. The increased heart rate and contractility lead to a further increase in cardiac output. In the case of muscular exercise, increased sympathetic activity may occur prior to the increase in venous return as the cerebral cortex 'anticipates' the activity.

Cardiac contractility

The force of contraction is determined by the initial fibre length (Frank-Starling mechanism) and by the ability of the cardiac muscle to contract at a given initial fibre length (*contractility*). These relationships are usually illustrated as a curve relating force of contraction to fibre length (Fig. 3.16), changes in contractility being shown as displaced but parallel curves.

Starling's law, as stated above, is almost impossible to validate in man because the two parameters (force of contraction and fibre length) cannot be measured.

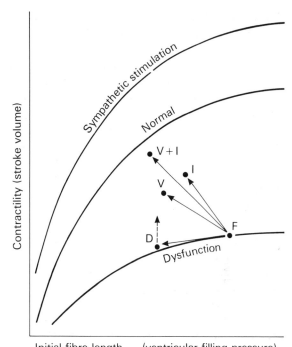

Fig. 3.16 Starling's Law of the heart and changes in myocardial contractility. Letters and arrows signify effects of different treatments in cardiac failure. I = inotropic drugs, V = vasodilator drugs; V + I = combined use; D = diuretics. Broken arrow indicates that ventricular function may improve later.

As a result parameters such as stroke volume, speed of contraction, maximum rate of rise of ventricular pressure, peak ventricular pressure, ejection fraction (stroke volume/end-diastolic volume) and stroke work (SV × [MAP − MVP]) have been used. All these parameters are indirect measures of the force of contraction and must be interpreted with care. For example, a leaking mitral valve results in a reduction in forward stroke volume despite an increase in left ventricular work.

Similarly, alternative parameters have been used to reflect initial fibre length. End-diastolic volume and pressure have been used widely. End-diastolic pressures, particularly right and left atrial pressures, require careful interpretation since the change in pressure with a given volume change depends upon the compliance of the chamber. Thus the pressure change in a stiff ventricle is greater than in a flabby ventricle for the same volume change.

Ventricular function curves based on the indirect parameters mentioned above are clinically useful in plotting the response to treatment but may be of limited value in determining deviations from normality.

Sympathetic stimulation is the most significant extrinsic factor which increases myocardial contractility. The effect may be induced by neuronal activity or by circulating endogenous or exogenous catecholamines. Both heart rate and contractility increase, with a parallel effect on cardiac output and myocardial oxygen consumption.

Calcium ions increase contractility, as do digoxin and insulin as well as all the sympathomimetic amines. Conversely, contractility is reduced by β-adrenergic blocking drugs, antiarrhythmic agents, the majority of general anaesthetics (vide infra) and an elevated extracellular potassium ion concentration.

Control of heart rate

Heart rate is determined by the rate of spontaneous depolarisation of the sino-atrial node. The resting heart rate is approx. 75 beat/min, and increases to 110 beat/min after total denervation, indicating the importance of inhibitory vagal parasympathetic activity. Thus cardiac acceleration may be achieved either by a decrease in vagal activity or an increase in sympathetic activity.

Increases in heart rate occur largely as a result of shortening of diastole. Excessive increases in heart rate impair ventricular diastolic filling such that stroke volume and cardiac output decrease. Similarly cardiac output decreases if an increasing stroke volume is unable to compensate for a decreasing heart rate. In a normal heart, cardiac output is unimpaired between 40 and 150 beat/min although this range may be considerably reduced by disease.

Assessment of cardiac function

The best indication of cardiac function is the state of the peripheral circulation. Simple methods of assessment, as discussed previously, are often adequate, and should be employed before more invasive techniques are contemplated.

Ventricular filling pressures

The pressure in the central veins (CVP) is equated with the right ventricular end-diastolic pressure. The pressure measured depends on venous return, the ability of the heart to respond, the state of filling of the circulation, and venous tone. Because CVP measurement is influenced by many factors and because the value noted depends critically on the zero point chosen, isolated readings are of little value. With any control system, the maximum information can be obtained by observing the effect of small perturbations. Thus the response of the CVP to small fluid challenges is more valuable than single readings. This is illustrated in Figure 3.17 where the upper panel illustrates the course of a young traumatised hypovolaemic patient who, with vigorous sympathetic activity, has induced such venoconstriction that CVP is elevated. Fluid challenges *decrease* the CVP as cardiac output increases and vasodilatation occurs. In contrast, the lower panel illustrates a patient with cardiac impairment. Fluid challenges produce a sustained elevation of CVP which on the second occasion exceeds the ability of the heart to respond, and active intervention is required.

In the examples given above it is assumed that right and left ventricular function is comparable and that changes in CVP reflect changes in left atrial pressure (LAP) both in direction and magnitude. Clinically there is often a marked disparity between the function of the two ventricles, and left ventricular filling pressures must be measured more directly. This is usually achieved by floating into the pulmonary artery a balloon-tipped catheter which is then wedged in a branch. Since there is no flow through that segment of the pulmonary circulation, the pressure at the tip of the catheter (PCWP) equilibrates to a value close to LAP.

Cardiac output

The measurement of cardiac output is useful as part of an overall assessment of the circulation. Isolated measurements are of little value. For example, a cardiac output of 5 litre/min indicates excellent function after myocardial infarction but indicates failure in severe sepsis or major burns. Again, this measurement is most useful in assessing the response to therapy. The standard method of measurement is the Fick principle, namely that oxygen consumption ($\dot{V}_{O_2}$) equals the arteriovenous oxygen content difference $(A-V)C_{O_2}$ multiplied by cardiac output ($\dot{Q}$).

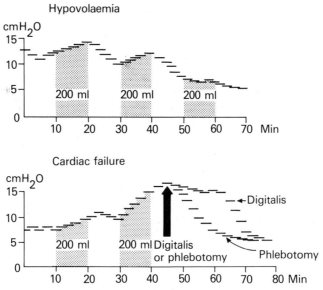

Fig. 3.17 Changes in central venous pressure with fluid replacement. Upper panel: hypovolaemia in a young patient. Lower panel: cardiac failure. See text for details.

$$\dot{Q} = \frac{\dot{V}_{O_2}}{(A-V)_{CO_2}} = \frac{250 \text{ ml/min}}{5 \text{ ml/100 ml}} = 5 \text{ litre/min}$$

This method is time-consuming and has been replaced in clinical use by thermal- or dye-dilution methods. The principal of these techniques is that a bolus of indicator is injected into blood entering the heart, where it mixes in the venous return. The concentration of indicator is measured downstream and plotted against time. Since the mass of indicator is known, integration of the concentration curve can be used to derive the volume in which the indicator was distributed, the cardiac output. Cold dextrose, the indicator in the thermal technique, is injected into the right atrium, and the decrease in blood temperature is sensed in the pulmonary artery by a thermistor, which is usually incorporated into a balloon catheter. Estimations may be repeated at frequent intervals.

Indocyanine green is the indicator used in the dye method. Sampling is usually from the radial artery through a detector cuvette. The initial dye has usually recirculated before the last dye has cleared the heart, thus obscuring the latter part of the decay curve. Modern cardiac output computers extrapolate from the first part of the curve, thus avoiding the problem of recirculation.

CARDIOVASCULAR RESPONSE TO DISEASE AND ANAESTHESIA

Hypovolaemia (Fig. 3.18)

Hypovolaemia is a common clinical problem. It is a result of imbalance between the blood volume and the capacity of the circulation and causes impaired tissue perfusion. It may be caused by loss of fluid, e.g. haemorrhage, or excessive vasodilatation, e.g. high spinal anaesthesia.

Loss of fluid reduces venous return, decreasing right atrial filling pressure and thus cardiac output. The resulting hypotension is countered by the baroreceptors, which increase heart rate and induce vaso- and venoconstriction. These measures maintain arterial pressure and minimise the decrease in cardiac output. Cardiac output is redistributed away from skin, muscles and viscera, and blood flow is maintained to heart and brain. Arterial pressure is usually maintained until approx. 20% of the blood volume is lost and cardiac output has diminished by 30%. Thereafter it decreases progressively. Any drug which attenuates vasoconstriction or tachycardia, for example anaesthesia and β-blockers, results in earlier hypotension.

Increased ADH and aldosterone secretion retain water and sodium, compensating for the fluid loss in the longer term. Reduction in capillary pressure

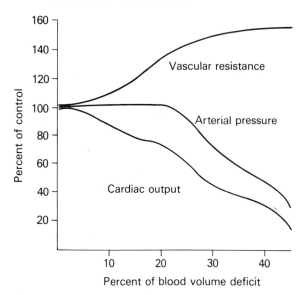

Fig. 3.18 Cardiovascular changes with progressive hypovolaemia.

results in a translocation of fluid from extracellular space into the circulation as a result of the oncotic pressure of plasma, further compensating for the hypovolaemia.

Severe or prolonged reduction in perfusion may lead to organ failure, for example renal failure. In addition accumulation of tissue metabolites may result in local vasodilatation, overcoming the vasoconstriction and exacerbating the hypotension. This phase has been termed 'irreversible shock' and represents clinically the phase when simple fluid replacement is inadequate to restore a normal circulation.

The initial management of hypovolaemia consists of replacement with the appropriate fluid. It is important that fluid is not given blindly but a cycle of assessment, therapy, reassessment, further therapy and so on is initiated to ensure optimum replacement. This cycle is emphasised in Figure 3.19, which shows a suggested plan of management of circulatory failure.

Cardiac failure

The heart may fail as a pump for many reasons, e.g. ischaemia, trauma, drugs and sepsis. As the ventricles fail, stroke volume is reduced and baroreceptor activity increased. The resulting venoconstriction increases ventricular filling pressures, initial

myocardial fibre length, and restores stroke volume towards normal. The reduced cardiac output also results in fluid retention. Eventually the myocardial fibres are unable to generate any further increase in contractility, and cardiac output diminishes rapidly. Venous pressures become so high that pulmonary and/or peripheral oedema occur.

Management of cardiac failure can be approached in three ways: optimisation of ventricular filling pressures, enhancement of contractility, and reduction of cardiac work. A reduction of filling pressure is necessary in most patients in right or left ventricular failure. This may be achieved by diuretics, venesection or venodilator drugs. Contractility may be enhanced by a variety of drugs (vide supra) but usually at the expense of increased myocardial oxygen consumption. Cardiac work is determined by the volume of blood pumped (cardiac output) and the resistance against which it is pumped (vascular resistance). The former is already reduced but reduction of the latter with vasodilators may enhance cardiac performance considerably. Such treatment must be given with care since excessive vasodilatation may result in severe hypotension and impairment of perfusion of vital organs. Filling pressures are often reduced by vasodilatation and may require adjustment.

Once again the need for a cycle of assessment therapy and reassessment is emphasised. Figure 3.16 shows the effect of various therapies on ventricular function.

Anaesthesia

All anaesthetic agents depress myocardial function in the isolated heart, but clinically the depressant effect may be countered or exacerbated so that the resultant effects on cardiac output may vary greatly (Fig. 3.20).

Sympathetic activity

Ether, cyclopropane and ketamine increase sympathetic activity, with maintenance of cardiac output during light anaesthesia. In contrast, other agents such as halothane depress sympathetic activity, leading to reduced contractility and peripheral vasodilatation. Halothane also enhances parasympathetic activity, resulting in bradycardia.

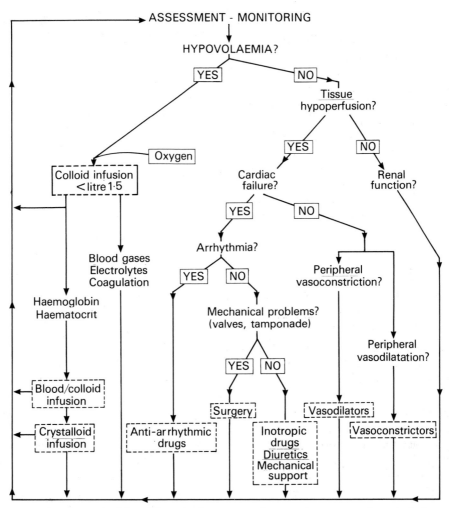

Fig. 3.19 Management of cardiovascular failure. The cycle of assessment, therapy and reassessment is emphasised.

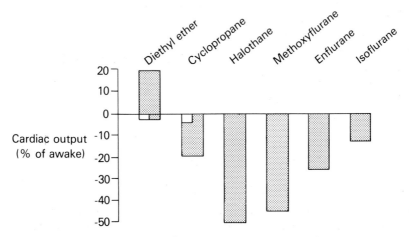

Fig. 3.20 Effect of different anaesthetic agents at 1 MAC on cardiac output in the intact dog.

Respiration

Artificial respiration may reduce venous return by increasing mean intrathoracic pressure. However, lighter planes of anaesthesia are usually used, and may offset the reduction in cardiac output.

Changes in Pa_{CO_2} may have profound effects. Hypercapnia increases cardiac output by sympathetic stimulation and by peripheral vasodilatation. However, hypercapnia may induce ventricular arrhythmias in the presence of volatile anaesthetics, e.g. halothane. Hypocapnia induces peripheral vasoconstriction, an increased vascular resistance and thus a reduction in cardiac output. Arterial pressure is usually maintained.

Surgical stimulation

Surgical stimulation generally results in increased sympathetic activity, counteracting the depressant effects of anaesthesia. Variations in arterial pressure with anaesthesia and surgical stimulation are often more pronounced in the elderly and hypertensive. Certain surgical stimuli such as distension of viscera or traction on peritoneum may induce vasodilatation and bradycardia, markedly reducing arterial pressure and cardiac output.

Other drugs

Many drugs, e.g. opioids and muscle relaxants, cause peripheral vasodilatation by direct action on the vessels, histamine release or ganglion blockade. These actions may be unwelcome in some circumstances, while in others they may be used deliberately to induce arterial hypotension.

Spinal and extradural anaesthesia

Spinal and extradural anaesthesia block the sympathetic outflow causing arteriolar and venous dilatation. Bradycardia also results if the cardiac fibres are involved (T_1–T_4). In general, providing arterial pressure is prevented from decreasing excessively by the judicious use of volume replacement and vasopressors, the circulation is well maintained.

FURTHER READING

Braunwald E 1974 Regulation of the circulation (two parts). New England Journal of Medicine 290: 1124, 1420
Cohn J N, Franciosa J A 1977 Vasodilator therapy of cardiac failure. New England Journal of Medicine 297:27
Gordon R J, Ravin M B, Daicoff G R 1979 Cardiovascular physiology for anaesthetists. Charles C Thomas, Springfield, Illinois
Guyton A C 1967 Regulation of cardiac output. New England Journal of Medicine 277: 805
Guyton A C 1981 The relationship of cardiac output and arterial pressure control. Circulation 64: 1079
Prys-Roberts C (ed) 1980 The circulation in anaesthesia. Blackwell Scientific Publications, Oxford
Rollason W N 1975 Electrocardiography for the Anaesthetist, 3rd edn. Blackwell Scientific Publications, Oxford
Scurr C, Feldman S (eds) 1982 Scientific foundations of anaesthesia, 3rd edn. Heinemann, London
Shimosato S 1981 Anesthesia and cardiac performance in health and disease. Charles C Thomas, Springfield, Illinois
Smith J J, Kampine J P 1980 Circulatory physiology — the essentials. Williams and Wilkins, Baltimore
Stuart J, Kenny M 1980 Blood rheology. Journal of Clinical Pathology 33: 417

4

Outlines of renal physiology

The kidney plays a vital role in maintaining homeostasis in order to ensure a stable internal environment necessary for each of the cellular components to function efficiently, despite a variable fluid and solute intake by the organism as a whole. Homeostasis is achieved by a combination of complex processes: excretion of the waste products of metabolism, production of hormones which influence other organs in the body and most importantly, control of the extra cellular fluid (e.c.f.) thereby indirectly influencing intracellular composition in terms of volume, osmolality and acid–base status. Before discussing the various components and functions of the kidney, it is necessary to consider briefly the body fluids and their compartments.

BODY FLUIDS AND COMPARTMENTS

In man total body water is approx. 60% of total body weight, i.e. 42 litre of water for a 70 kg man. In females, total body water is approx. 10% less, because of the greater proportion of fat in females compared with males, fat cells having a lower water content than other cells of the body. The water is distributed in various spaces or compartments.

Intracellular fluid

This is the largest water compartment in the body, representing two-thirds of total body water (approx. 28 litre).

Extracellular fluid

This constitutes the remaining one-third of total body water (14 litre) and may be further subdivided into two compartments:

1. Intravascular, i.e. within the plasma (4 litre).
2. Interstitial. This fluid (approx. 10 litre in volume) is outside the intravascular compartment and serves to 'bathe' individual cells.

The composition of the various fluids differs with the requirements of each compartment (Table 4.1). It may be seen that sodium is the main cation in the extracellular compartment, whereas potassium is the principal cation of the intracellular compartment.

Table 4.1 Composition and volume of body fluids according to compartment

	Intravascular (Plasma) 4 litre	Interstitial 10 litre	Intracellular 28 litre
Sodium (mmol/litre)	142	142	10
Potassium (mmol/litre)	5	5	150
Chloride (mmol/litre)	103	113	10
Bicarbonate (mmol/litre)	25	26	10
Protein (g/litre)	60–80	0	25
Osmolality (mosmol/kg H_2O)	285	285	285

This is achieved by the different permeability of cell membranes for certain cations; the cell membrane is approx. 50 times more permeable to potassium than to sodium. Intracellular protein carries a negative charge which attracts the positively charged potassium ions. Most importantly, however, the sodium pump actively extrudes sodium from the cell in exchange for potassium with the use of Na-K-ATPase as the energy source.

It is worth noting that the water content of plasma is 93%, the remainder of plasma being made up by proteins, lipids and other large molecular weight substances. Therefore, the actual value for sodium concentration in intravascular water should be approx. 153 mmol/litre. In clinical practice, if the proportion of water is reduced, e.g. by large increments in protein, lipid or glucose, the plasma sodium value is spuriously lowered; this is termed pseudohyponatraemia.

Water is permeable across cell membranes and there is a continual flux of fluid from the different body compartments at different rates of exchange. Two main mechanisms are responsible for these fluid shifts:

1. *Osmotic pressure.* Osmotic pressure is the pressure exerted by the number of particles in a solution. Osmolality, the usual term used in clinical practice, is defined as the number of milliosmoles per kg of water (mosmol/kg). Ions, being in greater abundance, exert a greater osmotic pressure. For example, sodium chloride, being composed of 1 sodium and 1 chloride ion, exerts 2 mosmol. Proteins, although of a larger molecular mass, exert less osmotic pressure. Water moves freely across a semipermeable membrane and does so from an area of low osmolality to that of higher osmolality, i.e. the increase in osmotic pressure attracts water. This movement continues until the osmotic pressure is equal on both sides of the membrane. This mechanism is in effect between the intracellular and interstitial compartments. As shown in Table 4.1, the osmolality in the three compartments is identical. Any increase in intracellular osmolality increases water transport into the cell, thereby increasing its volume, and vice versa.

2. *Hydrostatic pressure.* The main mechanism for fluid movement from the intravascular to the interstitial compartment, across a capillary bed, is hydrostatic pressure. Figure 4.1 shows the various pressures exerted as the hydrostatic pressure decreases from 32 mmHg at the arterial end to 12 mmHg at the venous end of the capillary. A constant 'negative' pressure drawing fluid into the capillary is the oncotic pressure exerted by plasma proteins. Hence, fluid moves out of the capillary at the arterial end and is withdrawn at the venous end. These hydrostatic pressures are known as Starling's forces. There is a small interstitial pressure, estimated to be approx. 2–5 mmHg, although it appears to have little or no effect on this mechanism unless the capillary, which may be damaged by some pathological process, leaks protein into the interstitium. If this occurs, then the interstitial pressure is increased and the existing balance of forces altered.

Renal blood flow

Before considering renal blood flow, it is necessary to understand the gross anatomy of the kidney. There are two populations of nephrons in the mammalian kidney.

1. *Cortical.* These nephrons (approx. 85% in man) lie within the cortex of the kidney and have short loops of Henle which dip only into the outer medulla.

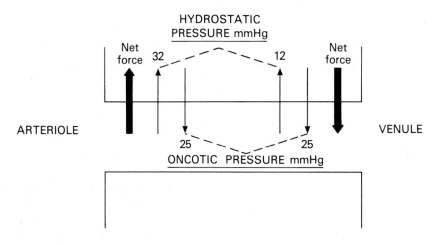

Fig. 4.1 Hydrostatic forces across a capillary wall (Starling's forces).

2. *Juxtamedullary*. These nephrons, which constitute the remaining 15% in man, lie in the juxtamedullary area of the cortex, and are distinguished from their outer cortical neighbours by having long loops of Henle entering the inner medulla to participate in the diluting and concentrating mechanisms of the kidney.

The blood supply to the kidney is from the renal artery, which, having entered the renal pelvis, divides into a number of interlobar arteries. These further divide into the arcuate arteries and supply the small interlobular arteries from which the glomerular vessels arise. Each glomerulus is supplied by a single afferent arteriole which branches into a network throughout the glomerulus. It then reforms into a single vessel, the efferent arteriole. The efferent arteriole in turn forms branches around the proximal tubule (pars recta) and around the loop of Henle to form the vasa recta. It is possible for the efferent arteriole from one glomerulus to form the vasa recta of an adjacent tubule. The mesh of vessels then reforms into a single vessel which drains into the interlobular vein and hence to the renal vein.

Considering its size in relation to other organs of the body, the kidney is unique in receiving an extremely high blood flow; approx. 20–25% of cardiac output. This amounts to 500–600 ml/min to each kidney. Such a flow rate is necessary to carry sufficient oxygen for the high energy requirements of tubular processes, especially cellular reabsorption.

Renal plasma flow (RPF) can be measured using the Fick principle:

$$\text{RPF} = \frac{U_x V}{RA_x - RV_x}$$

where $U_x V$ = rate of excretion of a substance

RA_x = renal artery concentration of the substance

RV_x = renal vein concentration of the substance

The commonest substance used is para-aminohippuric acid (PAH) which is almost completely cleared in one passage through the kidney. It is both filtered by the glomerulus and secreted by the renal tubule. In this instance RV_x should be negligible and, as there is no extrarenal clearance of PAH, the expression may be modified as follows:—

$$\text{RPF} = \frac{U_{PAH} V}{P_{PAH}} \text{ ml/min,}$$

where V = urine volume in ml/min

U_{PAH} = urine PAH concentration in mg/ml

P_{PAH} = plasma PAH concentration in mg/ml

Renal blood flow (RBF) may be calculated by adjusting the RPF for the haematocrit.

$$\text{RBF} = \frac{\text{RPF}}{1\text{-Hct}} \text{ ml/min,}$$

where Hct = haematocrit

As PAH is only 90% extracted by the human kidney, the clearance of PAH (C_{PAH}) underestimates RPF by approx. 10%. In order to improve the accuracy of measurement it is possible to estimate RPF from the disappearance curve of intravenously injected ^{131}I-labelled PAH, hence eliminating the potential error introduced by timed urine collections.

The extrinsic control of RBF is influenced by the sympathetic nerve outflow from T4 to L2. Increases in sympathetic tone such as those produced during haemorrhage, shock, pain, cold or severe exercise produce vasoconstriction.

Certain hormones (adrenaline, noradrenaline, antidiuretic hormone (vasopressin) in large nonpharmacological doses, serotonin and angiotensin) also reduce renal blood flow.

Within the kidney, RBF is redistributed to various anatomical areas. This has been demonstrated in animals using radioactive labelled tracers or microspheres and in man by the injection of radiolabelled inert agents (such as xenon or krypton) and measurement of their rate of disappearance over the kidney. From such studies in man, it has been shown that the cortex receives approx. 500 ml/min per 100 g of tissue, the outer medulla receives approx. 100 ml/min per 100 g and the inner medulla only 20 ml/min per 100 g. The lower medullary flow rate is necessary for the working of the countercurrent mechanism

There are two other properties that give the renal circulation distinguishing features. The first is that the mean glomerular capillary pressure is maintained at 45 mmHg, which is approx. 20 mmHg greater than other capillary networks in the body. This is necessary for glomerular filtration (vide infra). The mean peritubular capillary pressure is only 15 mmHg and lower than intratubular pressure, thereby enhancing tubular reabsorption.

The second feature is autoregulation, which occurs in the cortex but not in the medulla and allows constant blood flow when renal perfusion pressure is altered. It is an intrinsic property of the renal vasculature, i.e. it is independent of nerves or hormones, and occurs over a range of systemic arterial pressure from 90–180 mmHg. Over this range glomerular filtration rate (GFR) parallels RPF, but ceases when systolic arterial pressure decreases below 60 mmHg. The effects of autoregulation are achieved by changes in resistance in the afferent and efferent arterioles. When arterial pressure decreases, there is relative vasodilatation of the afferent arteriole and vasoconstriction of the efferent arteriole. This results in an increase in the fraction of plasma filtered (filtration fraction) and glomerular filtration is maintained. If arterial pressure increases, the vasoconstriction occurs in the afferent arteriole, with the opposite effects on filtration fraction.

The autoregulatory mechanism may be dampened by vasodilator drugs which act on smooth muscle vasculature, e.g. acetyl choline, dopamine, prostaglandins and the calcium antagonist group of drugs.

The exact mechanism of autoregulation is still a matter of debate. Originally it was believed to result either from mechanical factors, i.e. skimming of red blood cells and an increase in blood viscosity within the renal vasculature or a response to overall increase in intrarenal pressure generated by changes in systemic arterial pressure. Current evidence now favours the 'myogenic theory' which states that the increase in smooth muscle contraction is produced by increase in the intraluminal pressure, or by increase in the tangential tension of the vascular wall. The role of locally generated vasoactive substances, e.g. angiotensin II, remains controversial.

Glomerular filtration

The process of glomerular filtration allows 180 litre/24 h or 120 ml/min of fluid and solutes to pass through the glomerular capillaries via the endothelial fenestrations, the glomerular capillary basement membrane and the pedicles of the podocyte into Bowman's space. The fluid in Bowman's space which enters the proximal tubule is an ultrafiltrate of plasma, i.e. it is virtually protein free. Small amounts

of albumin pass through the glomerular basement membrane but are almost entirely reabsorbed in the proximal tubule so that the final urinary concentration of albumin is less than 120 mg/24 h. The ease with which solutes pass through the glomerular basement membrane depends on their size, charge and possibly shape.

The filtering process is extremely efficient for substances of low molecular weight, i.e. the ratio of solute concentration between the plasma within the glomerular capillary and the fluid in Bowman's capsule is 1. As molecular weight increases, the amount of solute filtered decreases until a cut-off point at a molecular weight of 70 000 is reached, above which no further molecules pass. It should be noted that this range allows for a small quantity of albumin (mol. wt 69 000) to be filtered. The constituents of the glomerular basement membrane are mainly negatively charged sialoproteins which repel the negatively charged protein particles in plasma. It has been demonstrated that dextrans, with a molecular weight similar to some small proteins but with no charge, pass through the glomerular basement membrane 10 to 20% more efficiently. There is also some evidence that changes in molecular shape may facilitate the passage of some molecules through the membrane.

The forces required to drive glomerular filtration are similar to the Starling forces across capillary networks elsewhere in the body, although of a higher magnitude. The mean arterial pressure in the glomerular capillary is 45 mmHg compared with 20 mmHg elsewhere. As discussed previously, this is a result of the presence of a second resistance vessel, the efferent arteriole. Also, this pressure remains relatively constant over a wide range of systolic arterial pressure as a result of the process of autoregulation. Glomerular filtration rate (GFR) is a product of the forces driving filtration minus the forces opposing filtration and may be expressed thus:

$$\text{GFR} \propto (P_{CAP} + \pi_{BC}) - (P_{BC} + \pi_{CAP}),$$

where
P_{CAP}	=	hydrostatic pressure in the glomerular capillary
P_{BC}	=	hydrostatic pressure in Bowman's capsule
π_{BC}	=	oncotic pressure in Bowman's capsule
π_{CAP}	=	oncotic pressure in glomerular capillary.

However, as π_{BC} is negligible, i.e. ultrafiltrate is virtually protein free, the relationship may be rewritten:

$$GFR \propto P_{CAP} - P_{BC} - \pi_{CAP}$$

To convert this relationship into an equation, the sieving coefficient (K_f), i.e. the resistance to flow across the glomerular basement membrane, is introduced:

$$GFR = K_f\,(P_{CAP} - P_{BC} - \pi_{CAP})$$

Measurement of glomerular filtration rate

In clinical practice the measurement of GFR is one of the commonest assessments of renal function. It is measured by determining the clearance of a substance which is filtered by the glomerulus but not reabsorbed or secreted by the renal tubule. The polyfructose inulin (mol. wt 5 000) is such a substance. Using the standard clearance formula,

$$C_{IN} = \frac{U_{IN}\,V}{P_{IN}} = 120\ \text{ml/min}$$

where
C_{IN} = inulin clearance in ml/min
U_{IN} = inulin concentration in urine (mg/ml)
P_{IN} = inulin concentration in plasma (mg/ml)
V = urine volume (ml/min)

There are two major disadvantages to this technique. Firstly, as inulin does not occur naturally in the body, it is necessary to infuse inulin intravenously to achieve a steady plasma level. To overcome this, it is customary to measure creatinine clearance using plasma creatinine, a byproduct of muscle metabolism. Although there is a slight diurnal variation of plasma creatinine levels and creatinine is secreted by the renal tubules at very low GFRs, creatinine clearance values are adequate for clinical practice and relate reasonably closely to inulin clearance.

The other disadvantage is the accuracy of timed urine collections. As with measurement of RPF, it is possible to use a radioactive labelled substance to measure GFR. Chromium-labelled ethylene diamine tetracetic acid (^{51}Cr-EDTA) is injected intravenously, and the disappearance rate calculated from blood samples obtained at two and four hours postinjection. This avoids urine collection, may be standardised for body surface area (as should all measurements of GFR), and may be used as an accurate reference method.

Filtration fraction

Although RPF is quite large, only a proportion is filtered and that proportion is called the filtration fraction (FF). It is derived as follows:

$$FF = \frac{GFR}{RPF} = \frac{C_{IN}}{C_{PAH}} = \frac{120\ \text{ml/min}}{600\ \text{ml/min}} = 0.2\ (20\%)$$

FF may alter as a result of autoregulation. For example, if RBF decreases there is an increase in efferent arteriole vasoconstriction and FF increases in order to maintain glomerular filtration.

Tubular function

The role of the renal tubule is to modify the volume and composition of the glomerular filtrate according to the needs of the organism. This is an enormous task. 180 litre of filtrate are produced per day and it is necessary to reduce this volume by 99% to achieve a final 24-h urine volume of approx. 1.8 litre. Similarly, approx. 25 000 mmol of sodium are filtered per day, the vast majority of this being reabsorbed to provide a urinary output of 100 to 200 mmol/24 h. In addition, it is necessary to conserve other filtered substances essential for the maintenance of homeostasis, e.g. glucose, bicarbonate, phosphate, etc. The renal tubule is also responsible for excretion of waste products of ingestion or metabolism, e.g. potassium, urea, creatinine, etc. The final regulation of acid–base status and of the concentration or dilution of the urine are also performed along the renal tubule.

Although each nephron acts as a single unit, it is possible for ease of understanding, to divide tubular function into the individual portions of the tubule, i.e. proximal tubule, loop of Henle, distal tubule and collecting tubule. In simple terms the proximal tubule may be considered the 'bulk reabsorber' and the remainder, the 'fine regulator' (Fig. 4.2).

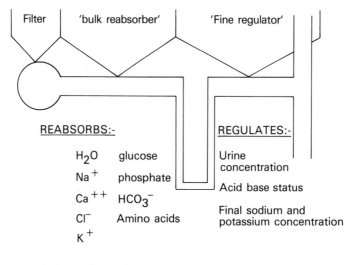

Fig. 4.2 Simple schema of tubular function.

Proximal tubule

In many ways, the proximal tubule is considered the bulk reabsorber as it is responsible for reducing the volume of glomerular filtrate by 80%. Seventy per cent of sodium and chloride, 90% of calcium, bicarbonate, magnesium, and 100% of glucose, phosphate and amino acids are reabsorbed during their passage through the proximal tubule. The fluid entering the proximal tubule from Bowman's space has a similar composition to that of plasma except for the absence of protein (Table 4.1). As the reabsorptive process is isosmotic, the osmolality remains identical at the beginning and end of the proximal tubule (290 mosmol/kg). The main ion to be reabsorbed in terms of concentration, energy requirements and its effect on other reabsorptive processes is sodium.

Sodium reabsorption. Sodium is reabsorbed through the proximal tubular cell both passively and actively.

Passive reabsorption. There are two forms of passive reabsorption for sodium:

1. Chemical. The intracellular sodium concentration in the proximal tubular cell is 30 mmol/litre. This is considerably less than the concentration of 140 mmol/litre in the tubular fluid. Sodium travels down the chemical gradient from the lumen to the cell.

2. Electrical. The potential difference within the tubular cell is -70 mV. This creates an electrical gradient for the positively charged sodium ions to travel from the lumen into the cell. Chloride, although negatively charged, travels with sodium in linked transport.

Active transport. Once sodium is within the cell it is pumped out (actively) in two directions. The first is into the intercellular space behind the so-called 'tight junction' (Fig. 4.3). This is an active energy-requiring pump which appears to be Na-K-ATPase independent. The effect of increased sodium concentration in the intercellular space is to increase the osmolality, and thus water passes from the cell into that space. The sodium and water within the intercellular space are then available for reabsorption by the peritubular capillary. In conditions of extracellular fluid expansion, the tight junction may open, and sodium together with water flows back from the intercellular space into the tubular lumen (back flow).

There is a second sodium pump situated on the contraluminal surface of the tubular cell. This is a Na-K-ATPase-dependent pump which exchanges sodium for potassium. Potassium, however, is freely permeable through the cell wall and may diffuse passively out again into the peritubular space. Again, the sodium in the peritubular space is available for reabsorption into the peritubular capillary.

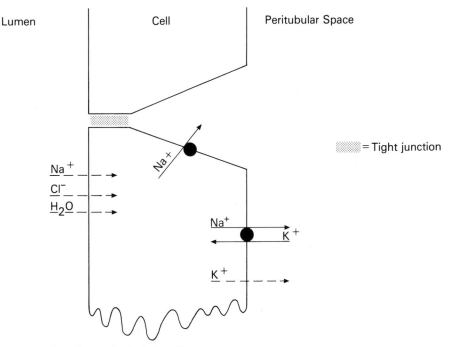

Lumen   Cell   Peritubular Space

= Tight junction

Na^+

Cl^-

H_2O

Na^+

Na^+ K^+

K^+

Fig. 4.3 Sodium transport through a proximal tubular cell.

The movement of sodium, chloride and water into the peritubular capillary is governed by Starling's forces. The driving forces are hydrostatic pressure in the peritubular space with capillary oncotic pressure and the opposing forces are capillary hydrostatic pressure with oncotic pressure in the peritubular space. However, as peritubular space oncotic pressure is negligible, and the peritubular space hydrostatic pressure is small, the main controlling factor is peritubular oncotic pressure. The sodium, chloride and water which are not taken up into the peritubular capillary re-enter the tubular lumen via the tight junction, i.e. there is an increase in back flow.

Having described the mechanisms of sodium reabsorption within the proximal tubular cell it is also necessary to consider sodium reabsorption and excretion by the kidney as a whole. As previously stated, the daily fractional excretion of sodium (the amount of sodium excreted in the final urine relative to the filtered load of sodium) remains relatively constant at approx. 1 to 2%. Filtered load is the product of GFR and plasma sodium concentration expressed in mmol/min. However, the sodium intake varies, and various mechanisms are required to cope with states of relative hypo- and hypervolaemia. There are three main mechanisms responsible.

1. Glomerulo-tubular balance. Although glomerular filtration rate remains relatively constant despite changes in systemic arterial pressure because of the autoregulatory mechanism, small changes in GFR produce large changes in the filtered load of sodium. When these occur, sodium reabsorption must alter in order to prevent large alterations in final sodium excretion. The anatomical arrangement of the peritubular capillaries, originating from the efferent arteriole, provides the ideal situation for a compensatory mechanism. When GFR decreases, there is a decrease in filtration fraction. This reduces the normally occurring increase in peritubular capillary oncotic pressure which in turn decreases reabsorption of sodium, chloride and water from the peritubular space. Conversely, if GFR increases, there is an increase in filtration fraction producing a greater increase in peritubular capillary oncotic pressure which enhances reabsorption. This mechanism is known as 'glomerulotubular balance'.

2. Aldosterone. Aldosterone has its main site of action in the distal tubule and is considered later.

3. Third factor. It has been known for over 20 years that when blood of a volume expanded animal is perfused into a normal animal, avoiding volume expansion in the recipient, there is a modest increase

in fractional sodium excretion, despite no change in renal haemodynamics. This phenomenon has been demonstrated in both isolated perfused kidneys and denervated kidneys and has led to the postulate that during volume expansion there is secretion of a so called 'natriuretic factor'. However, at the present moment, efforts to isolate such a hormone or factor have not been successful. The opposing view to the natriuretic factor is that all changes occurring during volume expansion may be explained by 'physical forces', e.g. changes in plasma proteins and therefore peritubular capillary oncotic pressure.

The possibility of a redistribution of intrarenal blood flow exerting an influence on overall sodium balance has yet to be evaluated fully. It is known that in cardiac failure, when a state of positive sodium balance occurs from increased sodium reabsorption, blood flow is directed away from the short outer cortical nephrons (salt losing) and directed to the longer juxtamedullary nephrons (salt retaining). It is not known if a similar modified mechanism plays a significant role in daily sodium balance.

Rate limited tubular transport

As shown in Figure 4.2, glucose, phosphate, bicarbonate and amino acids are almost totally reabsorbed in the proximal renal tubule. The mode of reabsorption differs from that described for sodium, chloride and water. The basic mechanism, as obtained in a titration study, is shown in Figure 4.4 using glucose as the example. During such a study the plasma glucose is slowly increased, avoiding extracellular fluid volume expansion. Plasma glucose, urinary glucose and GFR are measured. As the plasma glucose increases, glucose appears in the urine when the point of the renal threshold for glucose has been reached. This occurs when the plasma glucose is approx. 10 mmol/litre in man. The tubular reabsorption of glucose continues to increase with increments in plasma glucose until a plateau is reached when no further increase in glucose reabsorption rate can be achieved despite an increase in the filtered load of glucose. At that point, the transport mechanisms for glucose reabsorption by the tubular cells have been saturated. Thereafter, glucose excretion increases in parallel with the filtered load of glucose as plasma glucose increases. The 'plateau' at which maximal glucose reabsorption occurs is termed 'the tubular maximal reabsorption for glucose' (Tm_g). In man the value is 20 mmol/min. It should be noted from Figure 4.4 that the point at which glucose reabsorption reaches its maximum is not a fine 'cut off' but a small curve entitled 'splay'. Splay is caused by the heterogeneity of the nephron population in respect of glucose reabsorption. Some nephrons reabsorb maximally at a lower plasma glucose level than other nephrons within the kidney. A large splay is the cause of one type of renal glycosuria.

The same mechanism applies for phosphate reabsorption in the proximal tubule although this differs slightly from glucose in that the excretion of phosphate follows closer to the filtered load and the Tm for phosphate is much lower at 0.125 mmol/min.

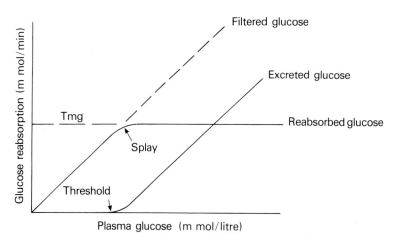

Fig. 4.4 The mechanism of glucose reabsorption in the proximal tubule.

The Tm for bicarbonate is approximately 3 to 3.5 mmol/min but may be altered by hydrogen ion secretion. There are five identified individual transport processes for the different groups of amino acids but their reabsorptive kinetics are similar to that of glucose. The reabsorption of sulphate in the proximal tubule also follows a similar pattern. Many of the above substances share a cotransport system with sodium. It is known that when proximal tubular reabsorption of sodium decreases with an increased fractional excretion of sodium, the Tm for glucose, phosphate and bicarbonate is decreased.

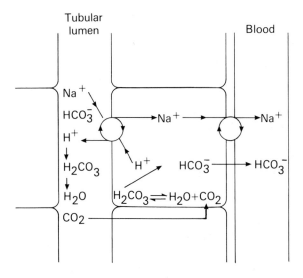

Fig. 4.5 Bicarbonate reabsorption in proximal tubule.

The mechanism of bicarbonate transport through the tubular cell (Fig. 4.5) is of particular importance because of its role in the renal regulation of acid–base balance. This mechanism may be summarised in three equations:

$$NaHCO_3 \rightleftharpoons Na^+ + HCO_3^- \qquad (1)$$

$$HCO_3^- + H^+ \rightleftharpoons H_2CO_3 \xrightarrow[\text{ANHYDRASE}]{\text{CARBONIC}} H_2O + CO_2 \qquad (2)$$

$$H_2O + CO_2 \xrightarrow[\text{ANHYDRASE}]{\text{CARBONIC}} H_2CO_3 \rightleftharpoons H^+ + HCO_3^- \qquad (3)$$

Bicarbonate enters the tubular lumen as sodium bicarbonate and dissociates into bicarbonate (a relatively impermeable anion) and sodium (1). The sodium passes into the cell in exchange for a hydrogen ion. The hydrogen ion combines with the bicarbonate in the tubular lumen to form carbonic acid. The enzyme carbonic anhydrase, present on the brush border of the proximal tubular cell, splits carbonic acid into carbon dioxide and water (2), both of which are freely permeable and enter the tubular cell. Here, intracellular carbonic anhydrase reforms carbonic acid which in turn, dissociates into free hydrogen and bicarbonate ions (3). The bicarbonate ion passes through the basal cell membrane and into the peritubular space and is available for reabsorption by the peritubular capillary. The hydrogen ion can be extruded from the cell in exchange for sodium and the cycle repeated. The enzyme carbonic anhydrase participates in both the dissociation and formation of carbonic acid depending on its site of action.

Another substance to be reabsorbed in the proximal tubule is uric acid. This is a small molecule which is filtered freely, and over 90% is reabsorbed in the proximal tubule. Uric acid homeostasis, however, is regulated by secretion of uric acid in the distal tubule. Another small molecule which is freely filtrable is urea, and approx. 50% of the filtered load is passively reabsorbed in the proximal tubule, the remainder passing down into the distal tubule to participate in the osmolar regulatory mechanisms of the inner medulla.

In addition to hydrogen ions, certain other substances such as organic acids and bases are secreted (i.e. moved from the peritubular capillary into the tubular lumen) in the proximal tubule. These include a number of drugs, e.g. penicillin, PAH. The secretory processes may be either active or passive and some have tubular maximal secretory capacities.

The loop of Henle, distal tubule and collecting tubule (Fig. 4.6)

The tubular fluid entering the loop of Henle is isosmotic and finally leaves the collecting duct as urine varying in volume, osmolality and composition according to the needs of the body. The fine regulatory mechanisms are situated in this portion of the nephron. The loops of Henle of the juxtamedullary nephrons dip deeply into the medulla whereas the collecting tubules of all nephrons pass through the medulla. There is an increase in osmolality passing from the cortex to the medulla which is essential for the concentration and dilution of tubular fluid. The main mechanism for this is the counter current multiplier situated in the loop of Henle (Fig. 4.6).

Counter current mechanism

The loop of Henle consists of a thin descending limb, and a thin first part followed by thick part of the ascending limb. The volume of fluid entering the loop of Henle is approx. 15% of the glomerular filtrate and only one-third of this leaves the cortical part of the collecting tubule. The tubular fluid enters the loop with an osmolality of 290 mosmol/kg and leaves at 100 mosmol/kg. The loop is the active part (a counter current multiplier) and the vasa recta surrounding the loop of Henle are the counter current exchanger. There are two main transport processes responsible for the work of the counter current mechanism.

1. Sodium and water reabsorption. The thick ascending part of the loop is impermeable to water but both sodium and chloride are transported into the interstitium. Although this is an active transport process there is much debate as to whether it is sodium or chloride which is transported. Current opinion favours chloride with sodium moving by a cotransport mechanism (see above). This results in an increase in the osmolality of the interstitium ranging from 300 mosmol/kg in the cortex to 1200 mosmol/kg at the tip of the loop. The descending limb is freely permeable to water, sodium and chloride, and all three move into the interstitium. Fluid enters the descending limb at an osmolality of 290 mosmol/kg and the osmolality slowly increases until it is equivalent to that at the tip of the loop, i.e. 1200 mosmol/kg. On passing up the ascending limb, sodium and chloride are removed but water is retained, and the osmolality decreases from 1200 to 100 mosmol/kg.

The vasa recta provide an important role in this osmolar transport. Although there is no active transport present in these vessels, water and solutes are freely permeable. The osmolality of blood entering the vasa recta is the same as that of the fluid

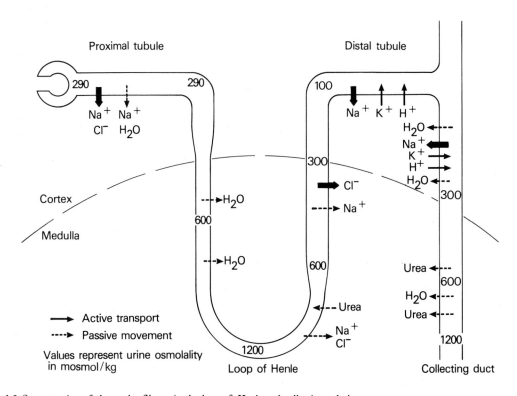

Fig. 4.6 Concentration of glomerular filtrate in the loop of Henle and collecting tubule.

entering the descending limb, i.e. 290 mosmol/kg and slowly increases to 1200 mosmol/kg as it passes down to the tip of the loop. This is achieved by the passage of water and solutes across its surface. The blood flow is significantly slower in the lower parts of the vasa recta, thus improving the efficiency of this exchange. As the vasa recta move from the medullary tip back towards the cortex, the same process occurs and the osmolality is returned to 290 mosmol/kg. As a consequence of the low flow rate in these vessels, oxygen content and energy requirements are markedly reduced.

2. Urea recycling. Urea, a waste product of protein metabolism, contributes up to 50% of the osmolality of the medullary interstitium. Because it is a small molecule it is filtered freely at the glomerulus and approximately half is reabsorbed during passage through the proximal tubule. As the tubular fluid passes down the descending limb the urea concentration is increased, firstly by the passage of water out of the descending limb, and secondly at the tip of the loop by the addition of urea, which moves freely from the medullary interstitium, an area of high urea concentration. The high concentration of urea at the tip of the medulla is achieved by the collecting tubule. The cortical part of the collecting tubule is impermeable to urea but permeable to water, resulting in an increase in urea concentration within the tubule. However, in the medullary portion of the collecting tubule, both water and urea pass into the interstitium. Hence, urea is recycled through the medulla and plays an important part in maintaining the high medullary osmolality essential for the counter current mechanism.

Sodium–potassium exchange.

More than 90% of filtered potassium is reabsorbed in the proximal tubule, and potassium which appears in the final urine is secreted in the distal tubule by a transport process loosely coupled to active sodium transport. As sodium is reabsorbed from the tubular lumen, a negative potential is created within the lumen which allows potassium to move passively down an electrochemical gradient. In this region, hydrogen ions are also secreted and compete with potassium to a degree dependent on the acid–base status. The control of sodium reabsorption in the distal tubule is primarily hormonal and probably controlled via the renin-angiotensin system.

Renin-angiotensin system

The renin-angiotensin system is an important part of the complex mechanism responsible for controlling extracellular fluid volume, the other 'effector' parts being plasma proteins (vide supra) and osmolar control (vide infra). Renin is a proteolytic enzyme secreted from the juxtaglomerular apparatus situated in the afferent arteriole. The secretion of renin is a matter of some debate. It has been suggested that a baroreceptor mechanism situated in the afferent arteriole detects a decrease in renal blood flow and responds by increasing renin production. The alternative hypothesis is that changes in sodium concentration in the distal tubule are detected by the macula densa situated in the early part of the distal tubule, increases in sodium concentration causing an increase in renin secretion. However, there is conflicting evidence on this latter point. The renin acts on an α_2 plasma protein (angiotensinogen) and splits off a decapeptide, angiotensin I. A converting enzyme found both in plasma and various tissues of the body, including lung, converts angiotensin I to angiotensin II. This agent has three main actions. It is a potent vasopressor which may act on the glomerular arterioles and thereby contribute to glomerulotubular balance. It has a direct action on the brain, stimulating the thirst centre. Of most importance is the effect of stimulating secretion of aldosterone from the zona glomerulosa of the adrenal gland. Plasma aldosterone levels are also affected by plasma potassium levels, an increase in potassium reducing the aldosterone level. The converse happens with plasma sodium levels, i.e. a decrease in plasma sodium increases aldosterone. The main action of aldosterone is to increase sodium reabsorption in the distal tubule. Potassium and/or hydrogen ions are then secreted into the tubule in exchange for reabsorbed sodium. The renin angiotensin system has its own feedback control, angiotensin II suppressing further secretion of renin.

Renal regulation of acid–base balance

The distal tubule participates both qualitatively and quantitatively in acid–base control. As described previously the majority (up to 80%) of filtered bicarbonate is reabsorbed in the proximal tubule and the remainder by the distal tubule. The absorptive mechanism for bicarbonate reabsorption in the distal tubule is similar to that of the proximal tubule, namely the formation and dissociation of carbonic acid by the enzyme carbonic anhydrase. Conversely, although there is some hydrogen ion secretion in the proximal tubule, the bulk is secreted in the distal tubule.

Hydrogen ions are excreted in the final urine in combination with either ammonia or phosphates. Approx. 60 mmol of hydrogen ion are excreted per day, of which two-thirds are combined with ammonia (NH_3) to form ammonium ion (NH_4^+) and one-third with sodium phosphate salts, often referred to as titratable acids (TA).

Ammonia (NH_3) is generated within the tubular cell mainly from the metabolism of the amino acid glutamine. When glutamine is converted to either glutamate or alpha ketoglutarate, which enters the citric acid cycle, a free ammonia molecule is generated. This is freely permeable through the cell wall and passes down the concentration gradient into the tubular lumen. Here it combines with free hydrogen ions to form NH_4^+ which is an impermeable anion and is therefore unable to re-enter tubular cells and so is excreted in the final urine.

The remaining one-third of hydrogen ions are excreted when combined with phosphate. Disodium hydrophosphate enters the distal tubule and dissociates. One sodium ion is reabsorbed leaving a negatively charged molecule. The positive hydrogen ion in the tubular lumen combines to form sodium dihydrophosphate which is excreted in the final urine.

Hydrogen ions for both ammonium and TA formation come from the intracellular dissociation of carbonic acid, and the net effect is the intracellular generation of a bicarbonate ion which passes through the basal border of the cell into the peritubular capillary. The amount of hydrogen ion secretion and bicarbonate regeneration depends predominantly on the acid base status. The total hydrogen ion secretion may be expressed by the following formula:

$$\text{Total } H^+ \text{ excretion} = NH_4^+ \text{ excretion} + TA$$
$$\text{excretion} - HCO_3^- \text{ excretion}$$

Osmolar regulation

By the time the glomerular filtrate enters the collecting tubule, its original volume has been reduced to 5% and when it leaves the collecting tubule it is reduced to 1%. Final urine volumes depend in part on the extracellular fluid volume and its regulation via sodium excretion, and in part on the regulation of plasma osmolality. The osmolar regulation system has a detector (osmoreceptors), a messenger (antidiuretic hormone ADH) and an effector (the collecting tubule).

The osmoreceptors situated in the hypothalamus detect changes in plasma osmolality, the major contribution being from plasma sodium. An increase in plasma osmolality stimulates the synthesis of ADH (vasopressin) in the supraoptic nuclei of the hypothalamus. The hormone is an octapeptide (8 arginine vasopressin) which passes along the nerve fibres to the posterior pituitary. After the appropriate stimulation, the hormone is released from storage granules in the posterior pituitary and secreted into the systemic circulation. Its action on the peritubular cell membrane is to increase the permeability of water. This involves activation of the cylic 3' 5' AMP system. Water is then reabsorbed from the collecting tubule and passes into the peritubular capillary to return the plasma osmolality to normal and reduce the urine volume. The reverse situation occurs if plasma osmolality decreases; ADH secretion ceases and the collecting tubule becomes impermeable to water, more water is excreted, urine volume increases and plasma osmolality increases towards normal levels. By this mechanism, it is possible that urine osmolality may vary from a hypotonic urine with a minimum value of approx. 60 mosmol/kg to a maximal value of 1200 to 1400 mosmol/kg. It should be noted that the final urine osmolality of hypertonic urine is equivalent to the tonicity at the tip of the renal medulla. ADH also increases the amount of urea reabsorbed in the cortical part of the collecting tubule thereby contributing to the counter current mechanism by increasing medullary tip osmolality.

It is possible to equate the action of ADH by determining the amount of water excreted or reabsorbed compared with the amount of solutes excreted. Osmolar clearance (C_{osm}), an expression of solute excretion is determined by using the standard clearance formula:

$$C_{osm} = \frac{U_{osm}V}{P_{osm}}$$

where U_{osm} = osmolar clearance in ml/min.

P_{osm} = plasma osmolality in mosmol/kg.

V = urine excretion rate in ml/min.

If urine is dilute, i.e. hypotonic, V is greater than C_{osm}. The difference is termed free water clearance (C_{H_2O}) and may be expressed as follows:

$$V - C_{osm} = C_{H_2O}$$

where C_{H_2O} = free water clearance in ml/min.

Conversely, if urine is concentrated, i.e. hypertonic, more water is reabsorbed and C_{osm} becomes greater than V. The term free water clearance then becomes negative.

Another way of explaining negative free water clearance is to consider that water is being reabsorbed, i.e. solute free water reabsorption, and may be expressed as follows:

$$V = C_{osm} - T^c_{H_2O}$$

or, $$T^c_{H_2O} = C_{osm} - V$$

where $T^c_{H_2O}$ = solute free water reabsorption in ml/min.

By varying the amount of water reabsorbed in the collecting tubule and influencing the plasma sodium concentration it may be seen that osmolar regulation plays a vital part in controlling body fluid status. The two systems, i.e. osmolar regulation and volume regulation are inter-related and in considering overall fluid balance it is not possible to dissociate the two.

In summary, the kidney plays a vital role in maintaining the 'milieu interieur'. It does so by variable adjustments to glomerular filtration rate, tubular reabsorption and secretion to produce a final urine which varies in volume, composition and acid–base status.

FURTHER READING

Bevan D R 1979 Renal function in anaesthesia and surgery. Academic Press, London

Davenport H W 1975 The ABC of acid–base chemistry, 6th edn. University of Chicago Press, Chicago

5

Physiology of the nervous system

STRUCTURE AND FUNCTION

The function of the human nervous system is the acquisition of information from the external environment and its computation to produce an integrated response. The central nervous system (c.n.s.) comprises the brain and spinal cord. The peripheral nervous system is composed of 43 pairs of nerves which contain afferent sensory fibres, conducting impulses to the central nervous system from the periphery, and efferent motor fibres conducting in the reverse direction. There are 10 000 000 000 neurones, each surrounded by neuroglial cells in the c.n.s. These cells are of two types: (1) oligodendrocytes which form myelin, and (2) microglia which phagocytose degenerating neurones.

The physiology of the nervous system is related intimately to membrane physiology and cell excitation. Excitability results from specialisation of excitable cell membranes. The intracellular environment is controlled by cell membranes which

exhibit selective permeability by virtue of membrane pumps. Excitable membranes undergo rapid reversible changes in permeability to certain charged molecules or ions (i.e. to a specific stimulus). For example, at a pressure receptor the membrane ionic permeability alters as a response to mechanical deformation, and flow of ions occurs across the membrane.

A cell membrane is composed of lipids and protein (Fig. 5.1). Lipid forms the major part of the cell membrane, which may be considered as a lipid bilayer arranged such that a polar head is located on the outside of the cell membrane and 1–2 hydrocarbon chains, which are hydrophobic, constitute the inner part of the bilayer. Cell membrane proteins are composed of chains of amino acids with different side chains, either hydrophilic or hydrophobic, which by folding can 'hide' their hydrophobic amino acids on the interior.

A lipid bilayer is very *impermeable* to small ions, therefore cell membrane permeability must reside in other structures, probably membrane proteins. The

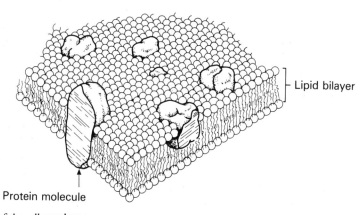

Lipid bilayer

Protein molecule

Fig. 5.1 Structure of the cell membrane.

proteins confer specific ionic permeability on the membrane whilst only a small part of the membrane appears to be involved directly in ion flow.

Membrane protein as ion pump

Ion movement across a cell membrane occurs against the electrochemical gradient and is therefore active. Membrane proteins which achieve active transport are termed ion pumps. All cell membranes contain a sodium pump (Fig. 5.2). Ionic permeability is of two kinds: (i) constant resting ionic permeability to ions including potassium (K^+) and chloride (Cl^-) not affected by physiological stimuli, (ii) nonconstant permeability, which changes rapidly due to the action of a stimulus on an appropriate membrane protein. Permeability is 'gated' by the stimulus. This is a characteristic feature of excitable membranes.

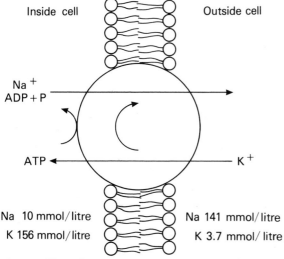

Fig. 5.2 The sodium pump.

Several possibilities exist for the actual transport of an ion across the cell membrane. A protein may act as carrier and ferry the ion across or it may span the bilayer and produce a pore (Fig. 5.3). This latter mechanism produces much more rapid transport.

Electrochemical gradient

This is a measure of the force driving a specific ion into or out of the cell. It comprises an electrical component, which is the potential difference between the inside and outside of the cell (-60 mV). The

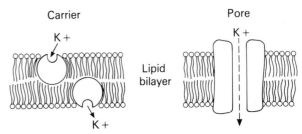

Fig. 5.3 Mechanisms of ion transport by proteins.

chemical gradient is a simple concentration gradient. In certain conditions these two components may oppose and cancel each other out, at which point the ion is in electrochemical equilibrium across the membrane and the Nernst equation applies. This is dependent upon the unequal distribution of ions across membranes. If at the resting potential of biological membranes, permeability to sodium (Na^+) and Cl^- are assumed to be zero, then

$$V = \frac{RT}{F} \log_e \frac{K_o^+}{K_i^+}$$

where:

V = potential difference
R = the gas constant
F = Faraday's constant
T = temperature
K_o^+ = concentration of K^+ in extracellular fluid (e.c.f.)
K_i^+ = concentration of K^+ in intracellular fluid (i.c.f.)

Nerve impulse and conduction

Characteristic changes in membrane potential on passage of a nerve impulse constitute an action potential. The passage of a stimulating current to this nerve axon produces first a stimulus artefact and then an action potential (Fig. 5.4).

Action potential. This is an all or none phenomenon. The least stimulus strength required to produce an action potential is termed the threshold stimulus. The transient reversal of the membrane potential propagates along an axon at constant velocity in a non-decremental manner. The refractory period is the period during which a second stimulating current does not elicit a second action potential. The absolute refractory period occurs

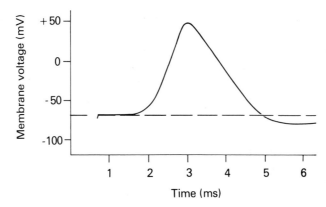

Fig. 5.4   The action potential.

immediately after the initial stimulus and lasts for approximately the same duration as the action potential itself. At this time, it is not possible to initiate a new impulse (Fig. 5.5). Thereafter the relative refractory period requires an increased threshold to initiate an impulse.

In the giant squid axon the resting membrane potential (-70 mV) is close to the Nernst potential for K^+ and results from selective permeability to K^+ in the axon membrane.

A change in resting potential is produced by changes in external and internal K^+ concentration.

The resting potential is the result of:

1. Ionic gradients produced by the sodium pump.
2. Selective permeability of the resting axon to K^+ with respect to Na^+.

As an action potential passes, the axon membrane becomes active and the membrane voltage is reversed from negative to positive. This corresponds to depolarisation with an overshoot to $+40$ mV. The action potential results from an increase in membrane *conductance* to Na^+, resulting in an increase in membrane potential towards the Nernst potential for Na^+. Thus, if the external Na^+ concentration decreases, the action potential becomes smaller in amplitude and eventually is reduced to zero. Selective block of Na^+ ion current can be produced experimentally with tetrodotoxin and of K^+ with tetraethylammonium. Such studies show that:

1. The sodium channel is opened rapidly by depolarisation of membrane voltage and closes slowly (inactivates) even if depolarisation is maintained. The open phase is always transient.

2. The potassium channel is opened slowly by depolarisation of the membrane and does not close during the short time scale of the action potential, i.e.

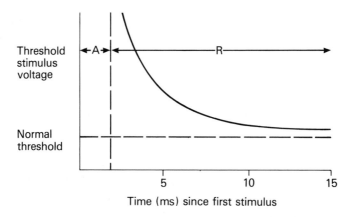

Fig. 5.5   Refractory period following an action potential.

there is late outward K^+ current whilst depolarisation is maintained.

A threshold stimulus produces an all or nothing response. The Na^+ channel is opened by membrane depolarisation, Na^+ ions pass through into the axon, producing more depolarisation, thereby opening more channels and further increasing Na^+ ion influx with outward flux of K^+, which resists depolarisation. Na^+ channels do not open until the membrane voltage has changed by 20 mV from the resting potential. Inactivated Na^+ channels take a few milliseconds to become functional again and therefore are not opened again by immediate depolarisation. These are the underlying events of the refractory period. The increase in K^+ conductance always tends to increase K^+ ion current which resists any change of membrane voltage away from the resting level.

Propagation of impulse (Fig. 5.6). Large axons have high conduction velocities. For fibres of a given diameter, conduction is increased greatly by myelination. Axons from 1 to 25 μm in diameter are myelinated. Those less than 1 μm are non-myelinated. Nerve fibres have a structure akin to a shielded electrical cable, in other words a central conducting core with insulation and an external conducting area which is e.c.f. In vertebrate myelinated fibres, a Schwann cell lays down myelin in concentric layers. Between neighbouring segments of myelin there is a very narrow gap termed the node of Ranvier, which is less than 1 μm wide, where there is no obstacle between the axon membrane and the extracellular fluid. This accounts for conduction occurring in a saltatory manner. The myelin sheaths act as high resistance barriers to current flow and excitation occurs only at the nodes of Ranvier. Hence the impulse is propagated from node to node. The events are summarised in Table 5.1.

Table 5.1 Summary of nerve impulse propagation

1. Resting membrane has a low ionic permeability, therefore electrochemical gradients are not readily dissipated
2. Membrane contains a sodium pump which requires ATP for energy to create and maintain ion concentration gradients
3. The resting membrane is selectively permeable to K^+, so a resting potential of -70 mV is set up, which is close to the Nernst equilibrium potential for potassium
4. Two types of gated ion channel exist within the membrane, which are opened or closed by changes in the membrane voltage

The synapse

A synapse occurs where the membranes of two excitable cells are closely apposed and allows transmission of information. The transmitter is usually chemical, is released in a controlled amount by the cell, and diffuses rapidly to bind to a receptor site on the second cell, producing rapid changes in ion flux. Presynaptic fibres divide into numerous fine branches, producing presynaptic knobs. A single anterior horn cell may receive 30 000 knobs from a large number of axons. The presynaptic membrane releases transmitter from dense, spherical synaptic vesicles (50 nm diameter) into a synaptic cleft of some 20–25 nm to the postsynaptic membrane (Fig. 5.7).

Transmission of impulses across a synapse is strictly unidirectional (in a nerve it is bidirectional)

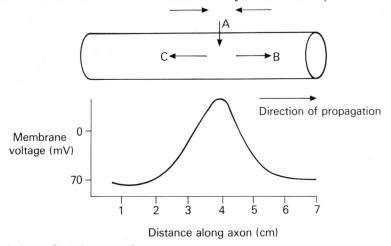

Fig. 5.6 Local circuit theory of impulse propagation.
A = influx of Na^+ ions at active membrane. B, C = current flow. B propagates the impulse. C finds the membrane refractory.

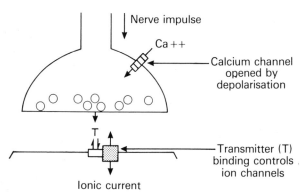

Fig. 5.7 Chemical synaptic transmission.

and involves a time delay. In the spinal motor neurone this amounts to 0.4 ms. A knowledge of total delay in a reflex pathway is useful in determining the number of synapses involved. Synapses operate in a graded fashion which allows the neurone to carry out integration and sifting of information. Enzymes break down the transmitter released, thereby reducing their duration of action at the postsynaptic membrane.

Control of transmitter release

The arrival of an action potential produces depolarisation of the terminal membrane, which opens voltage-sensitive calcium (Ca^{++}) ion channels with flux of Ca^{++} into presynaptic areas. This in turn stimulates transient exocytosis of the transmitter into the synaptic gap, where it diffuses rapidly to specific protein binding sites (receptors) on the postsynaptic membrane. Ionic currents through these sites then alter the membrane potential of the postsynaptic cell in a direction determined by the ion selectivity of the channels concerned. Depolarisation causes excitation, and hyperpolarisation inhibition. When nerve terminal Ca^{++} is increased, 100 vesicles are released within 1 ms. The postsynaptic membrane channels are gated by specific chemical stimuli. In the absence of nerve stimulation, miniature end-plate potentials (mepp) may be recorded (due to arrival of single transmitter vesicles). A propagative end-plate potential requires 100 transmitter vesicles. For example at the neuromuscular junction 1 impulse produces 100 vesicles, each containing 50 000 molecules of acetylcholine. Of the 5 000 000 transmitter molecules released, only 100 000 open a postsynaptic channel, but this is sufficient to cause

10 000 000 000 Na^+ ions to enter muscle in 1 ms. Both excitatory and inhibitory postsynaptic potentials can be recorded intracellularly. Presynaptic inhibition may also occur from inhibitory terminals situated on excitatory presynaptic nerve endings, which reduce the amount of neurotransmitter released.

It is well known that antibiotics may interfere with neuromuscular conduction, often by decreasing end plate transmitter. High concentrations of Mg^{++} and some antibiotics decrease evoked release of ACh mainly by competition for Ca^{++} binding sites on the nerve terminal. Postjunctional effects include receptor or end-plate ion channel blockade. There is considerable variability between antibiotics in their neuromuscular blocking mechanisms but this is an area of potential clinical importance.

Information processing by nerve networks shows:

1. Spatial summation. This occurs when stimulation of two afferent nerves together produces a response which neither alone can elicit. Both synapses may be excitatory for that particular nerve.

2. Temporal summation. Stimulation of the same nerve twice in rapid succession produces a response where a single stimulus elicits none.

There are also electrical synapses, e.g. in the retina, and synapses where transmitter release is controlled by graded depolarisations. There is, in fact, an immense variety of types of synapse between different classes of cell which use different transmitters and different polysynaptic channels.

Neurotransmitters

The number of putative central nervous system transmitters now exceeds 40. This suggests that synaptic transmission is more complex than simple transfer of excitation or inhibition from presynaptic neurone to the postsynaptic cell. There is a great range of synaptic connections and the possibility of chemical coding exists. It is already known that axo-axonal synapses may regulate the amount of transmitter released from presynaptic terminals; other inputs may trigger very long-lasting postsynaptic events (lasting for minutes) and therefore control the excitability of a target cell, rather than directly controlling its firing.

Fast chemical signalling in the central nervous system. This is the function of amino acid transmitters:

1. *Gamma amino butyric acid (GABA).* This transmitter occurs in all regions of the brain and spinal cord, mainly in local inhibitory interneurones. GABA rapidly inhibits virtually all c.n.s. neurones when applied locally, by virtue of increased cell permeability to chloride ions, thereby stabilising the membrane potential at or near the chloride equilibrium level. Most of these responses are mediated by GABA receptors. GABA may be used by as many as one-third of all synapses in the mammalian brain.

2. *Glycine.* This amino acid predominates as the inhibitory transmitter in the spinal cord.

3. *L-Glutamate and L-aspartate.* These produce excitatory depolarisation by activating membrane sodium channels.

Diffuse regulatory systems: monoamines. These are associated with diffuse neural pathways, mainly in the brain stem. Much of the monoamine release may be at nonsynaptic sites.

Neuropeptides. Virtually all peptide hormones of the endocrine and neuroendocrine systems also exist in distinct systems of the central nervous system neurones.

Membrane receptor function in anaesthesia

A receptor is an integral membrane protein which is recognised selectively by a precise hormone or neurotransmitter termed a ligand (Fig. 5.8). A ligand is an agonist if it activates a receptor to transduce a response, or an antagonist when the substance interacts with a receptor causing it to remain inactive and, by occupying the receptor, diminishes or aborts the effect of an agonist. The interaction between ligand and receptor is specific, reversible, saturable and a high affinity binding process.

Adrenergic receptors (ARs). Agonists at β ARs in order of potency include: isoprenaline, adrenaline, noradrenaline and dopamine. β_1-Receptors are found in the heart and are equally sensitive to adrenaline and noradrenaline. β_2-Receptors are found in smooth muscle and are more sensitive to adrenaline than noradrenaline. The effects are mediated by intracellular cyclic AMP (cAMP), the second messenger, which activates protein kinases (Fig. 5.9). Thus the β-adrenergic agonist receptor complex

diffuses laterally among the membrane until it couples to adenylate cyclase (the effector molecule which is then activated and catalyses synthesis of cAMP which is subsequently hydrolysed by phosphodiesterase).

Alpha adrenoreceptors mediate control of smooth muscle of the vasculature of the uterus and gastrointestinal tract. The order of potency of agonists is: adrenaline, noradrenaline, isoprenaline. There are two classes of α-receptors (Fig. 5.10); α_1 are postsynaptic and mediate constriction of smooth muscle. These are selectively blocked by prazosin and phenoxybenzamine. α_2-Receptors are presynaptic and mediate feedback inhibition by noradrenaline of further neurotransmitter release. These are blocked selectively by yohimbine. α_2-Receptors are found also on platelets where they mediate aggregation. Methoxamine and phenylephrine are selective α_1 agonists and clonidine is an α_2 agonist.

Within the central nervous system adrenaline is found in small groups of cells in the pons and medulla which project to the hypothalamus and brain stem and to the nucleus tractus solitarius, which may be important in central arterial pressure control. Noradrenaline is found in all areas of the brain and spinal cord, with a high density in the hypothalamus.

Dopamine receptors. Dopamine receptors occur in basal ganglia, substantia nigra, corpus striatum and limbic system. In the basal ganglia, dopamine is antagonistic to acetylcholine. Absence of dopamine is an important aetiological factor in Parkinsonism. In the hypothalamus, dopamine is concerned with release of prolactin. Dopamine suppresses prolactin secretion and dopamine antagonists, e.g. metoclopramide increases hyperprolactinaemia.

A dopaminergic system connects the limbic cortex, basal ganglia and hypothalamus and is concerned with behaviour. This system is involved in the pathogenesis of schizophrenia (phenothiazines block dopamine receptors). Dopaminergic fibres are concerned in the chemoreceptor trigger zone; stimulation produces nausea and vomiting. Dopaminergic and sympathomimetic receptors have been identified in the coronary, renal, cerebral and mesenteric vessels. Dopamine receptors occur also on the presynaptic membrane of postganglionic sympathetic nerves and sympathetic ganglia where their physiological role is unclear.

Acetylcholine (ACh) is found in motor neurones of the spinal cord and cranial nerve motor nuclei,

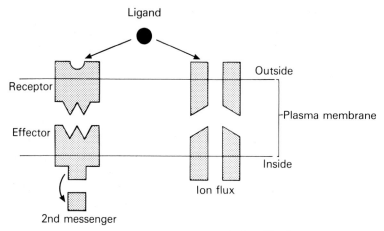

Fig. 5.8 Receptor-effector mechanisms: release of second messenger or promotion of ion flux.

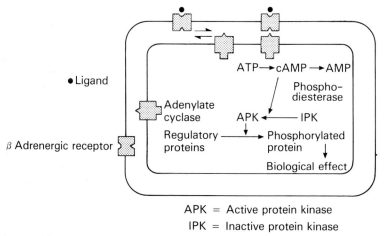

APK = Active protein kinase
IPK = Inactive protein kinase

Fig. 5.9 Beta adrenergic receptor.

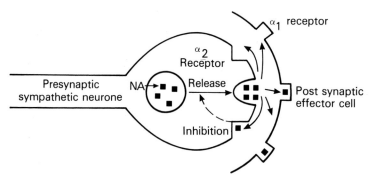

Fig. 5.10 Types of α-adrenergic receptors.
NA = noradrenaline.

where it acts as a *fast* chemical transmitter for neuromuscular transmission. In intrinsic pathways in the central nervous system it probably acts as a modulator in basal ganglia, the hippocampus, and the diffuse ascending pathways to the cortex, probably representing what was known as the ascending reticular activating system. ACh probably plays an important part in cortical arousal and e.e.g. changes of r.e.m. sleep. The effects of ACh are terminated by hydrolysis by cholinesterase. Its peripheral effects may be classified into: (i) muscarinic effects at postganglionic parasympathetic fibres; (ii) nicotinic effects at sympathetic and parasympathetic ganglia and the neuromuscular junction. Denervation of skeletal muscle enhances its sensitivity to ACh by development of a diffuse distribution of ACh receptors over postjunctional surfaces. Administration of suxamethonium in these circumstances results in severe hyperkalaemia.

Histamine receptors. H_1 receptors are responsible for contraction of smooth muscles (e.g. in the gut, and bronchi). H_2 receptors stimulate acid secretion by the stomach and increase heart rate. These effects are not prevented by H_1 antihistamines, but by H_2 receptor blockers, e.g. cimetidine and ranitidine. The vascular effects of histamine are mediated by both types of receptor. In some instances H_1 and H_2 have opposing actions, e.g. H_1 produces pulmonary vasoconstriction, H_2 pulmonary vasodilatation. Both H_1 and H_2 and perhaps other receptors exist in the brain.

Benzodiazepine. These act at specific synapses in the cord and central nervous system at which the transmitter is GABA. Benzodiazepines selectively facilitate GABA action at the synapses.

5 Hydroxytryptamine (5 HT, serotonin). This has been isolated from the brain stem, many forebrain sites and the dorsal horns of the spinal cord. It may represent one of the descending control pathways which modulate sensitivity of the spinal cord to pain input from the periphery, and therefore plays a key role in mediating analgesic actions of morphine and related opioid analgesics. In the forebrain, this system may be responsible for control of sleep and waking, central temperature regulation and control of aggressive behaviour.

Increasingly, neurotransmitters are found to be concerned with disease states. Anxiety probably involves many brain neurotransmitters, e.g. GABA, serotonin, noradrenaline and dopamine. Benzodiazepines exert their effects via a GABA/benzodiazepine receptor/chloride channel complex (Fig. 5.11), which may also mediate anxiety, and is enclosed in the lipid bilayer of cell membranes. There are strong indications that central monoamine metabolism is disturbed in depression and that the disturbance is *causal*.

Tricyclic antidepressants inhibit the presynaptic uptake of 5HT and noradrenaline (Fig. 5.12). The disturbances appear to be specific for endogenous depression. Research continues on the monoamine precursors, selective reuptake inhibitors and postsynaptic antagonists and the correlation between disturbances of 5HT, catecholamines and endocrine dysfunction.

In schizophrenia it has been noted that increased catecholamine activity may worsen symptoms. Neuroleptics in small doses dramatically reverse amphetamine induced psychoses whereas amphetamine induces schizophrenic exacerbations. This is further support for a dopaminergic abnormality. Some symptoms of schizophrenia are reduced by naloxone, suggesting that opioid peptides, e.g. enkephalins, are involved, although naloxone also blocks GABA receptors.

Epilepsy. A binding site for phenytoin, which interacts with the GABA/chloride ionophor/

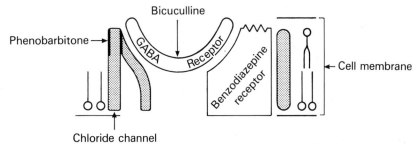

Fig. 5.11   GABA receptor, benzodiazepine receptor and chloride channel.

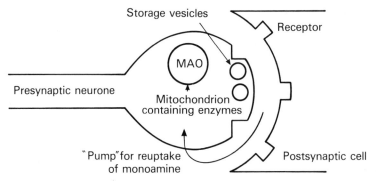

Fig. 5.12   Tricyclic antidepressants inhibit presynaptic uptake of 5HT and noradrenaline. MAO = monoamine oxidase.

benzodiazepine complex and an endogenous compound which binds to this site have been isolated from the brain. It is thought that one or more components of the GABA inhibitory system may be concerned with maintenance of a normal state (Fig. 5.13). It may be that in epilepsy there is a lower threshold for seizure, but inhibitory systems within the brain terminate the seizure.

Classification of nerve fibres

In 1943 Gasser produced a classification of nerve fibres which is still valid (Table 5.2).

The sensory system

Detection of mechanical stimuli

Peripheral receptors exist in excitable tissues. Skin receptors appreciate touch, cold, warmth and pain,

Table 5.2   Classification of nerve fibres (Gasser 1943)

Description of nerve fibre	Group		Diameter (µm)	Conduction velocity (m/s)
Myelinated somatic	A	alpha beta gamma	20	120
		delta	3–4	6–30 (pain fibres)
		epsilon	2	5
Myelinated visceral (preganglionic autonomic)	B		<3	3–15
Unmyelinated somatic	C		<2	0.5–2 (pain fibres)

and deeper receptors appreciate pressure and proprioception.

There are large numbers of different receptors and end-organs and although end-organs are specialised

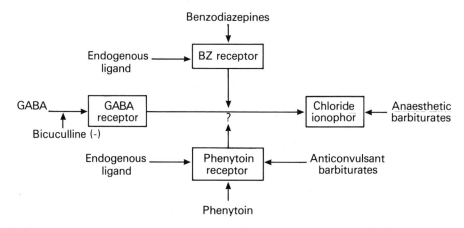

Fig. 5.13   Postulated receptor interactions in epilepsy. BZ = benzodiazepine.

for one form of sensation, the quality of sensation does not depend on the type of stimulus arousing it. Information is transmitted to the central nervous system by varying the frequency and patterns of action potentials. There is often extensive branching of axons and a single fibre may be said to have a 'peripheral receptive field'.

Adaptation

A sustained, mechanical stimulus produces only a transient response, i.e. there is processing of information at receptor level, so that the brain is not constantly informed of an unchanging stimulus. Adaptation is said to be a function of the 'onion skin' of Pacinian corpuscles, where the accessory structure added to the nerve ending is visco-elastic and deformation of the surface has only a transient effect on the core of the corpuscle. There is an electrical component of accommodation. A direct current applied to cause a sustained, artificial generator potential produces only a short burst of action potentials. Pacinian corpuscles show rapid adaptation so that steady state stimulus does not produce continuous activity. Muscle stretch receptors, on the other hand, show less adaptation.

Mechanical transduction

This consists of transfer of a mechanical stimulus through accessory structures to the nerve terminal itself (Fig. 5.14). A graded electrical response is then produced equivalent to the generator or receptor potential with initiation of an action potential.

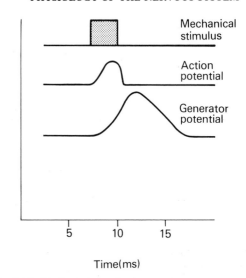

Fig. 5.14 Mechanical transduction.

A generator potential is produced by a mechanical stimulus and is a transient depolarisation of the nerve terminal membrane, independent of the ion channels. The potential appears to be created by the nerve terminal itself and the important stimulus is distortion of the terminal.

Modalities of cutaneous sensation

There are four main modes of cutaneous sensation: touch, cold, warmth, pain.

Touch. Touch provides information on shape, texture and hardness of the object. Tactile sensation (Fig. 5.15) is distributed in a punctate fashion, with variability from day to day. The smallest pressure

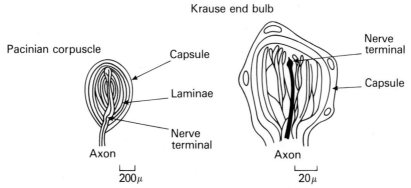

Fig. 5.15 Tactile receptors. Pacinian corpuscles are subcutaneous structures with receptive field 100 mm^2 which respond to vibration (40–600 Hz). Krause end bulbs are found in the dermis and respond to vibration (10–200 Hz) and movement from a field of 2 mm^2. They are concerned with spatial and intensity aspects of touch.

required to excite a sensation varies over the body surface. Touch spots are more frequent around hair follicles, the hair acting as a lever to transmit deformation to nerve endings around the shaft. Afferent fibres innervating these receptors have a large receptive field. Tactile sensation shows adaptation, localisation (which is also dependent on experience), discrimination between two points, and projection.

Temperature. Both warm spots and cold spots may be isolated on the skin. The latter are more numerous and there is daily variation in their distribution. This cutaneous sensation also shows adaptation. Sensitivity of the exposed skin varies with the area of the body, but at ordinary skin temperatures a temperature difference of 0.2°C can be detected by the forearms.

Pain. Pain registered by stimulation of the skin has a pricking, itching quality and is well localised. The pain threshold may be increased by one-third by distracting the subject's attention and reduced by half in sunburnt skin. The first sensation of pain arises abruptly and is carried by moderately large fibres, conducting impulses at 10 m/s. The second sensation is slower and of a burning nature, probably being carried by unmyelinated fibres.

Pain nerve endings are distributed in a punctate fashion independent of the end-organs concerned with touch and temperature. Further aspects of pain are considered separately later in this chapter.

Sensations from viscera and vessels travel in autonomic nerves and are often projected to a definite position on the surface of the body with the corresponding dermatome. This is relevant when considering referred pain (Fig. 5.16).

Spinal cord pathways

These may be divided into afferent (sensory), motor, cerebellar and autonomic.

Sensory afferent

Impulses arise in muscles, tendons, joints or skin. Dorsal root sensory ganglia and cranial nerve ganglia comprise primary neurones whose peripheral processes run with spinal nerves and whose central processes run into the cord. Some dorsal root fibres on entering the cord pass directly to motor neurones, constituting a monosynaptic reflex arc. Others synapse with cells in the dorsal horn of the grey matter and influence ventral horn cells by a reflex arc involving several neurones. The majority, however, form synapses with dorsal horn cells, cells in thoracic nuclei, the base of the dorsal horn or the nuclei gracilis and cuneatus (second order sensory neurones) (Fig. 5.17). These cross to the opposite side and end in the ventrolateral nucleus of the thalamus where they synapse with third order sensory neurones, the fibres of which pass through the posterior end of the internal capsule to the postcentral gyrus of the cerebral cortex. There are two major sensory systems:

1. The dorsal column-medial lemniscus system, which conducts proprioception, fine touch, vibration and some autonomic fibres.

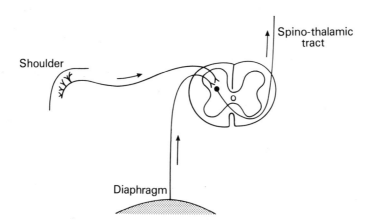

Fig. 5.16 Referred pain; irritation of the diaphragm is felt in the shoulder tip. Nerves from these areas synapse with common neurones in the spinal cord.

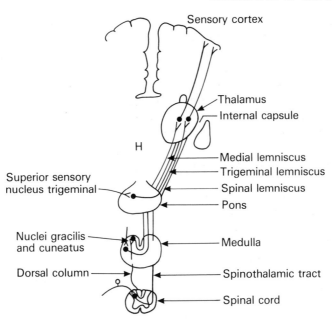

Sensory cortex

Thalamus

Internal capsule

H

Medial lemniscus

Trigeminal lemniscus

Superior sensory
nucleus trigeminal

Spinal lemniscus

Pons

Nuclei gracilis
and cuneatus

Medulla

Dorsal column

Spinothalamic tract

Spinal cord

Fig. 5.17 Major somatic afferent, sensory pathways. H = hypothalamus.

2. The spinothalamic tract; crude touch and pressure are conducted along the anterior spinothalamic tract, and pain and temperature in the lateral spinothalamic tract.

Both the sensory systems decussate before they reach the sensory cortex. The dorsal column system decussates in the medulla and the lateral spinothalamic tract close to its site of entry in the cord.

Descending control of sensory pathways is by efferent nerves acting at synaptic junctions of the relay nuceli of the ascending pathways, e.g. the dorsal horn, dorsal column and thalamic nuclei. These may be either facilitatory or inhibitory.

In the medulla, the two spinothalamic tracts blend to form the spinal lemniscus which is closely associated with corresponding fibres from the fifth cranial nerve. The thalamus acts as a relay station for sensory pathways. Ultimately somatosensory impulses from one side of the body are represented on the contralateral cerebral cortex only. Removal of the cerebral cortex results in the thalamus undertaking crude appreciation of sensation. The sensory cortex, however, is responsible for perception of sensation including the full appreciation of pain. If this sensory gyrus is completely obliterated, there is impairment but no abolition of sensation, although agnosia and disturbances of body image occur (vide infra).

Motor efferent

Lower motor neurones (l.m.n.) are anterior horn cells of the spinal cord grey matter and certain cranial nerve nuclei whose axons innervate voluntary muscle. Upper motor neurones run from the cortex or brain stem to l.m.ns and comprise the pyramidal and extrapyramidal tracts which are concerned with control of movement.

The pyramidal tract (Fig. 5.18) is so named because it forms the pyramid of the medulla. It originates mainly in the precentral gyrus of the cerebral cortex and runs first to cranial nerve nuclei (corticonuclear fibres) and then to the anterior columns of the spinal cord (corticospinal fibres). As these fibres descend from the cortex they traverse the internal capsule in an orderly arrangement. Most corticonuclear fibres cross the midline in the brain stem, terminating in the motor cranial nerve nuclei (cranial nerves III–VII, IX and X). Some uncrossed fibres remain and the tract continues through the pons in a dispersed fashion. Fibres become grouped together in a pyramid on the ventral aspect of the medulla oblongata. In the lower half of the medulla, 90% of fibres cross to the opposite side to descend in the posterior part of the lateral columns as the lateral pyramidal tract. A few fibres pass down on the same side in the anterior white column as the ventral pyramidal tract. A lesion of pyramidal fibres above the decussation produces a

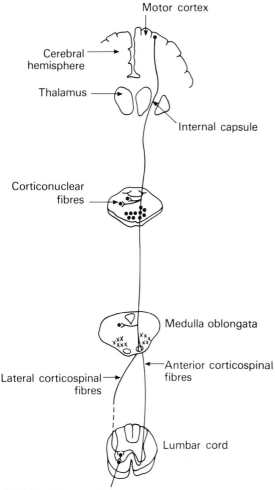

Motor cortex

Cerebral hemisphere

Thalamus

Internal capsule

Corticonuclear fibres

Medulla oblongata

Lateral corticospinal fibres

Anterior corticospinal fibres

Lumbar cord

Fig. 5.18 The pyramidal tract.

contralateral paralysis of voluntary muscles, impairing especially precise movements of the distal aspect of the limbs.

The extrapyramidal system is concerned chiefly with regulation of muscle tone, thus influencing posture and more stereotyped movements. It comprises a series of tracts connecting various areas of cerebral cortex, subcortical nuclei and brain stem nuclei. These tracts descend to the lower brain stem and spinal cord to influence l.m.ns through intermediate neurones.

Descending extrapyramidal tracts include the rubrobulbar and reticulospinal (Fig. 5.19). These accompany the pyramidal tracts to interneurones in the cord. Both systems influence the final, common pathways (l.m.ns) which are also influenced reflexly by sensory impulses.

The net result of extrapyramidal activity is inhibitory, so that lesions in the midbrain nuclei associated with this system may result in increased postural tone, and spasticity with uncontrolled tremors or movement. Two other descending pathways influence motor activity; the tectospinal and vestibulospinal tracts. These two tracts account for the influence of stimuli from the eye and the ear produced by movement.

Cerebellar pathways

Afferent and efferent pathways traverse via the cerebellar peduncles. The afferent pathways contain information from muscle spindles, Golgi tendon organs, and other proprioceptors, and reach the cerebellum in three main ascending pathways in each half of the spinal cord: the posterior and anterior spinocerebellar tracts and the posterior external arcuate fibres.

Efferent fibres from Purkinje cells in the cerebellar cortex ultimately traverse the superior cerebellar peduncles and cross to the opposite side in the lower half of the midbrain, ending mainly in the contralateral red nucleus. They project to the cerebral cortex, brain stem, reticular, vestibular and other nuclei.

Autonomic pathways

The sympathetic system (Fig. 5.20). This is a two-neurone system. Preganglionic sympathetic fibres have their cells of origin in the lateral horns of the grey matter in segments T1 to L2, and fibres leave the cord with motor nerves to voluntary muscle via the ventral nerve root. Preganglionic fibres run to the sympathetic trunk which lies a few centimetres from the vertebral column on each side from the level of the superior cervical ganglion downwards to the pelvis. Postganglionic fibres arise from these ganglia and usually join spinal nerves. Those to the head accompany the carotid artery. Sympathetic fibres to the gut do not relay in the sympathetic trunk, but in midline ganglia in front of the aorta (coeliac, superior and inferior mesenteric plexus). The function of the sympathetic nerves are described in Chapter 12, page 179.

Parasympathetic system (Fig. 5.21). This comprises a craniosacral outflow via cranial nerves III, VII, IX

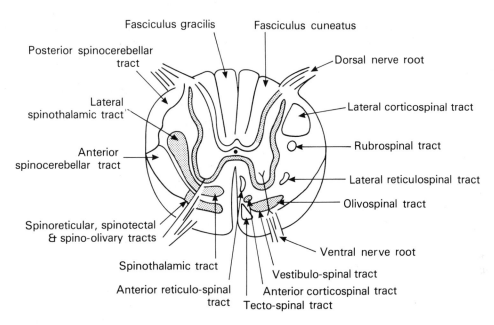

Fig. 5.19 Transverse section of the spinal cord to show major nerve tracts.

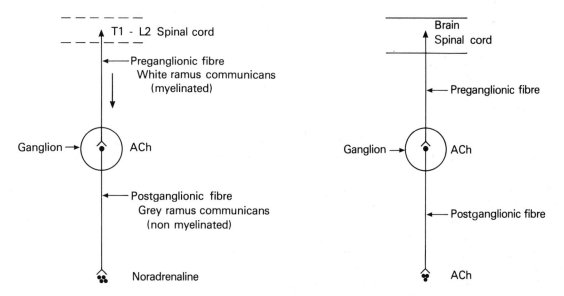

Fig. 5.20 Sympathetic nervous system. ACh = acetylcholine.

Fig. 5.21 Parasympathetic nervous system. ACh = acetylcholine.

and X, and S2–4. The actions are described in Chapter 12, page 177, and Table 12.1.

Central representation. Integration of autonomic and somatic activity maintains stable internal conditions despite a changing environment. Central nervous system areas concerned with autonomic activity (Fig. 5.22) include nuclei in the hypothalamus around the third ventricle, particularly the supraoptic, paraventricular, dorsal and ventral medial hypothalamic, posterior hypothalamic and mamillary.

There is, therefore, close association with the frontal lobes and the posterior pituitary. The hippocampal circuit (hippocampus, fornix, mamillary body, anterior thalamic nuclei, cingulate gyrus, hippocampus) represents a continuous relationship between the cortex, thalamus, hypothalamus and hippocampus and is influenced by pathways ascending from the spinal cord and brain stem and descending from the cortex. This area is involved in emotional reactions which are often the result of somatic and emotional interactions (nausea, flushing) and with memory. The hypothalamus is also important in temperature regulation, the sleep/wake rhythm, and endocrine and cardiovascular systems. Autonomic afferent fibres ascend through the cord and brain stem with somatosensory pathways to the hypothalamus, which acts as a relaying and redistributing centre from which impulses are projected onwards to the thalamus and frontal cortex.

Cranial nerves

These are situated on the base of the brain (Fig. 5.23). Cranial nerve I, the olfactory, is a special, visceral, afferent nerve, conveying impulses from the olfactory area of the nasal mucous membrane which traverses the cribriform plate of the ethmoid to the olfactory bulbs on the orbital surface of the frontal lobe.

Cranial nerve II, the optic nerve, is a special, sensory, afferent carrying visual impulses from the retina to the optic chiasma.

Cranial nerve III, the oculomotor, is a general, sensory, afferent and efferent nerve and constitutes the most important motor supply to extrinsic voluntary and intrinsic eye muscles.

The trochlear nerve (IV), is a general, sensory, afferent and efferent nerve and the only nerve to arise from the dorsal aspect of the brain stem. It supplies the superior oblique muscle.

Nerve V, the trigeminal nerve, is a general, sensory, afferent and special visceral efferent nerve, concerned with facial sensation. It also supplies the muscles of mastication. Its cutaneous distribution (Fig. 5.24) is of great clinical importance in the management of trigeminal neuralgia. This nerve may be involved in a tumour arising in the cerebello-pontine angle, e.g. an acoustic neuroma, together with involvement of cranial nerves VII and VIII.

The abducent nerve (VI), is a general, somatic,

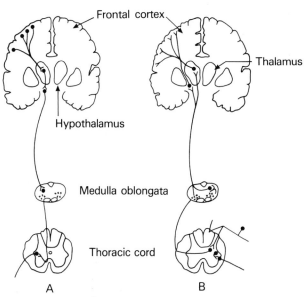

Fig. 5.22 Autonomic pathways between spinal cord and brain (not to scale) showing: A: probable efferent autonomic pathways from brain to spinal cord; B: probable afferent autonomic pathways from cord to brain.

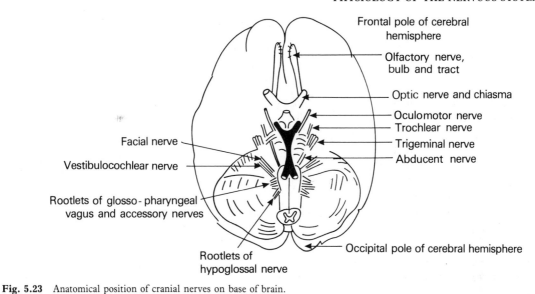

Frontal pole of cerebral hemisphere

Olfactory nerve, bulb and tract

Optic nerve and chiasma

Oculomotor nerve

Trochlear nerve

Trigeminal nerve

Abducent nerve

Facial nerve

Vestibulocochlear nerve

Rootlets of glosso-pharyngeal vagus and accessory nerves

Occipital pole of cerebral hemisphere

Rootlets of hypoglossal nerve

Fig. 5.23 Anatomical position of cranial nerves on base of brain.

afferent and efferent nerve, supplying the lateral rectus muscle. It has the longest intracranial course and may be damaged in conditions which raise intracranial pressure.

Nerves III, IV and VI can be tested by comparing eye movements and examining for ptosis and diplopia.

Cranial nerve VII (facial) is a general and special visceral, afferent and efferent nerve, which provides the main motor nerve supply to the face.

Cranial nerve VIII, the auditory, is a special

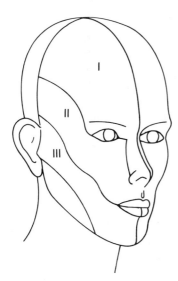

Fig. 5.24 Cutaneous divisions of the Vth nerve. I. ophthalmic; II. maxillary; III. mandibular.

afferent nerve, concerned with hearing and equilibrium, which may be tested by audiometry and caloric testing. The glossopharyngeal nerve (IX) is a general and special visceral, afferent and efferent nerve, which subserves one-third of taste and provides the motor supply to the pharynx.

Cranial nerve X, the vagus, is the major motor nerve to the viscera, palate and vocal cords and supplies most sensory modalities. Its function may be tested by examination of palatal movement, the voice and the ability to cough. Nerve XI, the spinal accessory, is a general and special visceral efferent, which supplies the sternomastoid and the upper part of the trapezius muscle.

The hypoglossal nerve (XII) is a general, somatic afferent and efferent nerve which is motor to the tongue.

Because of the close proximity of the last four cranial nerves, they may be involved jointly in pathological lesions, producing a weak, hoarse voice, nasal speech, difficulty in swallowing and regurgitation with production of an aspiration pneumonia. This constitutes a bulbar palsy and the airway should be protected.

Brain stem and midbrain function

The functions of the brain stem have been highlighted in recent years by the concept of brain stem death. An understanding of the functions requires some knowledge of the anatomy of this area.

Medulla (Fig. 5.25). 1. Motor pathways are situated ventrally. Corticospinal fibres traverse the internal capsule via the genu. They are situated medially in the cerebral peduncle, crossing the midline to supply the relevant cranial nerves of the opposite side. The motor nucleus of V, controlling the muscles of mastication, derives only half its innervation from the opposite hemisphere, i.e. there is bilateral innervation. Nerve VII has similar innervation for the forehead muscles, but the muscles of the lower face are innervated mainly by crossed fibres. Cranial nerve nuclei are situated in the dorsal areas of the medulla.

2. Sensory pathways constitute the intermediate layer of the brain stem. The gracile and cuneate nuclei are situated in the dorsal medulla. Spinothalamic sensation is associated closely with descending sympathetic pathways.

The trigeminal sensory system is very complex. Information from one side of the face enters the brain stem in the fifth nerve at the level of the midpons. Fibres concerned with the corneal reflex and touch decussate to the opposite side. Pain and temperature fibres descend parallel to the descending nucleus of the fifth nerve, relay to the opposite side in the lower medulla and become the secondary ascending tract of the fifth nerve adjacent to the medial lemniscus.

3. The brain stem contains cranial nerve nuclei of cranial nerves III to XII.

4. Control of respiration, heart rate and blood pressure. Within the medulla are the so-called vital centres, which are concerned with the automatic reflex control of the heart, lungs and circulation.

Afferent fibres originate in highly specialised visceral receptors, e.g. the carotid sinus and receptor cells within the medulla itself, which are responsive, for example, to Pa_{CO_2}. Control of swallowing, coughing and vomiting are also integrated in the medulla.

5. The fourth ventricle is situated within the brain stem.

Pons. A major feature of the pons is its peduncular connections. The medial lemniscus is the continuation upwards of the dorsal column sensory system.

Midbrain. (Fig. 5.26) This lies between the cerebrum and the pons. It contains the cerebral peduncles and the tectum. The cerebral aqueduct runs through the midbrain and connects the third and fourth ventricles. The tectum contains the colliculi, and receives some retinal fibres via the optic nerves, descending fibres from the optic cortex and ascending fibres from the cord. It is responsible for co-ordination of input from the auditory areas of the temporal cortex and cervical cord. The colliculi are also responsible for visual, auditory and vestibular reflexes.

The cerebral peduncles consist of a ventral aspect (which becomes continuous with the internal capsule), the substantia nigra, and a dorsal tegmentum. The corticonuclear, corticospinal and corticopontine fibres traverse the ventral aspect. The peri-aqueductal grey matter contains nuclei of cranial nerves III and IV and the mesencephalic nucleus of V. The red nucleus, which is an important relay

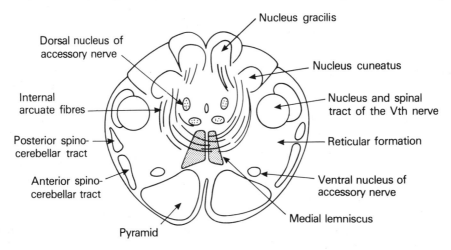

Fig. 5.25 Transverse section of medulla at level of sensory decussation.

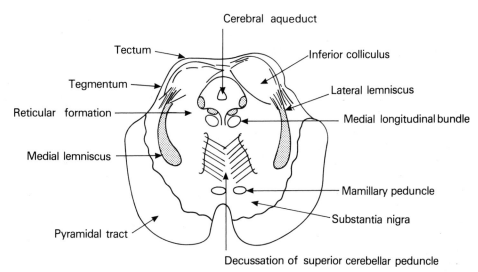

Fig. 5.26   Transverse section of midbrain at level of inferior colliculi.

station in paths between cerebellum, corpus striatum and spinal cord, is situated in the tegmentum.

The reticular formation. This constitutes the central core of the brain stem, projecting widely to the limbic system and cortex with many ascending and descending connections. Stimulation activates the cortex, initiating an arousal reaction, i.e. this area is responsible for generating the capacity for consciousness. Attention and circadian rhythms are also dependent upon the correct functioning of the reticular formation.

Brain stem function tests

1. Activity of nerves II to XII may be tested individually to permit localisation of a lesion.

2. Transmission of all motor information from the cortex to the spinal cord and all sensory information in the opposite direction. Although spinal reflexes may be active when the brain stem is destroyed there should be no abnormal posture, either decorticate (flexed forearms and extended legs) or decerebrate (extended hyperpronated forearms and extended legs), nor trismus.

3. Control of respiration. In the absence of brain stem activity there is apnoea. Loss of vasomotor control also occurs.

4. Brain stem reflexes:
(i) Oculocephalic. In the absence of brain stem function, when the head is rotated to one side and

held there for 3–4 s and then rotated through 180° in the opposite direction, the head and eyes move together. In a patient with damaged cerebral hemispheres and an intact brain stem, there is deviation of the eyes to the opposite side as the head is rotated, followed by realignment of the eyes with the head.

(ii) Vestibulo-ocular. If the clear, external auditory canal is irrigated with ice-cold saline and the brain stem is intact, there is nystagmus. When the brain stem is totally destroyed there are no eye movements.

The cerebral cortex

The surface anatomy of the cerebral cortex with underlying functions is illustrated in Figure 5.27. The dominant hemisphere is that opposite the dominant hand in right-handed individuals, but variable in those who are left-handed. If the dominant hemisphere is destroyed early in life then the other may slowly but incompletely assume intellectual functions. The cerebral cortex is concerned with higher intellectual functions: memory, learning and language. In the human, there are three major association areas, (i) the frontal, in front of the motor cortex; (ii) the temporal, between the superior temporal gyrus and limbic cortex; (iii) the parieto-occipital, between the sensory and visual cortex. These areas have complex connections from the thalamus, to each other and to the deeper cortex.

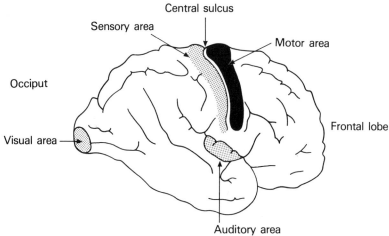

Fig. 5.27   Lateral aspect of cerebral cortex.

Coning

Brain swelling may be evident anatomically as midline shift. Displacement may cause part of a cerebral hemisphere, usually the temporal lobe, to become impacted under the falx cerebri or tentorial hiatus. Any expanding supratentorial lesion, e.g. middle meningeal haemorrhage, forces the medial aspect of the temporal lobe into the tentorial hiatus. Compression of the cerebral peduncle and oculomotor nerve causes pupillary changes (dilatation) with contralateral hemiparesis. Later, brain stem compression produces apnoea.

An expanding posterior fossa lesion may push the cerebellum into the tentorial hiatus. Medullary coning from high ICP forcing the medulla and cerebellar tonsil down into the foramen magnum is rapidly fatal by compression of the respiratory and vasomotor centres.

Cerebrospinal fluid (c.s.f.)

C.s.f. is formed by secretory cells of the choroid plexus, which project into the lateral and third ventricles (Fig. 5.28). C.s.f. then flows via the third ventricle through the aqueduct and fourth ventricle to escape by two lateral foramina of Luschka and median foramen of Magendie into the subarachnoid space around the brain and spinal cord.

C.s.f. is produced at approx. 0.5 ml/min. Its total volume is 120 ml and it is therefore turned over approx. every 4 h. Production must match absorption to prevent an increase in pressure. Obstruction to the flow of c.s.f. increases pressure, with dilatation of the ventricles upstream from the obstruction.

Resorption is mainly into the venous system via arachnoid villi, which are areas where the arachnoid invaginates into large venous sinuses. If the c.s.f. pressure is less than venous, the vacuoles collapse. Some c.s.f. is also probably absorbed around spinal nerves into spinal veins and through the ependymal lining of the ventricles. C.s.f. acts as a cushion between the skull and the brain. It may accommodate a certain change in brain volume by displacement into the lumbar region. In conditions producing cerebral atrophy there is an increase in c.s.f. volume.

C.s.f. is a clear, colourless liquid of specific gravity 1005, with less than 5 lymphocytes/mm^3 and pH 7.33 (Table 5.3). C.s.f. is probably produced from plasma by a combination of secretion and ultrafiltration. The high concentration of chloride arises because carbon dioxide passes into glial cells where, by the action of carbonic anhydrase, it is hydrated to carbonic acid

Table 5.3   Composition of plasma and cerebrospinal fluid

	Plasma (mmol/litre)	Cerebrospinal fluid (mmol/litre)
Urea	2.5–6.5	2.0–7.0
Glucose (fasting)	3.0–5.0	2.5–4.5
Sodium	136–148	144–152
Potassium	3.8–5.0	2.0–3.0
Calcium	2.2–2.6	1.1–1.3
Chloride	95–105	123–128
Bicarbonate	24–32	24–32
Protein	60–80 g/litre	200–400 mg/litre

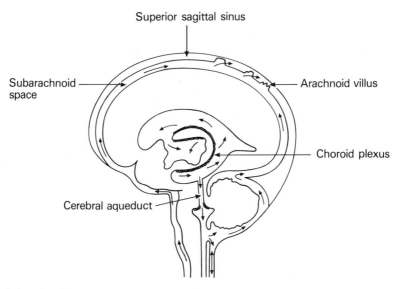

Fig. 5.28 The circulation of c.s.f.

(H_2CO_3). Resulting bicarbonate ions (HCO_3^-) are exchanged for chloride which passes into the c.s.f. against a concentration gradient. C.s.f. is slightly hypertonic; Na^+ and Mg^{++} ions are actively transported into c.s.f. Lipophilic substances pass readily from blood to brain, but dissociated hydrophilic substances pass only very slowly.

The blood brain barrier (Fig. 5.29) is composed of a lipid membrane of capillaries, the endothelial cells of which are joined by tight junctions around the entire periphery of each cell. Solutes at higher concentration in the e.c.f. of the brain diffuse into c.s.f. and are carried into blood at the arachnoid villi. Some substances are transported actively by cells of the choroid plexus from c.s.f. into blood.

Electrophoresis of c.s.f. proteins is now possible.

C.s.f. proteins are derived by filtration of plasma, from brain interstititial fluid and brain cells, and from cells of the c.s.f. compartment itself.

These proteins may reflect abnormalities of the filtration mechanism, of barrier function, brain metabolism or activities of the c.s.f. Electrophoresis has clinical application for investigation of certain neurological conditions, e.g. multiple sclerosis, Guillain Barré syndrome and neurosyphilis.

PAIN

Pain is a combination of severe discomfort, fear, autonomic changes, reflex activity and suffering.

Unmyelinated, peripheral, afferent fibres terminate

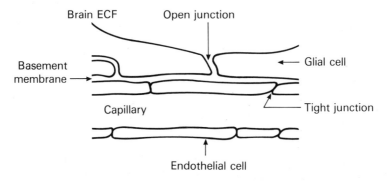

Fig. 5.29 Blood-brain barrier.

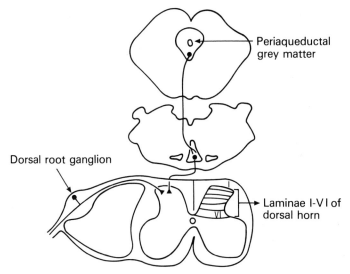

Fig. 5.30   Pain pathways.

in the substantia gelatinosa of the dorsal horn (Fig. 5.30) and smaller, myelinated afferents (group 3) terminate in the nucleus proprius (lamina V). Spinothalamic fibres arise at this layer.

In 1952 Rexed showed that cells of the grey matter of the spinal cord are arranged in nine laminae, I to IX, from the dorsal to the ventral cord, the tenth lamina lying around the central zone. Lamina I comprises the marginal zone, laminae II and III the substantia gelatinosa, and laminae IV, V and VI the nucleus proprius (Fig. 5.31). Small myelinated fibres activated by pin prick, and hot and cold receptors, terminate here. Laminae VII and VIII correspond to the nucleus intermedius, and give rise to spinoreticular fibres. Lamina IX is the ventral horn, and the output from this constitutes the ventral root.

Gate control theory of pain

Nociceptive impulses activate:

1. Nerve fibres which stimulate the substantia gelatinosa and nucleus proprius.
2. Large myelinated axons of the dorsal column fibres.

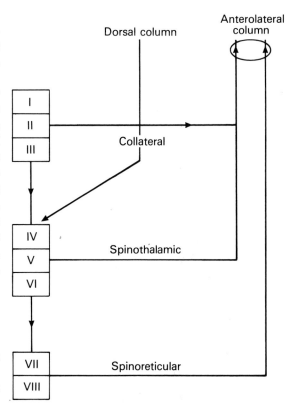

Fig. 5.31   Connections of Rexed laminae.

Segmental collaterals from the dorsal column fibres synapse in lamina IV. These exert an inhibitory influence on transmission of impulses from the substantia gelatinosa, with a reduction in painful sensation. Descending impulses control sensory input by direct and indirect modulation at every level of the brain stem and spinal cord, including the dorsal horn of the cord where they form part of the gate control mechanism. It is known that pain may be suppressed by stress, hypnosis, electrical stimulation and trance-like euphoria.

The gate control theory of pain as illustrated in Figure 5.32, was developed originally by Melzack and Wall in 1965. They postulated that large diamater A fibres (Aα) and small diameter A fibres (Aδ) and C fibres are all activated during noxious stimulation of

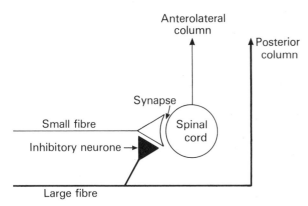

Fig. 5.32 Gate control mechanism.

peripheral receptors. At cord level, a gate exists which, under certain circumstances, opens to permit pain stimuli to pass through to higher centres. Small nerve fibre stimulation opens the gate, and large nerve fibre stimulation closes it by depression or facilitation of synaptic transmission. Two possible mechanisms of afferent synaptic inhibition have been described: (i) via a glycine transmitter site; (ii) via a GABA site with a longer latency.

In postherpetic neuralgia the pain results from loss of large fibres. In polyneuropathy, there is a relative increase in the small fibres without an increase in pain, i.e. selective inhibition of supraspinal origin, which can shut down transmission from nociceptors, leaving mechanoreceptor conduction almost un-impaired.

Endogenous opioids and pain

The opioid molecule is stereospecific, which supports the concept of specific binding sites. Sites of opioid receptors in the spinal cord include the marginal zone and substantia gelatinosa of the dorsal horn and the descending spinal trigeminal nucleus. At higher levels they are found in the palaeospinothalamic pain pathway and limbic system related to emotional behaviour. They are also found in the gut. In 1975

two related pentapeptides were isolated — methionine and leucine enkephalin. Met-enkephalin (methionine enkephalin) is formed by breakdown of pituitary beta lipotropin and is destroyed very rapidly. These features suggest its role as a neurotransmitter and, indeed, many enkephalin-containing neurones and nerve terminals are concentrated in laminae I and II of the dorsal horn.

There are three subclasses of opioid receptor: mu, delta and kappa. The spinal distribution of mu opiate receptors parallels that of enkephalins. The mu receptors are those most likely to be associated with pain pathways. A descending projection from neurones of the peri-aqueductal grey matter is responsible for stimulus-produced analgesia and opioid analgesia, but these neurones do not project directly to the spinal cord. There is a possibility that there may be an excitatory neurotransmitter between the two, e.g. glutamate or aspartate. Evidence points, however, to enkephalin being the transmitter at the inhibitory synapse depicted in Figure 5.32 in the gate control mechanism of pain.

The most likely substance to be concerned with transmission of pain is substance P. Transmission from substance P-containing primary afferents is blocked by morphine or enkephalin and pretreatment with naloxone prevents this. The inhibitory enkephalinergic synapses are probably activated by segmental collaterals of large myelinated primary afferents of the dorsal columns, explaining the value of transcutaneous and dorsal column stimulation in pain relief. Additionally, descending control pathways in neurones from the raphe nuclei which are unmyelinated and serotoninergic are closely related anatomically to enkephalinergic neurones. It seems probable, therefore, that both systems are concerned with pain suppression.

Electrical stimulation of the brain, in particular the peri-aqueductal grey matter, releases endorphins which are the precursors of enkephalins, and it is well known that pain relief by acupuncture is antagonised by naloxone. Direct administration of small amounts of opioid peptide into the brain elicits a variety of behavioural responses, and neuropeptides may be neuromodulators rather than neurotransmitters. It is becoming apparent that neurones may secrete more than one biologically - active substance, e.g. noradrenaline plus enkephalin. This leads to an increasing variety of chemically coded signals within c.n.s. neurones.

MECHANISMS OF GENERAL ANAESTHESIA

The underlying mechanism of general anaesthesia still awaits elucidation. Research is concentrated on the following questions:

1. What is the interaction of the anaesthetic agent with the receptor at molecular level?
2. What precisely is the disorder of cellular function produced by the anaesthetic?
3. What is the action of the anaesthetic at the synapse?

The well-known correlation between anaesthetic potency and lipid solubility indicates that anaesthetics have a hydrophobic mechanism of action. Originally developed in 1901, by H.H. Meyer and E. Overton as the lipid solubility theory, this is illustrated in Figure 5.33 as the correlation of anaesthetic potency (MAC) with oil/gas partition coefficient.

Against this is the aqueous theory of anaesthetic action suggested by the relationship between anaesthetic partial pressure and the decomposition pressure of the gas hydrates (clathrates) formed by the anaesthetics. It was suggested that anaesthetics affect water molecules in such a way as to reduce the conductance in the brain, perhaps by expanding the lipid membrane to occlude its microchannels. However, some potent volatile agents do not form clathrates under the relevant conditions. Some anaesthetics, e.g. fluorocarbons, do not fit this

correlation and there is no mechanism for the additivity of anaesthetic potencies. Therefore the lipid region of the cell membrane or the hydrophobic region of protein molecules is most likely to be the site of a common anaesthetic mechanism.

Pressure reversal and the critical volume hypothesis

If mice are placed in a pressure chamber and anaesthetised with halothane, the addition of helium to the chamber to increase the pressure to 50 atmospheres allows the mice to wake up, although the partial pressure of halothane and oxygen are unaltered. The critical volume hypothesis proposes that there is a critical hydrophobic molecular site which is expanded by an anaesthetic and contracted by pressure. The percentage reduction in anaesthetic potency is related linearly to the total increase in pressure and the slope is the same for all agents. However, at very high pressures, this relationship no longer pertains and, in addition, not all agents behave in the same way at high pressure.

Anaesthetic action on the axonal membrane

Anaesthetics may block conduction by preventing channels opening, altering the ability to pass Na^+ or by favouring the inactive state. In addition, any agent which chronically depolarises a membrane favours the inactive state, preventing channels opening.

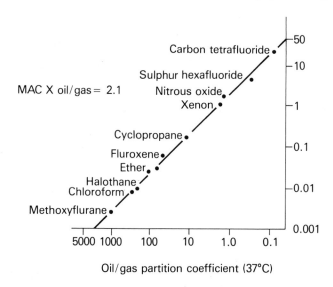

Fig. 5.33   Correlation of anaesthetic potency (MAC) with oil/gas partition coefficient. Standard deviations are omitted.

However K^+ channels may be blocked completely and an action potential may still be produced. Although relevant experimental evidence is lacking, anaesthetics might act by depolarising the membrane thereby reducing the absolute magnitude of the action potential and favouring persistence of Na^+ channels in the inactive state.

Role of conduction block in anaesthesia

General anaesthetics may act by reducing synaptic transmission whilst the impulse in presynaptic terminals remains unimpaired. There are two possible mechanisms:

1. Anaesthetic agents may, by inducing chronic depolarisation, reduce the amount of transmitter release per impulse by a mechanism similar to presynaptic inhibition. This may be mediated by a specific effect of anaesthetics on Ca^{++} entry.
2. Anaesthetics may interfere with the movement of the vesicle to and its fusion with the postsynaptic membrane.

Depression of the postsynaptic response

It is highly likely that this occurs in the anaesthetised patient. There is some evidence that anaesthetics may be selective for a specific type of synapse. In the invertebrates, volatile general anaesthetics preferentially depress excitatory rather than inhibitory transmission. Some analgesic properties of anaesthetics may be related to interactions with endorphin and enkephalin systems. Conductance changes to Na^+ can be detected at postsynaptic membranes and it seems likely that this neuronal function is altered by anaesthesia.

The critical volume hypothesis should permit temperature reversal of anaesthesia but this is difficult to test. Intravenous anaesthetics show considerable variation of pressure reversal between agents and this does not support the critical volume hypothesis for a single site of action for all anaesthetic agents. The concept, therefore, of a multisite expansion hypothesis has been developed by Halsey (1979).

Multisite expansion hypothesis

Much of this is controversial but the hypothesis may be summarised as follows:

1. General anaesthesia may be produced by the expansion of more than one molecular site; the sites may have different physical properties.
2. The physical properties of the molecular sites may be influenced by the presence of anaesthetics or pressure.
3. The molecular sites have a finite size and limited degree of occupancy.
4. Pressure need not necessarily act at the same site as the anaesthetic.
5. Molecular sites for anaesthesia are not perturbed by a decrease in temperature in a manner analagous to an increase in pressure.

Lipids in membranes move and rotate within the bilayer and influence the activity of proteins which control ionic and neurotransmitter fluxes. Perhaps the presence of a general anaesthetic in the membrane increases the movement of lipid and is associated with an increase in its volume. This might therefore effect conformational changes in the protein. The Na^+ channel protein requires an annulus of lipid in the more solid gel state to allow activity (i.e. the open state). Anaesthetics fluidise lipid causing protein to relax into the inactive (closed channel) state. Other studies suggest that anaesthetic agents increase the thickness of the lipid bilayer so that the protein pore cannot expand the membrane adequately.

Protein change

Nuclear magnetic resonance studies of volatile agents on haemoglobin have provided the first evidence that anaesthetic agents interact with hydrophobic pockets within proteins at sites which appear to behave as bulk solvents. Conformational changes are then transmitted and detected in nonhydrophobic areas of the protein. Conformational changes specific to an individual anaesthetic have been observed in the same protein.

Sensory-motor modulation systems

Anaesthetic action on sensory-motor modulation systems switches off excitation and turns on inhibition such that messages between the periphery and brain are blocked mainly at thalamic level with loss of motor control. Loss of consciousness occurs by a mechanism similar to an exaggerated sleep state.

The number of synapses in such pathways is irrelevant but the degree of supraspinal modulation of postsynaptic membrane excitation is important.

Miscellaneous

It is well known that inhalational agents produce a dose-dependent toxic effect, e.g. depression of cell multiplication, mitotic abnormalities, reduced synthesis of DNA with perhaps mutagenic and carcinogenic effects. In some way these may be related to anaesthetic mechanisms.

Other areas of study have included the effect of anaesthetic agents on the microtubules which give rigidity to cytoplasm. These are rings of protein molecules bound longitudinally. Cold and hydrostatic pressure both reversibly depolymerise these microtubular proteins, and produce narcosis. There remains the possibility that general anaesthetics reversibly depolymerise microtubular proteins by binding to nonpolar sites on globular proteins.

Proton pump leak theory

Anaesthetic agents increase leakiness in presynaptic vesicles which reduces pH gradients, in turn affecting release and uptake of neurotransmitter. This concept is dependent primarily on intracellular pH. Cooling and high pressure produce reduction of proton pump activity and reduce neurotransmitter concentration. Anaesthetic effects of high concentrations of CO_2 (30%) in animals are not related to lipid solubility but to a direct action on intracellular pH. Complete anaesthesia occurs at a c.s.f. pH of 6.7.

NEUROPHYSIOLOGICAL INVESTIGATIONS

Background electrical activity of the brain may be recorded from the intact skull by scalp electrodes which may be unipolar or bipolar, the latter measuring the potential difference fluctuations between two electrodes. The electroencephalogram (e.e.g.) (Fig. 5.34) is a continuous recording of the immediate electrical responses from the underlying brain and represents excitatory and inhibitory postsynaptic potentials in the larger dendrites of neurones of the superficial cortex.

In the resting adult, with the mind wandering and eyes closed, the most prominent component is alpha rhythm, 8–13 Hz, 50 μV amplitude, recorded best in the parieto-occipital region. Beta activity is 18–30 Hz, of lower voltage, and is found mainly over the frontal region. Theta activity occurs in normal children at 4–7 Hz and is composed of large regular waves. Delta activity is very slow — less than 4 Hz. If the eyes are open, fast, irregular low voltage activity occurs with no dominant frequency. This is termed alpha block or desynchronisation and occurs with any form of sensory stimulation.

Deep sleep induces large, irregular delta waves interspersed with alpha-like activity. Rapid eye

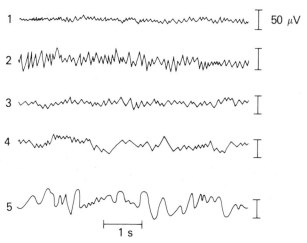

Fig. 5.34   E.e.g. 1: excited; 2: relaxed; 3: drowsy; 4: asleep; 5: deep sleep.

movement (r.e.m.) or paradoxical sleep occurs with rapid low voltage, irregular e.e.g. activity, resembling arousal. Wakening during this period is associated with reports of dreaming. R.e.m. periods occur approximately every 50 min and occupy a total of 20% of the young adult's normal sleep time. They are associated with a marked reduction in skeletal muscle tone. Repeated awakening during r.e.m. sleep produces anxiety and irritability with an increased percentage of r.e.m. sleep in subsequent undisturbed nights.

Characteristic changes in the e.e.g. occur in anaesthesia and other forms of coma. Increasing depth of anaesthesia with more potent agents produces slowing of the basic frequency of activity with a progressive increase in amplitude. Periods of iso-electricity appear, interspersed with bursts of activity. This is known as 'burst suppression'. With progressive depth of anaesthesia, there is increasing distance between bursts, resulting finally in an iso-electric line.

Characteristic changes with spike formation in the e.e.g. occur during epilepsy. Hypoxia produces an acute increase in the amplitude of the e.e.g. initially and then a marked reduction in amplitude with the appearance of slow waves as hypoxia worsens.

There are problems with using the e.e.g. to monitor the brain continuously. These are related largely to the cumbersome equipment, problems of interpretation, and interference from other electrical equipment. The unprocessed e.e.g. is still used by some anaesthetists in cerebrovascular surgery, including carotid artery surgery, as an indication of cerebral ischaemia, when it shows good correlation with cerebral blood flow.

Processed e.e.g. techniques

These offer no improvements in diagnostic sensitivity, but are simpler to use and clarify the display of information. Such techniques may be of limited value in evaluation of a complex situation, e.g. hypoxic changes occurring during hypothermia. There are numerous reports of the relationship between the processed e.e.g. and anaesthetic depth indicating that small changes are detectable which would be missed in the absence of processing.

Cerebral function monitor (c.f.m.)

This compresses all frequency and amplitude information in the e.e.g. into a single value. It uses two parietal electrodes, the signal from which is passed through a wide-band frequency filter to remove frequencies of less than 2 Hz, and more than 15 Hz (to reduce artefact and interference). The signal is amplified, rectified, integrated and compressed to produce a slow-running chart recording as a line, the height (above base line) of which indicates total power (Fig. 5.35). Undulations reflect fluctuations in power from one moment to the next, upward movement indicating increased activity. The machine also monitors electrode impedance to detect artefacts from incorrect function of the electrodes.

Such a monitor requires supplementing at regular intervals by a full e.e.g. because of the loss of information by processing. The main objection to the c.f.m. is that the record is neither one of frequency nor amplitude but a mixture of the two. It does, however, permit continuous monitoring of electrical activity.

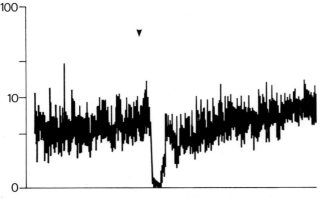

Fig. 5.35 Cerebral function monitor. This trace shows interruption of the circulation at the arrow causing a transient absence of cerebral activity.

Power spectrum analysis

This technique retains all information from the original e.e.g. Analysis of the e.e.g. occurs as follows:

1. The e.e.g. is digitised at frequent intervals known as epochs (2–16 s).

2. The epoch of data is subjected to Fourier analysis, separating the total e.e.g. wave form into a number of component sine waves of different amplitudes, the sum of which is equal to the original wave form, i.e. conversion into a number of standard waves for easy comparison.

3. The power spectrum is calculated by squaring the amplitudes of each individual frequency component, and displayed for each epoch graphically, so that patterns may be identified by examination of a number of epochs in succession. If the epochs are short, i.e. 2–4 s, this constitutes almost a continuous monitor.

Advantages. 1. All information is retained and small changes may be identified readily.

2. Each frequency band may be considered separately so that changes in one part of the spectrum cannot balance out changes elsewhere, as with the c.f.m.

3. Generation of the power spectrum minimises baseline drift by converting all low frequency components (0.05 to 0.50 Hz) to a single point.

4. Predictable changes may be detected, e.g. during halothane anaesthesia, there is less power at high frequencies and increased low frequency activity.

The currently available Berg analyser has the facility to switch from compressed data to raw data. It uses two pairs of electrodes and displays each hemisphere separately.

Display. A sophisticated, graphical display is essential because one of the main disadvantages of this technique is the vast amount of data generated (2000 data points per minute for each e.e.g. channel processed). The printed output consists of a graph of relative power versus frequency at each epoch of the analysis (Fig. 5.36). Time is presented vertically to produce a three dimensional graph, with a hill and valley appearance. Hills constitute those frequencies making a large contribution and valleys occur at frequencies containing less power. The points behind the hill are not printed.

Disadvantages. 1. High amplitude activity obscures

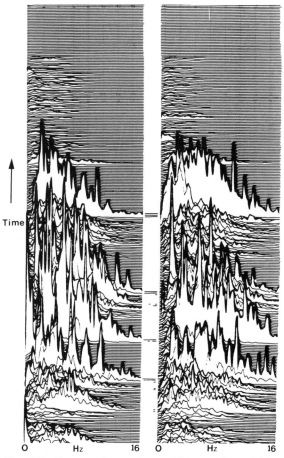

Fig. 5.36 Compressed spectral array. This trace shows fitting followed by electrical silence in a patient with meningoencephalitis.

subsequent lower amplitude activity at the same frequency.

2. Both time and power are displayed vertically and therefore output requires a two-dimensional XY plotter. Another technique for displaying power spectrum of the e.e.g. uses density modulation which produces a grey scale display.

Power spectrum techniques can detect differences between the two hemispheres and monitor changes during cerebral sedation techniques. Such therapy may require reduction in e.e.g. activity to the level of burst suppression or reduction of activity in the c.f.m. to 5 μV.

The c.f.m. is the simplest, automated, e.e.g. processor for intra-operative use but is less sensitive than the multilead e.e.g. for detection of focal ischaemia. It can detect severe global cerebral ischaemia from hypoxia and hypotension, and to some extent indicates depth of anaesthesia. Gross anaesthetic overdose and severe global hypoperfusion are detectable. The c.f.m. has proved useful in predicting the outcome of severe coma; patients with activity greater than 10 μV have survived whereas all those with less than 3 μV died.

Evoked potentials

Electrical events occurring in the cortex after stimulation of the sense organs may be detected by an exploring electrode over primary receiving areas for that particular sense. Evoked potential recordings constitute a noninvasive, objective, and repeatable supplement to clinical examination. Uses include assessment of functional integrity of specific cortical areas and pathways within the central nervous system. Visual, auditory and somatosensory evoked potentials are used widely in diagnosis. In order to detect the low amplitudes involved, an electronic averaging technique must be used to exclude the larger amplitude background electrical noise, composed largely of e.e.g. activity, with some nonneuronal electrical activity. Some form of plotter is also required. The signal varies with body size, position of the applied stimulus, conduction velocity of axons, number of synapses, location of neural generators of the evoked potential (EP) component, (i.e. either cortex or brain stem) and the presence of pathology.

Evoked potential recording is not yet a clinical tool for routine use, but subclinical lesions in multiple sclerosis may be detected by the combined use of auditory, visual and somato-sensory EPs which show an abnormality in 80% of patients with a definite history of multiple sclerosis and in up to 50% of those without any sign of a brain stem lesion.

Clinical applications of evoked potentials

1. Multiple sclerosis. As demyelination increases, complete conduction block occurs at lower temperatures.

2. Other demyelinating diseases. In general, in demyelination, dissociation may occur of the EP peak latency and amplitude abnormalities. Latency prolongation with preservation of peak amplitude results from axon demyelination, but a reduction in peak amplitude occurs as more fibres die.

3. Intracranial tumours. EPs may be used in intraoperative monitoring of involvement of specific neural pathways. Auditory brain stem EPs have been used in the early diagnosis of posterior fossa tumours where there is an inverse relationship between operability and detectability for acoustic neuromas.

4. Head injury. Somatosensory EPs are sensitive to hypoxia and ischaemia. With a reduction in cerebral blood flow, there is a reduction in amplitude of somatosensory EPs, but the wave form is unchanged. Compressive lesions, e.g. subdural haematoma, increase the latency of the wave form. The number of wave peaks recognised in a finite period of time correlates well with outcome, but not with CAT scan findings (i.e. gives information on functional rather than anatomical lesions).

5. Disease of the spinal cord and brachial plexus.

Central conduction time (CCT)

This is the time delay between an action potential generated in brain stem structure and the first cortical potential recordable (normally less than 6.4 ms). Other times are also described, for example the dorsal column to cortex conduction time. Central conduction time is independent of body size and peripheral nerve conduction velocity and is probably independent also of body temperature and barbiturate levels. Changes result from cortical dysfunction, abnormal synaptic delay in the thalamus or cortex (or both) and slowed axonal conduction. At 10 and 35 days, CCT correlates well with outcome in head injury. Changes in brain electrical activity vary with cerebral blood flow, and CCT has been used as an index of reduction of cerebral blood flow in subarachnoid haemorrhage. It may be used also as a monitor of developing ischaemia in association with surgery for subarachnoid haemorrhage.

For prediction of outcome in severe head injury, multimodality EPs are more accurate than clinical neurological signs, or the Glasgow coma scale.

CEREBRAL CIRCULATION

The circle of Willis (Fig. 5.37) comprises an arterial circle at the base of the brain, supplied by the two internal carotid and two vertebral arteries. In man, there is almost no anastomosis between the internal

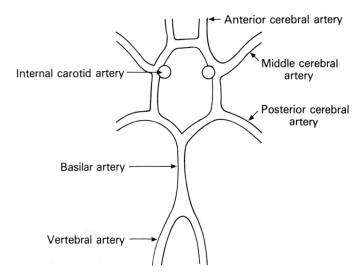

Fig. 5.37 The circle of Willis.

and external carotid arteries but stenosis of one supplying vessel to the circle of Willis may be accommodated by an anastomotic collateral flow from other supplies. The branches of these four arteries communicate with each other over the surface of the cortex. Watershed areas between areas of major vessel supply are those most likely to suffer in hypoxia and ischaemia. Venous drainage is into sinuses which also receive c.s.f. from arachnoid villi.

Cerebral blood flow

In dealing with the damaged brain, there are many circumstances in which it is important to obtain information on both global and regional blood flow. Autoregulation of cerebral blood flow and manipulation of intracranial pressure are discussed in Chapter 27, page 352. These two important aspects are therefore not considered further here.

Other clinical aspects of neurophysiology may be investigated quantitatively, e.g. Glasgow coma scale (see p. 362). The increasing sophistication of peripheral nerve stimulators now makes it possible to monitor nerve conduction during neuromuscular blockade and this technique is also discussed in a separate chapter (p. 173).

FURTHER READING

Bell G H, Emsley-Smith D M 1980 In: Patterson C R (ed) Textbook of physiology, 10th edn. Churchill Livingstone, Edinburgh
Greenburg R P, Ducker T P 1982 Evoked potentials in clinical neurosciences. Journal of Neurosurgery 56: 1
Hendry B 1981 Membrane physiology and cell excitation. Croom Helm, London
Larsson S J, Sauces A Jr, Ackman J J et al 1973 Noninvasive evaluation of head trauma patients. Surgery 74: 34

Levy W J, Shapiro H M, Maruchak G, Meathe E 1980 Automated e.e.g. processing for intraoperative monitoring. Anesthesiology 53: 223
Lipton, Sampson 1979 Current topics in anaesthesia series no 2, Control of chronic pain. Arnold, London
Marshall B E 1981 Clinical implications of membrane receptor function in anaesthesia. Anesthesiology 55: 160
McDowall G D 1976 Monitoring the brain. Anesthesiology 45: 117
Wardley-Smith B, Halsey M J 1979 Recent molecular theories of anaesthesia. British Journal of Anaesthesia 51: 619

6

Maternal and neonatal physiology

The physiology of pregnancy and the neonatal period involves a 10-month period during which two (or more) individuals, the mother and the fetus/neonate, undergo more dramatic changes in the 'milieu interieur' than at any other time in their respective lives. The adjustments in maternal homeostasis which accompany the development of the products of conception frequently precede the demands which they appear to supply. The rapid change in maternal organ size and function during pregnancy is surpassed by the even more rapid regression to nonpregnant norms after delivery. The neonate then exhibits an independent anabolic capacity unequalled in any later period.

PREGNANCY

The cardiovascular system

Clinical examination in normal pregnancy may reveal evidence of slightly increased heart size and increased flow with a loud first heart sound, reduced splitting of the second sound and an early or mid-diastolic murmur at the left sternal border. Changed position alters the e.c.g. axis; altered electrical complexes with more than the usual number of ectopic beats may be normal. Cardiac output, myocardial contractility, heart rate and stroke volume are increased; the increase in cardiac output (approx. 1.5 litre/min) commences in the first trimester, and is more marked in twin pregnancy. The arteriovenous oxygen content difference is reduced until the final month. When correlated with the reduced haemoglobin in pregnancy, the oxygen flux (see Chapter 2) is little altered from the nonpregnant state by these combined effects.

Through the combined effects of reduced peripheral vascular tone and the formation of new vascular beds, peripheral resistance is decreased during pregnancy particularly in the midtrimester, returning towards normal at term. The effect on arterial pressure is offset partly by the increase in cardiac ouput during pregnancy. Pre-eclampsia is associated with raised peripheral resistance, reduced cardiac output and relative hypovolaemia.

As pregnancy progresses, venous pressure is raised particularly in the lower limbs where oedema is seen in up to 40% of normotensive subjects. Central venous pressure may decrease dramatically in the supine position in late pregnancy predominantly from mechanical obstruction of venous return by the gravid uterus with inadequate collateral circulation through vertebral and splanchnic venous channels. The decrease in venous return reduces cardiac output and, if compensatory vasoconstrictor reflexes are obtunded, e.g. during general anaesthesia or a spinal nerve block, may cause severe hypotension.

There is no change in pulmonary arterial pressure during pregnancy though pulmonary blood flow, and thus pulmonary vascularity on chest X-ray, are increased corresponding to the increase in cardiac output. Where raised pulmonary vascular resistance pre-exists as in Eisenmenger's syndrome, pregnancy may lead to a rapid deterioration in the clinical state.

Although circulation time is not altered greatly in pregnancy, changes occur in regional distribution, with additional flow to uterus and placenta. The cardiovascular changes of pregnancy precede rather than follow formation of significant intervillous circulation. Renal blood flow rises to 400 ml/min above the nonpregnant level at the beginning of the second trimester and continues around this level until parturition. Increased skin blood flow results in subjective feelings of warmth and reduced heat tolerance due in part to increased peripheral blood flow and affected by posture and smoking. Capillary dilatation is demonstrable in pregnancy as is an increase in capillary numbers. Epistaxis and snoring in pregnancy coincide with nasal mucosal congestion and capillary dilatation. Breast engorgement and dilated veins on the breast surface may be part of the early signs of pregnancy. These multisystem changes may reflect partly the increasing functional demands and contributions of maternal and fetal metabolism at this time. Exercise tolerance is reduced largely as a result of increased body mass.

In addition to the overall tendency to vaso-dilatation, certain paradoxical responses are seen where vasoconstriction would be expected normally. The pressor response to angiotensin is less than normal. Blocking the autonomic system may result in a dramatic decrease in systemic arterial pressure during pregnancy suggesting a chronically active sympathetic tone.

Extradural nerve block is associated with increased venous capacity and decreased peripheral resistance in the lower limbs where pooling reduces venous return and effective circulating blood volume. Uterine contractions may mask the effective reduction in uterine perfusion by causing transient increases in systemic pressure as a result of iliac or aortic compression by the gravid uterus. In the hypertensive patient, uterine hypoperfusion may result from the combined reduced circulating blood volume of pre-eclampsia and hypotension associated with an extradural block. In heart disease, e.g. mitral stenosis, the use of extradural anaesthesia with resultant reduced venous return helps avoid pulmonary oedema, though cardiac output must be adequate to compensate for the effect of reduced peripheral resistance.

The respiratory system

Although some aspects of respiratory function have been inadequately studied in pregnancy because they necessitate invasive procedures or unrealistic demands on the pregnant woman, alterations in basic lung function throughout pregnancy have been well demonstrated.

In pregnancy inspiratory capacity gradually increases by approx. 300 ml while residual and expiratory reserve volumes decrease by some 200–300 ml. As a result of a 200 ml increase in tidal volume and unchanged respiratory rate, the minute ventilation increases from approx. 7.5 litre/min to 10.5 litre/min in late pregnancy with a 30–40 ml/min increase in oxygen consumption. The main stimulation to overbreathing in pregnancy is a change in central respiratory control but mechanical factors contribute. Forced expiratory volume remains at the normal 80–85% of vital capacity. Because of the greater reserve capacity of the respiratory than the cardiovascular system, significant functional deterioration of respiratory disease is less common in pregnancy.

Arterial carbon dioxide tension is reduced, the change being most marked in early pregnancy in advance of the CO_2 transfer needs of the fetus. Breathlessness is a common complaint in pregnancy and relates more to changes in Pa_{CO_2} than in respiratory function, being maximal up to 20 weeks gestation. The low maternal Pa_{CO_2} allows transfer of CO_2 from fetal to maternal blood for excretion while maintaining fetal P_{CO_2} at a tolerable level. Arterial pH is maintained at 7.4 by a reduced plasma bicarbonate and sodium.

The haematological system

The increased blood volume of pregnancy is seen from the first trimester and consists of increased red cell mass and, to a greater extent, plasma volume with consequent reduction in haemoglobin concentration despite a raised total haemoglobin content. The red cell concentration falls from around 4.2×10^{12}/litre to 3.7×10^{12}/litre in the third trimester. The lowest haemoglobin of approx. 1.5 g/dl below nonpregnant levels in those with adequate iron intake occurs at about 34 weeks gestation.

There is an increased demand for iron in pregnancy to meet the maternal increase in red cell volume and the requirements of the fetus and placenta. Some 700–1400 mg are required for this total demand. Blood loss at delivery of 200–500 ml is equivalent to 100–250 mg iron while subsequent breast feeding puts further demands on the mother's iron stores. The requirement for approx. 2.8 mg iron per day in early pregnancy increasing to 6.6 mg per day in excess of normal needs may be provided by maternal iron stores if the diet is adequate and absorption of dietary iron is maximal. However, in many countries iron supplementation is recommended for the pregnant woman. Iron absorption increases in pregnancy from the normal 5–10% to 40% by late pregnancy. The World Health Organisation recommends supplements of 30 to 60 mg iron per day to pregnant women with iron stores and 120 to 240 mg to women with no iron stores.

Folate requirements increase in pregnancy and the placenta transports folate actively to the fetus even when the mother is folate deficient. The first sign of folate deficiency is a low serum folate concentration, which precedes megaloblastic anaemia by months. With the difficulty in confirming folate deficiency by laboratory means, a poor haematological response to, or macrocytosis following, iron therapy should raise the suspicion of folate deficiency.

Increased folate intake should continue into the puerperium and signs of folate deficiency may appear first during breast feeding. A daily supplement of 300–500 mg of folate adequately covers the extra demands of pregnancy if the diet is suspect. Folate deficiency may be associated with abortion, fetal deformity, premature delivery and antepartum haemorrhage. The possible role of folate and vitamin deficiency at the time of conception in predisposing to neural tube defects in a susceptible group is now being investigated.

Vitamin B_{12} levels diminish during pregnancy especially in smokers, though maternal B_{12} stores are little affected. There is preferential transfer to the fetus. Deficiency of vitamin B_{12} is associated with subfertility or in-utero fetal death but inadequate B_{12} intake is rare in all but strict vegans who require supplementation at all times, including pregnancy.

The neutrophil count increases in pregnancy, related partly to oestrogenic stimulation, reaching a plateau by 30 weeks. The peripheral white cell count may increase dramatically, even during uncomplicated labour. The lymphocyte count is affected little but function appears suppressed, particularly with regard to cell-mediated immunity. Immunoglobulin and humoral immunity remain normal. These changes are thought to be crucial for the survival of the fetus although they result in decreased resistance to viral infection, to some bacteria and to malaria in susceptible populations. The platelet count shows a slight decrease in pregnancy.

Blood clotting and fibrinolysis alter during pregnancy when factors VII, VIII, X and fibrinogen are increased. The placenta plays a major role as a source of the specific lipoprotein thromboplastin whose action accelerates coagulation, bypassing the series of reactions involved in the contact system. Changes in coagulation factors are present from the third month. Low grade coagulation may be demonstrated in the intervillous spaces of the placenta and walls of the spiral arteries. At placental separation there is contraction of the myometrium and rapid closure of terminal spiral arteries, with a fibrin mesh covering the placental site.

Fibrinolysis in pregnancy is reduced until approx. 1 h after placental delivery, an inhibition thought to be mediated through the placenta while the increase in fibrin degradation products during labour may stem from the uterus. To accommodate the need for rapid coagulation following delivery, there is throughout pregnancy a state of hypercoagulability and a potential for thrombotic complications. Low-grade intravascular coagulation with altered clotting factor activity is reported in pre-eclampsia from 24 weeks. The coagulation changes, but not the cause of the pre-eclampsia, may be counteracted by use of low-dose heparin.

The alimentary system

Increased appetite and thirst are common in pregnancy, as are food cravings and aversions, highly flavoured foods being favoured as taste threshold rises. The gums often swell and soften under the influence of oestrogen.

Gastro-oesophageal reflux and its symptoms occur more frequently as gastro-oesophageal sphincter pressure decreases. Gastric secretion diminishes in the first and second trimesters, increasing towards term. Gastric motility is reduced in pregnancy, particularly in labour or when opioid analgesics have been administered.

Small intestinal function shows changes compatible with increasing demand for nutrients such as iron and calcium. Gut motility is reduced and, with the angiotensin/aldosterone-induced increase in water and sodium absorption from the large intestine, constipation is a common complaint.

Liver function has been studied extensively in animals but less so in humans. Temporary cholestatic jaundice occurs in some women with increased bile viscosity and canalicular dilation; the changes reverse after parturition. Liver blood flow and carbohydrate metabolism alter little in pregnancy. Serum bilirubin concentration is moderately raised in up to 15% of pregnant women leading to pruritus in some. The smooth muscle of the gall bladder becomes hypotonic and bile is discharged less efficiently than normal.

Nutrition in pregnancy must supply adequate protein, fat and carbohydrate for growth of the products of conception and of the uterus. The increased maternal energy needs are balanced partly by reduced activity. An estimate of total nutrients of fetus and mother amassed over pregnancy is 1 kg protein and 3.5–4 kg fat which, with ongoing metabolic activity approximates to an energy cost of 75–85 000 kcal. Energy is supplied by fat and carbohydrate, the latter mainly for the maternal brain and fetus with a small added requirement for structural material. Fat provides a fuel source apart from a small requirement for structural lipids and carrier substances. The new tissues laid down in the second half of pregnancy account for much of pregnancy's energy demands. Over the middle weeks maternal fat stores accumulate but in the final weeks before term the fetus, not the mother, stores fat. Overall some extra 250 kcal per day throughout pregnancy (or the equivalent in reduced energy expenditure) provide for increased demands. Calcium for the fetal skeleton includes approx. 30 g drawn from the maternal store. The general recommendation that an adequate mixed diet will provide all the necessary nutrients for pregnancy appears to hold true though iron and folate supplements are often advisable.

Plasma protein and albumin concentrations decrease in pregnancy; total lipid concentration, including phospholipids and nonesterified fatty acids rises. Amino acids show cyclical changes during the menstrual cycle with a decrease after menstruation. Only glutamic acid and alanine/valine increase in concentration over the course of pregnancy. In general, vitamins change in pregnancy according to their type; fat soluble vitamins increase with plasma fat concentrations while water-soluble vitamin concentrations decrease.

The needs for, and changes in, nutritional supplies during pregnancy cannot be estimated simply by measuring maternal plasma concentrations. There is a two-way exchange of metabolic products between mother and fetus and the homeostasis of pregnancy is only now being studied.

The renal system

Renal blood flow and glomerular filtration rates rise in pregnancy. Renal glucose handling is altered in pregnancy, reflecting the increased GFR, changes in plasma volume, sodium and potassium reabsorption and possibly the action of sex steroid hormones. Mild to moderate glycosuria is common in the normal healthy pregnant woman. In pregnant diabetics, diabetic control must be based on blood glucose measurement.

Renal handling of bicarbonate is altered little in pregnancy but there is a lower steady state plasma bicarbonate concentration and lower $P\text{CO}_2$, i.e. a reduced buffer pool. Potassium is conserved progressively throughout pregnancy in order to supply the cellular needs of the developing fetus and maternal tissues. There is a relative resistance to action of mineralocorticoids during pregnancy. The altered water balance results in a reduced plasma osmolality. A net accumulation of some 9–15 mmol sodium occurs in pregnancy and sodium homeostasis occurs about the newly determined pregnant norms. Because of the increased GFR, renal tubular reabsorption must increase in pregnancy, and there is increased aldosterone secretion.

Routine tests of renal function in pregnancy must be related to the pregnant norm. Serial creatinine clearances are useful and there are standards for urinary sediment findings in pregnancy. In the presence of renal disease, deteriorating renal function associated with hypertension is of grave significance.

The genital system

The corpus luteum of the ovary secretes progesterone which allows maintenance of early pregnancy prior to establishment of placental progesterone output, a function stimulated by human chorionic gonadotrophin (hCG) in association with luteinising hormone (LH).

The role of the uterus in pregnancy is to relax and contain the developing fetus and placenta with its associated tissues until the time of parturition when it must contract in a co-ordinated fashion to expel the uterine content. As pregnancy progresses mild myometrial hypertrophy and possibly some hyperplasia occur.

Uterine activity progresses from high frequency low amplitude inco-ordinate activity prior to 20 weeks, to lower frequency, higher amplitude contractions as term approaches. In the early months the uterus is insensitive to oxytocin. In contrast, prostaglandins E_2 and F_2 alpha cause uterine contraction throughout pregnancy. The cervix softens and dilates during pregnancy to the end-point of full effacement and dilatation at delivery. The timing of cervical changes shows marked interindividual variation.

The factors controlling the onset of labour in the human remain uncertain despite intensive investigation. Pregnancy may continue to term and labour occur in women who have had ovariectomy or hypophysectomy during pregnancy. Fetal brain plays a part in the precise control of length of gestation; anencephalic pregnancies are often prolonged. In the sheep, the fetal pituitary and adrenal have a central role in initiating labour, but evidence for a similar mechanism in man is not conclusive. The changes in prostaglandin levels during labour have suggested their possible role in its induction and maintenance.

During labour itself, prostaglandin secretion is likely to be crucial with fetal and maternal posterior pituitary hormones playing their part in the second stage of labour. Local reflexes such as the stimulation of oxytocin and prostaglandin secretion by cervical dilatation, natural or artificial, may be affected by extradural anaesthesia. Following parturition the uterus and cervix regress to near prepregnancy dimensions.

The endocrine system

Pituitary gland

The size of the pituitary gland increases in pregnancy with a dramatic increase in the number of prolactin-secreting cells and a decrease in growth hormone-secreting cells. The hormones of the pituitary show varying responses to pregnancy and lactation. Plasma prolactin concentrations increase progressively through pregnancy as its secretion responds to oestrogen stimulation. Its action leads to changes in the mammary gland, may influence fetal fluid and electrolyte balance, and may have a role in maintaining calcium balance. After parturition the level of prolactin declines but remains above nonpregnant levels while it acts to maintain lactation and prevent ovulation and conception during breastfeeding.

Growth hormone levels diminish during pregnancy and response to stimulation is reduced. ACTH, cortisol and metabolically inactive cortisone levels are higher in pregnancy than normal, possibly indicating a metabolic contribution from the placenta and fetus; the fetus may depend upon cortisol for lung maturation. Concentrations of thyrotrophin are altered little by pregnancy though its effects may be mimicked weakly by hCG.

Antidiuretic hormone is not known to play a specific role as normal pregnancy can occur in the presence of diabetes insipidus. Conversely pituitary tumour expansion during pregnancy may lead to diabetes insipidus which is usually temporary. Oxytocin is secreted during labour and exogenous oxytocin, particularly if administered intermittently, augments labour. During lactation oxytocin is released during suckling, causing myometrial cell contraction and milk ejection, actions independent of vasopressin secretion.

Thyroid gland

Thyroxine and tri-iodothyronine have a primary role in cellular metabolism. Their secretion is controlled by thyroid stimulating hormone synthesised in the anterior pituitary in response to hypothalamic thyrotrophin releasing hormone which is secreted in the presence of low thyroid hormone levels. Where iodine intake is borderline, the increased demand of pregnancy may stimulate compensatory follicular hyperplasia and goitre.

Thyroxine binding globulin (TBG) is raised in pregnancy associated with increased T_4 and, in the last trimester, T_3. However, the free thyroxine index gives a result within or at the upper end of the normal range.

Clinical features of hyperthyroidism may occur in normal pregnancy as heat intolerance, tachycardia, emotional lability and goitre. However, when these features are combined with poor weight gain or lid lag they should raise the suspicion of hyperthyroidism, which, if untreated, carries a significant risk of perinatal mortality. Known autoimmune hyperthyroidism may remit in pregnancy with its relative immune suppression but is then likely to be exacerbated postpartum. If Graves' disease is associated with raised long-acting thyroid stimulator (LATS) neonatal hyperthyroidism is likely and raised fetal heart rate may be recorded. Mild hypothyroidism is commoner than hyperthyroidism during pregnancy. Its diagnosis is important, carrying a risk, if untreated, of stillbirth or reduced infant IQ at follow-up.

The placenta

The placenta forms a physical barrier between maternal and fetal tissues but contributes actively to the maintenance of pregnancy in both. The human placenta is of the syncytiotrophoblastic type, separating maternal and fetal tissue with a single cell matrix. Renin is secreted by the placenta and may have a role in regulating placental blood flow. Fibrin deposition on the placental villi is a common finding and may act in the immunological processes of pregnancy. The immune system is active in both mother and fetus yet is modified in such a way as to allow the fetus to develop within the mother without the expected stimulation of host rejection. The mechanism by which this occurs over nine months with subsequent return to normal immune responsiveness in both organisms is understood poorly. The mother may modify the antigenic activity of the fetus as the fetus may influence permanently the maternal response to its antigens.

The respiratory function of the placenta must ensure adequate oxygen transfer to the fetus and extraction for its own needs. Placental blood flow and the characteristics of adult and fetal blood allow these functions to be fulfilled. Because 2, 3-diphosphoglycerate is less bound to fetal than adult haemoglobin there is less competition for oxygen binding sites. Fetal blood takes up oxygen more avidly than adult while maternal blood has reduced oxygen affinity. On reaching the tissue the steep oxygen dissociation curve allows release of oxygen for a relatively small decrease in P_{O_2}.

Carbon dioxide diffuses readily from fetus to mother down the concentration gradient provided by the mother's hyperventilation. The placenta allows free diffusion of CO_2 from the fetus but buffers him from the effects of maternal acidosis. Carbon monoxide diffuses across the placenta and is taken up avidly by fetal haemoglobin causing reduced oxygen-carrying capacity and supply to the fetus; this is of importance when mother smokes heavily in pregnancy.

Water diffuses freely among maternal and fetal tissues but net transfer is approx. 20–25 ml/day from mother to fetus. Any overhydration or dehydration of the mother affects the fetus in a similar way. Clinically this has occurred when women, given low sodium fluids plus oxytocin in labour, develop an antidiuresis with fetal and maternal hypo-osmolality and hyponatraemia leading to convulsions or death. Sodium and potassium exchange far in excess of the 6–7 g incorporated by the term fetus occurs during pregnancy.

The fetus is supplied with some 25–30 g glucose per day. The transfer is by facilitated diffusion stereospecific for D-glucose and there is a close correlation between maternal and fetal glucose levels. The placenta itself utilises glucose for glycolytic and hexose monophosphate pathways. A small glycogen store occurs in the placenta, but its availability and purpose are uncertain.

Amino acids are transferred actively from mother to fetus with the highest amino acid levels in the placenta. Relative concentrations vary and some amino acids, e.g. glutamic acid, may play a carrier role. Only immunoglobulins are transferred as proteins to the fetus; these are mainly IgG, but include abnormal antibodies such as those against platelets, leucocytes, red cells and long-acting thyroid stimulator (LATS).

Free fatty acids cross the placenta freely, the fetus synthesising lipids actively. Most lipids reflect maternal plasma levels but the concentration of arachidonic acid is higher in fetal plasma, possibly due to placental action on linoleic acid. Cholesterol transfers only slowly, most being synthesised by the fetoplacental unit.

Vitamins transfer by several methods, e.g. vitamin C crosses the placenta as dihydroascorbic acid and is converted to ascorbic acid which cannot recross the placenta. Folic acid occurs in different major forms in mother, placenta and fetus. Other water-soluble vitamins are thought to be transferred to the fetus in similar fashion.

Iron is transferred actively to the fetus with preferential placental uptake in situations of iron deficiency. Calcium, iodine and chromium are transported actively to the fetus emphasising the danger of radio-iodine studies in pregnancy. Most toxic metals reach the fetus poorly but mercury and, to a lesser degree, lead may be transferred freely.

Viruses may cross to the fetus, especially cytomegalovirus (CMV), rubella, herpes simplex, varicella, variola, hepatitis B, enteroviruses, Echo, polio and sometimes HBSAg (large particles of surface antigen). Listeria, treponema, Group B streptococci, toxoplasma and, in some countries, malaria parasites are the most common bacterial pathogens to infect the fetus. The gestational age at which the fetus is exposed to teratogenic infection determines the extent to which he is likely to be affected. Viruses such as rubella and CMV which can disrupt development have their most profound effect in the first trimester while varicella is of greatest danger when it infects the late third trimester fetus.

The placenta forms part of the fetoplacental unit and neither fetus nor placenta is complete as an endocrine organ. Placental steroids form part of a two-way traffic between mother and fetus, while its protein hormones appear to affect the mother while responding to fetal needs. Human chorionic gonadotrophin (hCG), placental lactogen (hPL) and pregnancy-associated plasma proteins are described. Its early appearance allows detection of hCG to be used as a test for pregnancy; its role appears to be to stimulate ovarian and possibly placental steroidgenesis.

Progesterone is the major progestogen in pregnancy. Progesterone has an overall catabolic nitrogen-losing effect on maternal metabolism. Although progesterone levels in the fetus are higher than those in the mother its fetal role is unclear.

THE NEONATE

The cardiovascular system

Fetal blood is oxygenated via the placenta from which venous blood flows through the umbilical vein with a Po_2 of 4 kPa. About half of this flow bypasses the hepatic capillary system via the ductus venosus to the i.v.c. and thence to the right (40%) and left (60%) atria, the latter by the streaming effect of the crista dividens and foramen ovale. Right atrial blood mixes with blood returning via the s.v.c. from the head and neck and with coronary sinus blood. At least 97% of s.v.c. blood enters the right ventricle and pulmonary artery while the left atrium and left ventricle receive better oxygenated umbilical vein blood and eject it to the ascending aorta, carotid and cerebral circulations, head, neck and upper limbs. The less oxygenated right ventricular output supplies the lungs (10%) and, via the ductus arteriosus, the descending aorta. The high pulmonary vascular resistance, widely patent ductus arteriosus and low pressure placenta allow approximately half of total cardiac output to return to the placenta for oxygenation. Redistribution of blood flow in the fetus may occur in response to changes in demand.

During the early weeks of postnatal life there is a gradual readjustment of blood flow through the cardiac chambers and major vessels as supply matches the new demands. Initially the ventricles are of equal thickness, the pulmonary arteries are relatively small and the ductus arteriosus may be widely open or a large ductal diverticulum may be present. Cardiac output is relatively high in the neonate. The systolic arterial pressure of the term neonate is 70–90 mmHg. The normal preterm infant's arterial pressure is slightly lower.

Pulmonary vascular resistance is high in the fetus as a result of the low Po_2 in utero. The pulmonary vessels constrict in response to hypoxia, low pH and hypercapnia, dilating after birth when the Po_2 and pH rise and Pco_2 falls. Pulmonary expansion also adds to the effect of pulmonary vasodilatation. Pulmonary arterial pressure decreases dramatically over the first three days then more slowly to reach adult levels by two weeks as thinning of the medial layer of the pulmonary vessels follows the early release of vasoconstrictor tone. Problems arise if pulmonary vascular resistance (PVR) remains high after birth, a situation which may accompany the hypoxia of lung disease or central hypoventilation or as a primary disorder (persistent pulmonary hypertension). A left to right shunt defect may lead to cardiac failure in the preterm infant in the early neonatal period, but after full term delivery the risk is greatest after the first month when PVR has fallen.

Autonomic responsiveness of the cardiovascular

system may be demonstrated from an early stage of fetal development though the balance of parasympathetic and sympathetic tone may change at different gestational ages. There may thus be unpredictable effects on the fetal heart rate of any autonomic stimulants or suppressors which cross the placenta after administration to the mother, e.g. to suppress labour or treat hypertension.

By full term, normal reflex control is present and significant baroreceptor function seems to be present in the premature infant. The specialised conducting tissues of the heart are present from early in the first trimester of pregnancy. By the time of delivery, the entire conducting system is fully formed.

The electrocardiogram differs markedly in the neonatal period from later infancy and childhood. Recording of V_4R is essential to allow interpretation of the childhood e.c.g. The QRS axis is normally right-sided at birth approaching the adult left-sided pattern from the end of the neonatal period onwards. The T-wave changes rapidly after birth from upright to isoelectric or inverted in left chest leads while right chest leads show positive waves for the first 2–3 days. The changes in e.c.g. complexes in the neonatal period are not fully explained by known anatomical changes, for dramatic haemodynamic changes occur mainly in the first two days.

The respiratory system

The fetus thrives at a PO_2 of 4 kPa, PCO_2 6.5–7 kPa and pH 7.2. Irregular fetal breathing movements may be detected from the second trimester, becoming more vigorous and occupying longer periods as pregnancy advances. These movements appear to coincide with r.e.m. sleep; their significance is unknown but they are associated with movement of liquor and may influence lung development. They are affected by maternal smoking and may give some indication of fetal well-being.

At birth the neonate must establish spontaneous pulmonary ventilation within seconds to maintain oxygenation. The stimuli to breathing appear to be sensory, involving touch, proprioception and the effects of cord occlusion. The mechanism of readjustment of respiratory control which resets the sensors to maintain more 'adult' blood gas values first involves changes in carotid chemoreceptor activity.

The importance of pulmonary surfactant in the establishment of normal respiration in the neonate is now accepted. The surface tension lowering effect of surfactant reduces the work needed to re-expand the lung with inspiration. Levels of surfactant are low in the idiopathic respiratory distress syndrome (IRDS) and may also diminish after prolonged exposure to pure oxygen, or after such stresses as hypothermia and infection.

The stimulus to synthesis of surfactant is not known but its production by the fetus can be deduced from the study of amniotic fluid lipids. Attempts to hasten surfactant production by use of exogenous steroids given to the mother have not been consistently successful though they may be effective in some cases. Use of continuous positive airway pressure to mimic the 'splinting' effect of surfactant may improve ventilatory function in IRDS while recent trials have aimed to correct the respiratory abnormality by administration of artificial surfactant into the airway.

If the infant fails to establish spontaneous respiration at birth, the sequence of events leads from primary apnoea through gasping irregular respiration to the 'last gasp' followed by secondary or terminal apnoea, when the heart continues to beat but spontaneous respiration will occur only after effective resuscitative intervention. Neonatal asphyxia may follow intrauterine or intrapartum hypoxia, exposure to maternal opioids, acute blood loss, trauma, particularly intracranial injury or massive aspiration. Hypoxia stimulates ventilation transiently in the neonate; in infants under two weeks hypoxia results in respiratory depression. The neonate withstands hypoxia for longer than the adult but prompt intervention with IPPV, external cardiac massage and restoration of blood volume where indicated are required. Heat loss, particularly from wet exposed skin, acidosis and hypoglycaemia, may exacerbate the neurological effects of asphyxia and should be corrected.

The gas exchanging capacity of the lungs in utero is unknown but is likely to be small. Major gas exchange occurs via the placenta. The first breath requires a large negative intrathoracic pressure of -40 to -100 cmH$_2$O with a volume of 30–40 ml. Thereafter compliance of the lungs increases and much smaller pressures are required. The tidal volume of a 3 kg infant is approx. 19 ml, his minute ventilation 530 ml/min and respiration rate 28/min.

Total pulmonary resistance including airway and nasal resistance is approx. 27.4 cmH$_2$O/litre/s of which almost 50% results from nasal resistance, emphasising the importance of any nasal obstruction in the obligatory nose-breathing neonate. Lung tissue resistance is approx. 30% of total resistance.

Oxygen consumption in the neonate is approx. 7 ml/min/kg in a thermoneutral environment. CO$_2$ output is proportional to O$_2$ consumption, and depends on the respiratory quotient, which is low initially as brown fat is metabolised (0.7 day 1–0.8 day 7).

Ventilation perfusion $(\dot{V}/\dot{Q})$ mismatching in the neonate results from perfusion of poorly ventilated lung (dead space) assessed as 35% of each breath, and from poor perfusion of ventilated areas (venous admixture) or right to left shunting which decreases in the normal from 24% at birth to 10% by the end of the first week. This shunt is increased when fetal channels including the foramen ovale or ductus arteriosus are open, a situation which is likely in hypoxia. The neonatal Pa_{O_2} is approx. 10 kPa by 5 h, Pa_{CO_2} is normal by 20 min and pH by 24 h. Over the first two days, Pa_{CO_2} continues to decrease to approx. 4.5 kPa then returns to normal, reflecting the respiratory compensation of the initial metabolic acidosis accompanying the elevated lactate levels at birth. The normal neonate has a slightly lower Pa_{O_2} than the adult but his haemoglobin is 97% saturated by day 2 as he has 60–70% HbF; this is replaced gradually with HbA over the first 3 months.

The haematological system

The full term infant has a red cell count of 4.6–5.3 $\times$ 10^{12}/litre and a haemoglobin of 13.7–20.2 g/dl, varying greatly with the extent of placental transfusion which may be up to one-third the neonatal blood volume. Over the second month marrow activity, though present, is much reduced and is outstripped by the growing neonate's blood volume, resulting in a fall in haemoglobin to approx. 11 g/dl by the ninth week; the fall in haematocrit is even greater because MCV decreases simultaneously, attaining the adult range by age 1 yr. Supplementary haematinics do not prevent this 'physiological anaemia' but the preterm infant, who has foregone the normal accumulation of iron stores in the third trimester, may require supplementary iron in addition to vitamins, folic acid and in some cases vitamin E.

Various red cell antigens develop during fetal life, their perinatal importance being their potential for crossing the placenta and inducing an immune reaction in the mother. If the maternal antibody so formed is of the IgG class and in sufficient quantity it may cross to the fetus and induce significant haemolysis with the risks of hyperbilirubinaemia and anaemia before or after birth. This occurs with the Rhesus Rh(D) antigen formed early in fetal life, other Rhesus antibodies being rare. In the 10% of Rhesus negative pregnancies where a mother carries a Rhesus positive infant there is a 1 in 15–20 chance of that infant suffering haemolytic disease of the newborn. Sensitisation has usually occurred during an earlier pregnancy (recognised or not) or following transfusion of Rhesus positive blood.

The administration of anti-D immunoglobulin to the Rhesus negative mother following first exposure to Rhesus antigen (i.e. after delivery of a first D-positive infant or termination of a D-positive pregnancy) removes the circulating antigen and prevents or reduces the stimulation of the immune response, minimising the risk for the next Rhesus positive fetus.

The ABO system antigens develop early but remain relatively ineffective as immune stimulants until after birth so that the risk of haemolytic disease of the newborn from ABO incompatibility is much less than that from rhesus disease. In addition, much of the anti-A and anti-B antibody is IgM and therefore does not cross the placenta. The IgG form does cross and may cause neonatal haemolysis with early jaundice and subsequent anaemia. The other blood group antigens develop at different times and with varying antigenicity. The Kell antibody is a rare but well recognised cause of haemolytic disease.

At term, HbF constitutes some 80–90% of the total haemoglobin though γ-chain synthesis is already on the decline. This proportion falls rapidly during the first four months to approx. 10–15% as HbF-containing red cells leave the circulation. Adult β-chain HbA concentration rises as HbF falls, eventually constituting more than 90% of the total. Clinically the thalassaemias are of importance in this period firstly as regards prenatal diagnosis (now reliably available by study of trophoblast aspirates during early pregnancy) and secondly, as the lethal homozygous γ- thalassaemia resulting in Hb_{Barts} (γ_4) which presents as a stillborn or grossly hydropic preterm infant.

By term the normal granulocyte count is approx. 8×10^9/litre with a wide range of normal (6–26). Lymphocytes appear in the blood at the tenth week increasing to approx. 4.0×10^9/litre by term (range 2–11). Although chemotaxis of granulo- and monocytes is less efficient in the healthy neonate, phagocytosis and killing are normal. Humoral factors (e.g. complement) are reduced especially in the preterm infant, while the stress of illness reduces granulocyte bactericidal activity.

The alimentary system

The functions of the gut include swallowing, digestion, absorption and onward propulsion of ingested nutrients. Swallowing occurs first at approx. the twelfth fetal week, increasing in frequency until, by the twenty-third week approx. 5 ml/kg/h of amniotic fluid is swallowed. The co-ordination of swallowing involves tongue, palatal and pharyngeal muscles with the reflex response then allowing laryngeal elevation and glottic closure.

The oesophagus provides a transit route for swallowed material; absorption does not occur there though salivary amylase is already initiating digestion of starch. The gastro-oesophageal sphincter is variable in action in the neonate and may permit gastro-oesophageal reflux.

While gastric mixing involves all areas of the stomach, onward propulsion requires co-ordination of antral, pyloric, duodenal and thence intestinal activity. Rates of gastric emptying show marked individual variation in the newborn and may be slowed by any coexisting systemic illness, effects of some maternal drugs and extreme prematurity.

In common with the adult, the neonate absorbs fat as chylomicra after its digestion by pancreatic lipase, action of bile salts, hydrolysis and re-esterification. Although deranged exocrine pancreatic function affects fat absorption, this is rarely a significant problem in the neonate. Bile salt abnormalities may affect fat absorption with associated malabsorption of the fat soluble vitamins A, D, E and K; these must therefore be supplemented parenterally if fat absorption is reduced. In the neonate, vitamin K deficiency may present as haemorrhagic disease of the newborn with spontaneous bleeding, usually into the gut, the renal tract or the central nervous system. This disorder occurs in wholly breast-fed infants since breast milk contains very much less vitamin K than the artificial formula feeds. A single dose of vitamin K given enterally or parenterally after birth prevents this potentially serious problem.

Water and electrolyte absorption is one of the major roles of the large intestine. Osmotic gradients play an important role in facilitatory reabsorption of water and electrolytes and severe diarrhoea can result in the neonate from inappropriate use of hyperosmolar feeds. Colonic fluid absorption is associated with a prostaglandin-mediated mechanism.

Passage of meconium normally occurs within the first 24 h in the term infant. Delayed passage beyond 48 h or associated with abdominal distension raises the suspicion of Hirschsprung's disease. Meconium is an alkaline mixture of swallowed debris, desquamated cells and bile. Meconium staining of the amniotic fluid indicates fetal distress and an infant born from such an intrauterine environment risks meconium aspiration. Rigorous aspiration of the oro- and nasopharynx before the first breath with direct aspiration of the trachea if necessary minimises the risk of the potentially life-threatening meconium aspiration syndrome. This syndrome results from mechanical obstruction of airways and chemical pneumonitis and may lead to respiratory distress, hypoxia, risk of pneumothorax and the need for prolonged IPPV.

Neonatal jaundice

Jaundice is common in the neonatal period. Up to half of all neonates become noticeably icteric. Pathological processes may explain the development of jaundice by excess haemoglobin breakdown, e.g. Rhesus disease, ABO incompatibility, red cell fragility in hereditary spherocytosis, red cell enzyme defects in glucose-6-phosphate dehydrogenase and pyruvate kinase deficiencies, systemic infection, polycythaemia following a large placental transfusion or resorption of extravasated blood caused by bruising at delivery. Much less commonly, metabolic or hepatic defects may give rise to jaundice. However, in the majority of neonates no specific cause for jaundice is identified and the label 'physiological jaundice' may be applied. This jaundice is thought to result from a combination of reduced red cell lifespan, increased haem breakdown and limited hepatic enzyme capacity for conjugation. The hyper-bilirubinaemia is thus unconjugated, appears after the first 2 days, rises to a peak around day 4–5, then decreases over a similar period as the liver enzymes increase in activity.

The most significant risk of unconjugated hyperbilirubinaemia is deposition of bilirubin in the cells of the basal ganglia, midbrain and brain stem leading to kernicterus with later deafness, low IQ and dyskinetic cerebral palsy. There is no absolute level of bilirubin at which this occurs but levels of unconjugated bilirubin much above 350 μmol/litre in a well, full-term infant are avoided by use of exchange transfusion or phototherapy; the latter induces photodegradation of bilirubin in the skin to water-soluble products excreted in the urine. The risks of hyperbilirubinaemia are increased by coexisting hypothermia, hypoglycaemia, acidosis, dehydration and prematurity.

Drugs in the neonate may affect jaundice by displacing bilirubin from albumin, e.g. sulpho-namides, by increasing red cell breakdown in the G-6-PD deficient subject or by affecting hepatic enzyme activity, e.g. phenobarbitone. The handling of drugs by the neonate may be very different from the adult and may change rapidly as enzyme activity alters. As in pregnancy the risks may outweigh potential benefits in many cases. Exposure of the fetus to drugs in early pregnancy may interfere with normal growth and differentiation, e.g. thalidomide, phenytoin, warfarin. Use of drugs in late pregnancy may produce postpartum effects, e.g. sedation by opioid analgesics, profound hypotonia, hypotension and hypoglycaemia by benzodiazepines whose half-life is several days in the neonate.

The renal system

Renal function in utero differs from that after birth in that the placenta regulates water and electrolyte transport until parturition. The fetal kidneys regulate production of amniotic fluid by producing large volumes of urine with a relatively low sodium concentration. Intra-uterine renal blood flow is low relative to postnatal rates due to higher renal vascular resistance.

At birth the neonate continues to show a high urine flow rate with little sodium reabsorption over the early hours, rising after the first week. Neonatal plasma osmolarity is influenced profoundly by osmolarity of the mother's plasma and later by administered enteral and parenteral fluids. Renal bicarbonate handling shows a pattern of maturation reflecting changes in the neonatal capacity for handling sodium. Urine pH may therefore remain inappropriately high in the presence of acidaemia.

The endocrine system

Pituitary gland and the adrenal glands

The adrenal cortex in the fetus functions as part of the so-called fetoplacental unit. Placental pregnenolone offers the fetal adrenal zone its required precursor for cortisol and corticosterone synthesis. As term approaches, the adult zone expands with the necessary 3-β-hydroxy-dehydrogenase for independent conversion of pregnenolone to progesterone.

The fetal pituitary is sensitive to feedback inhibition by excess maternal corticosteroids administered at high dose therapeutically or resulting from excessive maternal synthesis in Cushing's syndrome. Following delivery such infants are at risk of hypoadrenalism. Normally fetal pituitary ACTH stimulates the fetal and adult areas of the adrenal from the end of the first trimester. Growth hormone is secreted by the neonatal pituitary gland but at this stage it appears to affect insulin action and glucose metabolism rather than acting as a primary determinant of somatic growth.

Thyroid gland

Neonatal thyroxine concentration is very nearly equal to maternal levels with a rapid increase in thyroid activity associated with TSH secretion over the first 2 days, then a fall by 5 days. TSH levels are higher in cord than maternal blood, peak at 15–30 min after birth then fall to childhood levels by 2 to 3 days. This peak may be influenced by body and environmental temperature changes at delivery.

The thyroid hormones affect total energy expenditure, primary physiological functions including cardiac output, heart rate, glomerular filtration rate, renal plasma flow and water secretion, and c.n.s. function. The hypothyroid neonate may be diagnosed clinically at birth or in the early weeks, or may be identified by high TSH levels on neonatal screening with no signs or symptoms, presumably with some residual thyroid responding to increased TSH stimulation. An ectopic or lingual thyroid may produce this biochemical picture. Early detection and treatment improves prognosis for development and growth.

Neonatal hyperthyroidism is rare but may occur in an infant whose mother has been hyperthyroid due to LATS action. The infant may be irritable, jaundiced with hepatosplenomegaly, thrombocytopenia, exomphalos, goitre and congestive cardiac failure. Signs may appear only after some days or weeks and, although treatment may be required to control symptoms, the disorder is self-limiting.

The endocrine pancreas

The normal term infant has a normal insulin response to ingested carbohydrate from birth. The blood glucose levels of neonates are often found to be lower than those of adults without causing apparent symptoms of hypoglycaemia, particularly in preterm infants. Treatment of hypoglycaemia is indicated if symptoms are present or if it is persistent despite feeding.

Pancreatic hypersecretion of glucagon and insulin with hypoglycaemia may occur in neonates with erythroblastosis fetalis particularly if preterm. There are marked changes in glucagon levels though the details of these interactions are not yet fully understood. Infants of poorly-controlled diabetics may likewise risk neonatal hypoglycaemia.

Parathyroid glands and calcitonin producing cells in the thyroid

The fetus maintains higher serum concentrations of calcium and phosphorus than the mother as a result of an active placental transport system. Abnormalities of maternal calcium homeostasis may affect the fetus secondarily. Maternal parathyroid hormone does not cross the placenta to the fetus. The hypercalcaemic fetal norm is associated with high phosphate levels and high renal tubular reabsorption of phosphorus, suggesting chronic parathyroid inhibition or calcitonin activation.

FURTHER READING

Comline R S, Cross K W, Dawes G S, Nathanielsz P W 1975 Fetal and neonatal physiology. Proceedings of the Sir Joseph Barcroft Centenary Symposium. Cambridge University Press, Cambridge

Davis J A, Dobbing J 1981 Scientific foundations of paediatrics, 2nd edn. William Heinemann, London

Godfrey S, Baum J D 1979 Clinical paediatric physiology. Blackwell Scientific Publications, Oxford

Hytten F E, Chamberlain G 1980 Clinical physiology in obstetrics. Blackwell Scientific Publications, Oxford

Hytten F E, Leitch I 1971 The physiology of human pregnancy, 2nd edn. Blackwell Scientific Publications, Oxford

MacDonald R (ed) 1978 Scientific basis of obstetrics and gynaecology, 2nd edn. Churchill Livingstone, Edinburgh

Mirkin B L 1975 Perinatal pharmacology: placental transfer, fetal localisation and neonatal distribution of drugs. Anesthesiology 43: 156

Shearman R P (ed) 1979 Human reproductive physiology. Blackwell Scientific Publications, Oxford

Smith C A, Nelson N M (eds) 1976 The physiology of the newborn infant. Charles C Thomas, Springfield, Illinois

Stern L 1972 Drug interaction, part II: drugs, the newborn infant and the binding of bilirubin to albumin Paediatrics 47: 916

7

Principles of general pharmacology and pharmacokinetics

Pharmacokinetics comprises the study and characterisation of the time course of drug absorption, distribution, metabolism and excretion in addition to the relationship of these processes to the time course of desirable and toxic effects of drugs. Pharmacodynamics comprises the study of the pharmacological effects of a drug determined by its action on specific receptors and the concentration of the drug at the receptor site. In simple terms this reduces to:

pharmacokinetics — what the body does to a drug
pharmacodynamics — what the drug does to the body (Fig. 7.1).

Recently, very sensitive, accurate and reproducible methods have become available for measuring drug concentrations in plasma. This has produced a remarkable increase in the number of pharmacokinetic studies. Many of these articles provide no data concerning the relationship between kinetic measurements and the pharmacological effects of the drug. Pharmacokinetics is a technique and not an end in itself. Clinical pharmacology is concerned with the biological effects of a drug. Thus in the selection of a drug for use, pharmacokinetics is of importance in selection only if two or more drugs are available with very similar effects and toxicity.

However, pharmacokinetics generally and the study of drug absorption, distribution, metabolism and excretion have a great contribution to make in anaesthesia and clinical pharmacology.

PHARMACODYNAMICS — BASIC CONCEPTS OF DRUG ACTION

Drugs may exert their effect in one of three ways:

1. *Action dependent on chemical or physicochemical properties.* Some drugs act by combining with a small molecule or ion (e.g. neutralisation of gastric acid by antacids or chelation of ferrous ion by desferrioxamine). Local anaesthetics and inhalation anaes-

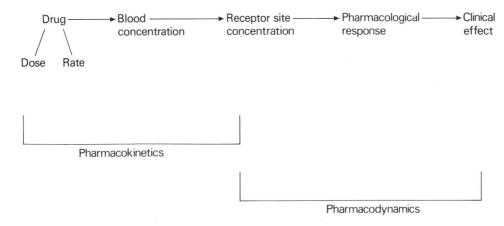

Fig. 7.1 Factors concerned in drug responses.

thetics may produce nonspecific changes in the lipid or protein components of nerve membranes and thus change the diameter of the pores that are concerned with ion transport and nerve conduction (see Chapter 5).

2. Enzyme inhibition. Many drugs act by inhibiting naturally occurring enzymes. They are often related chemically to natural substrates and may be metabolised by the enzyme system. Examples include allopurinol which inhibits xanthine oxidase and sulphanilamide which inhibits folate synthetase. Reversible enzyme inhibitors compete with natural substrates for enzymes and their action does not depend on the formation of stable chemical bonds. Their effects are usually of short duration. Edrophonium, neostigmine and pyridostigmine inhibit cholinesterase by formation of a covalent chemical bond resulting in carbamylation of the enzyme. The covalent bond is hydrolysed slowly and the enzyme is regenerated slowly.

Enzyme inhibition may be irreversible as a result of the formation of a stable chemical bond between enzyme and its inhibitor. Subsequent recovery from enzyme inhibition depends upon regeneration of the enzyme (e.g. monoamine oxidase inhibitors, organophosphorus insecticides). These drugs have a very long duration of action and may produce effects lasting for weeks.

3. Receptors. In most instances, drug action is produced by a physicochemical interaction between the drug and macromolecular components of tissues (receptors). These receptor sites are not readily identifiable physical entities but usually are related closely to tissue cells which mediate the effects. Normally they are areas of cell membranes. In some instances, 'second messengers' (e.g. cyclic AMP or calcium ions) may be released as a result of drug receptor interaction and mediate the response to the drug.

Receptors are very sensitive to low concentrations of drug and the magnitude of the response depends on the concentration of the free drug at the receptor site which in turn depends on the dose and the continuing processes of drug absorption, distribution and elimination. Other normal characteristics of drug-receptor interactions include saturability, reversibility and specificity. The L-form of a stereo-isomer may be pharmacologically active while the D-form is inactive (e.g. narcotic analgesics).

Relationship between drug dose and response

A drug response results from the reversible combination between drug and receptor, the magnitude of the response depending on the amount of drug-receptor complex formed. A drug which 'fits' the receptor well binds strongly and thus has a high *affinity* for the receptor. Pharmacological effect is usually related to drug dosage or concentration by a dose-response curve (Fig. 7.2). The shape of this curve reflects the extent of occupancy of receptor sites by the drug. The maximal response should correspond to occupancy of all receptor sites. However, if 'second messengers' are involved, they may be the limiting factor in the production of the maximal response. The relative affinity of a drug for a receptor may be defined as the concentration required to produce half the maximal response. In some instances, the magnitude of the pharmacological response may not be related predictably to the proportion of receptors occupied by the drug. Very potent drugs may produce a maximal response when

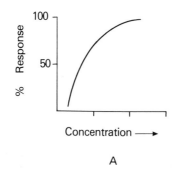

A

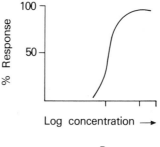

B

Fig. 7.2   The relationship between drug concentration and response. In A, the concentration is plotted on a linear scale and the shape is hyperbolic. In B, the concentration is plotted on a logarithmic scale and the shape is sigmoid.

occupying a small proportion of the total population of receptors. The presence of these 'spare receptors' ensures that adequate pharmacological effects may be produced by relatively low concentrations of drugs or transmitters. Spare receptors probably occur at the neuromuscular junction (e.g. only 25% of the receptor population is required to produce a maximum twitch response). Thus competitive antagonists, e.g. D-tubocurarine, may require to occupy a significant number of receptors before any effect is obvious on neuromuscular transmission.

In addition to the affinity of the drug for the receptor, the *intrinsic activity* of the drug is important. This may be defined as a measure of the maximal response that the drug can produce when given in very high concentrations. Thus, two similarly acting drugs with similar affinity for the receptor site but with different intrinsic activities require a different extent of receptor occupation to produce the same response. The drug with high intrinsic activity requires less receptor occupancy and thus a lower dose (Fig. 7.3).

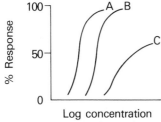

Fig. 7.3   Log concentration - response curves. A — agonist with high affinity for receptor. B — agonist with lower affinity than A but still achieving 100% response. C — partial agonist. The drug does not achieve a maximal response.

Agonists, partial agonists and antagonists

A drug with high affinity and high intrinsic activity is termed an *agonist*. An agent with high affinity but no intrinsic activity is an *antagonist* since it prevents a drug that does have activity from interacting with the receptor site. *Partial agonists* are drugs which cannot produce a maximal response in spite of very high concentrations. Morphine, naloxone and buprenorphine are examples of agonist, antagonist and partial agonist respectively.

Antagonists are competitive if they combine *reversibly* with the same receptor as the agonist. Because of this reversibility, the maximal response to the agonist may still be obtained if the concentration

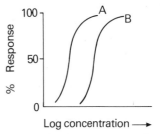

Fig. 7.4   Log concentration - response curves. A — agonist alone. B — agonist A in the presence of a competitive antagonist.

of the agonist is high enough, i.e. the dose response curve shifts to the right and is parallel to that of the agonist in the absence of the antagonist (Fig. 7.4). There are many examples (Table 7.1).

Table 7.1   Some examples of competitive antagonism

Drug	Drug or transmitter antagonised
naloxone	morphine and other opioids
atropine	acetylcholine (muscarinic)
D-tubocurarine pancuronium	acetylcholine (neuromuscular junction)
hexamethonium trimetaphan	acetylcholine (ganglia)
propranolol	adrenaline (β receptors)
cimetidine	histamine (H_2 receptors)

Antagonists are noncompetitive if they *inactivate* the receptor. The effect is to reduce the intrinsic activity of the agonist without changing its affinity so that a maximal response cannot be obtained by increasing the concentration of the agonist (Fig. 7.5). This effect may be reversible or irreversible.

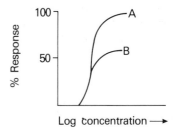

Fig. 7.5   Log concentration - response curves. A — agonist alone. B — agonist A in the presence of a noncompetitive antagonist.

Non-competitive antagonists often have a long duration of action and their effects are usually unrelated to their plasma concentration. An example is phenoxybenzamine antagonism at α-adrenoceptors.

Desensitisation, tachyphylaxis and tolerance

Repeated or continuous use of drugs may lead to a progressive decrease in the observed response. This process may be called desensitisation, tachyphylaxis or tolerance. *Desensitisation* is a decrease in cellular sensitivity or responsiveness to the repeated use of a drug. Acute desensitisation occurs quickly and is reversible. This may be explained by receptors existing in the resting, activated and desensitised state. Chronic desensitisation occurs slowly and is less readily reversible. It may result from loss of receptors from effector cells (e.g. in myasthenia gravis or after chronic use of sympathomimetic bronchodilators in asthma). *Tachyphylaxis* is a rapid decrease in pharmacological response. One example is a drug which acts by releasing endogenous transmitters for nerve endings (e.g. ephedrine). The response to repeated doses declines rapidly because of transmitter exhaustion. *Tolerance* occurs classically with opioid analgesics. Larger and larger doses are required to produce a pharmacological response. It may result from altered responsiveness of cells of the central nervous system and this may be similar to chronic desensitisation. For barbiturates, induction of hepatic microsomal enzymes may play an important part.

DRUG ABSORPTION

Unless a drug is applied directly to its site of action (e.g. local anaesthetic drugs or antacids) or is given intravenously, it must be absorbed from the site of application before being carried in the circulation to its site of action.

Drugs may be given:

1. Via the gastrointestinal tract: oral, rectal, sublingual.

2. Parenterally: intramuscular, subcutaneous.

3. By inhalation.

4. Transdermally.

Oral administration

Most drugs are given orally and there are very many factors which influence the rate and the amount of drug absorbed (Table 7.2). In acute situations, e.g. analgesic, sedative and antiarrhythmic therapy, the rate of absorption is more important than the amount of drug absorbed and delayed absorption may result in therapeutic failure. In chronic therapy, e.g.

Table 7.2 Factors affecting drug absorption after oral administration

Factor	Notes
Drug characteristics	
Tablet disintegration Dissolution time	Solution is absorbed more rapidly than tablets
Chelation or formation of insoluble complex with another drug	e.g. Fe^{++} and tetracycline
Patient characteristics pH	For some drugs, changes in pH will change the solubility or the degree of ionisation
Gastric emptying rate	Usually the most important factor affecting rate of absorption. It is influenced by posture, drugs, food and disease
Intestinal transit time	Diarrhoea may decrease the amount of drug absorbed
'First pass' metabolism	Occurs in the small intestine or the liver and reduces the amount of drug that reaches the systemic circulation
Gastro-intestinal disease	e.g. Pyloric stenosis delays gastric emptying and drug absorption

warfarin, digoxin and corticosteroid administration, the amount of drug absorbed is more important than the rate.

There are four possible mechanisms of absorption:

1. Passive diffusion — by far the most important process. The drug must be in solution and be lipid soluble (i.e. unionised). Absorption occurs because of a concentration gradient across the small intestinal mucosa. Theoretically, acidic drugs, e.g. aspirin, should be absorbed better in the stomach where the pH is low and the drug is unionised but in practice, because the gastric mucosa has a small surface area compared with the small intestine, it is absorbed better in the small bowel. Drugs are almost all absorbed by passive diffusion in the small intestine and the rate of gastric emptying is an important rate limiting factor.

2. Active transport — this mechanism is highly specific and requires energy expenditure. Some amino acids, sugars and vitamins are absorbed by this mechanism. Methyldopa and L-dopa may be absorbed by this process.

3. Filtration through pores — these pores are so small that only compounds with a molecular weight less than 100 can be absorbed. This is unimportant for drug absorption.

4. Pinocytosis — some macromolecules may be absorbed thus but it is unimportant for drug absorption.

Drugs including lignocaine, glyceryl trinitrate, propranolol and opioid analgesic drugs undergo extensive 'first pass' metabolism. This tends to inactivate the drug before it reaches the systemic circulation. Thus the intravenous dose is much smaller than an oral dose and pharmacological effects after oral administration may be unpredictable.

Sublingual administration of a drug avoids the phenomenon of 'first pass' metabolism since the drug is absorbed directly into the systemic circulation. Variation in absorption occurs if a varying amount of the drug is swallowed with saliva.

Rectal administration is popular in some cultures. Part of a dose of drug given rectally is absorbed systemically and part into the portal circulation. Thus absorption may vary. However, this route avoids gastric irritation, e.g. with aspirin administration by mouth.

Intramuscular and subcutaneous administration

Drugs may be administered parenterally because they are destroyed in the stomach (e.g. benzylpenicillin), or poorly absorbed from the gut (e.g. gentamicin or quaternary amines), or have significant 'first-pass' metabolism (e.g. opioid analgesics). However, intramuscular administration does not guarantee rapid or complete absorption. Diazepam is absorbed more rapidly and predictably after oral administration than after intramuscular injection.

The major factor affecting absorption is regional blood flow — the better the perfusion, the faster the absorption. Reduced cardiac output may result in delayed absorption. Water solubility of the drug is also a major determinant of the rate and the completeness of absorption. The drug should be sufficiently water soluble at physiological pH to remain in solution in the interstitium of the muscle until absorption occurs. Drugs including diazepam, phenytoin and digoxin may precipitate at the site of injection and absorption is slow and erratic.

Inhalation

Drugs given by inhalation usually have a rapid onset of action since there is an extremely large epithelial surface available for absorption. Many anaesthetic agents are given by this route.

General anaesthesia occurs when the partial pressure (tension) of agent in the central nervous system (which is assumed to be related to that in the alveoli) is sufficiently great to induce loss of consciousness. The factors which affect alveolar concentration are shown in Table 7.3. The three major factors are alveolar ventilation, drug uptake and concentration. Ventilation raises the alveolar concentration by bringing anaesthetic into the lungs and uptake decreases alveolar concentration by removing the agent.

Table 7.3 Factors affecting rate of absorption of inhalation anaesthetics

1. Apparatus
   Dead space
   Solubility of drug in rubber
   Concentration of drug
2. Alveolar ventilation
3. Uptake of agent into blood
   Cardiac output
   Solubility of drug in blood
   Ventilation/perfusion
   Tissue uptake

Factors which determine the uptake of the agent by the blood are solubility, cardiac output and the concentration gradient between the alveoli and venous blood. The higher the solubility of the anaesthetic agent *in blood* the greater the uptake and the more slowly will the necessary alveolar concentrations (and thus anaesthesia) occur. Less soluble agents have a more rapid onset of anaesthesia. The same is true in reverse on withdrawing anaesthesia. Less soluble agents are eliminated from the body more rapidly.

Increased cardiac output increases uptake from the alveoli and slows the onset of anaesthesia. Conversely, shock reduces uptake and accelerates the onset of anaesthesia or may lead to overdosage, especially with more soluble agents (Fig. 7.6).

The concentration gradient between the alveoli and blood is maximum at the beginning of induction of anaesthesia and is zero at equilibrium.

The inspired concentration of the anaesthetic agent influences the rate at which alveolar concentration rises (concentration effect). A higher inspired concentration results in a more rapid approach of alveolar concentration to the inspired concentration (Fig. 7.6).

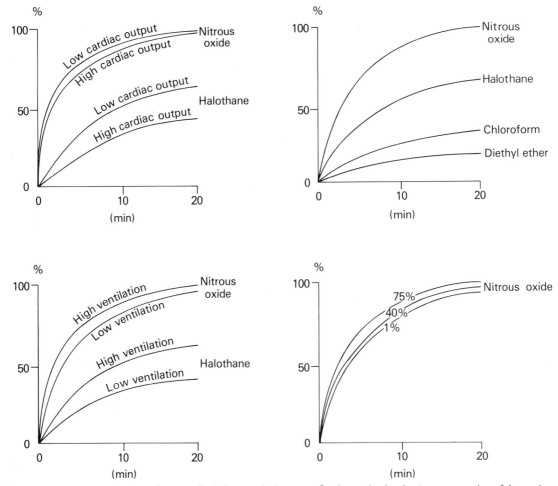

Fig. 7.6 Factors affecting the rate of uptake of volatile anaesthetic agents. On the y-axis, the alveolar concentration of the gas is expressed as a percentage of the inspired concentration.

Changes in ventilation have a small effect on the less soluble anaesthetics, e.g. nitrous oxide, cyclopropane or enflurane, but they have a profound effect on the very soluble agents, e.g. ether, methoxyflurane or chloroform. Doubling ventilation may almost double the alveolar concentration for the soluble agents.

Ventilation/perfusion abnormalities affect less soluble agents more than soluble agents. In one lung anaesthesia, doubling the ventilation to one lung doubles the alveolar partial pressure of the soluble agent in that lung. This compensates for the unventilated lung. No such compensation occurs with less soluble agents.

The anaesthetic system may influence the uptake of agents. If it is large then changes occur slowly. If the

agent is soluble in rubber (e.g. halothane and methoxyflurane) concentrations rise more slowly at induction. In practice, therefore, high concentrations of anaesthetic agents are given at induction of anaesthesia followed by a rapid reduction to maintenance inspired concentrations. This mirrors the high initial uptake which reduces rapidly in 5 to 15 min. Uptake continues to decrease at a much slower rate.

After total body equilibration, elimination of anaesthetics occurs as an inversion of uptake. The output of less soluble agents is initially high and declines rapidly to a lower level. The output of soluble agents is high initially but decreases gradually over a period of time. Recovery parallels this output and is rapid with less soluble agents and slow with soluble agents. Increasing alveolar ventilation accelerates recovery while depressed ventilation slows recovery.

Transdermal absorption

Most drugs are well absorbed when applied to the skin surface and up to 10 mg of drug can be administered by this route in 24 h. Examples are hyoscine for travel sickness and glyceryl trinitrate for angina.

DISTRIBUTION

Drug distribution throughout the body depends largely on physicochemical properties (e.g. lipid solubility and protein binding) and blood flow. Ionised water-soluble drugs, e.g. penicillin or myoneural blocking drugs, cannot penetrate cell membranes readily and therefore have a small apparent volume of distribution. Lipid soluble drugs have a large volume of distribution and are distributed widely in tissues.

Plasma protein binding

Drug distribution may be affected by reversible binding to plasma proteins (e.g. albumin, α_1 acid glycoprotein or globulin) since only the unbound fraction is immediately available for diffusion into tissues. Protein binding is primarily a method for the rapid distribution of drugs from their site of absorption to their site of action. The binding of highly lipid soluble drugs (e.g. thiopentone) is essential for transport in plasma because of their low solubility in plasma water. During perfusion of the tissues, the concentration of unbound drug in plasma decreases and the protein-bound drug dissociates.

Protein binding is of relevance only if drugs are more than 80% bound. Two drugs may compete with each other for the same binding site and thus increase the free concentration of one or both agents. Enhancement of the therapeutic effect may occur (e.g. aspirin displaces warfarin from its protein-binding sites and increases its anticoagulant effect). Binding to plasma proteins may be decreased in renal and hepatic disease.

Blood–brain barrier

Ionised drugs (e.g. myoneural blocking drugs) do not cross the blood–brain barrier and drugs which are extensively protein bound (e.g. warfarin) cross in very small amounts. Drugs with a high molecular weight do not cross readily. In contrast, low molecular weight, lipid-soluble drugs cross into the brain rapidly.

Placenta

Low molecular weight, lipid-soluble drugs are transferred readily across the placenta. Thus all sedative drugs used in anaesthesia cross into the fetus. Some metabolites of these drugs which are active may then accumulate in the fetus and result in neonatal depression (e.g. desmethyl-diazepam, norpethidine).

Intravenous anaesthetic agents

After intravenous administration, anaesthetic agents (e.g. thiopentone) induce sleep in one arm–brain circulation time because the brain has a rich blood supply and because the drug is lipid soluble and crosses the blood–brain barrier rapidly. All tissues with a rich blood supply (vessel-rich group: brain, heart, kidney, glands and gastrointestinal tract) achieve high concentrations of drug very rapidly. As the plasma concentration decreases by distribution, the drug leaves these tissues and is distributed to other tissues which have not yet achieved equilibrium because of a poorer blood supply (muscle group and then fat group). Because of this distribution, the drug leaves the brain, the drug effect wears off and the patient awakens. At the time of recovery from the drug's effects, virtually no drug has been broken down in the body. Thus thiopentone, in common with almost all anaesthetic agents, has a short duration of action because of its rapid distribution throughout the body. Of the commonly used agents only propanidid is destroyed rapidly in the body (by plasma cholinesterase).

If thiopentone is given repeatedly to maintain anaesthesia, its duration of action becomes more prolonged with each injection. After four or five administrations it is possible that recovery from the drug no longer occurs because of distribution but occurs only when the drug is broken down in the body. This is a very much slower process and the effects of the drug may be prolonged and unpredictable with repeated administration.

METABOLISM

Most drugs are lipid-soluble and therefore cannot be excreted unchanged in the urine or bile. They must undergo a process of biotransformation known as metabolism. The main purpose of metabolism is to make the drug more water soluble so that it can be excreted. It results usually in inactivation of the drug.

Some drugs used in anaesthesia are esters and are hydrolysed in the plasma by cholinesterase. Their breakdown is very rapid (e.g. procaine, suxamethonium, propanidid). For some drugs a significant amount is metabolised in the kidney (dopamine), bowel mucosa (isoprenaline) or lung (prilocaine). However, the liver is the major site of drug metabolism in man. Drugs may undergo phase 1 or phase 2 reactions or both. Phase 1 reactions are simple chemical reactions including oxidation, reduction, hydroxylation or acetylation. Phase 2 reactions are conjugations with glucuronide, sulphate or glycine. Both reactions make the drug more water soluble.

Drugs which undergo phase 1 reactions include benzodiazepines, barbiturates, halothane, rifampicin, anticonvulsants and corticosteroids. Many of the reactions are catalysed by a group of nonspecific enzymes in the endoplasmic reticulum (known as hepatic microsomal enzymes) or the mixed function oxidase system which includes the enzyme cytochrome P450. The most important of the phase 2 reactions is glucuronidation which depends also on the enzyme systems in the endoplasmic reticulum.

Enzyme induction

Drugs which are substrates for the mixed function oxidase system have the capacity to enhance the enzyme system such that they and other drugs which share this route of metabolism are metabolised more rapidly. This results in a very profound change in metabolising capacity which reaches a maximum after 1–2 weeks of therapy. Drugs which are known to induce enzymes include phenobarbitone, phenytoin, carbamazepine, rifampicin, griseofulvin, inhalation anaesthetics and alcohol. Drugs whose effects are reduced or abolished by this increase in metabolism include the oral contraceptive pill, warfarin and anticonvulsants. All these drugs have a long duration of action which terminates because of drug metabolism. Drugs which are given as a single bolus intravenous injection and the effects of which normally diminish because of distribution (e.g. thiopentone, diazepam, morphine) are not affected by enzyme induction unless they are given repeatedly. Sometimes, phase 1 metabolism does not result in inactivation of the drug and the metabolites of a drug are active pharmacologically. Examples of this phenomenon include diazepam, pethidine, chlorpromazine, lignocaine, chloral hydrate and trichloroethylene. For other drugs, the metabolites may be toxic (e.g. halothane, paracetamol, methoxyflurane). In these instances, enzyme induction may enhance drug activity or toxicity.

Enzyme inhibition

Some drugs may inhibit hepatic microsomal enzymes in a competitive or noncompetitive manner (e.g. tolbutamide, cimetidine, phenylbutazone, chloramphenicol). Other drugs compete for an enzyme system, e.g. plasma cholinesterase (propanidid and suxamethonium) or monoamine oxidase. The net result is usually a prolongation of drug action.

EXCRETION

Relatively few drugs are water soluble and therefore excreted unchanged by the kidney. However, almost all metabolites are eventually eliminated from the body in urine or bile. Small amounts appear in saliva or milk. Compounds with a low molecular weight are excreted in urine and drugs with a larger molecular weight (e.g. tubocurarine) appear in the bile.

Renal excretion

The processes involved in renal excretion include:
1. Glomerular filtration.
2. Active tubular reabsorption.
3. Passive reabsorption.
4. Active secretion.

Glomerular filtration

All nonbound drug is filtered at the glomerulus. Since the glomerular perfusion time is much longer than the drug-protein dissociation time, a significant amount of protein bound drug may also be filtered.

Active tubular reabsorption

Some ions and physiological compounds (e.g. lithium, amino acids and glucose) are reabsorbed in the proximal tubule by an active process. This is relatively unimportant for drugs.

Passive reabsorption

The reabsorption of water along the nephron results in a reduction of urine flow from 125 ml/min at the glomerulus to 1 ml/min in the collecting duct. This concentration of nonreabsorbed solute in the lumen by a factor of 125:1 encourages passive diffusion of lipid soluble drugs across the tubules to be reabsorbed in the blood stream.

Since most drugs are weak acids or weak bases and thus exist in both ionised and unionised forms at physiological pH, the pH of the luminal fluid alters the proportion of the drug that is unionised and therefore absorbed passively from the tubules. Acidification of the urine results in ionisation of basic drugs and thus enhances excretion by reducing the amount reabsorbed. Ephedrine, fenfluramine and amphetamine excretion is enhanced by acidification of the urine. Conversely, alkalinisation of the urine results in enhanced excretion of acidic drugs such as aspirin and phenobarbitone. Alkalinisation of the urine is often induced in aspirin poisoning in an attempt to increase the rate of renal excretion.

Active secretion

This is the usual mechanism by which the kidney excretes drugs. Proximal tubular secretion results in the elimination of penicillins, aminoglycosides, antibiotics, digoxin, practolol and neuromuscular blocking drugs. This process requires energy; it acts against a concentration gradient; protein-binding of drugs does not inhibit it and drugs may compete with each other for the process (e.g. probenecid and penicillin).

Biliary excretion

Biliary excretion is the major route of elimination for water-soluble compounds with high molecular weight (400–500). Drugs or their metabolites are usually eliminated from the liver cells by active transport. The mechanism is similar to that described for active renal tubular secretion. Radiographic dyes, penicillins and neuromuscular blocking drugs are secreted into bile. In particular, monoquaternary ammonium compounds (e.g. D-tubocurarine) are more rapidly eliminated than bisquaternary ammonium compounds (e.g. dimethyltubocurarine.)

Some compounds eliminated as the glucuronide in the bile are hydrolysed within the lumen of the bowel and are then reabsorbed. This is known as the enterohepatic circulation.

PHARMACOKINETICS

One compartment model

Many processes in pharmacology may be described satisfactorily by 'first order' kinetics — the rate of change of concentrations or of transfer between compartments is proportional to the drug concentration in the particular compartment. For example, if plasma concentrations of drug are plotted against time (Fig. 7.7a) a single exponential curve is obtained. If the logarithm of the concentration is plotted against time, a straight line results (Fig. 7.7b).

If the natural logarithm is used, the slope of the line is K, the rate constant for the system. If the logarithm to base 10 is used

$$K = \text{slope} \times 2.3$$

K has the units of reciprocal time and represents the proportion of drug eliminated from the system in unit time. Thus $K = 0.1/h$ means that 10% of the drug is removed from the system each hour. The half-life ($T_{\frac{1}{2}}$) is defined as the time required for the concentration of drug to decline by 50%. It is inversely related to K thus

$$T_{\frac{1}{2}} = \frac{0.693}{K}$$

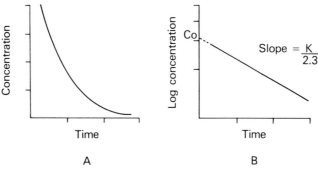

Fig. 7.7   A one-compartment model — monoexponential decline in plasma concentration. A — linear scale. B — logarithm (to the base 10) scale.

The total apparent volume of distribution (V) of the compartment may be calculated from the equation

$$V = \frac{dose}{\text{Concentration at time 0}} = \frac{D}{C_0}$$

The clearance (Cl) of a drug is the volume of plasma that is cleared of the drug in unit time. Total body clearance represents the sum of all clearances (e.g. renal, hepatic, pulmonary etc.).

It follows from the definitions given above that

$$\frac{clearance}{\text{Volume of distribution}} = K$$

i.e.

$$\frac{Cl}{V} = K$$

By substitution,

$$T_{1/2} = \frac{0.693 \times V}{Cl}$$

Although this one-compartment model approximates to the clinical situation some time after intravenous administration of a drug (when distribution is complete and only elimination processes need be considered) a model with two compartments provides a more adequate description of plasma concentrations after intravenous injection of a drug.

Two-compartment model

This approximation assumes that the body may be resolved into a central compartment of small apparent volume and a peripheral compartment of larger volume. The compartments do not necessarily correspond to specific anatomical entities. The decrease in plasma concentrations of many drugs after intravenous injection is consistent with this concept and one observes a biexponential decline in plasma concentrations. An initial rapid decline (resulting from drug distribution) is followed by a slower phase (drug elimination) (Fig. 7.8). Hybrid values for volume of distribution (V_β) and the slow half-time ($T_{\frac{1}{2}\beta}$) may be calculated as described for the one-compartment model. By substraction of an extrapolation of the β slope from the data points, similar calculations may be performed for the rapid phase (Fig. 7.8).

Total body clearance (Cl) can be calculated from

$$Cl = \frac{dose}{AUC \text{ from } t = 0 \text{ to } t = \infty}$$

(AUC = the area under the plasma concentration time curve)

Intravenous infusion

Constant rate intravenous infusion results in gradually increasing plasma concentrations until steady state concentrations are achieved. At steady state,

amount of drug in = amount of drug out

i.e., infusion rate = plasma concentration × clearance

$$I = C_{ss} \times Cl$$

From the start of infusion, half the steady state plasma concentration is achieved in one half-life of the drug. Following an infusion equal to four times

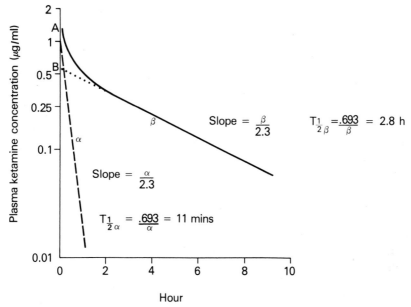

Fig. 7.8 A two-compartment model — biexponential decline in plasma ketamine concentration (after intravenous injection of 2 mg/kg) represented by solid line.

By extrapolating the β slope back to the Y axis and subtracting the values on the line from the measured concentration at each time point, the α slope is obtained.

The β and α slopes meet the Y axis at B and A respectively. The equation that best fits the data is:

$C_t = Ae^{-\alpha t} + Be^{-\beta t}$

C_t = Concentration at time t

Table 7.4 Mechanisms of drug interactions

	Example	Effect
1. Pharmaceutical incompatibility	Thiopentone and suxamethonium	Precipitate
2. Interference with drug absorption	Opioid analgesics and orally administered drugs	Delayed absorption
3. Changes in drug distribution (e.g. displacement from plasma protein binding sites)	Aspirin and warfarin	Bleeding
4. Competition at receptor sites	Adrenaline and propranolol	Antagonism
5. Change in hepatic metabolism		
a) enzyme induction	Phenobarbitone and warfarin	Reduced effect of warfarin
b) enzyme inhibition	Cimetidine and many other drugs	Prolonged effect
c) changes in liver blood flow	Halothane and ketamine	Delayed elimination of ketamine
6. Interference with excretion		
a) renal	Probenecid and penicillin	High penicillin concentration
b) biliary	—	—
7. Antagonism or potentiation by drugs acting on the same physiological system or at the same time	Alcohol and barbiturates	Potentiation
8. Changes in fluid and electrolyte balance	Diuretics and digoxin	Digoxin toxicity
9. Miscellaneous		
a) monoamine oxidase inhibition	—	—
b) antagonism of antibiotics	—	—

the half-life, concentrations are within 10% of the eventual steady state concentration.

Oral administration

When the drug reaches the mucosa of the small intestine and absorption rate (assumed to be a first order process also) is greater than elimination rate, plasma concentrations rise. When the amount of drug at the absorption site is sufficiently reduced so that elimination rate exceeds absorption rate, plasma concentrations decrease with time.

The bioavailability of a drug is the extent of its absorption. It is usually calculated by comparing the areas under the plasma concentration time curves (*AUC*) after oral and intravenous administration of the same dose of the drug and expressing the former as a percentage of the latter. Drugs with a high 'first-pass' metabolism have a low bioavailability.

Drug interactions

In modern therapeutic and anaesthetic practice, polypharmacy is the rule and drug interactions are likely. A classification with examples is given in Table 7.4.

FURTHER READING

Curry S 1977 Drug disposition and pharmacokinetics, 2nd edn. Blackwell Scientific Publications, Oxford
Dollery C T 1973 Pharmacokinetics — master or servant. European Journal of Clinical Pharmacology 6: 1
Eger E I 1981 Uptake, distribution and elimination of inhaled anaesthetics. In: Scurr C, Feldman S (eds) Scientific foundations of anaesthesia, 3rd edn. Heinemann, London
Gibaldi M 1977 Biopharmaceutics and clinical pharmacokinetics, 2nd edn. Lea and Febiger, Philadelphia
Greenblatt D J, Koch-Weser J 1975 Clinical pharmacokinetics. New England Journal of Medicine 702: 964

Meffin P J, Birkett D J, Wing L M H 1979 Fundamentals of clinical pharmacology 2. How drugs act. Current Therapeutics 20: 87
Prescott L F 1980 Clinically important drug interactions. In: Avery G S (ed) Drug treatment, 2nd edn. Churchill Livingstone, Edinburgh and London
Tognoni G, Bellantuono C, Bonati M, et al 1980 Clinical relevance of pharmacokinetics. Clinical Pharmacokinetics 5: 105
Tucker G T 1979 Drug metabolism. British Journal of Anaesthesia 51: 603

8

Inhalational anaesthetic agents

Oxygen

History

Joseph Priestley isolated oxygen in 1777 and speculated on both the beneficial effects of the gas and also its toxic effects. Lavoisier and Laplace demonstrated in 1780 that oxygen was taken into the body via the lungs and converted to carbon dioxide and water. Haldane popularised the use of oxygen in clinical practice during the first World War.

Preparation

Commercially, oxygen is manufactured by fractional distillation of liquid air. Before liquefaction of air, carbon dioxide is removed and liquid oxygen and nitrogen separated by means of their different boiling points (oxygen $-183°C$, nitrogen $-195°C$).

Presentation

Oxygen is supplied in cylinders at a pressure of 137 bar at 15°C. The cylinders are painted black with a white shoulder.

Many institutions use piped oxygen and this is supplied either by a 'bank' of oxygen cylinders ensuring a continuous supply, or as liquid oxygen. Premises using in excess of 5000 cubic feet of oxygen per week find the latter more economical. The pressure of oxygen in a hospital pipeline is approx. 4 bar which is the same as the pressure distal to the reducing valves of gas cylinders attached to anaesthetic machines.

Physical properties

Oxygen is tasteless, colourless and odourless with a specific gravity of 1.105 (air = 1) and a molecular weight of 32. At atmospheric pressure it liquefies at $-183°C$ but at 50 atmospheres the liquefaction temperature increases to $-119°C$.

Oxygen supports combustion although the gas itself is not flammable. Oxygen at high pressure may cause an explosion in the presence of oil or grease.

Physiological data

The physiological aspects of oxygen are dealt with predominantly in Chapter 2 and the clinical uses in Chapter 20. However, it should be noted that high concentrations of oxygen may induce undesirable effects. Clinically, the most important adverse effect of 100% oxygen is the tendency to produce absorption collapse in the lungs within 10–20 min. Even small concentrations of nitrogen exert an important 'splinting effect' and this accounts for the

Table 8.1 Important adverse effects of high inspired pressures of oxygen

Cardiovascular effects
  Myocardial depression and vascular constriction. These effects are not clinically significant with 100% O_2 in healthy patients but may be overt in patients with severe cardiac disease
Absorption atelectasis
  Collapse of lung units may occur in 6 min with 100% O_2, 60 min with 85% O_2 in the presence of airway closure
CO_2 narcosis
  Respiratory depression in patients with chronic chest disease and significant hypoxic ventilatory drive
Pulmonary toxicity
  Lung damage (capillary congestion, interstitial and alveolar oedema) is dependent on the partial pressure of oxygen and duration of exposure. Onset of oxygen-induced lung pathology occurs after approx 30 h exposure to P_{IO_2} of 100 kPa
C.n.s. toxicity
  Convulsions similar to grand mal epilepsy occur with exposure to hyperbaric pressures of O_2.

current avoidance of 100% oxygen in estimation of pulmonary shunt ratio ($\dot{Q}s/\dot{Q}t$) in patients with lung pathology (where a greater degree of airway closure would result in greater areas of alveolar atelectasis). The adverse effects of oxygen are summarised in Table 8.1.

Carbon dioxide

History

Carbon dioxide was discovered by Von Helmont and isolated by Joseph Black in 1757. Yandell Henderson in the United States in 1925 and J.S. Haldane in England in 1926 demonstrated the physiological significance of carbon dioxide. Before the disadvantages of high levels of Pa_{CO_2} were appreciated, anaesthetists frequently used CO_2 to stimulate respiration but more recently, attention has been directed towards prevention of rebreathing in anaesthetic circuits and maintaining normocapnia in the spontaneously breathing patient.

Preparation

In the laboratory:

1. Action of a strong mineral acid on a carbonate.
   $NaHCO_3 + HCl \rightarrow NaCl + H_2O + CO_2$
2. Fermentation of grain in the preparation of alcohol.
3. Commercially: carbon dioxide is produced by the action of heat on calcium or magnesium carbonate in the preparation of their oxides, e.g.

$$Ca\,CO_3 \xrightarrow{\text{HEAT}} CaO + CO_2$$

Presentation and physical properties

Carbon dioxide is supplied in the liquid state in grey cylinders at a pressure of 50 bar at 15°C.

There is 0.03% carbon dioxide in the atmosphere. It combines readily with water to form carbonic acid. The molecular weight is 44.

Carbon dioxide is nonflammable and does not support combustion.

Physiological data

The physiological aspects of CO_2 are dealt with predominantly in Chapter 2. Variations in cardiovascular state induced by alterations in Pa_{CO_2} may be similar to those induced by pain or lightness of anaesthesia and the differential diagnosis is described in Table 20.2. For completeness the cardiovascular effects of CO_2 are summarised here in Table 8.2

Table 8.2   Cardiovascular effects of CO_2

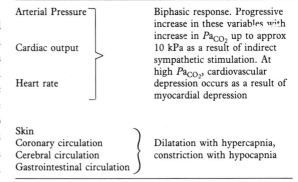

Arterial Pressure Cardiac output Heart rate	Biphasic response. Progressive increase in these variables with increase in Pa_{CO_2} up to approx 10 kPa as a result of indirect sympathetic stimulation. At high Pa_{CO_2}, cardiovascular depression occurs as a result of myocardial depression
Skin Coronary circulation Cerebral circulation Gastrointestinal circulation	Dilatation with hypercapnia, constriction with hypocapnia

Use of carbon dioxide in anaesthesia

1. During induction — carbon dioxide may be used to stimulate respiration during a gaseous induction after a heavy opioid premedication. Care should be taken to avoid undue hypercapnia.

2. To produce hyperventilation in order to facilitate blind nasal intubation.

3. To increase cerebral blood flow during carotid artery surgery. This is an area of some controversy since hypercapnia may induce 'stealing' of blood away from an ischaemic area of brain. Many prefer to maintain normocapnia during this surgical procedure (see Chapter 27).

4. To assist in reinstitution of spontaneous ventilation after a period of artificial hyperventilation.

The use of carbon dioxide in anaesthetic practice has declined as appreciation of its disadvantages has increased and as a result of the introduction of i.v. induction agents and relaxant anaesthetic techniques.

Nitrous oxide

History

Nitrous oxide was prepared first by Priestley in 1772. Its properties were investigated in 1799 by Sir

Humphrey Davy who recognised its potential for alleviation of pain and suggested that it may be used as an anaesthetic for surgical operations. In 1844 it was employed for the production of surgical anaesthesia by Horace Wells, an American dentist. Wells tried unsuccessfully to demonstrate the anaesthetic properties of nitrous oxide at Massachusetts General Hospital. Despite this setback Wells continued to use nitrous oxide in his practice but it was overshadowed subsequently by ether. It was not until Cotton reviewed its use in 1867 that the dental profession showed any interest and by 1868 nitrous oxide was supplied compressed in cylinders. Edmund Andrews in 1868 combined it with oxygen to give longer anaesthesia. Its use continued to be pioneered by Hewitt and McKesson and today it is used widely during balanced anaesthesia.

Manufacture

Commercially, nitrous oxide is produced by heating ammonium nitrate to between 245°C and 270°C.

$$NH_4NO_3 \xrightarrow[245-270°C]{HEAT} N_2O + 2H_2O$$

Produced with the nitrous oxide are a number of impurities:

Ammonia
Nitric acid
Nitrogen
Nitric oxide (NO)
Nitrogen dioxide (NO_2)

After cooling, ammonia and nitric acid are reconstituted to ammonium nitrate which is returned to the beginning of the process. The remaining gases then pass through a series of scrubbers. The purified gases are compressed and dried in an aluminium drier. Continuous sampling of the gas for analysis takes place as it leaves the scrubber. The resultant gases are expanded in a liquefier with the nitrogen escaping as gas. The nitrous oxide is then evaporated, compressed and passed through another aluminium drier before being stored in cylinders.

The higher oxides of nitrogen dissolve in water to form nitrous and nitric acids. All these substances are toxic and if inhaled produce methaemoglobinaemia, and pulmonary oedema leading to death (in severe conditions).

Presentation

Nitrous oxide is supplied in a liquid state in cylinders and the amount of N_2O may be determined by weighing the cylinder. The full and empty weights of the cylinder are stamped on the shoulder. Above the liquid level, nitrous oxide is in the gaseous phase and the pressure of the gas remains relatively constant until all the liquid has vaporised; the pressure then decreases rapidly as the remaining gas is used. Nitrous oxide cylinders should be kept in the vertical position during use so that the liquid phase falls to the bottom of the cylinder. During continuous use, the cylinder may cool as a result of the latent heat of vaporisation of the liquid and ice may form on the lower part of the cylinder.

Physical properties

Nitrous oxide is not inflammable but it does support combustion.

Nitrous oxide is colourless, non-irritant and slightly sweet smelling.

Molecular weight 44
Boiling point −88°C
Blood/gas solubility 0.47 at 37°C
Oil/water solubility 3.2
Critical temperature 36.5°C. (Temperature above which it is not possible to liquefy a gas with pressure alone.)
Critical pressure 72.6 bar.
MAC 105

Pharmacology

Nitrous oxide provides easy and pleasant induction of anaesthesia. However, it is a weak anaesthetic agent and in all but the seriously ill patient, does not produce adequate anaesthesia when used alone with O_2. Therefore, nitrous oxide is used usually in combination with other agents. When using nitrous oxide in a relaxant technique, awareness may be a problem, particularly during anaesthesia for Caesarian section where adjuvants are kept to a minimum.

Nitrous oxide is an excellent analgesic. This, together with its low blood/gas solubility coefficient and pleasant administration, make it useful in clinical practice. Good analgesia for postoperative physiotherapy and burns dressings may be achieved using up to 25% nitrous oxide without loss of consciousness. Entonox (premixed 50% nitrous oxide in oxygen) is used extensively to provide pain relief during childbirth.

Nitrous oxide is a relatively safe anaesthetic agent. It is excreted unchanged via the lungs.

1. Respiratory system — it is nonirritant and causes no increase in secretions or bronchospasm. It produces mild depression of respiration.

2. Cardiovascular system — nitrous oxide causes direct myocardial depression. Systemic arterial pressure is maintained by a baroreceptor-induced increase in systemic vascular resistance. These effects are difficult to detect clinically in healthy patients but they may assume importance in patients in cardiac failure.

3. Muscle tone — remains normal.

4. Smooth muscle including uterine muscle is unaffected.

5. Liver and kidney function are unaltered.

Nitrous oxide occupies an important place in most general anaesthetic techniques. It may be used in conjunction with oxygen as a carrier gas mixture for volatile agents or with opioids in a relaxant technique.

Entonox

Entonox is the trade name given by B.O.C. to a mixture of 50% nitrous oxide in oxygen. Under pressure, certain mixtures of nitrous oxide and oxygen remain in the gaseous phase at temperatures and pressures at which nitrous oxide is normally in the liquid phase (Poynting effect). If the cylinders are exposed to cold, the nitrous oxide may liquefy and fall to the bottom of the cylinder resulting in an uneven administration of nitrous oxide and oxygen; initially oxygen is delivered and, latterly, nitrous oxide. Entonox liquefies at $-7°C$. If there is any doubt regarding a cylinder which has been exposed to a cold environment, it should be rewarmed and inverted several times to ensure adequate mixing.

Entonox is used commonly for its analgesic properties in obstetrics and for burns dressings and other painful procedures.

Cyclopropane

History

Cyclopropane was synthesised by Von Freund in 1882. Its anaesthetic properties were discovered in 1929 by Lucas and Henderson in Toronto. It was used first as an anaesthetic by W. Easson Brown, but as the use of cyclopropane was not encouraged in the Toronto General Hospital it was developed in Madison, Wisconsin.

Manufacture

1. From natural gas found in the United States.
2. From trimethylene glycol, which is produced in the fermentation of molasses.

$$
\begin{array}{cccc}
CH_2OH & & & CH_2Br \\
| & & & | \\
CH_2 & + & 2HBr & \rightarrow & CH_2 & + 2H_2O \\
| & & & | \\
CH_2OH & & & CH_2Br \\
\text{Trimethylene} & \text{Hydrobromic} & \text{Trimethylene} \\
\text{Glycol} & \text{Acid} & \text{Dibromide}
\end{array}
$$

$$
\begin{array}{ccc}
CH_2Br & & CH_2 \\
| & & \diagup \diagdown \\
CH_2 & + \quad Zn \quad \rightarrow & CH_2 — CH_2 + ZnBr_2 \\
| & & \\
CH_2Br & & \text{(Trimethylene)} \\
& & \text{Cyclopropane}
\end{array}
$$

Presentation

Cyclopropane is stored as a liquefied gas in orange metal cylinders at a vapour pressure of 5 bar at 15°C. Thus the cylinder does not require a reducing valve. As with nitrous oxide, the pressure in the cylinder provides no indication of the volume of gas remaining.

Physical properties

Cyclopropane is a colourless gas with a characteristic pleasant, sweet smell.

Molecular weight 42.

Vapour density 1.42 (air = 1).

Boiling point $-33°C$.

Freezing point $-127°C$.
Blood/gas solubility 0.45 at 37°C.
Oil/water solubility 34.4.
Critical temperature 125°C.
Critical pressure 54.7 bar.
MAC 9.2.

Flammability: cyclopropane forms an explosive mixture with oxygen and nitrous oxide throughout the anaesthetic range of concentrations, and in air in concentrations between 3 and 10%.

Pharmacology

Uptake and distribution. Induction is pleasant with cyclopropane, and both induction and recovery are rapid. Cyclopropane is relatively insoluble in water. Therefore, little is carried in plasma, and because of the high lipid solubility, much is absorbed into red blood cells. Because of the high potency of cyclopropane it may be administered in high oxygen concentrations; as general rule, for healthy patients:

4% cyclopropane in oxygen → analgesia
8% cyclopropane in oxygen → light anaesthesia
20–30% cyclopropane in oxygen → deep anaesthesia.

Respiratory system. Cyclopropane is relatively nonirritant to the respiratory tract, though in concentrations exceeding 50% it may cause laryngospasm. However, it is a powerful respiratory depressant, causing a progressive decrease in tidal volume associated with increased rate of respiration as the depth of anaesthesia increases. The respiratory depressant effect of cyclopropane is accentuated by the use of heavy opioid premedication, and this combination may result in apnoea.

Cardiovascular system. In a heart-lung preparation, cyclopropane directly depresses the myocardium. However, in man this response is modified by its effect on both the parasympathetic and sympathetic nervous systems. Cardiac output increases during light anaesthesia as a result of the sympathomimetic action of cyclopropane. However, at concentrations in excess of 20%, or after an opioid premedication, a decrease in cardiac output occurs.

Arterial pressure is often well maintained as a result of increases in both cardiac output and peripheral resistance. Cyclopropane has both direct and indirect

effects (via sympathetic stimulation) on smooth muscle, causing vasoconstriction. Administration to spontaneously breathing patients, however, frequently causes an increase in Pa_{CO_2}, with subsequent capillary vasodilatation, which may cause oozing at the site of operation.

Heart rate. In the unpremedicated patient, cyclopropane causes a slight reduction in heart rate. Cyclopropane is thought to cause both vagal and sympathetic stimulation to the heart. If atropine is administered, the patient may exhibit unopposed sympathetic stimulation causing tachycardia, often associated with a high incidence of arrhythmias. After opioid premedication, sympathomimetic action is decreased and predominant vagal stimulation occurs, with a resultant bradycardia.

Cardiac rhythm. Cyclopropane is often associated with cardiac arrhythmias:

1. Vagal bradycardia < 50 beat/min
2. Ventricular ectopics (which may lead to ventricular fibrillation). This tendency is accentuated by:

  (a) Overdosage.
  (b) Hypercapnia.
  (c) Catecholamines — increased circulating sympathetic amines and sensitisation of the myocardium to exogenous adrenaline administration.
  (d) Hypoxia.
  (e) Atropine.

Other organs. Cyclopropane causes a reduction in renal blood flow proportional to the concentration administered. It also stimulates production of antidiuretic hormone. Hepatic blood flow is reduced in proportion to the depth of anaesthesia, and the resultant hypoxia to the liver may result in hepatocellular damage.

Cyclopropane depresses uterine contractions at deep planes of anaesthesia, though it has little effect at light planes.

Uses of cyclopropane

Before the introduction of halothane, cyclopropane was a popular agent both for induction and maintenance of anaesthesia. Because of its expense and its explosive properties, it is administered using a closed circuit. In skilled hands it is a safe and useful agent. However, because of its effects on the respiratory and cardiovascular systems, and also its flammability, it is falling into disuse.

Cyclopropane is useful as an induction agent since it is potent and has a low blood gas solubility providing rapid induction of anaesthesia. It is administered in a high concentration of oxygen, which may be beneficial in the sick patient. It is regarded by some as a good induction agent for the hypovolaemic patient, because cardiac output and arterial pressure are maintained. However, this is achieved at the expense of a reduction in splanchnic and renal blood flow, and peripheral perfusion.

Cyclopropane is safer if administered without opioid premedication and using controlled ventilation. Careful monitoring of the patient's colour, peripheral perfusion, pulse, arterial pressure, e.c.g. and response to surgical stimulation is essential

Cyclopropane shock

During cyclopropane anaesthesia, in the spontaneously breathing patient, carbon dioxide retention occurs and this, in combination with the sympathetic response to surgical stimulation, helps to maintain the patient's arterial pressure. During emergence, the patient's Pa_{CO_2} returns to normal, the surgical stimulus ceases and there may be a profound decrease in arterial pressure.

Emergence delirium

This may be seen in young, healthy patients undergoing relatively minor surgery, and may be avoided by the use of a dose of postoperative analgesia before the end of the operation.

VOLATILE ANAESTHETIC AGENTS

Diethyl ether

History

Ether was prepared first in 1540 by Valerius Cordus though it was not until three centuries later that its anaesthetic properties were recognised. It was used clinically for anaesthesia in New York by Clarke and in Georgia by Crawford Long in 1842. They did not publish their results until after Morton gave his

famous demonstration at the Massachusetts General Hospital. Shortly after this, ether gained popularity in Great Britain.

Manufacture

By heating together ethyl alcohol and concentrated sulphuric acid

$$C_2H_5OH + H_2SO_4 \rightarrow C_2H_5HSO_4 + H_2O$$
$$C_2H_5HSO_4 + C_2H_5OH \rightarrow C_2H_5OC_2H_5 + H_2SO_4$$

Concentrated sulphuric acid and ethyl alcohol are heated to 130°C in a still with a constant flow of alcohol. The vapour contains a mixture of ether, alcohol and water. Any sulphur dioxide is removed by sodium hydroxide, and the ether and alcohol are separated by fractionation. The ether is dried using calcium chloride, and distilled.

Physical properties

Ether is a colourless volatile liquid with a characteristic smell.

Molecular weight 74.

Vapour density 2.6 (air = 1).

Boiling point 35°C.

Saturated vapour pressure 425 mmHg (56.7 kPa) at 20°C.

Blood/gas solubility 12 at 37°C.

Oil/water solubility 3.2.

MAC 1.92.

Latent heat of vaporisation 89 cal/g.

Flammability: ether vapour is inflammable in air in concentrations of 1.8% to 36.5%, and in oxygen at 2–82%. When using ether it is essential to avoid diathermy and utilise an efficient ducting system.

Pharmacology

Uptake and distribution. The solubility of diethyl ether in oil is three times greater than in water. In comparison with other volatile anaesthetic agents (e.g. halothane with an oil/water solubility coefficient of 330) ether is more soluble in water and in blood. Since ether has a relatively high blood solubility, the rate of equilibration of alveolar with inspired concentrations is slow. In addition, ether is irritant to the respiratory tract, and so the inspired concentration must be raised slowly. Consequently, the net effect is that induction of anaesthesia is prolonged and recovery slow. Because of its high blood/gas solubility, inspired concentrations of ether are raised gradually to 20% for induction of anaesthesia, compared with 2–3% for halothane.

The other notable physical characteristic of ether is that it possesses a latent heat of vaporisation of 89 cal/g (c.f. halothane, 35 cal/g). These two factors have dictated the design of ether vaporisers. Provision is made to avoid significant cooling of the ether which would lead to decreased vaporisation (e.g. the use of a large water jacket as in the EMO apparatus). Ether vaporisers are often rather large in consequence.

Respiratory system. Since ether is very soluble, the rate-limiting factor in induction is alveolar ventilation. Ether stimulates respiration, and minute volume increases with depth of anaesthesia until surgical anaesthesia is achieved. Ether is irritant to the respiratory tract and if the concentration is increased too rapidly, coughing or breath holding occurs. Stimulation of salivary secretions occurs and premedication with atropine or hyoscine is recommended. Ether dilates bronchi and bronchioles and is therefore useful in patients with bronchospasm.

Respiratory stimulation caused by ether is a result of:

1. Direct stimulation of the respiratory centre.

2. Stimulation of receptors at the lower end of the respiratory tract.

3. Stimulation of pulmonary stretch receptors.

4. Stimulation of extrapulmonary stretch receptors.

5. Occasionally, development of a metabolic acidosis — usually in young children or associated with lactic acidosis secondary to liver disease.

Pa_{CO_2} is maintained at normal levels with ether until deep planes of surgical anaesthesia are achieved when respiratory depression occurs and precedes cardiovascular depression. However, if opioid premedication is used, the minute volume decreases during induction of anaesthesia and Pa_{CO_2} increases.

Cardiovascular system. In vitro, ether is a direct myocardial depressant. However, in vivo, more complex changes occur. Myocardial depression is counteracted by sympathetic stimulation. Ether should therefore be used with caution in patients who are receiving β-blocking or ganglion-blocking drugs or in combination with spinal or extradural anaesthesia. In general there is no decrease in cardiac output until deep levels of anaesthesia are attained or the patient's sympathetic system is compromised. Cardiac irregularities are seen rarely with ether as it does not cause sensitisation of the myocardium to catecholamines. It is safe to use ether when adrenaline is administered in combination with local anaesthetic agents.

Skeletal muscle. Ether relaxes skeletal muscle by two mechanisms:

1. Depression of spinal reflexes.
2. Antidepolarising action at the motor end-plate.

Ether therefore potentiates the effects of nondepolarising muscle relaxants.

Gastro-intestinal tract. Ether depresses the smooth muscle of the intestine; this is related directly to the blood concentrations of ether. The drug is emetic by two mechanisms.

1. Solution in saliva, which is swallowed and causes irritation to the stomach.
2. Stimulation of the vomiting centre.

Metabolism. Patients may develop respiratory acidosis if ventilation is depressed. Ether stimulates gluconeogenesis (glycogen $\rightarrow$ glucose) and hence induces hyperglycaemia. In those patients whose glycogen stores are impaired, ketone bodies may be formed, with consequent metabolic acidosis. 85–90% of ether is exhaled unchanged via the lungs. Approx. 4% is metabolised in the liver to acetaldehyde and ethanol.

The American National Halothane Study demonstrated that ether was one of the safest anaesthetic agents, with the lowest rates of hepatic damage and mortality.

Trichloroethylene

History

Trichloroethylene has been used as an industrial solvent and degreasing agent since its discovery in 1864. In 1934, Jackson of Cincinnati described its anaesthetic properties, though the toxic symptoms seen in those who worked with trichloroethylene had been known for some time. Its use in Britain was popularised by Hewer and Hadfield in 1941.

Manufacture

When acetylene is treated with chlorine, tetra-chloroethane is formed. This reacts in a calcium hydroxide slurry to form trichloroethylene, which is purified by distillation.

$$C_2H_2 + 2Cl_2 \rightarrow C_2H_2Cl_4$$
$$2C_2H_2Cl_4 + Ca(OH)_2 \rightarrow 2C_2HCl_3 + CaCl_2 + 2H_2O$$

Trichloroethylene

usually written
$$\underset{CCl_2}{\overset{CHCl}{\|}}$$

Physical properties

Trichloroethylene is a colourless liquid with a smell similar to that of chloroform. Because of its similarity to chloroform, trichloroethylene is coloured blue for anaesthetic use and marketed under the trade name 'Trilene'. It contains 0.01% thymol to retard decomposition.

Molecular weight 131.

Boiling Point 87°C — i.e. low volatility.

Saturated vapour pressure 60 mmHg (8 kPa) at 20°C.

Blood/gas solubility 9.0 at 37°C.

Oil/water solubility 400.

MAC 0.17.

Vapour density 4.35.

Flammability: trichloroethylene is not flammable in oxygen or air in the concentrations used in anaesthesia.

Stability

Trichloroethylene is converted into hydrochloric acid and phosgene on contact with heat or sunlight. The drug should therefore be stored in metal containers or brown glass bottles. Trichloroethylene must not be used with soda-lime since:

1. Heat decomposes trichloroethylene with the formation of phosgene and hydrochloric acid.

2. Heat in the presence of alkali converts trichloroethylene into hydrochloric acid and

$$\underset{CCl_2}{\overset{CHCl}{\|}} \quad \overset{NaOH}{\rightarrow} \quad \underset{CCl}{\overset{CCl}{\|\|}} + HCl$$

Dichloracetylene

$$\underset{CCl}{\overset{CCl}{\|\|\|}} + O_2 \rightarrow COCl_2 + CO$$

Phosgene

dichloracetylene, the latter combining with oxygen to form carbon monoxide and phosgene.

Pharmacology

Uptake and distribution. Trichloroethylene is relatively soluble in blood and therefore induction and recovery are prolonged. Because trichloro-ethylene is highly soluble in lipid, induction and maintenance are difficult, particularly in the obese patient. Recovery is also more prolonged than in the asthenic patient.

The high lipid solubility correlates with the high potency of the agent. However, because of its low SVP, it is difficult to administer trichloroethylene in useful concentrations and the drug is therefore frequently described (incorrectly) as a weak anaesthetic.

Respiratory system. Trichloroethylene is moderately irritant to the respiratory tract, though less so than ether. It causes rapid shallow respiration (tachypnoea) often associated with hypoxia and hypercapnia as a result of stimulation of lung stretch and deflation receptors.

Cardiovascular system. Arterial pressure, pulse rate and forearm blood flow remain stable during trichloroethylene anaesthesia. However, almost every type of arrhythmia has been described, particularly when high concentrations are used although supraventricular are more common than ventricular arrhythmias. The incidence of ventricular arrhythmias is increased by the use of adrenaline. Deaths have been reported from primary cardiac failure with trichloroethylene.

Gastro-intestinal tract. Trichloroethylene causes a high incidence of postoperative nausea and vomiting.

Skeletal muscle. Trichloroethylene causes little muscular relaxation.

Uterine muscle. In analgesic concentrations (<0.5% in air) trichloroethylene has no effect on uterine contractions. However, in higher concentrations it depresses myometrial contractility.

Metabolism. Trichloroethylene is metabolised extensively. 20–30% of the drug is metabolised to trichloroethanol (which is conjugated with glucuronic acid) and trichloroacetic acid, which is excreted in the urine.

The place of trichloroethylene in clinical practice

Trichloroethylene is a good analgesic and is often used for its analgesic rather than hypnotic properties. It therefore retains a place in obstetric analgesia. The Emotril and Tecota inhalers are designed to administer between 0.35%–0.5% trichloroethylene in air, and their use was approved by the Central Midwives Board until 1983.

In anaesthetic practice, the good analgesic effect of trichloroethylene has made it useful as an adjunct to a relaxant technique. It is particularly useful in obstetric anaesthesia for Caesarian section, where low concentrations may be used to avoid awareness in the mother, and to produce analgesia.

Trichloroethylene may also be useful when nitrous oxide is contraindicated, e.g. pneumothorax.

Although trichloroethylene has disadvantages

(i) respiratory depression
(ii) cardiac irregularities
(iii) forms phosgene with soda-lime
(iv) slow induction and recovery

it still has a useful place in clinical practice as it is:

(i) noninflammable
(ii) safe — in the ventilated patient
(iii) good analgesic
(iv) cheap.

In the spontaneously breathing patient trichloroethylene anaesthesia is reserved for minor surgery since it is difficult to achieve a deep level of anaesthesia, and muscle tone is well maintained.

Methoxyflurane

History

The first use of methoxyflurane in man was described by Artusio and colleagues in 1960. After its introduction, it was used widely but its popularity declined after the description of toxic reactions. It is still available for clinical use.

Formula

$$H - \underset{\underset{Cl}{|}}{\overset{\overset{Cl}{|}}{C}} - \underset{\underset{F}{|}}{\overset{\overset{F}{|}}{C}} - O - \underset{\underset{H}{|}}{\overset{\overset{H}{|}}{C}} - H$$

2,2-dichloro-1,1-difluoroethyl methyl ether

Physical properties

Methoxyflurane is a clear, almost colourless, volatile liquid with a characteristic fruity odour. The B.P. and U.S.P. preparations contain 0.01% w/w butylated hydroxytoluene as an antioxidant.

Molecular weight 165.
Boiling point 105°C.
Saturated vapour pressure 23 mmHg (3 kPa) at 20°C.
Blood/gas solubility 13 at 37°C.
Oil/water solubility 400.
MAC 0.16.

Methoxyflurane has a noncorrosive vapour. It is compatible with soda-lime.

Flammability: nonflammable under ordinary conditions, but burns in oxygen at higher temperatures and concentrations.

Pharmacology

Uptake is extremely slow due to its low potential alveolar concentrations and high blood/gas solubility. Its low MAC indicates high potency.

Metabolism. Like enflurane and isoflurane, methoxyflurane is a halogenated ether. Some of the inhaled dose is excreted unchanged through the lungs. A significant amount (perhaps 50–70%) is metabolised to oxalic acid, fluoride ion, carbon dioxide, dichloracetic acid and methoxyfluoracetic acid. The two of these metabolites (especially fluoride ion) have been held responsible for the occurrence of 'high output renal failure' where the distal convoluted tubule becomes insensitive to the effects of antidiuretic hormone. Concentrations of fluoride ion reach a peak on the second to fourth post anaesthetic day. The incidence of renal toxicity seen with this agent is small, possibly as low as 0.03% of administrations. It is now recommended that total dose be restricted to less than 2 MAC-hours to maintain fluoride ion concentrations below toxic levels.

Respiratory system. Increased respiratory frequency and decreased tidal volume are seen at light levels of anaesthesia. This is particularly evident in the absence of opioid premedication. At deeper levels of anaesthesia there is a marked reduction in expired minute volume and assisted or controlled ventilation is required.

Cardiovascular system. Arterial pressure decreases with increasing depth of anaesthesia. This is due mainly to a reduction in cardiac output, with peripheral resistance being relatively unchanged. Pallor of the face and extremities is a feature of deep anaesthesia, even in the presence of hypercapnia. There has been no report of increased endogenous catecholamine secretion during methoxyflurane anaesthesia, nor is there evidence that methoxyflurane sensitises the myocardium to the effects of exogenous catecholamines.

Uterine muscle. Contractions of the uterus are not inhibited by methoxyflurane.

Central nervous system. Slowing of cerebral function has been seen following administration of this agent. Cerebral blood flow is increased by inhalation of methoxyflurane.

Muscle relaxation. There is no evidence of potentiation of neuromuscular blockade by methoxyflurane. Muscle relaxation is good, but can be variable.

Uses/advantages

1. Now rarely used in clinical anaesthesia, but does provide profound analgesia during the recovery phase.

2. Occasionally used for analgesia. In childbirth 0.35% methoxyflurane in air may be administered by midwives. This is provided by the Cardiff Inhaler — a draw over fixed output version of the Cyprane 'TEC' vaporiser used on anaesthetic machines.

3. Chemically stable at clinical concentrations.

4. Cheap agent, cf new halogenated ethers and halothane.

Disadvantages

1. Toxicity associated with prolonged use.
2. Long postanaesthetic 'hangover'.
3. Very slow induction.

Halothane

History

With the increased use of diathermy and other electrical apparatus in operating theatres in the 1940s there was a need for a safe, potent, nonflammable, nonexplosive, volatile anaesthetic agent. In 1951 Suckling manufactured halothane, which was released into clinical practice in 1956 in the U.K. and in the U.S.A. in 1958.

Formula

$$F - \underset{\underset{F}{|}}{\overset{\overset{F}{|}}{C}} - \underset{\underset{Cl}{|}}{\overset{\overset{Br}{|}}{C}} - H$$

2-bromo-2-chloro-1,1,1-trifluoroethane

Physical properties

Halothane is colourless and has a sweet, pleasant smell.

Molecular weight 197.

Boiling point 50°C.

Latent heat of vaporisation at boiling point 35.2 cal/g.

Saturated vapour pressure 243 mmHg (32.4 kPa) at 20°C.

Oil/water solubility 220.

Blood/gas solubility 2.5 at 37°C.

MAC 0.75.

Flammability: mixtures of halothane in air and in oxygen are nonflammable in the concentrations used in anaesthetic practice.

Halothane is mixed with 0.01% w/w thymol as a stabilising agent. It should be stored in a closed container away from light and heat.

Halothane is safe to use with soda-lime. In the presence of a naked flame, halothane decomposes to form bromine though under normal conditions this is unlikely to be a hazard. Halothane does not damage metals when dry but in the presence of moisture may corrode aluminium, tin, lead, magnesium and alloys including solder or brass. Rubber and certain plastics expand and deteriorate in the presence of halothane.

Pharmacology

Uptake and distribution. Since it is relatively insoluble in blood (blood/gas solubility 2.5) alveolar concentration equilibrates rapidly when inspired. As alveolar concentration may be assumed to be equivalent to brain tension, induction of anaesthesia is relatively rapid and recovery is also rapid.

Halothane is a potent anaesthetic agent (MAC 0.75). Because of its potency, safe administration requires fine control of the vapour concentration. Specially designed temperature and flow controlled vaporisers are essential.

Metabolism. Approx. 20% of halothane is metabolised in the liver normally by oxidative pathways, and the end products excreted in the urine. Metabolism of halothane is of particular interest because it is generally held that the extremely rare liver damage occurring after halothane anaesthesia is related to metabolites formed by reductive pathways. The major metabolites are bromine, chlorine, trifluoroacetic acid and trifluoroacetylethanol amide. These metabolites, and halothane itself, are not hepatotoxic.

Respiratory system. Halothane is nonirritant and pleasant to breathe during induction of anaesthesia. During induction there is rapid loss of pharyngeal and laryngeal reflexes and this, associated with inhibition of salivary and bronchial secretions, ensures that an airway may usually be well maintained without endotracheal intubation.

Five to ten minutes after the introduction of halothane, there is an increase in respiratory rate, and reduction in tidal volume, resulting in an unchanged or decreased minute volume. The Pa_{CO_2} does not increase as much as would be expected from the decrease in minute volume, probably because of decreases in metabolic rate and carbon dioxide production. Oxygen uptake is decreased.

Tachypnoea may be associated with halothane administration, but unlike trichloroethylene, halothane does not increase either the resistance of the lungs to inflation, or the tone of abdominal muscles.

Clinically, halothane has been shown to be a useful agent in patients with chronic bronchitis or emphysema. There is a decrease in bronchomotor tone, and halothane may be used to relieve bronchospasm associated with anaesthesia.

Cardiovascular system. The effect of halothane on the cardiovascular system is a complex inter-reaction of peripheral and central effects. In isolated preparations, profound myocardial depression occurs. In patients under controlled ventilation at normocapnia, the systemic vascular resistance is unchanged and hypotension results almost entirely from a reduction in cardiac output. However, in spontaneously breathing patients, some degree of hypercapnia occurs with a reduction in systemic vascular resistance, and some improvement in cardiac output.

There is a reduction in myocardial oxygen demand associated with reductions in myocardial contractility, left ventricular wall tension, heart rate and cardiac work. However, decreased myocardial contractility results in a lower mean aortic pressure and an increased left ventricular end-diastolic pressure (LVEDP), which may impair oxygen supply and result in decreased subendocardial perfusion. Though there is both myocardial depression and decreased myocardial blood flow, the coronary arteries remain reactive to vasodilator or constrictor influences. Provided that undue elevations in LVEDP and hypotension do not occur, halothane may be advantageous in patients with coronary artery disease because of the reduced oxygen demand caused by bradycardia and decreased contractility.

Heart rate 1. Vagal effect — halothane produces a bradycardia readily reversed by atropine.

2. Arrhythmias — almost all types of ventricular arrhythmia may occur during halothane anaesthesia; the incidence is increased in the presence of hypercapnia or hypoxia. Unlike other anaesthetic agents halothane does not produce an increase in circulating catecholamines.

During local infiltration with adrenaline-containing local anaesthetic solutions, multifocal extrasystoles and sinus tachycardia have been observed and cardiac arrest has been reported. Thus caution should be exercised when these solutions are used during halothane anaesthesia and the following recommendations have been made in respect of safe use:

(i) avoid hypoxia and hypercapnia

(ii) avoid concentrations of adrenaline greater than 1 in 100 000

(iii) avoid a dose in adults exceeding 10 ml of 1 in 100 000 in 10 min or 30 ml/h.

The use of β-blocking agents either prophylactically or for therapy of arrhythmias is only partially effective. Beta-blocking drugs must be used with great caution in the presence of halothane if severe myocardial depression is to be avoided. The newer agents, enflurane and isoflurane are safer than halothane as the dose threshold for catecholamine-induced arrhythmias is greatly elevated.

Arterial pressure. There is a reduction in arterial pressure during halothane anaesthesia. This results particularly from depression of myocardial contractility and bradycardia and may be antagonised partly by atropine.

Gastro-intestinal tract. The incidence of nausea and vomiting is small. Halothane depresses gastro-intestinal motility.

Uterus. Halothane relaxes uterine muscle in direct proportion to the concentration used. It is safe in low concentrations (< 0.5%) and reduces the likelihood of awareness during anaesthesia for Caesarian section. Halothane should be used with caution in higher concentrations as increased uterine bleeding unresponsive to oxytocics may occur.

Skeletal muscle. Halothane produces a useful clinical degree of skeletal muscle relaxation and it potentiates the nondepolarising muscle relaxants. Shivering during the early postoperative period is not uncommon, and may increase oxygen requirements, resulting in hypoxia. Methylphenidate is useful in treatment of shivering caused by halothane.

Liver. Halothane itself is not hepatotoxic although there have been reports of extensive liver damage associated very rarely with its use. It is now known that halothane has a reductive metabolic pathway with intermediate hepatotoxic metabolites. The reductive pathway is stimulated by hypoxia. The risk of postoperative liver dysfunction associated with halothane is increased in the presence of:

1. Obesity — as a result of increased tissue hypoxia and greater storage capacity for the anaesthetic.

2. Hypoxaemia.

3. Short interval between administration — four weeks to three months.

4. Enzyme induction by drugs, e.g. phenobarbitone, phenytoin.

In summary, halothane is a very useful inhalational anaesthetic agent. Its main advantages are:

1. Rapid smooth induction
2. Minimal stimulation of salivary and bronchial secretions
3. Bronchodilation
4. Muscle relaxation
5. Rapid recovery

The disadvantages are:

1. Poor analgesia
2. High cost
3. Arrhythmias
4. Postoperative shivering
5. Possibility of postoperative liver dysfunction.

Enflurane

History

Enflurane was synthesised first by Ohio Medical Products and underwent animal experiments in 1963. It was first evaluated clinically in 1966. Enflurane has been used in the USA since 1971.

Formula

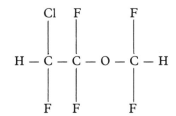

2-chloro-1,1,2-trifluoro-ethyl difluoromethyl ether

Physical properties

Enflurane is clear and colourless with a pleasant ethereal smell.

Molecular weight 184.5

Boiling point 56°C

Saturated vapour pressure 175 mmHg (23.3 kPa) at 20°C

Specific gravity 1.52 at 20°C

Blood/gas solubility 1.9 at 37°C

Oil/water solubility 120
MAC 1.68
Flammability: enflurane is nonflammable.
Enflurane is a stable solution. The vapour is noncorrosive and compatible with soda-lime.

Pharmacology

Uptake and distribution. Because of the low blood/gas solubility coefficient of enflurane there is rapid equilibration between alveolar and arterial partial pressures. Therefore, induction is rapid. Enflurane is less fat soluble than halothane, and emergence is more rapid. The MAC value is twice that of halothane; it is therefore half as potent.

Metabolism. All fluorinated ethers are metabolised in the liver to nonvolatile products which are excreted in the urine. Methoxyflurane, another fluorinated ether, is known to produce inorganic fluoride ions during its metabolism in quantities sufficient to cause nephrotoxic damage in man. To date, extensive trials have not demonstrated toxic levels of fluoride ions after administration of enflurane.

Enflurane has undergone extensive trials to examine its effect on the liver and so far, no major problems have been detected.

Evidence suggests that there is little risk of teratogenesis associated with the use of enflurane in clinical practice.

Respiratory system. Enflurane vapour is nonirritant and does not increase salivary or tracheobronchial secretions. Therefore, induction is pleasant and smooth. Reduction of laryngeal reflexes is not as great as with halothane.

Enflurane causes more profound respiratory depression than halothane in equipotent concentrations. In common with halothane, enflurane is suitable for patients with obstructive lung disease, as it causes bronchodilation and no increase in secretions.

Cardiovascular system. Enflurane is directly depressant to the myocardium, and more so than halothane. At equal MAC concentrations, enflurane causes greater depression of myocardial contractility and cardiac output than halothane and a small reduction in systemic vascular resistance at normocapnia (no change with halothane). Con-

sequently there is a greater degree of hypotension than halothane produces. In contrast with halothane, enflurane causes a reflex tachycardia.

Arrhythmias are uncommon and there is less sensitisation of the myocardium to catecholamines than with halothane. Enflurane appears to be the agent of choice when there are high circulating levels of endogenous or exogenous catecholamines.

Uterus. Enflurane relaxes uterine musculature in a dose-related manner. Initially, it was suggested that it caused a diminished response to oxytocics though in a therapeutic dosage this has been found not to be so. Enflurane is useful for reducing the incidence of awareness at Caesarian section.

Central nervous system. Enflurane produces a dose-dependent depression of e.e.g. activity but at moderate to high concentrations ($>3\%$) it produces epileptiform paroxysmal spike activity and burst suppression. These are accentuated by hypocapnia. Twitching of the face and arm muscles may be seen. It is therefore avoided in the epileptic patient.

Muscle relaxation. Enflurane produces dose-dependent depression of neuromuscular transmission. It potentiates nondepolarising neuromuscular blocking drugs (to a greater extent than halothane) and dosage must be reduced accordingly.

Enflurane is a useful agent in clinical practice. Its particular advantages are:

1. Rapid recovery
2. Pleasant induction
3. Little biotransformation (less than 1–2%, implying little risk of hepatic dysfunction)
4. Inhalational agent of choice with high circulating levels of endogenous or exogenous catecholamines.

Isoflurane

History

Isoflurane was developed in 1965 by Ohio Medical Products, New Jersey. Although clinical studies were undertaken in 1970, because of early laboratory reports of carcinogenesis which were not subsequently confirmed, it was only approved by the United States Food and Drug Administration in 1980.

It is a fluorinated chlorinated ether and is an isomer of enflurane.

F   H   F

H — C — O — C — C — F

F   Cl   F

1-chloro-2,2,2-trifluoro-ethyl difluoromethyl ether

Isoflurane is chemically stable.

Physical properties

Molecular weight 184.5

Boiling point 49°C

Saturated vapour pressure 250 mmHg (32 kPa) at 20°C

Blood/gas solubility 1.4 at 37°C

Oil/water solubility 174

MAC value 1.15

Flammability: isoflurane is nonflammable

From its physical characteristics isoflurane should produce a more rapid induction than halothane. Unfortunately, it is more irritant and this limits its usefulness.

Pharmacology

Metabolism. Negligible quantities of isoflurane undergo biotransformation and therefore the likelihood of the drug producing hepatic dysfunction is also negligible.

Respiratory system. Respiratory depression occurs in a dose-related manner similar to that for enflurane.

Cardiovascular system. Whilst isoflurane is also a myocardial depressant in vitro, the drug causes less reduction in cardiac output than either halothane or enflurane (Table 8.3).

Central nervous system. Because isoflurane is a structural isomer of enflurane it was thought that it might produce similar e.e.g. changes but this is not so.

Table 8.3 Comparison of cardiovascular effects of volatile anaesthesic agents

	Mean arterial pressure	PVR	HR	RAP	CO
Halothane	↓	↔	↓	↑↑	↓↓
Enflurane	↓↓	↓	↑↑	↑↑	↓↓↓
Isoflurane	↓↓↓	↓↓	↑	↑	↓

FURTHER READING

Adams A P 1981 Enflurane in clinical practice. British Journal of Anaesthesia 53: 275
Churchill-Davidson H C 1978 A practice of anaesthesia. Lloyd-Luke, London
Farman J V 1981 Some long established agents — a contemporary review. British Journal of Anaesthesia 53: 115
de Jong R H, Eger E 1975 MAC expanded AD 50, AD 95 values in common inhalational anesthetic agents in man. Anesthesiology 42: 384

Medishield 1967 General information on gases and cylinders. British Journal of Anaesthesia 39: 343
McCaughey W 1972 A summary of the National Halothane Study. British Journal of Anaesthesia 49: 371
Nitrous oxide death 1967 Editorial, Lancet 2: 930
Parbrook G D 1968 Therapeutic uses of nitrous oxide. British Journal of Anaesthesia 40: 365
Smith G 1981 Halothane in clinical practice. British Journal of Anaesthesia 53: 17S

9

Intravenous anaesthetic agents

CHARACTERISTICS OF AN IDEAL INTRAVENOUS ANAESTHETIC AGENT

The physical properties of an ideal i.v. induction agent include stability in solution, a long shelf-life, and water solubility. Lipid-soluble drugs require solutions which are viscous, occasionally produce pain on injection and frequently cause side effects.

The drug should be nonirritant if injected extravascularly. A low incidence of venous thrombosis following injection is an important requirement. Pain on intra-arterial injection of a small amount is a useful property if further harmful injection is to be avoided.

The drug should produce its action in one arm–brain circulation time. In addition, it should produce a rapid recovery with little hangover effect. Redistribution to non-nervous tissue and rapid detoxication to inert metabolites is ideal. However, a drug with an ultrashort duration of action may increase the incidence of awareness.

Analgesic properties are very useful. Excitatory effects (tremor, spontaneous involuntary muscle movements and hypertonus) on induction are undesirable, as are coughing, hiccup and laryngospasm.

The ideal i.v. anaesthetic agent should have a negligible effect on the cardiovascular system and should not depress respiration.

Intravenous anaesthetics should not interact with neuromuscular blocking drugs and should not depend on cholinesterases for inactivation. An ideal agent should have a very low incidence of hypersensitivity reaction and histamine release even in atopic patients and those who show a sensitivity to other drugs. Exposure to the drug should not sensitise the patient to subsequent administration. An agent which produces postoperative nausea and vomiting is undesirable, as is one which causes emergence delirium or unpleasant dreams and hallucinations.

No currently available i.v. induction agent matches the characteristics of an ideal drug (Table 9.1).

BARBITURATES

The barbiturates include both rapidly and slowly acting drugs (Table 9.2).

Structure-activity relationship

Barbituric acid (Fig. 9.1) is constituted from malonic acid and urea and is inert hypnotically, but substitutions in the 1, 2, or 5 positions of the ring produce compounds which are suitable for i.v. anaesthesia.

The anaesthetically active barbiturates are classified into four chemical groups (Table 9.3).

Substitution of a sulphur atom for the oxygen at position (2) produces a thiobarbiturate. These compounds are lipid soluble and are invariably rapidly-acting.

Substitution of a methyl group for the H atom at position (1) produces a rapidly acting drug with a shortened duration of action. The methyl group also confers convulsive activity, of which tremor, involuntary movement and hypertonicity are manifestations.

Increasing the number of carbon atoms in substituted groups at position (5) increases the potency of the agent. The presence of an aromatic nucleus in an alkyl group which is attached directly at position (5) produces compounds with convulsant properties. Direct substitution with a phenyl group confers anticonvulsant activity.

Table 9.1 Main actions of intravenous anaesthetics (after Dundee 1979)

Physical properties	Thio-pentone	Metho-hexitone	Propa-nidid	Althe-sin	Keta-mine	Etomi-date
Water soluble	+	+	−	−	+	+*
Stable in solution	−	−		+	+	+
Long shelf life	−	−		+	+	+
No pain on intravenous injection	+	−	+	+	+	−
Nonirritant on subcutaneous injection	−	±	+	+	+	
Painful on arterial injection	+	+		−		
No sequelae from intra-arterial injection	−	±	+	+		
Low incidence of thrombosis	+	+	−	+	+	−
Small volume	−	+(2%)	±	+	+	−
Effects on body						
Rapid onset	+	+	+	+	−	+
Recovery due to:						
redistribution	+	+		+	+	
detoxication		+	+	+		
Induction:						
excitatory effects	−	+ +	+	+	+	+ + +
respiratory complications	−	+	−	−	−	−
Cardiovascular:						
arterial pressure reduction	+	+	−	+ +		+
Analgesic	−	−	+	±	+ +	−
Antanalgesic	+	+	−	−	−	?
Interaction with relaxants	−	−	+	−	−	−
Hypersensitivity not uncommon	−	−	+	+ +	−	−
Postop. vomiting	−	−	+ +	−	+ +	
Emergence delirium	−	−	−	−	+ +	−

* Aqueous solution not commercially available.

Table 9.2 Classification of induction agents (Dundee 1975)

Rapidly acting	*Slower acting*
Thiobarbiturates	Phencyclidines (ketamine)
Methylbarbiturates	Tranquillizers (diazepam etc)
Eugenols	Neuroleptic drug combinations
Althesin (steroid)	and i.v. analgesics
Etomidate sulphate (imidazole)	Others: sodium oxybutyrate
	chlormethiazole
	barbiturates

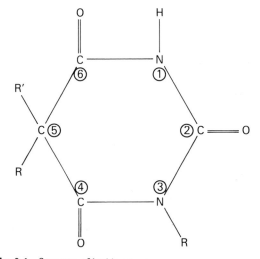

Fig. 9.1 Structure of barbiturate ring.

Table 9.3 Relation of chemical grouping to clinical action of barbiturates

Group	Substituents Position (1)	Position (2)	Group characteristics when given i.v.
Oxy barbiturates	H	O	Delay in onset of action degree depending on 5 and 5′ side chain. Useful as basal hypnotics. Prolonged action
Methyl barbiturates	CH₃	O	Usually rapidly acting with fairly rapid recovery. High incidence excitatory phenomena
Thio barbiturates	H	S	Rapidly acting, usually smooth onset of sleep and fairly prompt recovery
Methyl thio barbiturates	CH₃	S	Rapid onset of action and very rapid recovery but with so high an incidence of excitatory phenomena as to preclude use in clinical practice

Substitution at position (3) on the ring is usually with a sodium salt.

Thiopentone

This is the most commonly used i.v. induction agent and is a rapidly acting thiobarbiturate.

Physical properties

Thiopentone is a yellowish-white hygroscopic powder with a bitter taste and a faint smell of garlic. Anhydrous sodium carbonate 6% is added to the powder to prevent formation of free acid by carbon dioxide from the atmosphere and the powder is contained in an atmosphere of nitrogen. The mixture is readily soluble in water. Thiopentone sodium should be stored in a well-closed container and the solution prepared freshly. The oil water solubility coefficient is 4.7 and the pH of the 2.5% solution is 11.

Pharmacokinetics

Following the administration of a bolus of the drug, mixing in the blood volume occurs, with subsequent diffusion into brain. The anaesthetic effect is determined by the following factors:

1. Blood flow to the brain.
2. pH: only the non-ionised fraction is able to penetrate the lipid barrier between blood and brain and the potency of the drug is dependent on the degree of ionisation at the pH of e.c.f. At a pH of 7.4, 61% of thiopentone is nonionised (pKa 7.6).
3. The relative solubility of the nonionised drug in lipid water.
4. Protein binding: depending on pH, 70–80% of thiopentone is bound to plasma albumin. Hyperventilation increases the nonbound fraction and increases the anaesthetic effect, as a result of increased plasma concentration of free drug. Decreased plasma protein binding occurs in malnutrition and other severe wasting illnesses, with increased sensitivity to thiopentone.

Distribution to other tissues

Figure 9.2 describes the expected distribution of the drug following a single i.v. injection. Thiopentone is injected into the central blood volume from which it is carried rapidly to well-perfused tissues referred to in Figure 9.2 as viscera. (Also termed: vessel-rich

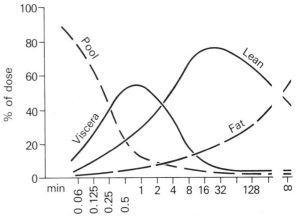

Fig. 9.2 Distribution of thiopentone following bolus i.v. administration.

group, e.g. brain, liver, kidneys and other well perfused viscera.) Equilibrium with muscles is not obtained until approx. 15 min after injection and thereafter the concentration in tissues and viscera declines at a rate parallel to the decrease in plasma concentration. Thiopentone leaves the brain within 1 min. Despite its affinity for fat, uptake by adipose tissue is slow as a result of its poor blood supply. The maximum uptake by fat does not occur until 1 h after uptake by muscles has ceased. Ninety minutes after injection, 50% of the thiopentone should be in fat depots. Twenty-four hours after administration 65–75% of a dose of thiopentone which is still in the body is in the fat depots.

Table 9.4 shows the potential capacity of various organs for the drug as determined by size and tissue/blood partition coefficients. The time constant indicates the time taken for the tissues to become saturated with thiopentone.

Table 9.4 Factors influencing the distribution of thiopentone in the body

	Viscera	Muscle	Fat	Others
Relative blood flow	Rich	Good	Poor	Very poor
Blood flow (litre/min)	4.5	1.1	0.32	0.08
Tissue volume (litre) (A)	6	33	15	13
Tissue/blood partitition coefficient (B)	1.5	1.5	11.0	1.5
Potential capacity (A × B)	9	50	160	20
Time constant (capacity/b.f.) (min)	2	45	500	250

It seems that early awakening following a single injection of thiopentone results primarily from redistribution from viscera and blood to muscle and fat, although there is in addition a small and as yet unknown contribution by metabolism.

Metabolism

Barbiturates are highly lipid soluble and the main mode of detoxication is oxidation and reduction in the endoplasmic reticulum by cytochrome P450. The liver has the largest amount of endoplasmic reticulum and is therefore the major site of metabolism. Hepatic dysfunction prolongs the action of thiopentone.

Excretion

The degree of ionisation governs renal excretion of barbiturates. Unionised drug in the glomerular filtrate diffuses back into the circulation through the renal tubules and even after administration of large doses, only small amounts are present in urine.

Placental transfer

There is no appreciable barrier to the passage of thiopentone to the fetus. Equilibrium between maternal and fetal concentrations occurs in 2–3 min.

Cumulative action

The return of consciousness occurs some time before the return of full mental faculties. An appreciable amount of thiopentone (30%) may remain in the body 24 h after administration and if a patient requires a further anaesthetic within 24 h there is an increased effect from the second dose. This applies to other drugs given during the early recovery period, e.g. alcohol, sedatives. When intermittent doses of thiopentone are given, less drug is necessary after 20–30 min and the duration of action is prolonged.

Factors affecting the distribution of thiopentone

A. Hypovolaemia. Hypovolaemia may result in increased adverse haemodynamic effects. Thiopentone produces vasodilatation resulting in hypotension and alteration in organ perfusion. This decrease in arterial pressure affects the distribution of thiopentone and produces increased intensity and duration of effect. In addition, haemodilution following haemorrhage results in low plasma protein concentrations which produce reduced plasma binding and more free (active) drug. Thus, shocked patients are very sensitive to thiopentone.

B. Anxiety. Larger induction doses of thiopentone are required in anxious patients and duration of action is reduced. In anxiety there is an increased muscle blood flow resulting in a more rapid redistribution of the drug to muscle, with a decrease in brain concentration and reduced duration of sleep.

C. Obesity. As thiopentone is not distributed initially to fat, there is little change in the depth of narcosis or duration of action when normal doses are given. However, when large doses are given over a prolonged period of time there may be a prolongation of narcosis.

Intra-arterial thiopentone

Accidental injection of thiopentone into an artery is a hazard of i.v. anaesthesia. The brachial artery lies in close proximity to the median cubital vein in the antecubital fossa. There may be anatomical variations in arterial supply to the arm, e.g. a superficial ulnar artery lying immediately beneath the median cubital vein without the protection of a bicipital aponeurosis (see Chapter 1).

Intra-arterial injection of thiopentone results in intense, burning pain and may cause gangrene of part of the forearm or fingers. It is produced by an initial intense arterial constriction followed by thrombosis. Intra-arterial injection of thiopentone produces local release of noradrenaline from the vessel wall causing transitory vascular spasm. However, intense chemical endarteritis may occur with stasis and intimal damage leading to thrombosis.

Many years ago, it was demonstrated that crystals of insoluble thiopentone form in the circulation and these may block small blood vessels. The release of ATP from damaged red cells and platelet aggregation initiate the process of thrombosis.

Treatment. The operation must be postponed. If the needle is still in the artery, an α-blocking agent, e.g. tolazoline, should ge given. Brachial plexus block or stellate ganglion block produces vasodilatation of the limb and is recommended. Heparin should be given i.v. and long-term anticoagulation commenced. Thiopentone 2.5% is much safer than 5% thiopentone following intra-arterial injection.

During induction of anaesthesia, it is important to pause after injection of 2 ml of thiopentone and ask the patient if there is pain in the arm or hand.

Extravascular injection

This may result in local tissue necrosis. Infiltration of the area with 1% procaine or hyaluronidase minimises this complication.

Acute tolerance

There is a relationship between the induction dose of thiopentone and the blood concentration at which the patient awakes. With larger induction doses, the patient awakes at a higher blood concentration. In addition the increments of drug required to maintain surgical anaesthesia are increased.

Dose

3–5 mg/kg of 2.5% solution. 5% solution should *not* be used. The dose required varies considerably according to the age and condition of the patient. Only the smallest dose necessary should be given to produce the desired effect. A fatal overdose is administered very easily. Rapid rate of injection produces a quicker and deeper response and a faster recovery.

Thiopentone may be administered rectally to provide basal narcosis. Five or 10% solutions are used, the dose being 1 g/22 kg body weight. The drug is effective 15 min after administration.

Induction characteristics

Induction is smooth and quiet. In some patients, there may be minor limb movements but these are not troublesome. They occur more frequently after the rapid injection of large doses of the drug and the incidence and severity are affected by the nature of the premedication, (reduced by opioids and increased by phenothiazines, hyoscine and other nonanalgesic drugs).

Recovery

Postoperative restlessness is rare and vomiting is infrequent.

Physiological effects

Nervous system. Thiopentone produces effects within 30 s of i.v. injection. It is a poor analgesic and in small doses is antanalgesic. This is responsible for some of the postoperative restlessness found in a small number of patients, especially those in whom pain is a prominent feature.

Reactions to stimuli including surgical incision may occur in the presence of apnoea and apparent deep depression of the central nervous system.

There is significant depression of cerebral utilisation of oxygen during thiopentone anaesthesia. This has led to the suggestion that thiopentone may provide protection of cerebral cells against hypoxia.

Cardiovascular system. Thiopentone causes reduction in cardiac output by peripheral vasodilatation and depression of myocardial contractility. Cardiac irritability is unaffected but arrhythmias may occur in association with hypercapnia or hypoxia. Transient hypotension is proportional to the rate and amount of drug injected.

Respiratory system. Thiopentone depresses the respiratory centre. Following a few deep breaths, a short period of apnoea is common; then respiration begins with a decreased rate and reduced depth of ventilation. Surgical and other stimuli increase the tidal volume during this period. There is a potential danger of respiratory depression in the recovery period as a result of withdrawal of stimulation.

Respiratory depression is dependent on dose, speed of injection and the presence of other central depressants, e.g. morphine. Thiopentone produces a mild degree of bronchoconstriction. Laryngospasm may occur during light thiopentone anaesthesia, although rarely in adequately atropinised patients. The spasm results from relative parasympathetic overactivity and is nearly always associated with stimulation in the region of the larynx, e.g. blood, mucus or gastric contents, or the presence of a laryngoscope blade. The sensitivity of the laryngeal reflexes disappears as the degree of central depression increases.

Musculature. There is a reduction in skeletal muscle tone with increasing central depression.

Indications

1. Induction of anaesthesia.
2. Sedation during local anaesthesia.
3. Control of convulsions during general or local anaesthesia, eclampsia, epilepsy etc.

Precautions

Care must be taken to avoid an overdose in sick and elderly patients and in those who have received opioids or other central depressants.

Contraindications

1. Porphyria. A lower motor neurone lesion may be produced.
2. Airway obstruction, e.g. Ludwig's angina
3. Fixed cardiac output disorders, e.g. mitral stenosis and constrictive pericarditis — vasodilatation may lead to severe hypotension. In addition, great care should be taken in any patient with severe cardiac disease (e.g. angina, cardiac failure), since severe hypotension may occur as a result of myocardial depression and peripheral vasodilatation.

In patients with coronary artery disease or coronary insufficiency, myocardial infarction may be precipitated if excessive hypotension is produced and patients with treated or incipient cardiac failure may be precipitated into cardiac failure.

4. Severe shock: in this situation, arterial pressure is maintained by peripheral vasoconstriction; vasodilatation produced by a normal dose of thiopentone may be fatal.

5. Adrenocortical insufficiency (Addison's disease). Unless there is adequate replacement with cortisone, patients with adrenocortical insufficiency are unable to respond to stress, and may develop profound hypotension.

6. Lack of apparatus to inflate the lungs with oxygen or to perform pharyngeal suction.

Methohexitone

Physical properties

Methohexitone is a white crystalline powder, which is mixed with anhydrous sodium carbonate. It is readily soluble in water to form a solution with pH 10–11. The pKa is 7.9 (75% is nonionised at pH 7.4). It has a low oil/water partition coefficient. In solution, it is stable at room temperature for 6 weeks.

Dose

1–1.5 mg/kg of 1% solution.

Induction characteristics

Loss of consciousness occurs in one arm-brain circulation time.

Methohexitone may cause mild pain on injection. There is a moderate incidence of excitatory phenomena in the form of abnormal muscle movement, coughing and hiccupping. The total dose of the drug and the speed of injection affect the incidence and severity of muscle movement. In addition, this involuntary movement is increased by premedication with promethazine or hyoscine and decreased with opioid analgesics. The incidence of coughing and hiccup is unaffected by premedication but decreased by parasympathetic antagonists, slow injection of the drug and the use of a small total dose.

There is a low incidence of hypersensitivity reactions to methohexitone.

Recovery

With doses of approx. 1 mg/kg, the immediate recovery of consciousness is rapid and occurs in 2–3 min. This is slightly shorter than with equipotent doses of thiopentone or Althesin but longer than after an equipotent dose of propanidid. The active drug circulates for several hours. A tendency for sleepiness is maximal around 4 h after administration and is potentiated by alcohol. Patients should not take alcohol for at least 12 h after day-care anaesthesia and should always be accompanied home.

Physiological effects

Nervous system. Methohexitone is antanalgesic, in common with thiopentone.

Cardiovascular system. Methohexitone produces hypotension of lesser degree and shorter duration than an equipotent dose of thiopentone. This leads to a reflex baroreceptor-mediated tachycardia.

Respiratory system. There is a dose-dependent respiratory depression, of greater magnitude than that following thiopentone.

Indications

Because of its short recovery time, methohexitone is used widely for outpatient anaesthesia, e.c.t. and dental extractions.

Contraindications

Methohexitone is contraindicated in epilepsy since convulsions may be induced in susceptible patients. It is also contraindicated in patients with porphyria, severe cardiac disease and respiratory tract obstruction.

EUGENOLS

Propanidid

Propanidid is an ultrashort-acting induction agent with a rapid recovery. Manufacture of this drug was discontinued in 1984.

Physical properties

Propanidid is a colourless or pale yellow oily liquid derived from oil of cloves. It is insoluble in water, but prepared as a 5% solution in Cremophor EL which is added as a solubilising agent. The mol. wt is 337.4, boiling point 210–212°C, and pH 7.8. The solution is viscous but may be diluted with normal saline.

Metabolism

Propanidid is bound temporarily to plasma proteins and is broken down rapidly by esterases in the liver and plasma. Important metabolic pathways involved in metabolism are: (a) splitting of the ester linkage; (b) splitting of the diethyl amino group.

Ninety per cent of propanidid is eliminated as inactive metabolites in urine within 2 h. Rapid injection produces higher blood concentrations and is associated with more rapid breakdown. There is competition between propanidid and suxamethonium for plasma cholinesterases and thus the effect of suxamethonium is potentiated.

Dose

6–7 mg/kg. It is approximately half as potent as thiopentone.

Induction characteristics

The incidence of venous thrombosis is 4% (approximately twice as great as with thiopentone or methohexitone). Accidental injection into an artery is not followed by vascular complications.

Sleep occurs in one arm–brain circulation time. Six per cent of patients show involuntary muscular movements and 8–9% cough or hiccup. This is a higher incidence than with thiopentone but less than with methohexitone. The incidence is reduced if analgesic premedication has been administered.

Recovery

Recovery is quicker than after thiopentone and occurs in 4–8 min. Propanidid is the least cumulative of all the i.v. anaesthetic agents. There is no potentiation of alcohol 2 h after return of consciousness from propanidid. Recovery is rapid as a result of detoxication by plasma cholinesterase to an acid metabolite with no anaesthetic properties. There is a higher incidence of nausea and vomiting than after i.v. barbiturates.

Physiological effects

Nervous system. The e.e.g. changes are similar to those produced by i.v. barbiturates. A fast, low-voltage activity gives way to progressively slower activity of high voltage (200 μV) followed by bursts of low voltage activity punctuated by periods of electrical silence. The e.e.g. returns to a normal pattern within 20 min of administration.

Cardiovascular system. There is a transient decrease of approx. 30% in arterial pressure resulting from central depression rather than peripheral dilatation. This is accompanied by reflex tachycardia. The decrease is more marked in hypertensive patients. There are a number of reports of acute hypotension or cardiac arrest following induction with a normal dose of propanidid in healthy patients as a result of hypersensitivity reactions.

Respiratory system. The onset of anaesthesia is marked by a period of hyperventilation lasting 15–30 s. This is followed by a variable degree of respiratory depression or even apnoea. This probably results from initial stimulation of the peripheral chemoreceptors, followed by slight depression. The Pa_{O_2} decreases during the period of hypoventilation.

Musculature. A small increase in resting muscle tension may be produced.

Indications

Short surgical procedures where rapid recovery is required. Therefore it is ideal for outpatient work. The hyperventilation facilitates blind nasal intubation. Propanidid may be used in patients with porphyria.

Precautions

The effect of suxamethonium is prolonged and may outlast the period of unconsciousness, leading to paralysis and awareness.

A number of reports of anaphylactic reactions suggest that the drug should be given only when there are positive indications for its use.

STEROIDS

Althesin

Althesin is a mixture of two steroids, alphaxalone and alphadolone acetate, both with a pregnane nucleus and possessing anaesthetic properties. Apart from a weak antioestrogenic action there are no hormonal actions of the steroid. A C—O group in the 3 and 20 positions are essential for anaesthetic activity whereas a double bond between carbon atoms 4 and 5 is essential for hormonal activity.

Manufacture of this agent was discontinued in 1984.

Physical properties

Althesin contains 9 mg/ml of alphaxalone and 3 mg/ml of alphadolone. Both steroids have anaesthetic activity. Alphadolone is approximately half as potent as alphaxalone and is included because it improves the solubility of the latter.

The two drugs are solubilised in 0.25% saline by the addition of 20% w/v polyoxyethylated castor oil (Cremophor EL). This may be diluted with normal saline before injection.

Metabolism

Protein binding is not extensive (50%). The half-life of the drug is 6–8 min. Redistribution is the principle mechanism in rapid return of consciousness following a single dose. The actions of the drug are terminated by active hepatic metabolism, and the breakdown products are excreted in the bile. Seventy per cent appears in faeces and 30% in urine following enterohepatic recirculation. There is little cumulation in tissues.

Dose

0.05–0.1 ml/kg. Althesin has a high therapeutic ratio (four times as great as i.v. barbiturates).

Induction characteristics

Althesin produces loss of consciousness in approx. 30 s with a duration of approx. 5–10 min, depending on dose. It is painless on i.v. injection, nonirritant to tissues, and thrombophlebitis is seldom a problem. Induction is not as smooth as with thiopentone but the small amount of muscle movements which occur are of little clinical significance and less than with methohexitone. Cough, hiccup and laryngospasm are rare after Althesin. Surgical anaesthesia persists for approximately half the duration of unconsciousness (approx. 2–3 min). After the onset of unconsciousness there is good muscle relaxation.

Recovery

Recovery is faster than following equivalent doses of thiopentone and there is less hangover effect. This results from the rapidity of both redistribution and breakdown. Recovery is similar to that following methohexitone. There is a low incidence of postoperative nausea, vomiting, excitement and venous thrombosis. Mild euphoria on recovery and uncontrollable weeping have been reported.

Physiological effects

Nervous system. The e.e.g. is different from that seen with i.v. barbiturates in that burst suppression is very commonly seen even in light planes of anaesthesia.

Some retrograde amnesia occurs with Althesin.

Cerebral blood flow, cerebral oxygen consumption and intracranial pressure are all reduced by Althesin.

Althesin is neither analgesic nor antanalgesic.

Cardiovascular system. Following injection there is peripheral vasodilatation with slight flushing of the skin. Central venous pressure decreases and hypotension of 10–20% results. Reflex tachycardia occurs and this is associated with an increase in threshold to adrenaline-induced arrhythmias. Cardiovascular changes revert to normal over a period of 2–3 min.

Respiratory system. Following induction there may be irregularity of ventilation or a short period of apnoea after which breathing is shallow and rapid. Respiratory rates of approx. 30 breath/min are common in unpremedicated patients. There is a small increase in Pa_{CO_2} and decrease in Pa_{O_2}.

Indications

Althesin may be used as an alternative to the rapidly acting barbiturates. It is useful for outpatient work (because of rapid metabolism) and may be used as the sole agent for short procedures.

Althesin may be used also as a continuous infusion to maintain light sleep in patients on intensive therapy units, and to provide total i.v. anaesthesia for surgical operations. Rapid recovery occurs even after prolonged infusion.

Precautions

The main disadvantage of Althesin as an induction agent is the frequency of anaphylactoid reactions which may occur either on first or subsequent administration. These reactions are manifest clinically as severe bronchospasm and circulatory collapse which may require treatment with adrenaline, antihistamines, corticosteroids and a plasma volume expander. The reported incidence varies from 1 in 11 000 to 1 in 1900. In most instances the complement system is activated to cause anaphylaxis but the initial trigger of either the classical or the alternate pathway of complement activation (see Chapter 19, p. 288) awaits elucidation. It is not known if the drug or the solubilising agent Cremophor EL is primarily responsible for these effects on the immune system. Cremophor EL is known to cause anaphylactoid reactions in cats, dogs and other susceptible species.

Althesin should be used with care in the presence of liver disease. It cannot be used in porphyria.

Minaxolone

Minaxolone is a new water-soluble steroid i.v. anaesthetic. The drug produces more prolonged recovery after short outpatient anaesthesia and infusions than Althesin.

Currently, minaxolone is withdrawn from use because of suspected toxicity.

BENZODIAZEPINES

Midazolam

Midazolam is a rapidly acting water-soluble benzodiazepine. It possesses the typical pharmacological properties of this group, i.e. hypnosis, anxiolysis, muscle relaxation and anticonvulsant activity.

Midazolam has an imidazole ring fused in position 1,2 with the benzodiazepine ring. It is supplied as a colourless solution of 10 mg midazolam base as the hydrochloride in 2 ml aqueous solution.

Dose and induction characteristics

The drug may be used for i.v. sedation or as an i.v. induction agent with total absence of excitatory effects. For sedation, 0.07 mg/kg by slow i.v. injection is given until the patient becomes drowsy (30–100 s). The total dose required is usually 2.5–7.5 mg. The elderly are more sensitive to the drug and require lower doses.

When used as an induction agent in a dosage 0.15–0.5 mg/kg, there is wide variation in response with sleep occurring in approx. 3 min. This variation is a disadvantage on a busy operating list.

Recovery

The mean elimination half-life of midazolam is 2 h and so recovery is significantly faster than with diazepam but slower than thiopentone. The metabolites are inactive and there are no 'hangover' effects.

The effects on the cardiovascular and respiratory systems are usually small. The incidence of venous sequelae is very low.

Indications

Midazolam is indicated for sedation during endoscopy procedures and dentistry. It may also be used as an induction agent for anaesthesia where speed of onset of action is not important.

OTHER DRUGS

Etomidate

Physical properties

Etomidate is a carboxylated imidazole compound unrelated to any other hypnotic. It is a white crystalline powder with a mol. wt of 342.4. It is unstable in aqueous solution but soluble in ethanol and propylene glycol. It is presented commercially in 10 ml ampoules containing 2 mg/ml of the drug dissolved in water with 35% propylene glycol at pH of 8.1. Seventy-eight per cent of the drug is bound to plasma albumin.

Dose

0.2–0.3 mg/kg. The drug is 4 times more potent than methohexitone and 12 times more potent than thiopentone.

Induction characteristics

Consciousness is lost within 10–65 s of administration depending on the rate of injection, dose of drug and type of premedication. Spontaneous involuntary muscle movement, tremor and hypertonus may occur following injection and the incidence is higher than with methohexitone. The frequency of cough and hiccup is similar to that with methohexitone. Pain on injection occurs in 25–50% of patients and this is reduced by fast injection, use of a large vein, or the addition of lignocaine.

Recovery

Recovery is rapid and arousal from a single dose occurs in 6–8 min depending on premedication. The quality of recovery is good with no hangover. Repeated doses are not cumulative. Only 2.5% of the injected dose remains in the circulation 2 min after administration, at which time peak concentrations are found in the brain and major organs. The drug is quickly broken down by hydrolysis by esterases in liver and plasma. Detectable amounts of etomidate persist in plasma for at least 6 h. Eighty-seven per cent of the total administered drug is excreted in the urine (3% in an unchanged form). Thirteen per cent of the drug is excreted in the bile.

There is a higher incidence of nausea, vomiting and venous sequelae than after thiopentone or methohexitone.

Physiological effects

Nervous system. The e.e.g. pattern of anaesthesia with etomidate is similar to that seen after barbiturates and propanidid. Muscle movements during induction with etomidate are not associated with epileptiform discharges, and therefore probably originate from deep cerebral structures or brain stem. Cerebral blood flow is decreased and in premedicated patients, intraocular pressure is reduced.

Cardiovascular system. Although cardiovascular stability is a feature in healthy individuals, hypotension occurs if etomidate is administered to the hypovolaemic patient. Large doses may produce tachycardia.

Respiratory system. Large doses may be associated with apnoea of up to 45 s duration, but respiratory depression is not a significant problem with clinical doses.

Indications

Etomidate is ideal for outpatients in whom cardiovascular stability and rapidity of recovery are important. The absence of histamine release makes it a suitable alternative to Althesin.

Contraindications

Prolonged i.v infusions may result in reduction in circulating corticosteroids and may increase the incidence of severe infection.

Diprivan

2,6di-isopropyl phenol (ICI 35868)

This is a new induction agent with a rapid recovery time which is faster than thiopentone but slower than propanidid.

The drug is virtually insoluble in water at room temperature and is presented in a concentration of 10 mg/ml in 16% Cremophor EL, or in a lipid emulsion. Plasma protein binding is high (>90%).

Dose

A dose of 2 mg/kg is recommended for induction in unpremedicated patients.

Induction characteristics

Induction time may be dependent on dose and speed of injection. Pain on injection and hypersensitivity reactions have been reported.

Recovery

Recovery is rapid with few side effects. The short duration of action is caused apparently by redistribution and rapid metabolism and thus the drug may be given by repeated injection or continuous infusion without cumulation.

Gamma hydroxybutyric acid

This is a derivative of gamma amino butyric acid, a naturally occurring neurohormone which is an inhibitory transmitter in the nervous system.

It has a slow onset of action (10–15 min) and lasts 60–90 min. It has been used for cardiac catheterisation in children. It is seldom used now in the United Kingdom.

Ketamine

Ketamine hydrochloride is an i.v. induction agent which is not classified as a rapidly acting agent. It is a derivative of phencyclidine and produces dissociation; complete analgesia is combined with only superficial sleep.

Physical properties

Ketamine is prepared in an acid solution and is given either i.v. or i.m. The preparations available are 10, 50 or 100 mg of ketamine base/ml. The 50 and 100 mg solutions contain 1/10 000 benzethonium chloride as a preservative. Ketamine is excreted by conversion to water soluble metabolites by N-demethylation and hydroxylation of the cyclohexanone ring. The breakdown products are excreted in the urine.

Dose

Two mg/kg i.v. produces sleep within 30–90 s, lasting 5–10 min. Repeated doses may be given if a longer effect is desired without significant cumulative effects. Ten mg/kg i.m. produces surgical anaesthesia within 2–8 min with a duration of 10–20 min. A continuous infusion of 50 μg/kg/min has been recommended for the production of analgesia without loss of consciousness for minor surgery.

Induction characteristics

Unlike thiopentone, there is a delay of between 30 and 90 s for onset of sleep when ketamine is given i.v., and between 2–8 min when it is given i.m.

The slow onset of anaesthesia is not a major disadvantage provided it is anticipated. Hypertonus may be a problem and it may be difficult to distinguish between hypertonus and light anaesthesia. Respiratory complications do not occur frequently during induction of anaesthesia with ketamine.

Although the laryngeal reflexes are not depressed markedly with clinical doses of ketamine, the extent to which protective reflexes remain intact is not as great as was originally suggested, particularly in the presence of depressant premedication.

Ketamine produces increased salivation and it is important that patients are given atropine beforehand.

Recovery

Recovery is slower after ketamine than other i.v. induction agents. It is often difficult to know when patients are awake. They may be deeply anaesthetised yet have open eyes and so the normal end-points are difficult to assess. Postoperative nausea and vomiting occur fairly commonly. There are two important aspects of recovery which merit attention:

1. *Emergence delirium or excitement.* This occurs in the immediate postoperative period and patients become disorientated, extremely restless and agitated. These signs are often accompanied by irrational talking or uncontrolled crying or moaning.

2. *Vivid dreams or hallucinations.* These may occur up to 24 h after ketamine. Frequently they have a morbid content and are often experienced in vivid colours.

Emergence disturbances are uncommon in children and the elderly. Females appear to be more prone than males. The absence of premedication and disturbing the patient during arousal increases the incidence. They are uncommon after prolonged surgery.

Heavy premedication with opioid-hyoscine, or opioid-hyoscine-droperidol is effective in reducing emergence delirium but has less effect in preventing unpleasant dreams. Intravenous droperidol, given towards the end of surgery, is also effective against delirium, but not dreams. In contrast, i.v. diazepam, although ineffective against delirium, reduces the incidence of unpleasant dreams. An oral mixture of 10 mg nitrazepam and 20 mg droperidol as premedication before ketamine is reported to reduce the incidence of all sequelae, as does premedication with lorazepam.

Physiological effects

Nervous system. The dual action of ketamine on cerebral activity has led to the use of the term 'dissociative anaesthesia'.

There are persistent marked changes in e.e.g. with dominant theta activity and abolition of alpha rhythm. An increase in cerebral blood flow may give rise to acute increases in intracranial pressure.

Amnesia persists for about 1 h after apparent recovery of consciousness but the drug does not cause retrograde amnesia.

Cardiovascular system. Ketamine stimulates the cardiovascular system causing tachycardia and hypertension. In the absence of depressant premedication, systolic arterial pressure increases by 20–40 mmHg with a slightly smaller increase in diastolic pressure. These changes occur also on subsequent injection. Cardiac output is unchanged or increased. These responses are blocked or attenuated by halothane.

The effects of ketamine are thought to result from veratrine-like facilitation of calcium ion transport across the cell membrane of cardiac muscle and Purkinje fibres, since they are blocked by verapamil.

Ketamine sensitises the heart to small doses of adrenaline and may precipitate arrhythmias in the presence of endogenous or exogenous catecholamines. Ketamine is not vagolytic and the oculocardiac reflex is not abolished in children.

Respiratory system. Respiration is not depressed, except by larger doses. There is better preservation of pharyngeal reflexes and patency of the upper airway than with other i.v. agents. However, obstruction of the airway, laryngeal spasm and inhalation of vomit *do* occur.

Other systems. Ketamine causes an increase in tone of striated muscle and elevation of intraocular pressure.

Adverse effects on the liver or kidneys have not been reported.

Indications

Ketamine may be used as the sole agent for minor operations which do not require muscular relaxation. It is also useful for inducing anaesthesia in poor-risk patients because of its stimulant effect on the cardiovascular system. It is useful in situations where there is difficulty in maintaining an airway (e.g. severe burns or trauma affecting the face or upper airway), and for repeated anaesthetic procedures in small children (e.g. change of burns dressings, ocular examination, radiotherapy, bone-marrow sampling, etc.).

Ketamine is an invaluable agent in the field situation, e.g. trapped casualties and for dealing with the mass disaster situation. In addition there are occasions when an i.m. agent is more useful than an i.v. agent. Ketamine has been used in a 0.1% solution in 5% dextrose as a slow i.v. infusion for postoperative pain relief and for analgesia in patients in the intensive care unit. In higher dosage it has been used for total i.v. anaesthesia.

Precautions

Ketamine is contraindicated in patients with hypertension, a history of cardiovascular accident, raised intracranial pressure, a recent penetrating eye injury or a history of psychiatric disorder.

TOTAL INTRAVENOUS ANAESTHESIA

Operating department pollution and awareness are two problems associated with established methods of anaesthesia. Alternative methods to avoid these problems include local anaesthetic techniques (which are not suitable for all patients) and total i.v. anaesthesia.

There is no i.v. anaesthetic drug which possesses all the characteristics of an ideal agent and so separate agents are used to provide hypnosis, muscle relaxation and analgesia.

The hypnotic should be effective, simple to administer, safe, and rapidly distributed and eliminated so that cumulation is unlikely to occur. Suitable agents for producing hypnosis are Althesin, methohexitone, etomidate and ketamine, the analgesic properties of the last being particularly useful. These are combined with an analgesic (e.g. morphine, fentanyl, alfentanil) and when artificial ventilation is to be employed, a muscle relaxant drug.

ADVERSE REACTIONS TO INTRAVENOUS ANAESTHETIC AGENTS

These may take the form of pain on injection of the agent, venous thrombosis, involuntary muscle movement, hiccup, hypotension and post-operative delirium. All these adverse reactions may be modified by the anaesthetic technique.

Hypersensitivity reactions, which resemble the effects of histamine release, are rarer and less predictable.

Anaphylactoid

Anaphylactoid reactions do not imply a specific mechanism for histamine release whereas *anaphylactic* reactions involve antibody (IgE)-antigen reactions and imply previous exposure to the drug.

Clinical features

The clinical features of a hypersensitivity reaction consist of a rapidly developing flush over the upper half of the body. There is usually hypotension (which may be so severe as to lead to impalpable pulses), and later the development of cutaneous oedema and possibly glottic oedema. Swelling of the eyelids may occur. This oedema may result in the loss of a considerable amount of circulating fluid. Bronchospasm occurs in less than 50% of instances. Rarely, abdominal pain and vomiting may occur.

Incidence

The highest incidence is for propanidid, varying from 1 in 800 to 1 in 1700.

The incidence for Althesin varies from 1 in 1900 to 1 in 11 000 although this is said to be an underestimate.

Reactions to thiopentone are rare (1 in 16 000), but when they occur are more dangerous.

The role of Cremophor EL

Cremophor EL is a mixture of higher fatty acids which is used for solubilising some of the i.v. anaesthetics. There are more adverse reactions to Cremophor-containing anaesthetics.

Mechanism of anaphylactoid reactions

1. *Type I hypersensitivity response.* This type of reaction occurs more commonly following thiopentone than Althesin.
2. *Classical complement mediated reaction.*
3. *Alternative pathway activation of C3.* The majority of Althesin reactions occur in this group.
4. *Pharmacological or chemical release of histamine.*

Predisposing factors

Patients with an atopic tendency (e.g. asthma, hay fever or eczema) or food allergies have a higher incidence of reactions. The chance of a reaction is also increased when the drug is administered on a second occasion, particularly within a short time.

Treatment

Replacement of circulatory blood volume is the most important aspect of treatment as 1–2 litre may be lost rapidly into tissue spaces. The most effective solution is PPF, since crystalloids are lost rapidly through a dilated vascular bed (with increased permeability). Tracheal intubation and oxygenation may be required. Vasoconstrictors may be used, but restoration of vascular volume is more important.

Aminophylline is used for bronchospasm and adrenaline or isoprenaline to increase cardiac output in more severe reactions. Steroids have been advocated, but the value of antihistamines is doubtful.

It is essential to note that i.v. anaesthetic agents must *never* be given in a location devoid of resuscitation equipment.

FURTHER READING

Churchill-Davidson H C 1978 A practice of anaesthesia, 4th edn. Lloyd-Luke, London
Clarke R S J 1982 Hypersensitivity reactions to intravenous anaesthetic drugs. In: Atkinson R S, Langton Hewer C (eds) Recent advances in anaesthesia and analgesia 14. Churchill Livingstone, Edinburgh
Dundee J W 1979 Intravenous anaesthetic agents. Arnold, London
Price H L, Kovnat P J, Safer J N, et al 1960 The uptake of thiopental by body tissues and its relation to the duration of narcosis. Clinical Pharmacology and Therapeutics I: 16
Saidman L J 1974 Uptake, distribution and elimination of barbiturates In: Eger E I (ed) Anaesthetic uptake and action. Williams and Wilkins, Baltimore
Savage T M 1979 New anaesthetic drugs and techniques — enflurane, etomidate and total intravenous anaesthesia. In: Atkinson R S, Langton Hewer C (eds) Recent advances in anaesthesia and analgesia 13. Churchill Livingstone, Edinburgh
Vickers M D, Schnieden H, Wood-Smith F G, 1984 Drugs in anaesthetic practice, 6th edn. Butterworths, London
Watkins J, Milford Ward A 1978 Adverse response to intravenous drugs. Academic Press, London
Whitman J G 1978 Adverse reactions to intravenous agents. British Journal of Anaesthesia 50: 677

10

Drugs used to supplement anaesthesia

This chapter describes the pharmacology of drugs used either for premedication or as an adjunct during anaesthesia.

OPIOIDS

The most commonly used drugs are those with analgesic properties. Formerly these were termed 'narcotics', but since some new drugs induce relatively little physical addiction, the term is inappropriate. The term 'opiate' is also inappropriate as it suggests a derivative of opium. The most appropriate description is 'opioid agonist/antagonist', and commonly used drugs may be classified as follows:

1. Opioid agonists
   a. natural opium alkaloids
      (i) morphine
      (ii) codeine
   b. semisynthetic opium alkaloid
      (i) heroin
   c. synthetic opioids
      (i) pethidine
      (ii) fentanyl
      (iii) alfentanil
2. Opioid agonist/antagonists
   a. pentazocine
   b. buprenorphine
   c. nalbuphine
3. Opioid antagonist
   naloxone.

Morphine and related opioid drugs produce profound analgesia, but there is a high incidence of undesirable side effects which occasionally have dangerous consequences. All the drugs in this group have similar actions and side effects; thus morphine may be discussed in detail and important differences in the other drugs discussed individually.

Mechanism of action

There is a 'spectrum' of analgesic activity ranging from those drugs with pure agonist activity (e.g. morphine) to pure antagonist activity (e.g. naloxone). The opioid antagonist, naloxone, possesses no analgesic properties and is capable of reversing the analgesic and other actions of morphine. Between the ends of this 'spectrum' are drugs which have both agonist and antagonist properties (e.g. pentazocine and buprenorphine). These compounds produce analgesia (i.e. agonism) if given alone, but antagonise analgesia produced by morphine and other pure agonists, and are therefore classified as 'partial agonists' or 'opioid agonist/antagonists'.

There are several peptide compounds (the enkephalins and endorphins) which are formed endogenously, and which possess properties similar to those of exogenously administered opioids. The enkephalins are found in high concentration in the central grey matter of the brainstem and areas of the spinal cord, whereas β-endorphin, structurally a much larger molecule with a longer duration of action, is present in high concentration in the pituitary and has similar endocrine actions to those of morphine.

These substances act by binding to specific 'opioid receptors' which are distributed widely throughout the central nervous system. There are probably several different types of 'opioid receptor' (see Chapter 5) and the reader is referred to the review by Schachter for further information.

Exogenously administered opioids have different

affinities for these receptor sites. Thus the initial mechanism of action of the different opioid-like drugs may be explained by differing degrees of receptor occupancy. Subsequently there is central depression of cholinergically mediated transmission and other types of neurotransmission concerned with analgesia within the central nervous system.

Morphine

Although it is possible to synthesise morphine, it is produced commercially from the dried juices of the seed capsules of the poppy *Papaver somniferum*. Chemically, morphine is a tertiary amine and a weak base, being therefore more water soluble than other opioid derivatives including pethidine and fentanyl which are more lipid soluble.

Actions (Table 10.1)

The actions of morphine may be classified as central and peripheral. Actions on the central nervous system are both depressant and stimulant.

Analgesia

All types of pain are relieved. However, morphine is more effective against dull and continuous than sharp and intermittent pain. In addition to elevation of pain threshold, the psychological (emotional) component of pain is diminished. This effect is augmented by a sensation of euphoria and drowsiness which, as the dose is increased, progresses to sleep and eventually to an anaesthetic state characterised by decreased reflex irritability, and profound respiratory and cardiovascular depression.

Respiratory system

Depression of respiration occurs as a result of direct depression of the medullary respiratory centre. The carbon dioxide response curve is flattened and shifted to the right (Fig. 10.1). Clinically, both respiratory rate and tidal volume are diminished, but the main effect is on rate and occurs within 2–5 min following i.v. injection, and more slowly after i.m. injection.

Cardiovascular system

There is little effect on arterial pressure in normal individuals in the supine position. However, peripheral arteriolar and venous dilatation occur as a result of central depression of the vasomotor centre, a reduction in vasoconstrictor tone, and release of histamine. Hypotension may therefore occur in individuals with a decreased blood volume or to

Table 10.1 Summary of the actions and side effects of morphine

Central	Depressant →	Analgesia
		Sedation
		Depression of cough reflex
		Depression of respiratory centre
		Depression of metabolic rate (hypothermia)
		Depression of vasomotor centre
	Excitatory →	Euphoria, hallucinations
		Convulsions (in high dosage)
		Miosis (stimulation of oculomotor centre)
		Vomiting ⎫ (stimulation of chemoreceptor
		Nausea ⎬ trigger zone)
		Bradycardia (vagal stimulation)
		Release of ADH & other pituitary hormones
Peripheral	Increase in smooth muscle tone	
	Histamine release →	Bronchospasm
		Hypotension
		Erythema
		Sensation of warmth, flushing

whom drugs with vasodilator properties (e.g. phenothiazines) have been administered.

Occasionally bradycardia may occur from stimulation of the vagal centre.

Emesis and nausea

This may be distressing and unpleasant and results from stimulation of the chemoreceptor trigger zone in the floor of the fourth ventricle. It appears to be related to a dopamine-like effect thereby explaining why drugs with powerful dopamine-blocking effects such as the neuroleptic agents (butyrophenones and phenothiazines) are effective antiemetics in opioid-induced vomiting.

Vomiting is a frequent occurrence in the postoperative period, often after several doses of opioid have been given. Persistence of symptoms may continue for some time after administration of the last dose of opioid.

In equianalgesic doses, there is no significant difference between the emetic effects of morphine and other opioid drugs.

Miosis

This results from stimulation of the Edinger-Westphal nucleus of the oculomotor centre. Pupillary constriction is a characteristic feature and may interfere with pupillary responses associated with depth of anaesthesia.

Depression of cough reflex

Depression of the cough centre occurs only with morphine and its derivatives, synthetic drugs (pethidine, etc.) having no direct action. Antitussive effect may impair the restoration of normal laryngeal activity in the immediate postoperative phase.

Other actions

Histamine release. This is responsible for the characteristic flush and sensation of warmth following i.v. injection and erythema at the site of injection.

Bronchospasm occurs occasionally. It may be preferable therefore to avoid morphine in asthmatic patients. Vasodilatation secondary to histamine release probably plays little role in the occurrence of hypotension following morphine.

Increase in smooth muscle tone. Reduced gastrointestinal motility and peristalsis produce delay in gastric emptying, which may be a factor in inducing postoperative vomiting. Slower absorption of orally administered drugs and a tendency to constipation are also features of morphine.

Smooth muscle contraction occurs in the sphincter

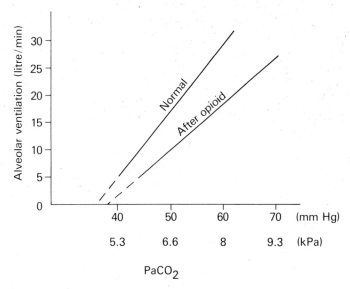

Fig. 10.1 The ventilatory response to arterial P_{CO_2} in the normal individual, and following administration of morphine. Note that not only is the response curve shifted to the right, but its slope is decreased.

of Oddi, ureter and bladder sphincter and therefore morphine should be avoided in biliary and renal colic.

Endocrine effects. These include release of ADH from the anterior pituitary and inhibition of release of ACTH, FSH and LH. These actions resemble those of the endogenous opioids, presumably reflecting their neuro-endocrine function.

Metabolic. Large doses of morphine may contribute to hypothermia by decreasing muscle activity and basal metabolic rate, and increasing heat loss through vasodilatation.

Fate

When administered orally, the bioavailability of morphine is approx. 20% of that following parenteral routes as a result of 'first-pass' metabolism in the liver. Following oral administration maximum effect occurs within 2 h and the duration of effect is approx. 6 h.

Following i.v. and i.m. injection, analgesia reaches a peak in 20 min and $1\frac{1}{2}$ h respectively and the duration is approx. 4 h.

Profound and prolonged analgesia may also be produced by administration of morphine via the extradural and intrathecal routes (see Chapter 23).

Following i.v. administration, one-third of a bolus of morphine is protein bound, the remainder diffusing rapidly and accumulating in paren-chymatous tissues. Plasma concentrations (Fig. 10.2) subsequently depend on metabolism, redistribution back into the vascular compartment, excretion and, to a certain extent, on enterohepatic circulation. Although morphine is regarded clinically as a drug with a longer duration of action than fentanyl, inspection of pharmacokinetic parameters (see Chapter 7) reveals that its clearance is more rapid (Table 10.2). Thus cumulation should present a greater problem with fentanyl than morphine.

Table 10.2

	Vd (litre/kg)	$T_{\frac{1}{2}}\beta$ (min)	Cl (ml/min per kg)
Fentanyl	4	219	13
Alfentanil	0.9	94	6
Morphine	3.2	210	11
Pethidine	4.1	222	11

Morphine is deactivated in the liver by dealkylation, oxidation and conjugation with glucuronide. Both free and conjugated morphine appear in the urine.

Morphine crosses the placental barrier and neonatal respiration may be profoundly depressed.

The dosage varies between 5 and 20 mg i.m. depending on individual circumstances. For i.v. use in supplementing inhalational anaesthesia, smaller doses may be used incrementally depending on the

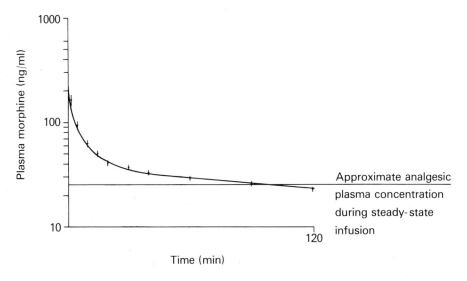

Fig. 10.2 Plamsa morphine concentration following administration of 10 mg morphine by i.v. injection. Initially, the concentration decreases rapidly due to distribution into tissues. The subsequent decline is slower as the drug is metabolised and excreted.

duration of surgery, type of premedication and general health of the patient, although under certain circumstances it is possible to use larger initial doses.

In order to evaluate the correct dose of any opioid, bearing in mind that it is important to avoid the risk of respiratory depression, the following factors must be considered.

1. Age: increased sensitivity to opioids in the elderly.

2. Duration of surgery: in relation to the known duration of the opioid.

3. Concurrent use of other depressant drugs: potentiation of depressant effects of opioids.

4. Concurrent respiratory disease: opioids may precipitate respiratory failure in chronic obstructive airways disease.

5. Conditions limiting respiratory movement: severe kyphosis.

6. Obesity: the risk of hypoventilation as a result of limited diaphragmatic movement

7. Endocrine abnormalities: increased opioid sensitivity in hypothyroidism and Addison's disease.

8. Liver disease: increased sensitivity especially in cirrhosis and infective hepatitis.

9. Miscellaneous:
   a. debilitation
   b. malignancy   } increased sensitivity
   c. chronic infection
   d. intracerebral pathology and head injury — further depression of conscious level and risk of further elevation of intracranial pressure resulting from hypercapnia.

Diamorphine

Diamorphine is a semisynthetic derivative of morphine, with similar actions and side effects. It has approximately twice the potency and a greater euphoric effect than morphine. Its onset of action is more rapid and its duration shorter. Being more lipid soluble it is absorbed more easily by the oral route than morphine.

There are clinical impressions that there is less associated respiratory depression, nausea and vomiting but more sedation than with morphine, although this has not been substantiated in clinical trials. It is, however, a more powerful antitussive agent than morphine.

Diamorphine undergoes rapid deacetylation first to monoacetylmorphine and then very rapidly to morphine and is excreted as the conjugated glucuronide. The average dose is of the order of 4–8 mg for healthy adult males.

Papaveretum

This is a partially purified extract of opium consisting of 50% morphine, the remaining 50% being composed of relatively ineffective opium alkaloids (codeine, thebaine, narcotine and papaverine). There is less interference with gastro-intestinal motility than with pure morphine which is accounted for by the papaverine fraction which is spasmolytic. Papaveretum 20 mg is equipotent with morphine 12.5 mg in terms of analgesia, but there is a greater degree of respiratory depression and sedation. The average dose in an adult is 15–20 mg. Occasionally larger doses are required, but elderly patients require considerably smaller doses.

Buprenorphine

This is a relatively new synthetic analgesic derived from the opium alkaloid thebaine and is closely related to morphine. It has powerful agonist actions and partial antagonist actions with a low potential for physical dependence and addiction. Currently it is not subject to controlled drug regulations.

Buprenorphine has a long duration of action of the order of 6–8 h, resulting from slow dissociation from the drug-receptor complex. The potency is much greater than that of morphine, 0.4 mg being equipotent to 10 mg of the latter.

Euphoria and dysphoria are not marked, but other side effects resemble those of morphine, vomiting and drowsiness being marked. Respiratory depression is similar to that following morphine but in high doses there is a 'ceiling' effect which becomes maximal 3 h after intramuscular injection.

A disadvantage of buprenorphine is that respiratory depression cannot be reversed easily by the use of naloxone. Nonspecific respiratory stimulants (e.g. doxapram) should therefore be used initially.

Dosage varies from between 0.3–0.6 mg for i.v. or i.m. use. Sublingual administration of buprenorphine in a dose of 0.4 mg produces effective analgesia which is more predictable than that following oral administration of other opioid drugs since 'first pass' metabolism in the liver is obviated.

Pethidine

Pethidine is a synthetic opioid with actions similar to morphine but differing in having mild anticholinergic actions.

The analgesic potency of pethidine is less than that of morphine, 100 mg being equipotent to 10 mg of the latter and there is a shorter duration of action, of the order of 2–3 h.

Pethidine produces sedative effects similar to those of morphine but euphoria is not as marked. Respiratory depression is of shorter duration and there is no specific action on cough reflexes other than that produced by sedation.

Actions on the cardiovascular system differ from those of morphine in that there is a mild quinidine-like effect which may reduce myocardial excitability and the incidence of ventricular arrhythmias. This may be related to and associated with the mild local anaesthetic action of pethidine.

Arterial pressure is normally unaffected, but as with morphine, hypotension may occur in patients with decreased circulating blood volume. This effect is related to a reduction in peripheral arterial and venous tone resulting from smooth muscle relaxation.

The actions of pethidine on the gastro-intestinal tract result in either little change in tone, or relaxation. Spasm is often relieved and constipation is less likely to occur than with morphine.

The incidence of nausea and vomiting may be slightly greater with pethidine than morphine, but these side effects are of shorter duration.

Pethidine produces less release of histamine than morphine and therefore it may be preferable for asthmatic patients.

In cases of overdose with pethidine, cerebral hyperexcitability and convulsions may occur. In patients receiving monoamine oxidase inhibitors, the inadvertent administration of pethidine may cause convulsions and coma associated with hypertensive crises. This may be related to inhibition of neuronal reuptake of 5 hydroxytryptamine.

Pethidine is well absorbed by most routes but higher oral doses are required because of 'first pass' hepatic metabolism. In common with all opioids, placental transfer occurs leading to severe fetal depression.

Dosage is of the order of 1–2 mg/kg by i.m. injection. For supplementation of anaesthesia,

boluses of 10 mg may be given i.v. at approx. 20 min intervals, although larger doses may be used depending on the type of premedication used and the size and general health of the patient.

Levorphanol

Levorphanol is 4–5 times more potent than morphine and it possesses the longest duration of action of all the commonly used opioid analgesics (6–8 h). If used i.v. for supplementation of anaesthesia sufficient time should elapse before opioids are used for postoperative pain relief because of persistent respiratory depression.

Levorphanol is much less sedative than morphine and is not effective in relieving anxiety. Nausea and vomiting are also less frequent.

The dosage is approx 0.5 mg/10 kg i.v. depending on patient size, but the dose should be reduced in elderly and frail patients.

Fentanyl

Fentanyl is a synthetic opioid related structurally to pethidine. In combination with droperidol, it forms the basis of neuroleptanalgesia. Analgesic potency is approx. 100 times greater than that of morphine and 1000 times greater than that of pethidine, but the duration of action is relatively short; of the order of 30 min. Repeated doses may be required at shorter time intervals if used as a supplement to inhalational anaesthesia.

The short duration of action is related entirely to rapid redistribution since clearance is slower than that of morphine. Only 10% is excreted unchanged. Provided that the total dose is limited, it is a particularly useful drug for short surgical procedures and possibly day-case surgery.

Fentanyl is much more fat soluble than morphine and crosses the blood–brain barrier more readily thereby having a more rapid onset of analgesia (1–2 min in comparison with 10–15 min for morphine by i.v. route).

Respiratory depression

This may be profound and is dose related, occurring within 1–2 min and becoming maximal in 5 min following i.v. administration.

There have been reports of late respiratory depression occurring following the use of fentanyl. An explanation for this phenomenon awaited elucidation of the pharmacokinetic parameters of fentanyl (Table 10.2). Clinically, the short duration of action is related to redistribution, but if the plasma concentration is maintained relatively high by a large total dose, the slow elimination time produces a prolonged duration of action outlasting that of naloxone or other opioid antagonists or respiratory stimulants.

Cardiovascular effects

Fentanyl has little effect on the cardiovascular system. A small reduction in arterial pressure may occur, but this is related to mild bradycardia from vagal stimulation and effects on peripheral resistance are of little importance.

Other side effects

Sedation is relatively small in comparison with morphine and pethidine. The incidence of nausea and vomiting is similar to that of other opioids.

Very occasionally the so-called 'wooden chest' effect, typified by chest wall rigidity, occurs. This is a feature of fentanyl and alfentanil in large doses, but it may occur with all opioid drugs. It is overcome easily by the administration of a muscle relaxant.

Fentanyl causes less release of histamine than pethidine and there appears to be freedom from constipation.

Dosage

This varies with the length and nature of surgery. For spontaneously breathing patients 0.1–0.2 mg may be given slowly i.v. (i.e. over 1 min). Larger doses (0.6–0.8 mg) may be given if ventilation is controlled following the use of a muscle relaxant.

Fentanyl has been used in 'high dosage', i.e. exceeding 50 μg/kg, in order to avoid the use of volatile anaesthetic agents. These large doses may suppress totally the metabolic effects of anaesthesia and surgery (elevation of plasma glucose, cortisol, GH, ACTH concentrations, etc). However, the duration of action is very prolonged and patients may require IPPV postoperatively; even if spontaneous ventilation appears adequate, observation is required in the intensive care unit for 24 h postoperatively.

Phenoperidine

Phenoperidine, is similar to fentanyl and is also related chemically to pethidine. A dose of 1 mg is equianalgesic with 100 mg of pethidine. It has a rapid onset of action and shorter duration of action (approx. 1–2 h) than pethidine.

The drug produces profound respiratory depression (1.5 mg of phenoperidine having a greater effect than 10 mg of morphine) but has little effect on the cardiovascular system.

The dosage for supplementation of anaesthesia is between 1–3 mg depending on the duration of surgery and mode of ventilation.

Phenoperidine may also be used with droperidol in neuroleptanaesthesia, but currently its major use is in intensive care for analgesia and sedation.

Alfentanil

Alfentanil is a derivative of fentanyl. It has a higher lipid solubility and therefore a faster rate of onset of action (within one circulation time). The smaller volume of distribution and more rapid elimination time $(T_\frac{1}{2}\beta)$ ensure that it has both clinically and pharmacokinetically a much shorter duration of action than fentanyl (Table 10.2). It is therefore more suitable than fentanyl for administration in continuous i.v. infusion since it has a lower potential for postoperative respiratory depression than fentanyl when used in high dosage.

Alfentanil, in common with fentanyl, has little effect on the cardiovascular system. It may occasionally produce muscular rigidity.

OPIOID ANTAGONISTS

The effects of opioid drugs are mediated through different specific receptor sites occurring throughout the central nervous system. The opioid antagonists act as competitive antagonists at these sites. Several of the drugs used as antagonists (e.g. nalorphine) also possess intrinsic agonist activity, having different affinities for different receptor sites. Thus they may behave as competitive antagonists at one site, but exert agonist actions at another. Naloxone is the only drug with pure antagonist actions, whereas nalorphine, levallorphan, pentazocine and buprenorphine possess partial agonist and· antagonist actions.

Naloxone

Naloxone, a derivative of oxymorphone, is the only commercially obtainable pure opioid antagonist.

The drug is extremely well tolerated and it may be given in many times the therapeutic dose without ill effect. It has a rapid onset of action (within 1 min. of i.v. injection) and a duration of action of approx. 30 min. The relatively short duration of action may cause return of respiratory depression induced by an opioid of longer action and patients should be monitored carefully for an appropriate length of time following its use.

All the effects of opioids are also reversed, so that arterial pressure may increase, sedation diminishes and (if awake) the postoperative patient may be in severe pain.

Naloxone reverses respiratory depression produced by pentazocine (in contrast to nalorphine which does not) but is ineffective against buprenorphine, and also against respiratory depression induced by other groups of drugs, e.g. barbiturates, although there have been occasional reports of reversal of the depressant effects of diazepam.

Naloxone is the drug of choice in opioid analgesic induced depression in the neonate.

The average dose for the adult is 0.2–0.4 mg i.v. although it is better to dilute the drug and to titrate dose against effect in order to avoid re-emergence of excessive pain.

It has been suggested recently that naloxone in high doses may be beneficial in certain types of shock.

Nalorphine

Nalorphine is a morphine-related drug possessing opioid antagonist and agonist properties. As a respiratory depressant and analgesic, nalorphine is almost as effective as morphine but unpleasant psychomimetic effects preclude its use for analgesia.

Only in the presence of opioid induced respiratory depression does nalorphine exhibit antagonist properties. The average dose is 5–10 mg i.v., but, unlike naloxone, care is needed not to administer too great a dose because of the risk of inducing further respiratory depression. It is ineffective against pentazocine (in contrast with naloxone) and depression from other groups of drugs.

The duration of action is 1–4 h.

It is no longer available in the U.K.

Levallorphan

This is an opioid antagonist with partial agonist actions and is related to the agonist drug levorphanol. As with nalorphine, its use has been superseded by naloxone.

Levallorphan has greater analgesic effects but produces less respiratory depression and psychomimetic effects than nalorphine.

Levallorphan antagonises opioid-induced respiratory depression in doses of 1–2 mg. The duration of action is shorter than the parent drug levorphanol. It has been suggested that in the absence of naloxone, levallorphan is preferable to nalorphine for reversal of respiratory depression.

BENZODIAZEPINES

These drugs, of which there are several now commercially available, constitute an important advance over the barbiturates as sedatives and hypnotics, with less serious side effects, and low addiction potential. In addition to their sedative and tranquillising effects, they also produce mild muscle relaxation and possess anticonvulsant activities.

Site and mode of action

The benzodiazepines affect polysynaptic pathways within the brain and spinal cord, particularly in the midbrain reticular formation (affecting wakefulness) and the amygdala area of the limbic system which is responsible for the relay of the expression of emotion (affecting anxiety).

The mechanism of action appears to be stimulation of the activity of an inhibitory transmitter, gamma aminobutyric acid (GABA), causing presynaptic inhibition within these areas.

Diazepam

Diazepam is relatively lipid soluble and water insoluble and so it has a more predictable effect when given by the oral or i.v. route in comparison with the i.m. route when absorption is slow, erratic, and incomplete.

For i.v. use, diazepam is available in a rather viscous solvent containing propylene glycol, ethanol and sodium benzoate. If this is diluted with water, a cloudy suspension is formed which should not be used for i.v. injection.

After a single oral or i.v. dose the clinical effects diminish fairly rapidly as a result of rapid tissue redistribution rather than metabolism. However, the drug has a prolonged half-life of 20–40 h and its metabolites are biologically active (the principal compound being oxazepam) with even slower metabolism. A secondary peak effect occurs after 6 to 8 h, as a result of enterohepatic recirculation.

Actions on central nervous system

Sedation. There is a progressive transition from sedation through hypnosis to unconsciousness as the dose is increased.

Generally with the benzodiazepines, analgesia is not produced, although the MAC value for inhalational agents is reduced. The drug may diminish requirements for opioids in the treatment of postoperative pain since the affective component of pain is decreased.

Amnesic effects. There is conflicting evidence on whether or not true retrograde amnesia occurs; however, anterograde amnesia occurs which is dose related and potentiated by other drugs used as premedicants. The effect appears to result from an action on the early consolidation phase of memory processing.

Anticonvulsant effects. Diazepam acts as a very useful 'broad spectrum' anticonvulsant. The site of action is not at the seizure focus, but the drug prevents subcortical spread of seizure activity. Tolerance to anticonvulsant activity occurs more rapidly than to sedative actions.

Respiratory system

Slight depression of respiration occurs with small doses but this may become significant in doses greater than 0.3 mg/kg i.v. as a result of direct depression of respiratory drive and decreased respiratory muscle efficiency (see *Muscle relaxation* below).

Complete apnoea has been reported following the administration of diazepam alone, and also after barbiturates and other respiratory depressants. Caution should be exercised in elderly or debilitated patients and those with obstructive airways disease.

Cardiovascular system

Larger doses decrease cardiac output and systemic arterial pressure, producing reflex tachycardia and an increase in peripheral resistance. In doses used for premedication, there is little effect on the cardiovascular system.

Muscle relaxation

There is a minor muscle relaxant action which is useful for the treatment of muscle spasm in tetany and other neuromuscular disorders. Muscle relaxation results partly from an action on polysynaptic pathways in the spinal cord and partly direct depression of motor nerve and muscle function.

The muscle relaxation produced is inadequate for surgery and there is no significant potentiation of depolarising or nondepolarising muscle relaxants at the neuromuscular junction. However, muscle relaxant requirements may be reduced by the action of diazepam on the spinal cord.

Other effects

1. Placental transfer occurs rapidly leading to neonatal depression.
2. Potentiation of hypotension induced by ganglion-blocking agents.

Uses in anaesthesia

Cardioversion. Intravenous injection at a rate of 5–10 mg/min until dysarthria occurs, produces good sedation and amnesia.

Endoscopy. Muscle relaxation, amnesia and sedation provide good conditions.

Dentistry. The drug may be used i.v. to produce sedation and amnesia but the dose must be restricted to avoid loss of laryngeal reflexes.

Premedication. The benzodiazepines are particularly useful as oral premedicants producing sedation, relief of anxiety and amnesia without the side effects of opioids (in particular nausea and vomiting). In adults a dose of 10–30 mg may be used.

Supplementation of intravenous anaesthesia. Diazepam should not replace the standard i.v. induction agents, since onset of sleep is slow and recovery is prolonged. However, it may be used i.v. to supplement balanced anaesthetic techniques to reduce the possibility of awareness.

Adverse effects

1. Persistence of drowsiness, impairment of mental functions, dysarthria and ataxia into the postoperative period.

2. Occasionally, muscle weakness, headache, nausea and vomiting, vertigo, joint and chest pains may occur.

3. Pain at the site of injection and subsequent thrombophlebitis. This is less likely to occur if injection is made into a large vein, or using a suspension of diazepam in Intralipid ('Diazemuls').

4. Increased sensitivity and confusion in the elderly.

Lorazepam

This drug has similar actions to diazepam, but it has a longer duration of action, persisting for up to 48 h. Its amnesic effect is greater than that of diazepam. It has no respiratory depressant actions.

Lorazepam may be used for premedication in doses of 1–4 mg orally $1\frac{1}{2}$ h before induction of anaesthesia. It may also be given i.v. with a lower incidence of thrombophlebitis than diazepam.

Other benzodiazepines

Nitrazepam has a shorter duration of action than diazepam and is used mainly as a hypnotic. There is no anticonvulsant activity and grand mal and petit mal attacks may be precipitated in susceptible subjects. The dose for night sedation is 5–10 mg orally.

Temazepam has a significantly shorter action than any of the above drugs and is also used for night sedation and premedication in doses of 10–30 mg.

Table 10.3 Properties of the neuroleptic drugs

	Butyrophenones	Phenothiazines
Neurolepsis	+ + + +	+
Antiemetic activity	+ + + +	+
Sedation	+	+ + +
α-blocking activity	+	+ + +
Antihistamine activity	–	+ +
Hypothermic effect	–	+
Antiarrhythmic effect	Strong protection against catecholamine induced arrhythmias	Weak protection
Anticholinergic effect	–	+
Analgesia	No direct analgesic action but potentiates other analgesics	Potentiation Slight direct effect (chlorpromazine) Slight antanalgesic effect (promethazine).

BUTYROPHENONES AND PHENOTHIAZINES (Table 10.3)

These may be classified together as drugs which possess 'neuroleptic' activity, which may be defined as having the following characteristics:

1. Inhibition of motor activity including spontaneous movement and learned responses.
2. Antagonism of apomorphine-induced vomiting.
3. Antagonism of arousal induced by amphetamine.

Clinically, the neuroleptic drugs produce a state of calmness and lack of awareness of the patient's surroundings.

The phenothiazines are weak neuroleptics with a wide range of activity including hypnosis, α-adrenergic blockade and histamine antagonism. Hypothermia and dyskinetic (Parkinson-like) effects may occur.

The butyrophenones are stronger neuroleptic drugs with minimal hypnotic and α-blocking effects.

Chemically all neuroleptic drugs are tertiary aromatic amines derived from methyl-ethylamine.

BUTYROPHENONES

Droperidol, haloperidol

These drugs act by decreasing cell membrane permeability by the formation of a 'monolayer' which acts as a lipid-water interphase.

The drugs are thought to act by occupying GABA receptors leading to an accumulation of transmitter (dopamine, noradrenaline, 5HT etc) in the intersynaptic cleft. There is a specific action at the chemoreceptor trigger zone where dopamine is an important transmitter and this accounts for the potent antiemetic effect of the butyrophenones.

When droperidol is administered alone, the patient appears tranquil and placid and apparently indifferent to the environment, but later may complain of having experienced unpleasant sensations of mental restlessness and agitation. Occasionally c.n.s. stimulation may occur, producing dyskinesia and possible Parkinsonian crises. This tendency is reduced if the drugs are given in combination with an opioid.

The neuroleptics have no specific analgesic actions but may prolong the effectiveness of opioids. The basis of neurolept-analgesia and anaesthesia is the administration of a neuroleptic drug in combination with an opioid. Usually, droperidol is given with either fentanyl or phenoperidine.

Cardiovascular system

Cardiovascular side effects are common with the phenothiazines, but minimal with the butyrophenones, which possess only a mild degree of α-blocking activity. When given i.v. in doses of 2.5–5 mg droperidol may produce a small transient decrease in arterial pressure. This effect may be augmented in the presence of other hypotensive drugs. There is significant protection against cardiac arrhythmias induced by catecholamines.

Other effects

There is mild cerebral vasoconstriction producing reduction in c.s.f. pressure. Total body oxygen consumption is reduced, whilst there is little effect on respiration.

Droperidol produces effects within a few minutes of i.v. administration and these persist for 6–12 h. Thus, there may be re-emergence of unpleasant subjective effects if given in conjunction with a short-acting opioid.

Haloperidol has similar actions to droperidol, but has a duration of action of 24–48 h.

Although both drugs possess little instrinsic sedative action, the effects of other sedative drugs may be potentiated leading to prolonged sedation.

Droperidol may be administered in doses of 2.5–10 mg by oral, i.v. or i.m. routes.

PHENOTHIAZINES

Chlorpromazine

Action on the central nervous system

1. There is a marked depression of the reticular activating system producing drowsiness and loss of interest in the environment.

The sedative effects of other drugs and anaesthetics are potentiated, but in contrast with other agents (e.g. the benzodiazepines) there is no anticonvulsant effect.

2. There is a powerful antiemetic action resulting from specific effects on the chemoreceptor trigger zone; in large doses there is direct depression of the vomiting centre. Chlorpromazine is therefore a useful agent to counteract vomiting induced by opioids.

3. Depression of the temperature regulating centre produces a tendency to hypothermia.

4. Central depression of sympathetic activity produces hypotension.

Cardiovascular system

Peripheral and splanchnic vasodilatation occur by an α-adrenergic blocking effect. In combination with central depression of vasomotor activity, this leads to hypotension which may be prolonged. Hypotension may often be 'unmasked' by the administration of a general anaesthetic which further depresses compensatory mechanisms especially in the elderly and those suffering from severe atherosclerosis.

The pressor response to catecholamines is reduced.

Respiratory system

In moderate doses, there is little effect, although there have been reports both of depression and of stimulation.

Laryngeal and bronchial reflexes are depressed. Secretions are reduced by an anticholinergic effect.

Hypothermic effect

There is a tendency for body temperature to decrease as a result of depression of the heat regulating centre, inhibition of shivering, and increased heat loss through peripheral vasodilatation.

Chlorpromazine may be used during rewarming from hypothermia to reduce shivering.

Analgesia

Chlorpromazine possesses mild analgesic actions and also potentiates the opioids. However, promethazine has antanalgesic properties.

Other effects

1. Voluntary muscle. There is no direct effect but the action of muscle relaxants may be enhanced.

2. Smooth muscle. The anticholinergic effect leads to a reduction in gastro-intestinal tone.

3. Liver. Occasionally jaundice occurs as a result of cholestasis resulting from a sensitivity reaction. The incidence is low (less than 0.5%) and occurs 1–4 weeks following administration unless there has been a previous reaction to the drug. The reaction is not dose dependent and recovery is usually slow but complete.

4. Antihistamine and local anaesthesia. These effects are mild, although other phenothiazines may possess more potent actions than chlorpromazine.

Fate

Considerable metabolism occurs in the gut wall and liver, but this is variable and accounts for wide variation in response to the drug when administered orally to different individuals.

Usage and dosage

1. Premedication. 25–50 mg i.m. alone or in combination with other drugs e.g. opioids.

2. Sedation. 50–100 mg orally, although larger doses are used in various psychiatric states.

3. Antiemesis. 25–50 mg 4–6 hrly i.m.

4. As a constituent of the so-called 'lytic-cocktail' used for sedation. This mixture has been superseded by newer drugs, e.g. diazepam. It comprises a mixture of chlorpromazine 50 mg, promethazine 50 mg and pethidine 100 mg diluted in water and administered slowly i.v.

5. Postoperative analgesia. The dosage of opioid analgesics may be reduced.

Other phenothiazines

Perphenazine (Fentazin). This drug is used mainly for its powerful antiemetic action in doses of 2.5–5 mg i.m. It is less likely to cause hypotension than chlorpromazine.

Promazine (Sparine). In doses of 25 mg this produces effects similar to those of chlorpromazine, with fewer undesirable effects.

Promethazine. This possesses greater antihistamine and anticholinergic actions than chlorpromazine. Sedation is also more marked, but in contrast with chlorpromazine there is a slight antanalgesic effect. Hypotension is less likely to occur than with chlorpromazine.

The major use in anaesthesia is for premedication when its sedative, antiemetic and anticholinergic properties are useful. The normal dose is 25 mg or 50 mg by i.m. injection.

ANALEPTICS

Analeptics are drugs which stimulate the central nervous system without antagonising analgesia. Although they may cause arousal their major use is to stimulate respiration. They act by stimulation of either medullary centres or carotid and aortic bodies. Of the drugs currently available (nikethamide, vanillic acid diethylamide, methylphenidate and doxapram) only the last enjoys popularity.

Doxapram is useful when respiratory stimulation is required without reversal of other actions of the opioids. It may be given by slow i.v. injection in doses up to 50 mg or as an infusion at 3 mg/min in 500 ml dextrose containing 1.0 g. There is some evidence to suggest that given routinely at the end of upper abdominal surgery, it may reduce the incidence of postoperative chest infection.

Physostigmine is an anticholinesterase drug and not a classical analeptic. It crosses the blood–brain barrier and antagonises the adverse effect of hyoscine (prolonged drowsiness and confusion).

FURTHER READING

Bowman W C, Rand M J 1980 Textbook of pharmacology, 2nd edn. Blackwell Scientific Publications, Oxford

Bullingham R E S 1981 Synthetic opiate analgesics. British Journal of Hospital Medicine 25: 128

Dundee J W, Haslett W H K 1970 The benzodiazepines. British Journal of Anaesthesia 42: 207

Edmonds-Seal J, Prys-Roberts C 1979 Pharmacology of drugs used in neuroleptanalgesia. British Journal of Anaesthesia 42: 207

Goodman-Gilman A, Goodman L S, Gilman A (eds) 1980 The pharmacological basis of therapeutics, 6th edn. Macmillan, London

Parkhouse J, Pleuvry B J, Rees J M H 1979 Analgesic drugs. Blackwell Scientific Publications, Oxford

Schacter M 1981 Enkephalins and endorphins. British Journal of Hospital Medicine 25: 128

Vickers M D, Schnieden H, Ward-Smith F G, Stewart H C 1984 Drugs in anaesthetic practice, 6th edn. Butterworths, London

11

Neuromuscular blockade

Anaesthetists use neuromuscular blocking drugs to abolish skeletal muscle contractions which may occur as reflex responses to painful stimuli or to tracheal intubation, and also to abolish or reduce skeletal muscle tone which may hinder access to a surgical field or make artificial ventilation difficult. These requirements may be produced by other means, e.g. deep general anaesthesia, or local anaesthetic blocks placed to affect the specific motor nerves involved. However, the former method is usually accompanied by undesirable side effects whilst local anaesthetic techniques are time-consuming and may not be appropriate. The introduction of tubocurarine in 1942 produced an expansion in anaesthetic techniques and the number of neuromuscular blocking drugs now available is considerable.

PHYSIOLOGY OF NEUROMUSCULAR TRANSMISSION

Skeletal muscle rarely contracts in the absence of activity in the motor nerve supplying it. An exception is the contracture seen sometimes in patients with malignant hyperthermia. The link between nerve activity and muscle contraction was shown by Claud Bernard in his demonstration in 1857 that curare acts somewhere between the nerve and the muscle and in 1936 Sir Henry Dale established that acetylcholine is the transmitter involved.

The whole process whereby a nerve action potential leads to a contraction of the myosin and actin filaments in the muscle is complex. The stages may be summarised as follows:

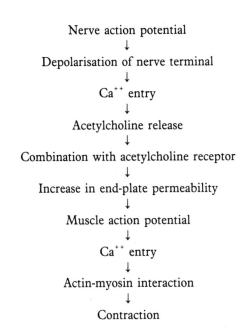

Nerve action potential
↓
Depolarisation of nerve terminal
↓
Ca^{++} entry
↓
Acetylcholine release
↓
Combination with acetylcholine receptor
↓
Increase in end-plate permeability
↓
Muscle action potential
↓
Ca^{++} entry
↓
Actin-myosin interaction
↓
Contraction

The following description is necessarily simplified: a detailed account may be found in Katz (1966), Bowman (1980) and Bowman & Rand (1980).

Release of acetylcholine by a nerve impulse

The nerve impulse arises in cells in the ventral horns of the spinal cord and the equivalent cells in the brain for the cranial nerves. Each impulse travels down the nerve axon as a wave of depolarisation, jumping in myelinated nerves from one node of Ranvier to the next (see Chapter 5). At its termination, each nerve fibre divides and may supply between 4 and 300 muscle fibres. The junction between nerve and

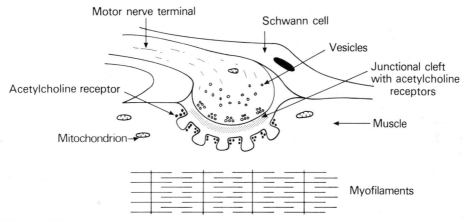

Fig. 11.1 Diagram of the neuromuscular junction.

muscle is termed the neuromuscular junction (Fig. 11.1).

The nerve action potential invades all the nerve terminals and depolarisation occurs as a transient initial increase in permeability to sodium ions followed by an increase in potassium permeability. In addition, there is an increase in calcium permeability. An increase in intracellular Ca^{++} concentration occurs and is essential for the next step — the release of acetylcholine. Low extracellular Ca^{++} leads to less release of acetylcholine. High magnesium concentrations antagonise entry of calcium and reduce the release of acetylcholine.

The central role of acetylcholine

Acetylcholine as the transmitter is the key to neuromuscular transmission. In skeletal muscle, the electrical forces produced by the nerve action potential are too weak to initiate a muscle action potential. Acetylcholine acts as a chemical amplifier to ensure transmission. It is synthesised, stored and released from the nerve terminal, diffuses across the junction to combine with a specific receptor and is destroyed finally by a specific enzyme.

Synthesis. Acetylcholine is synthesised in the cytoplasm of the nerve terminal from choline and acetyl coenzyme A under the control of a specific enzyme, choline acetyltransferase. Choline is taken up by a carrier system in the nerve terminal membrane from the amount present in the cleft both by diffusion from plasma and by breakdown of acetylcholine. Acetylcoenzyme A is generated initially

in the mitochondria. Blocking drugs similar to hemicholinium-3 are taken up into the cell in place of choline and may produce myoneural block by depleting the nerve terminal of acetylcholine.

Storage. Whilst there is some free acetylcholine present in the nerve terminal, the majority is packed into vesicles. Each vesicle is spherical with a bilayer wall. The concentration of acetylcholine in the vesicle greatly exceeds that in the cytoplasm. Whilst vesicles are present throughout the nerve terminal, many are concentrated in specific zones opposite the folds in the muscle membrane on the opposite side of the junction. The vesicles are formed from membrane material synthesised originally perhaps in the cell body but also recycled from the terminal membrane following exocytosis.

Release of acetylcholine. Acetylcholine is released from the nerve terminal in one of two ways. Although some is released from the acetylcholine in the cytoplasm of the nerve, release from vesicles is most important physiologically.

Some acetylcholine is released spontaneously. The effects can be detected as small voltage depolarisations of the muscle membrane — termed *miniature end-plate potentials* (m.e.p.ps) — but these are insufficient to generate a muscle action potential. They occur randomly but are approximately equal in size. Each one corresponds with the release of the contents of one vesicle in the nerve terminal. Release occurs as a result of exocytosis with the vesicle membrane fusing with that at the terminal.

Depolarisation produced by a nerve action potential and subsequent entry of calcium ion leads to a release of the contents of two to three hundred vesicles synchronously. This larger amount diffuses across the synaptic cleft and produces an *end-plate potential* (e.p.p.) in the adjacent muscle membrane.

Acetylcholine receptor is a specific protein present in maximum concentration on the crests of the folds opposite the local clustering of vesicles in the nerve terminal. It consists of a number of subunits. Acetylcholine binds to specific points of the receptor and initiates a chain of events. Firstly there is a change in the shape of the receptor molecule which in turn affects the shape of a protein in the membrane which acts as a channel through the membrane — an ionophore. Normally the channel is closed. When influenced by the union of acetylcholine with its receptor, it opens for approx. 1 ms during which time sodium ions flood into the muscle cell and potassium ions pass out. The normal resting muscle membrane potential (about -70 mV) is produced as a result of a relative impermeability to sodium ions and a relative permeability to potassium. The changes in permeability lead to a reduction in the transmembrane voltage — a depolarisation which changes the potential to about -15 mV. Normally, however, the depolarisation sets up local currents in the muscle membrane and produces a spreading depolarisation. Muscle membrane is similar to all excitable membranes and a depolarisation produces a wave of depolarisation spreading along the fibre by opening selective channels for sodium ions. These ionophores are opened electrically whereas those at the end-plate are driven chemically.

Destruction of acetylcholine. The acetylcholine released by the nerve impulse or spontaneously is destroyed by acetylcholinesterase present in the synaptic cleft. The enzyme is extremely efficient and virtually all the acetylcholine is metabolised before the ionophore has relaxed back into its normally closed state. The choline released may be taken up back across the nerve membrane to be rebuilt into acetylcholine.

Muscle excitation contraction coupling

Once an end-plate potential depolarises the adjacent muscle membrane sufficiently, a muscle action potential is generated which spreads to each end of the muscle. The spread is accompanied by an inward spread down into the T-tubule system and leads to a release of calcium ions from the sarcoplasmic reticulum. In turn, this activates myosin ATPase, which results in the creation of force in the cross bridges linking the thick myosin and thin actin filaments. Muscle shortening or force generation or both occur. The calcium release is transitory and calcium is taken up actively again into the sarcoplasmic reticulum and mitochondria. Once the normal low intracellular calcium ion concentration is achieved, muscle relaxation occurs. The muscle action potential lasts approx. 1 to 2 ms; the contraction evoked by a single *twitch* lasts about 100–200 ms.

Effect of repetitive nerve stimulation

The events described so far show how one nerve impulse may generate one muscle twitch. However, effective muscle contraction usually requires a combination of activity in many muscle fibres and repetitive activity to generate sustained tension. This latter is a *tetanic* contraction. A single nerve action potential leads to the release of more than enough acetylcholine to produce an end-plate potential of sufficient size to generate a muscle action potential. Only some 20% of the released acetylcholine is needed to generate the muscle action potential.

In order to tetanise muscle, it is necessary that nerve and muscle action potentials occur fast enough to abolish the fade of tension seen with a single twitch. The rates needed vary from muscle to muscle but are normally of the order of 25 Hz. Rates of up to 200 Hz produce sustained contractions; each nerve impulse evokes a muscle action potential. The amount of acetylcholine released by each nerve impulse in such a train is not the same. The first impulse releases most and then there is a decrement to a new steady level. With the release of the contents of the vesicles near the junction, a transport process comes into play to bring up new vesicles; time is required to reform and fill the old vesicles. However, although a decrement occurs, it is not sufficient to reduce the total amount of acetylcholine released per nerve impulse to an amount below the threshold required to generate an action potential.

This is the traditionally accepted view of the cause of the decrement in end-plate potentials seen during tetanus. Not all workers accept this explanation which has been derived largely from experiments in muscles partially or totally paralysed with a curare-like drug. An alternative hypothesis suggests the presence of additional acetylcholine receptors on the nerve terminal. Some of the acetylcholine released acts on these and produces an increased mobilisation of vesicles and hence improved release of acetylcholine on the next impulse (a type of positive feedback). Curare-like drugs act not only on the postjunctional but also on the prejunctional receptors and destroy this feedback. In consequence less acetylcholine is released on each impulse at the start of a tetanic train. A decrement occurs until the level of release matches the level of delivery of vesicles to the nerve terminal.

A second phenomenon occurs with tetanic rates of stimulation. During the tetanus there is a decrement in rate of release of acetylcholine. Immediately after the tetanus, single nerve impulses release a greater amount of acetylcholine than before as more vesicles discharge than normally. The exact mechanism is uncertain; it may involve a hyperpolarisation of the nerve terminal by the tetanic train of stimuli or an effect on intracellular calcium.

Both phenomena are important when normal transmission is impaired especially by curare-like drugs.

PHARMACOLOGY OF NEUROMUSCULAR BLOCK

Neuromuscular block may be produced by a variety of mechanisms. Only two are used therapeutically, but anaesthetists may be involved in resuscitation and intensive care of victims of other toxins. The following is a brief classification of the types of block:

Drugs preventing acetylcholine synthesis:
  hemicholiniums.
Prevention of acetylcholine release:
  botulinum toxin
  high magnesium concentration.
Depletion of acetylcholine stores:
  black widow spider venom
  funnel-web spider venom
  β-bungarotoxin
  tetanus toxin.

Block of acetylcholine receptors:
  α-bungarotoxin
  nondepolarising relaxants
  depolarising relaxants
  myasthenia gravis.
Block of cholinesterase:
  reversible agents
  organophosphorus compounds.

Nondepolarising acetylcholine antagonists

These drugs (of which tubocurarine was the first to be used clinically) act by combining with the postjunctional acetylcholine receptors without stimulation. Their actions may be overcome by increasing the acetylcholine concentration: thus they are competitive blockers.

The characteristics of a nondepolarising block are:

1. The block appears without any preceding stimulation

2. During a partial block a train of nerve impulses (which normally produces a sustained tetanus) shows an initial contraction which fades.

3. Following a tetanic train of stimuli, single shocks lead to a temporary increase in the strength of the muscle twitch. This is termed post-tetanic potentiation, or facilitation or decurarisation.

4. The block is antagonised by drugs which mimic the action of acetylcholine (e.g. suxamethonium) or by drugs producing an increased local concentration of acetylcholine (anticholinesterases).

Two explanations of tetanic fade have already been mentioned. There is a third possibility. Experimentally, it can be shown that tubocurarine acts not only on the postjunctional receptor but may slip into an open ionophore producing a block of ionic conductance. Obviously the channel in the ionophore has to be opened; this requires some acetylcholine-receptor interaction. Thus channel blocking becomes apparent during intense use and shows tetanic fade. It is uncertain if this mechanism occurs in humans in physiological conditions.

Depolarisation blocking drugs

Whilst the actions of drugs such as tubocurarine are relatively easy to explain, those of suxamethonium and decamethonium are less so. These drugs mimic the action of acetylcholine and result in an initial depolarisation and brief muscle contraction seen clinically as muscle fasciculations. The drugs are not destroyed by the cholinesterase present at the neuromuscular junction and the depolarisation persists. However, it is unable to trigger any more muscle action potentials at the zone of muscle membrane adjacent to the end-plate. There is a persistent current flowing into the end plate which does not trigger the explosive increase in sodium conductance necessary to fire the muscle action potential. A similar finding occurs if acetylcholine is kept at a high concentration by using large doses of anticholinesterases. Depolarisation block is characterised by:

1. An initial period of muscle fasciculation.
2. An absence of tetanic fade during partial block
3. An absence of post-tetanic facilitation
4. Anticholinesterases may make the block more intense.

With prolonged administration, the characteristics of depolarisation block change and come to resemble those seen with nondepolarising agents. In particular tetanic fade and post-tetanic facilitation develop gradually. The explanation of this altered pattern is by no means certain. It may be that the drugs *desensitise* the receptors and, in effect, reduce their numbers; or it may be a result of a prejunctional action. On occasion, this type of block may be antagonised by an anticholinesterase. Unfortunately this is not always so, and the block may be intensified. The safest therapy is to maintain artificial ventilation and wait. Testing with a nerve stimulator helps to determine when recovery has occurred.

CLINICAL PHARMACOLOGY OF NEUROMUSCULAR BLOCKING DRUGS

Nondepolarising drugs

Seven nondepolarising drugs are currently available in the United Kingdom. In order of introduction, they are tubocurarine, gallamine, alcuronium, pancuronium, fazadinium, atracurium and vecuronium. Each produces the characteristic block already described but they differ in potency, in duration of action and in side-effects.

All the drugs are ionised and water soluble and contain at least two charged nitrogen atoms. Most have two quaternary nitrogen groups. Tubocurarine and vecuronium have only one but they possess a second tertiary nitrogen group which at physiological pH attracts a hydrogen ion — thus they have two charged nitrogen atoms.

Table 11.1 summarises the doses used normally to initiate full neuromuscular block, and the average duration of effect expected. Being charged water-soluble compounds it may be expected they will have volumes of distribution similar to the e.c.f. volume. Because some bind to plasma proteins and other constituents of the body, some have higher volumes of distribution. Water soluble charged molecules are excreted by the kidney; thus the clearance values of these drugs are of the same order as glomerular filtration rate. Some clearances are greater, and liver uptake and biliary excretion play a part in eliminating tubocurarine, pancuronium, fazadinium and vecuronium. Renal failure and impaired liver perfusion and function impair the excretion of these drugs. Atracurium is unique in that, whilst it is stable at low

Table 11.1 Dosage and pharmacokinetics of non-depolarising drugs

Drug	Tubocurarine	Gallamine	Alcuronium	Fazadinium	Atracurium	Vecuronium	Pancuronium
Initial dose (mg/kg)	0.25–0.5	1–2	0.3	1	0.3–0.6	0.05–0.1	0.05–0.1
Duration of effect (min)	30–60	20–40	20–40	60	20–40	30–45	45–120
Maintenance dose (mg/kg)	0.1	0.5	0.1	0.25	0.15	0.015	0.015
Duration (min)	20–30	20–30	20–30	20	20	15	30
Volume of distribution, Vd_{ss} (l/kg)	0.61	0.24	0.32	0.19	0.16	0.27	0.31
Clearance (ml/kg/min)	2.9	1.2	1.4	4.0	5.5	5.1	1.8
$T\frac{1}{2}$ (min)	170	160	200	42	20	55	116

temperatures and a pH of 4, at body temperature and pH it spontaneously undergoes a Hofmann reaction which breaks it into inactive products. This action requires no catalytic enzyme and produces a drug half-life of approx. 20 min. Table 11.1 summarises the volumes of distribution, clearances and elimination half-lives. It also shows the size of incremental doses commonly used to maintain paralysis and the expected duration of effect of these doses.

The onset of block with these drugs depends on the dose used. With all drugs, if a dose is used which does not produce complete paralysis, it may take some 3–5 min to produce a maximal effect. Shorter onset times are seen with larger doses but with the penalty of prolonged recovery.

The duration of block with all drugs is variable. Coefficients of variation of 25% or more are usual even when doses are given standardised for body mass. Factors increasing the duration include:

1. Poor renal function — especially in the elderly.
2. Pre-existing liver disease.
3. The use of inhalational anaesthetics especially enflurane and diethylether. Halothane has a lesser potentiating effect.
4. The use of suxamethonium to facilitate tracheal intubation
5. Pre-existing disease especially myasthenia gravis and the myasthenic syndrome associated classically with carcinoma of the bronchus.
6. Hypokalaemia.
7. Acidosis: this may delay recovery. It is not clear if this is a direct action or an effect on excretion.

Side effects

The choice of a particular nondepolarising drug is often influenced by the side effects produced. Table 11.2 lists the common ones. It may be necessary to avoid the use of some of the drugs in some patients, but the side effects can be useful. For example the combination of ganglion block and histamine release with tubocurarine produces hypotension. This may help in producing a bloodless field. In contrast, when it is necessary to maintain arterial pressure, pancuronium is a better choice with its mild sympathomimetic effect. Vecuronium and atracurium were selected for introduction as agents devoid of significant cardiovascular action at doses which produce complete neuromuscular block.

In addition to these effects it is probable that all these drugs can initiate an anaphylactoid reaction featuring skin rashes, bronchospasm, laryngeal oedema and hypotension. The anaesthetist must have available all the necessary equipment and drugs necessary to cope with this life-threatening response.

Depolarising drugs

Suxamethonium, suxethonium and decamethonium are the three depolarising agents currently available. Of these suxamethonium is the most popular. Suxethonium is very similar and is available as a powder. Suxamethonium is available as a solution and some deterioration occurs if it is not stored at 4°C.

Dosage of suxamethonium

Tracheal intubation is usually carried out easily following an i.v. injection of 1 mg/kg. Half the dose is usually enough for electroconvulsive therapy. The drug may be given by i.m. injection in double these doses. Neonates also appear to need a somewhat greater dose.

In adults, 1 mg/kg produces apnoea which usually lasts approx. 5 min. Complete recovery of hand muscle paralysis takes another 5 min.

Table 11.2 Side effects of nondepolarising drugs

Drug	Tubocurarine	Gallamine	Alcuronium	Fazadinium	Atracurium	Vecuronium	Pancuronium
Histamine release	+ +		+		+	−	
Ganglion blockade	+ +					−	−
Vagal blockade		+ +		+ +	−	−	+
Sympathomimetic action					−	−	+

Paralysis may be maintained using further bolus i.v. injections of 0.25–0.5 mg/kg or using a continuous infusion with a solution of 1 or 2 mg/ml. The rate of infusion should be· adjusted by monitoring its effect using a nerve stimulator. Tachyphylaxis occurs commonly and the character of the block changes gradually from that traditionally seen with depolarising drugs to the pattern seen with competitive agents. The first signs of a change may be seen as early as 10 min following the initial injection.

Metabolism of suxamethonium

The ester links in the molecule are vulnerable and metabolism is catalysed by the enzyme plasma cholinesterase. This is normally present in sufficient concentration to ensure a half-life of approx. 4 min for suxamethonium. The production of the enzyme is controlled genetically and five variants of the enzyme are known. Patients homozygous for atypical enzymes do not destroy suxamethonium. These patients are sensitive and a normal dose may result in respiratory paralysis for 2 h or more. Recovery is associated with a desensitisation block.· Treatment is based on artificial ventilation until recovery occurs. Subsequently the patient and the family should be investigated to determine the nature and extent of the abnormality. Susceptible patients should carry warning cards to help prevent subsequent mishaps.

Low concentrations of normal plasma cholinesterase are also found in patients undergoing plasmaphoresis, in those using ecothiopate eye drops and in those with terminal liver cell failure. The normal half-life of plasma cholinesterase is approx. 2 weeks.

Side effects and dangers of suxamethonium

The muscle relaxation produced by suxamethonium is profound, of rapid onset and, usually, ephemeral. No other neuromuscular blocking drug matches these desirable properties and the drug is still in common use despite considerable disadvantages from the following side-effects:

Malignant hyperthermia. Suxamethonium is the most potent triggering agent to induce malignant hyperthermia in susceptible subjects (see p. 287).

Hyperkalaemia. The depolarisation produced by suxamethonium leads to reduction in intracellular potassium. Some patients may exhibit a very large potassium flux and develop dangerous increases in serum potassium concentrations. The following groups are susceptible:

1. Patients with severe burns.
2. Patients with extensive muscle damage.
3. Paraplegic patients.
4. Patients with peripheral neuropathies.

The patients in the first three groups develop the problem gradually; immediately following an injury there is no problem. Susceptibility develops one week later. Patients with hyperkalaemia and renal failure are less at risk unless they have peripheral neuropathy.

Arrhythmias. A bradycardia, which may lead to cardiac arrest, is common, especially in children given repeated i.v. injections. The slowing is usually maximal after the third or fourth injection. Atropine should be used before administering multiple doses of suxamethonium.

Muscle pain. Patients, especially young, ambulant women develop severe muscle pains on the day after receiving suxamethonium. The fasciculations may produce tearing of muscle fibres and local small haemorrhages. Up to 50% of patients experience pains after suxamethonium administration. The incidence is reduced if a small dose of a nondepolarising drug is given (e.g. gallamine 20 mg) 1–2 min before the suxamethonium. As many of the nondepolarising drugs have some protective action against depolarising drugs the dose of suxamethonium may need to be increased by 30–50%. Pancuronium, having a mild anticholinesterase action, is an exception.

Intraocular (and intracranial pressure). Suxamethonium causes a transient increase in intraocular and, to a lesser extent, intracranial pressure. Part of this effect results from increases in arterial and venous pressures. There is also prolonged contracture of the extraocular muscles. This effect is important if intraocular pressure is raised or if there is an open injury to the eye where there may be a loss of intraocular contents. If the use of suxamethonium cannot be avoided, pretreatment with a small dose of a nondepolarising drug attenuates the risk of extrusion of ocular contents.

Anaphylactoid reactions have been reported and may

prove fatal. Patients claiming to be sensitive to suxamethonium should be assessed to see if they have atypical cholinesterase as opposed to drug allergy.

Myotonia. Patients develop a contracture with suxamethonium.

Decamethonium

This produces a longer duration of effect than an equipotent dose of suxamethonium. The block commences with a depolarisation pattern and transforms slowly to the depolarising pattern. It has little effect on the cardiovascular system. A dose of 4–6 mg is suggested for adults, with a maximum dose of 10 mg.

Anticholinesterase drugs and reversal of block

The actions of nondepolarising neuromuscular blocking drugs normally are, and those of depolarising drugs given over a long period may be, antagonised by increasing the local concentration of acetylcholine at the endplate. Three reversible anticholinesterase drugs are used clinically: edrophonium, neostigmine and pyridostigmine. Neostigmine is the most potent and a dose of 0.03 to 0.05 mg/kg is usually sufficient. Pyridostigmine is used in a dose of 0.1–0.2 mg/kg. Edrophonium in a dose of 0.5 to 1 mg/kg is also effective and of sufficient duration of action not to lead to a loss of action before the concentration of blocker has decreased to a safe level.

All three drugs have muscarinic actions producing salivation, intestinal contraction and bradycardia. Treatment with atropine or glycopyrrolate (0.015 and 0.01 mg/kg respectively) given either before or with the anticholinesterase minimises these effects. In attempting to antagonise a nondepolarising block it is well to remember that the more intense the paralysis the slower is the effect of an anticholinesterase. Normally some 5 min is required for maximum effect. Attempting to reverse a block just induced with 0.1 mg/kg of pancuronium may prove impossible.

ASSESSMENT OF NEUROMUSCULAR BLOCK

At the end of any anaesthetic during which neuromuscular blocking drugs are used, the anaesthetist must be certain that there is no residual block before discharging the patient to the recovery room. The assessment of the nature and degree of block is therefore vital

Clinical assessment

It is relatively easy to ask a conscious patient to produce a tetanic contraction of a muscle group. Lifting the head above a pillow for 5 s, ability to cough, protruding the tongue, or sustaining a hand grip are examples of readily available methods (Table 11.3). Measurements available include monitoring

Table 11.3 Clinical assessment of adequacy of neuromuscular transmission

1. Grip strength ⎫
2. Adequate cough ⎬ subjective
3. Ability of the patient to sustain a head lift for at least 5 s
4. Ability to produce a vital capacity of at least 10 ml/kg body weight
5. Ability to produce a negative inspiratory effort of at least −20 cmH$_2$O against an obstructed airway

tidal and minute volumes and vital capacity. The last is preferable since many patients, even when partially paralysed, have enough muscle power to maintain a normal minute volume. In unconscious patients, the measurement of adequate tidal and minute volume are only guides that recovery is on the way as would be the finding of a normal arterial carbon dioxide tension. In addition it is useful to examine the pattern of breathing: partially paralysed patients often have an unco-ordinated pattern with the diaphragm contracting but the intercostal muscles paralysed giving a see-saw pattern of breathing (paradoxical respiration).

Nerve stimulators

The use of electrical nerve stimulators should ensure that no patient is left partially paralysed without adequate respiratory support.

The nerve stimulator uses an electrical pulse to depolarise all motor nerve fibres in a peripheral nerve and hence release acetylcholine at all the nerve terminals to produce maximum depolarisation at the muscle receptors (supramaximal stimulation). The evoked muscle response may be observed visually by the anaesthetist, palpated, or recorded as either the electrical activity (e.m.g.) or the force produced (force transducer). The electrical pulses may be delivered as single shocks, as a sequence of high frequency pulses to evoke a tetanic contraction or as trains at lower frequencies. Figure 11.2 shows a commercial instrument for delivering single twitches and trains of four.

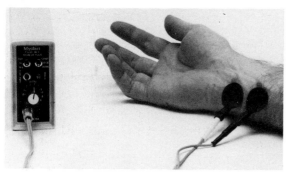

Fig. 11.2   The Myotest nerve stimulator.

Parameters for stimulators

In order to depolarise the nerve fibres, it is essential to apply sufficient current for a given period of time. Using stimuli applied through the skin, a current of up to 50 mA may be needed for between 0.2 and 1.0 ms. This requires a voltage of the order of 50–300 V. The current passed is unlikely to lead to any adverse cardiac effects.

Extending the duration of the pulse to longer than 2 ms may produce a double activation of the nerve because there is an 'off' effect when the duration exceeds the refactory period of the fibres.

Motor nerve fibres, being of the largest size, are the easiest to excite electrically. In conscious patients it is usually possible to evoke muscle contraction without undue pain. Tetanic stimulation rates are often an exception to this.

Patterns of stimulation

The correct use of a nerve stimulator should enable the anaesthetist to determine if neuromuscular transmission is normal, totally blocked or partially blocked. If partially blocked it is possible to estimate the type and degree of block. Three patterns of stimulation are useful and the effects may be observed visually (Fig. 11.3) or recorded on a chart recorder using a force transducer attached to the thumb (Fig. 11.4).

1. *Twitch–tetanus–twitch*. A train of single shocks given at a rate of not more than 1 every 3 s is followed by a tetanic train (at 50 Hz or more) for 3 s and the

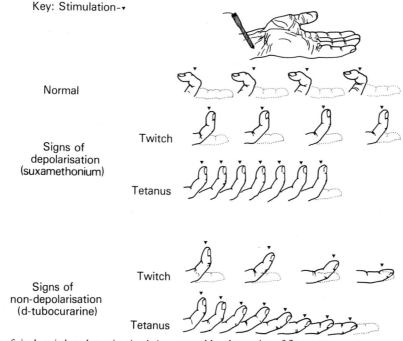

Fig. 11.3   Effects of single twitch and tetanic stimulation assessed by observation of finger movement.

train of single shocks is repeated. Four basic patterns of response are seen (Fig. 11.4).

    a. *Normal response:* twitch response followed by a strong sustained tetanic contraction and no potentiation of the post-tetanic twitches as compared with the pretetanic twitches.

    b. *Total block.* No responses.

    c. *Partial depolarising block.* The twitch responses are weak followed by a weak but sustained tetanic contraction. There is no post-tetanic potentiation.

    d. *Partial nondepolarising block.* The initial twitch responses are weak, the tetanic train evokes a contraction which fades rapidly and the post-tetanic twitches are markedly potentiated compared with the pretetanic twitches. A similar pattern is seen in myasthenia gravis.

    2. *Train of four.* The continued use of the twitch–tetanus–twitch sequence is not advisable in routine monitoring. Continual high frquency stimulation leads to some local reversal of block and in conscious subjects it is painful. However the

pattern of fade is seen at much lower stimulation frequencies without producing excessive local reversal. The train-of-four technique (Fig. 11.4) uses four stimuli given at 0.5 s intervals. It may be repeated every 10 s without significant loss of information. The results are interpreted in the same way as is the response to a tetanic burst.

    The train-of-four ratio can be calculated as the ratio of the force generated by the fourth force of contraction to the first when force transducers are used. Since transducers are not used widely, of more clinical relevance is the train-of-four count (Table 11.4). As recovery from total paralysis occurs, the first response seen is a twitch response with the first

Table 11.4   The train-of-four count

No. of twitches present (count)	Extent of block
1, 2, 3	75%
1, 2	80%
1	90%
None	100%

Note: The normal working range during anaesthesia is usually 75–95% block (see Fig. 11.5) with competitive blockers.

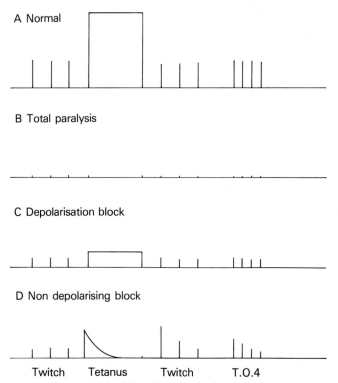

Fig. 11.4 Effects of single twitch, tetanus, and train-of-four (T.O.4) assessed by a force transducer recording contraction of the adductor pollicis muscle.

shock, then a response also to the second; later still the third and finally the fourth appear. The number of shocks which evokes contractions is the train-of-four count. The lower the count the more paralysed is the patient. The higher the count the more easily a nondepolarising block is antagonised. Abdominal surgery using a thiopentone–opioid–relaxant sequence is usually possible with train-of-four counts of one or two (Table 11.4 and Fig. 11.5).

3. *Post-tetanic twitch count.* Frequently the stimulation patterns described produce no response. If a nondepolarising blocking drug has been used, one further test is possible. The nerve is stimulated at a frequency of 1 Hz, and subsequently a tetanic train at 50 Hz is applied for 5 s followed by stimulation at 1 Hz. The number of post-tetanic shocks which evoke potentiated and detectable twitches is counted. There are usually about 12 to 20 before the train-of-four count detects the first response. Reversal of block is usually easy if the post-tetanic count is more than 10. (N.B. The absence of any response to a train-of-four does not necessarily imply that a block cannot be easily reversed.)

The first pattern of twitch–tetanus–twitch is useful for diagnosing block and the other two patterns help in the clinical administration of neuromuscular blocking drugs.

The successful use of nerve stimulators demands knowledge of the anatomical position of motor nerves. The ulnar at the elbow and the median and ulnar at the wrist are accessible as is the facial nerve and the lateral popliteal nerve. With surface electrodes, it is useful to clean the skin thoroughly with a degreasing agent and apply a conductive jelly electrode.

Clinical use of nerve stimulation

It can be argued that a peripheral nerve stimulator should be used in every patient when blocking drugs are used in order to detect abnormal responses and to act as a guide to the need for incremental doses. A stimulator is particularly useful in the following situations:

1. When prolonged anaesthesia is undertaken.
2. In patients with renal or hepatic dysfunction.
3. In patients with known sensitivities.
4. When infusion techniques are used.
5. Where there is doubt regarding antagonism of block.
6. When new drugs are being investigated.
7. In patients with myasthenia or myasthenic syndromes.
8. In the ICU to assess any residual block and especially if it is necessary to make a diagnosis of brain death.

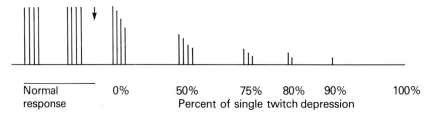

Normal response   0%   50%   75%   80%   90%   100%

Percent of single twitch depression

Fig. 11.5 Train-of-four stimulation observed with a transducer and recorder permitting assessment of both TO4 count (Table 11.4) and TO4 ratio. The TO4 ratio is the ratio of the height of the 4th to the 1st twitch. A ratio greater than 70% indicates adequate neuromuscular transmission following competitive blockers. The TO4 is more sensitive than single twitches: a TO4 count of two corresponds to 80% blockade of a single twitch response.

FURTHER READING

Bowman W C 1980 Pharmacology of neuromuscular function. John Wright and Sons, Bristol
Bowman W C, Rand M J 1980 Textbook of pharmacology, 2nd edn. Blackwell Scientific Publications, Oxford

Katz B 1966 Nerve, muscle and synapse. McGraw-Hill, New York
Katz R L (ed) 1975 Monographs in anesthesiology, vol 3: muscle relaxants. Excerpta Medica, Amsterdam
Zaimis E 1976 Neuromuscular junction: handbook of experimental pharmacology, vol 42. Springer Verlag, New York

12

Drugs affecting the autonomic nervous system

THE AUTONOMIC NERVOUS SYSTEM

The term autonomic nervous system (a.n.s.) refers to the nervous and humoral mechanisms which modify the function of the 'autonomous' or 'automatic' organs. These organs or functions include heart rate and force of contraction, calibre of blood vessels, contraction and relaxation of smooth muscle in gut, bladder and bronchi, visual accommodation and pupillary size, secretion from exocrine glands etc. The a.n.s. can be subdivided into two separate entities, the parasympathetic and sympathetic systems, on the basis of anatomical and pharmacological criteria. In order to understand the action of drugs in the a.n.s. it is necessary initially to review these subdivisions briefly.

Parasympathetic system

The neuronal components of the parasympathetic system arise from cell bodies of the motor nuclei of the cranial nerves, III, VII, IX and X in the brain stem, and from the sacral segments of the spinal cord. The preganglionic fibres run almost to the organ innervated and synapse in ganglia within the organ, giving rise to postganglionic fibres which innervate the relevant tissues. The ganglion cells may be well organised as in the myenteric plexus of the intestine or diffuse as in the bladder or blood vessels. The chemical transmitter both at pre- and postganglionic synapses is acetylcholine. The neurotransmitter is stored in the presynaptic terminal in agranular vesicles, released by neuronal depolarisation, and acts at specific receptor sites on the postsynaptic terminal. Its activity is terminated by diffusion from the site of action and more specifically by degradation by acetylcholinesterase.

Based upon the actions of the alkaloids muscarine and nicotine, the specific receptor sites within the parasympathetic nervous system have been subdivided pharmacologically. Thus, the actions of acetylcholine at the postganglionic neuro-effector site are mimicked by muscarine and are termed muscarinic, whereas preganglionic transmission is termed nicotinic. Acetylcholine is also the transmitter substance released from voluntary nerve endings at the neuromuscular junction. The receptor sites in this situation are also nicotinic; the pharmacology of drugs acting at this site is described in Chapter 11. Although it is possible to modify transmission at the preganglionic (nicotinic) site, drugs active at this site (ganglion-blocking drugs) are now rarely used clinically and we shall concentrate primarily in this chapter on drugs active at the postganglionic muscarinic site.

Sympathetic nervous system

The preganglionic fibres of the sympathetic nervous system arise in the cell bodies in the lateral horn of the spinal cord associated with spinal segments T1 to L2, the so called 'thoracolumbar' outflow. The first synapse occurs shortly after leaving the spinal cord in the sympathetic ganglionic chain giving rise to postganglionic fibres which innervate the effector organs. Acetylcholine is the transmitter, via a nicotinic receptor, at the preganglionic synapse (as in the parasympathetic ganglia). The adrenal medulla is innervated by preganglionic fibres from the thoracolumbar outflow, activation of which stimulates, via nicotinic acetylcholine receptors, the release of adrenaline from this gland. At the postganglionic sympathetic endings chemical transmission is mediated by noradrenaline which is present in the presynaptic terminals as well as the adrenal medulla. Adrenaline is found in only insignificant amounts in the nerve endings and is primarily released as a circulating hormone from the adrenal medulla. Adrenaline and noradrenaline are composed of a basic ring structure with -OH groups in the 3 and 4 position in relationship to a sidechain ending in an amine subgroup (Fig. 12.1). Both catecholamines are synthesised from the essential amino acid phenylalanine via a number of steps including the production of dopamine (Fig. 12.1) which may act as a precursor for both adrenaline and noradrenaline when administered exogenously (vide infra). The action of noradrenaline released from granules in the presynaptic terminals is terminated by diffusion from the site of action, reuptake back into the presynaptic nerve ending, and metabolism locally by the enzyme catechol-o-methyltransferase.

The actions of the catecholamines are mediated by specific postsynaptic cell surface receptors. Pharmacological subdivision of these receptors was first suggested by Ahlquist in 1948 into two groups (α and β) based upon the effects of adrenaline at peripheral sympathetic sites. These were originally termed excitatory and inhibitory receptors,

respectively, because of their general tendency to produce those effects when stimulated, but as many exceptions to this general rule have been found, they are referred to solely as α- and β-adrenoceptors. Since Ahlquist's original observations further subdivision of both these receptor systems has been proposed on both functional and anatomical grounds. Thus, β-adrenoceptor mediated events in the heart (β_1 effects) (increase in force and rate of contraction) have been differentiated from those producing smooth muscle relaxation in bronchi and blood vessels (β_2 effects). Similarly, α-adrenoceptor mediated post synaptic events (e.g. vasoconstriction) have been termed α_1 effects to differentiate them from the feedback inhibition by noradrenaline of its own release from the presynaptic terminals (mediated via an α_2-adrenoceptor on the presynaptic membrane). These various subdivisions are summarised in Table 12.1.

On the basis of more recent detailed pharmacological studies, it has become apparent that this anatomical subdivision of the adrenoceptor subtypes is an oversimplification. Thus, most organs and tissues contain both β_1 and β_2-adrenoceptors, which may even subserve the same function. Also both α_1 and α_2-adrenoceptors exist postsynaptically.

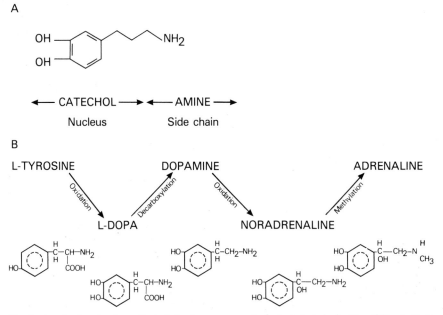

Fig. 12.1 A — Standard molecular structure of catecholamines, composed of a 'catechol ring' with −OH substitution in the 3 and 4 positions relative to the 'amine side chain'.
B — Intermediate metabolism of naturally occurring catecholamines from the essential amino acid L-tyrosine.

Table 12.1   Responses of major effector organs to autonomic nerve impulses

Organ	Receptor subtype	Adrenergic	Cholinergic
Heart	$\beta_1(?\beta_2)$	↑ Heart rate ↑ Force of contraction ↑ Automaticity and conduction velocity	↓ Heart rate ↓ Force of contraction ↓ Conduction velocity
Arteries	$\alpha_1\ (?\alpha_2)$ β_2	Constriction Dilatation	Dilatation
Veins	$\alpha_1\ (?\alpha_2)$ β_2	Constriction + + Dilatation +	
Lung			
bronchial muscles	β_2	Relaxation +	Contraction + +
bronchial glands	?	(?Inhibition)	Stimulation +
GI tract			
motility	$\beta_2\ (?\alpha_2)$	Decrease	Increase + + +
sphincters	α	Contraction	Relaxation
Kidney	β_2	Renin secretion	
Bladder			
detrusor	β	Relaxation	Contraction + + +
sphincter	α	Contraction	Relaxation + +
Liver	β_2, α	Glycogenolysis + + Gluconeogenesis +	? Glycogen synthesis
Uterus	β_2, α	Pregnant contraction (α) Nonpregnant relaxation (β)	

However, for the purposes of general discussion of drugs acting on the sympathetic nervous system, the original anatomical subdivisions will be used and important departures from this indicated where relevant. The important actions of the subdivision of the a.n.s. on various effector organs are summarised in Table 12.1

Second messenger systems

Stimulation of catecholamine receptors on the extracellular surface of the cell membrane leads to activation of intracellular events by the generation of so-called second messengers. Thus, stimulation of the β-adrenoceptor leads, via coupling to the enzyme adenylate cyclase, to the generation of intracellular cyclic adenosine monophosphate (cAMP). Cyclic AMP in turn, via activation of intracellular enzyme pathways, produces the associated alteration in cell function (e.g. increased force of cardiac muscle contraction, liver glycogenolysis, bronchial smooth muscle relaxation). The concentration of intracellular cAMP is modulated also by the enzyme phosphodiesterase which breaks down cAMP to its inactive form. The balance, therefore, between production and degradation of cAMP is an important

regulatory system for cell function. This somewhat simplified scheme is illustrated in Figure 12.2. The mechanism of transduction of the signal from the β-adrenoceptors across the cell membrane to the enzyme adenylate cyclase is incompletely understood, but almost certainly involves specialised intramembranous proteins that interact with guanine nucleotides.

Since β-adrenoceptor stimulation increases production of cAMP, its association with the enzyme adenylate cyclase is termed 'positive coupling'. The converse, receptor activation leading to reduction of intracellular cAMP, is termed 'negative coupling' to adenylate cyclase and this results from stimulation of the α_2-adrenoceptor (Fig. 12.2). An example of this 'negative coupling' is seen in α_2-adrenoceptor mediated platelet aggregation which is associated with a reduction in platelet cAMP content. The complex interactions between inhibitory (α_2) and stimulatory (β_1 and β_2) effects on cAMP in a single cell are still incompletely understood.

The α_1-adrenoceptor appears not to affect cAMP levels within the cell directly. Activation of this receptor produces changes in membrane transfer of Ca^{++} ions and alteration of intracellular calcium pools which lead, for example, to smooth muscle

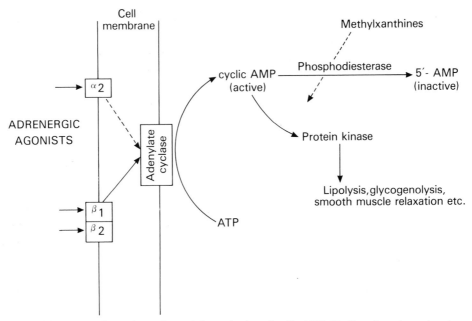

Fig. 12.2 Relationship between adrenergic agonists and the production of cyclic AMP. Binding of agonist to the adrenoceptors on the cell surface membrane activates either stimulation ($\rightarrow \beta_1$, β_2) or inhibition ($\rightarrow \alpha_2$) of the enzyme adenylate cyclase which catalyses the conversion of ATP to cyclic AMP and is, in turn, inactivated by the intracellular enzyme, phosphodiesterase. Cyclic AMP interacts with cytoplasmic protein kinase to initiate various cell functions.

contraction. The mechanism whereby the α_1-adrenoceptor alters transmembrane ionic flux is related probably to receptor activated changes in membrane phospholipid content and the modulation of calcium channels.

DRUG EFFECTS ON THE SYMPATHETIC NERVOUS SYSTEM

Drugs which partially or completely mimic the effects of sympathetic nerve stimulation or adrenal medullary discharge are termed sympathomimetic. A wide variety of drugs has sympathomimetic activity, and they may be classified into drugs which act: (i) directly on the adrenoceptor, e.g. the catecholamines adrenaline, noradrenaline and isoprenaline; (ii) indirectly, causing release of noradrenaline from the adrenergic nerve endings, e.g. amphetamine, ephedrine; (iii) by both mechanisms, e.g. dopamine.

The major clinical effects of these drugs are produced by action via α- or β-adrenoceptors or both (dopamine also acts via dopamine receptors — vide infra), and can be classified as follows.

Cardiovascular effects

Blood vessel calibre

Contraction and relaxation of smooth muscle in the blood vessel walls controls the calibre of the lumen and thus resistance to blood flow. Contraction of the smooth muscle produces vasoconstriction and increased peripheral resistance and is mediated via α-adrenoceptor stimulation. This comprises the normal physiological noradrenergic tone in the blood vessels. Conversely relaxation of arterial smooth muscle producing vasodilatation is via activation of β_2-adrenoceptors and is mediated physiologically by circulating adrenaline.

Cardiac contraction

Stimulation of the force and rate of cardiac contraction (inotropic and chronotropic effects respectively) is mediated via β-adrenoceptors in the heart muscle stimulated physiologically by both adrenaline and noradrenaline. Although the β_1-adrenoceptor is associated classically with this activity, recent functional and biochemical studies have indicated a role also for β_2-adrenoceptors in these actions of sympathomimetic drugs.

Cardiac output

The overall effect on cardiac output depends on the interaction of effects on cardiac rate and contractility with changes in peripheral vascular resistance. Thus, adrenaline and isoprenaline increase cardiac output via positive inotropism coupled with peripheral vasodilatation. However, noradrenaline, particularly in high dosage, may reduce cardiac output by intense vasoconstriction despite an equally effective action on cardiac contractility.

Arterial pressure

The effects on arterial pressure depend on the balance of cardiac output and peripheral resistance and vary with the effects of different sympathomimetic agents. Drugs which increase peripheral resistance, in addition to cardiac contractility, are most effective in increasing arterial pressure, but this may be at the expense of intense and possibly damaging vasoconstriction.

Nonvascular smooth muscle

In general, nonvascular smooth muscle is relaxed by sympathomimetic drugs. This effect is generalised and mediated by the β_2-adrenoceptor. Thus, bladder wall smooth muscle and, more importantly, uterine smooth muscle may be relaxed by these drugs. The latter effect is more pronounced in the oestrogen-dominated uterus and sympathomimetic agents are used to reduce uterine contractility in threatened premature labour. Most important in this group, however, is bronchodilation. Drugs specifically active at β_2-adrenoceptors (β_2-agonists) are potent bronchodilators (see Chapter 13), in addition to possessing vasodilating properties.

Metabolic effects

The metabolic effects of sympathetic nervous stimulation are related to effects on glucose and lipid metabolism. Insulin release is partially under sympathetic control and is stimulated via activation of a β_2-adrenoceptor. Likewise, adrenaline induced glycogenolysis in both the liver and muscles is β_2-adrenoceptor mediated. The physiological response to adrenaline release, therefore, includes an increase in insulin release and provision of sufficient substrate for its action.

Stimulation of β_2-adrenoceptors on adipocytes induces mobilisation and release of free fatty acids causing increased blood concentrations.

Type 1 hypersensitivity

The release of mediators of anaphylaxis (histamine, SRS-A) from mast cells is inhibited by drugs which cause an increase in mast cell cyclic AMP levels, including some sympathomimetic compounds active via the β-adrenoceptor on the mast cell surface. This effect may be relevant to the use of these drugs in acute asthma, and particularly anaphylaxis.

DRUGS ACTING ON THE SYMPATHETIC NERVOUS SYSTEM

We shall consider the most commonly used sympathomimetic agents in relationship to this classification of actions and to their most common clinical usage in shock, hypotension and cardiac failure. The use of β-agonists as bronchodilators is discussed in Chapter 13.

Catecholamines

This group comprises naturally occurring and synthetic compounds which have a common molecular configuration based upon the catechol nucleus and amine side-chain illustrated in Figure 12.1. Their effects are produced by interaction at specific catecholamine receptors (α, β and dopamine).

Adrenaline

Adrenaline has both α and β adrenergic effects. It is used mainly as a bronchodilator and in the treatment of acute allergic (anaphylactic) reactions. Except in emergency situations, i.v. injection is avoided because of the risk of inducing cardiac arrhythmias. Subcutaneous administration produces local vasoconstriction and a 'smoothed-out' effect by slowing absorption.

Adrenaline may be used by aerosol inhalation in bronchial asthma but its use in this context has been superseded largely by the newer β_2-agonists (Chapter

13). Intravenous and intracardiac adrenaline is used in cardiac arrest situations to provoke ventricular fibrillation if asystole has occurred, so that electrical defibrillation can be initiated.

The effect of adrenaline on arterial pressure and cardiac output are dependent on dose since, although both α and β-adrenoceptors are stimulated, β_2 vasodilatory effects are most sensitive. Thus, in large doses, direct stimulatory effects on cardiac output plus potent vasoconstriction (particularly in precapillary resistance vessels of skin, mucosa and kidney), produce a rapid increase in systolic arterial pressure. Diastolic arterial pressure is less affected because of β_2 vasodilatation in muscle beds (the characteristic physiological redistribution of the circulation associated with adrenaline) and, therefore, pulse pressure widens. In low dosage, adrenaline may produce no overall effect on arterial pressure or a slight decrease with an increase in cardiac output. However, its use as a positive inotropic agent at low doses has been superseded by newer drugs.

Noradrenaline

In contrast to adrenaline, noradrenaline acts almost exclusively on α-adrenoceptors, although it is less potent at these receptor sites than adrenaline. Infusions of all doses of noradrenaline therefore increase both systolic and diastolic arterial pressure by vasoconstriction of arteriolar and venous smooth muscle. Despite some stimulatory effects on cardiac contraction, the intense vasoconstriction leads either to no change or a decrease in cardiac output at the cost of increased myocardial oxygen demand. In high dosage the universal vasopressor effects reduce renal blood flow and glomerular filtration rate.

The problems of induction of cardiac arrhythmias, adverse effects on renal function and intense vasoconstriction (leading to ischaemia in the periphery) have limited the clinical use of this agent in hypotension and shock.

Isoprenaline

Isoprenaline has virtually no activity at α-adrenoceptors. Its main actions are via β-adrenoceptors in the heart, smooth muscle of bronchi, skeletal muscle vasculature and the gut. Intravenous infusion reduces peripheral resistance mainly in

skeletal muscle but also in renal and mesenteric vascular beds. Cardiac output is raised by an increase in venous return to the heart, combined with the positive inotropic and chronotropic actions of the drug. This may result in an increase in systolic arterial pressure.

Bronchial smooth muscle is relaxed and this effect, combined with other β_2 effects on release of mast cell mediators, has led to its widespread use in asthma, although newer specific β_2-agonists are probably preferable because of less cardiac stimulation.

Isoprenaline is absorbed unreliably by sublingual or oral routes and is administered usually by i.v. infusion or aerosol. As a direct cardiac stimulant, its most important use is in increasing the rate of cardiac contraction in heart block, by direct chronotropic action on the subsidiary pacemaker, often as an interim measure following acute myocardial infarction prior to insertion of a temporary pacing wire. Its use as a positive inotropic agent in septicaemic and cardiogenic shock has been superseded by newer agents.

Dopamine

Dopamine stimulates both α- and β-adrenoceptors in addition to specific dopamine receptors present in renal and mesenteric arteries. The balance of agonist properties exhibited by dopamine is related closely to dosage. It is administered only by the i.v. route.

Dopamine has a direct positive inotropic action on the myocardium via β-adrenoceptors and also by virtue of causing release of noradrenaline from noradrenergic nerve terminals. In low dosage (2–5 μg/kg/min) the major effects of dopamine are reduction of regional arterial resistance in renal and mesenteric vascular beds by an action on specific dopamine receptors. The result is an increase in renal blood flow, glomerular filtration rate and sodium excretion. Slightly higher doses (5–10 μg/kg/min) lead to inceasing direct inotropic action with little or no peripheral vasoconstrictor effects. This combination of increased cardiac output and renal vasodilatation is useful particularly in the management of cardiogenic, traumatic, septic and hypovolaemic shock, where excessive use of direct sympathomimetics associated with a major increase in physiological sympathetic activity may lead to severe compromise of renal blood flow and peripheral circulation. At these low and intermediate doses, direct cardiac chronotropic action is usually minimal and, thus, tachyarrhythmias are less common than with other sympathomimetics. In addition, at these doses dopamine increases systolic and pulse pressure, and has little effect or slightly increases diastolic arterial pressure. Total peripheral resistance is usually unchanged.

In higher dosage (>15 μg/kg/min), pronounced α-adrenoceptor activity of dopamine is seen, with direct vasoconstriction and increased cardiac stimulation (simulating infusions of noradrenaline). In general, therefore, these higher dose rates should be avoided. Occasionally the combination of a direct acting vasodilator (e.g. nitroprusside) and high dose dopamine may be of use in cardiogenic shock, although results are generally not encouraging.

The half-life of dopamine is very short and therefore its effects are controlled readily by alteration of infusion rate.

Dobutamine

Dobutamine resembles dopamine chemically, but is primarily a β_1-agonist with little or no indirect activity. It has less β_2-agonist action than isoprenaline and almost no α-adrenergic effects. It has no action at specific dopamine receptors. Dobutamine appears to be relatively more effective in enhancing cardiac contractile force than in increasing heart rate. Its effects on increasing sinus node automaticity, atrial and ventricular conduction velocity and enhancing A-V nodal conduction are less than those of isoprenaline.

Infusion of dobutamine at rates ranging form 2.5–15 μg/kg/min produce progressive increases in cardiac output with increased systolic arterial pressure, as peripheral resistance does not decrease. Decrease in pulmonary artery wedge pressure also occurs, indicating reduced diastolic filling pressure of the left ventricle. Urine output and sodium excretion are increased, presumably secondarily to the improvement in cardiovascular status, as the drug has no direct effect on renal vascular resistance.

Since the effects of dobutamine on heart rate and systolic arterial pressure are minimal in comparison with other catecholamines, oxygen demands on the myocardium may be increased to a lesser degree. Thus, dobutamine appears theoretically to have some advantages over other catecholamines for improving myocardial function in heart failure when peripheral resistance and heart rate are high; in this circumstance, combination with vasodilator drugs may increase efficacy.

Noncatecholamines

This group of drugs includes a large number of synthetic amines which have a wide variety of clinical actions mimicking those of the catecholamines in different combinations. These drugs may have direct actions at adrenergic receptors or may produce effects by causing release of catecholamines after first being taken up into sympathetic nerve terminals.

Those compounds which cause release of catecholamines (e.g. amphetamine, ephedrine) have considerable effects within the c.n.s. and their use has been superseded largely by newer drugs with more specific and less unpredictable actions.

Compounds with a direct action at adrenergic receptors may selectively affect α or β-adrenoceptors. Drugs with selective α-adrenoceptor effects are potent vasoconstrictors, e.g. phenylephrine, methoxamine. Their actions on the cardiovascular system are similar to noradrenaline, with its associated problems (vide supra). Phenylephrine is now used mostly as a nasal decongestant, a mydriatic or as a local vasoconstrictor in solutions of local anaesthetics. Absorption of phenylephrine from mucous membranes may occasionally produce systemic side effects. Drugs with a direct action at β-adrenoceptors have wider clinical use and will be considered in a little more detail.

Selective β_2-agonists

Compounds in this group include the drugs salbutamol, terbutaline, fenoterol and rimiterol. Because of their relative specificity for β_2-adrenoceptors these drugs relax smooth muscle of bronchi, uterus and vasculature whilst having much less stimulant effect on the heart than isoprenaline. However, these drugs are only partial agonists and their maximal stimulant activity even at β_2-adrenoceptors is less than that of isoprenaline.

The selective β_2-agonists are most widely used in the treatment of bronchospasm (see chapter 13), thereby avoiding the direct and possibly toxic effects of isoprenaline on the heart. High dosage of these drugs by oral, i.v. or inhalational routes, may still produce tachyarrhythmias.

The effects of these drugs on the cardiovascular system have been of interest recently in the treatment of cardiac failure. Intravenous administration of salbutamol causes a decrease in systemic vascular resistance and left ventricular filling pressure as a result of peripheral vasodilatation. Thus there is a consequent increase in cardiac output in patients with cardiac decompensation. In moderate doses (13 μg/min) the changes in systemic arterial pressure and heart rate are small. These indirect positive inotropic effects are supplemented by direct action of salbutamol on cardiac function probably via β_2-adrenoceptors, which are present in cardiac muscle. In high doses salbutamol is less selective and also has some stimulant activity on cardiac β_1-adrenoceptors which may limit its use because of tachycardia. Hypotension and reflex tachycardia produced by vasodilatation may also offset the advantages of decreasing myocardial work load. For these reasons salbutamol may be less useful in cardiogenic shock than dopamine or dobutamine.

Selective β_1 agonists

Drugs with selective β_1 partial agonist properties have been developed from the group of β-adrenoceptor antagonists with intrinsic sympathomimetic (partial agonist) activity (vide infra). Enhancing the intrinsic activity of the β-blocking drugs produces compounds which, in low dosage, have stimulant activity at the β-adrenoceptor equivalent to approx. 40–50% of that of isoprenaline. In higher dosage, however, the agonist effect reaches a plateau and the resulting action of the drug on the heart rate is less than isoprenaline. In theory, drugs of this class would be useful for their positive inotropic effect; no peripheral vasoconstrictor action, and a less direct chronotropic action on the heart than the catecholamines. The only compound with these effects presently available (for i.v. use only) is prenalterol, which has a chemical structure similar to practolol. Although originally considered to have pure β_1 effects, prenalterol has been shown to stimulate β_2-adrenoceptors in higher doses, possibly producing some vasodilatation. This pharmacological profile may be favourable in a drug for use in cardiac failure, i.e. positive inotropism (β_1) combined with afterload reduction (β_2 vasodilatation).

In practice, use of these drugs in cardiac failure should be limited to situations of mild to moderate failure with low sympathetic drive. When high sympathetic activity is present, these drugs may exhibit the β-blocking activity expected of a partial agonist and thus worsen the clinical condition. Intravenous prenalterol is of use in shocked patients with low cardiac output and low heart rates resulting from prior use of β-blockers. Orally active drugs of this class are in the process of development and may find a place in the chronic treatment of moderate cardiac failure.

β-adrenoceptor antagonists

In general, the β-adrenoceptor antagonists (β-blockers) are structurally similar to the β-agonists, e.g. isoprenaline. Alteration in molecular structure (primarily in the catechol ring), however, has produced compounds which will not activate adenylate cyclase and the second messenger system despite binding avidly to the β-adrenoceptor. These compounds possess high affinity for the receptor but little or no intrinsic activity and therefore inhibit competitively the effects of the naturally occurring catecholamines.

There is now a wide variety of β-blockers available for clinical use and choice of the appropriate agent is thus made more difficult. However, the general properties of these drugs are best reviewed collectively.

Pharmacodynamic properties of β-blockers

The properties of individual drugs are summarised in Table 12.2.

β-blocking potency. The relative potency of the β-blocking drugs (i.e. their ability to antagonise competitively the effects of catecholamines at the β-adrenoceptor) is not clinically of any general relevance. However, the relative ability of these drugs to antagonise selectively effects mediated by the β-adrenoceptor subtypes is more important. Compounds are available which block preferentially either β_1- or β_2-adrenoceptors, although in clinical practice the β_1 or so-called 'cardioselective' drugs are more important. The β_1 selectivity is, however, only a relative property and these drugs exert β_2 effects in higher doses. Practolol was the first drug developed

Table 12.2 Pharmacological properties of β-adrenoceptor blockers

Drug	β-Blockade potency ratio; propranolol = 1	Approx. equiv. oral doses	Relative Cardioselectivity	Partial agonist activity	Membrane stabilising effect
Acebutolol	0.3	100 mg	±	+	+
Atenolol	1	50 mg	+	0	0
Metoprolol	1	50 mg	+	0	±
Nadolol	2–4	20 mg	0	0	0
Oxprenolol	0.5–1	40–60 mg	0	+ +	+
Pindolol	6	5 mg	0	+ + +	+
Practolol	0.3	100 mg	+ +	+ +	0
Propranolol	1	40 mg	0	0	+ +
Sotalol	0.3	100 mg	0	0	0
Timolol	6	5 mg	0	±	0

with clinically useful cardioselectivity. More recent drugs are less cardioselective, e.g. atenolol, metoprolol and acebutolol. The clinical importance of cardioselectivity will be considered later.

Intrinsic sympathomimetic activity. The first drug shown to be capable of blocking β-adrenoceptors was dichloroisoprenaline. This compound has a very similar structure to isoprenaline, differing only in the substitution of two chlorine atoms for the -OH groups in the catechol ring. Because of this close similarity, it has some stimulant or agonist activity at the β-adrenoceptor equivalent approximately to 50% of that of isoprenaline, i.e. it exhibits partial agonist or intrinsic sympathomimetic activity (ISA). Thus, at low levels of sympathetic activity this stimulant effect is apparent, but at high levels of sympathetic discharge, blockade of endogenously released catecholamines is the major clinical effect. The clinical significance of ISA is largely theoretical, but may be of some practical importance as discussed later.

Membrane stabilising activity. Some β-blockers have a quinidine-like action on nerve and cardiac conducting tissue. This can be demonstrated in vivo as a stabilising effect on the cardiac action potential noticeably reducing the slope of phase 4, and thus decreasing excitability and automaticity of the myocardium (see Chapter 13). The membrane stabilising activity is thought to be unlikely to have clinical significance generally, since it occurs at drug concentrations very much higher than those ordinarily achieved in plasma after usual therapeutic doses.

Pharmacokinetic properties of β-blockers

The pharmacokinetic properties of β-blockers are summarised in Table 12.3. All β-blockers are weak bases and most are well absorbed to produce peak plasma concentrations 1–3 h after oral administration. The effect of food is to delay the rate rather than reduce the extent of absorption. This is

Table 12.3 Pharmacokinetic properties of β-adrenoceptor blockers

	Half-life (h)	Volume of Distribution (litre/kg)	Bioavail-ability (%)	% Unchanged in urine	Is first pass effect significant?	Active metabolites
Acebutolol	8	3.0	50*	35	Yes	Yes
Atenolol	6–9	0.7	40	40	No	No
Metoprolol	3–4	5.6	50	3	No	Yes
Nadolol	24	—	—	25	—	No
Oxprenolol	2	1.2	30	50	No	No
Pindolol	3–4	2.0	100	40	No	No
Practolol	6–12	1.6	100	Over 90	No	No
Propranolol	2–4	3.6	30	Under 1	Yes	Yes
Sotalol	5–13	2.4	100	90	No	No
Timolol	4	1.6	50	20	Yes	No

* includes active metabolites

unlikely to have any important effect on chronic equilibrium concentrations of the drugs in plasma. An important characteristic of the highly metabolised β-blockers (e.g. propranolol) is their tendency to be affected by first pass through the liver. This reduces the bioavailability of the drugs, but this is offset by the fact that the 4-hydroxylated metabolites so formed are also active. The first pass metabolism also tends to become saturated, so that proportionately higher plasma concentrations of the parent drug are achieved at higher oral doses. This adds an important complication to pharmacokinetic studies of these drugs which should include measurement of pharmacological effect to be useful. The first pass effect is also a source of wide interindividual variation in plasma concentrations achieved from the same dose. Other highly metabolised β-blockers, metoprolol and acebutolol, also produce active metabolites.

Atenolol, nadolol, practolol and sotalol are excreted largely unchanged in the urine and so are much less affected by impairment of liver function. All β-blockers are widely distributed throughout the body and this, it seems, produces higher concentrations in the central nervous system than in plasma. This is particularly true for the more lipid-soluble molecules (e.g. propranolol). Distribution is rapid over 5–30 min, so that after oral administration the β-blockers can be fitted to a one compartment pharmacokinetic model, the distribution phase being of little clinical importance.

Most β-blockers have a half-life of 2–4 h. The less lipid soluble drugs atenolol and practolol have longer half lives of 6–9 and 9–12 h respectively and nadolol has the longest — 24 h. Although propranolol and alprenolol depend less on the kidney for elimination than other β-blockers, the possible accumulation of active metabolites, which are excreted renally, should be considered when used in patients with renal failure. The plasma concentrations of unchanged propranolol have also been shown to be increased in uraemia.

Interindividual variation in plasma concentrations is less with drugs excreted renally than those primarily metabolised. The plasma concentration-response relationship also shows individual variation, possibly as a result of differences in level of sympathetic tone. β-blockers have a flat dose response curve so that large changes in plasma concentration may give rise to only a small change in degree of β-blockade. Differences in the formation of active metabolites amongst highly metabolised β-blockers further complicates plasma concentration–response relationships.

Cardiovascular effects of β-blockers

Antiarrhythmic activity. Although the mechanism of antiarrhythmic action of β-blockers is unknown, it appears to be a property inherent in β-blockade itself, i.e. antagonism of catecholamine effects on the cardiac action potential and muscle contractility. The result is a slowing of rate of discharge from the sinus and any ectopic pacemaker, and slowing of conduction and increased refractoriness of the A-V node. β-blockers also retard conduction in anomalous pathways of the heart. The membrane stabilising properties do not appear relevant to the anti-arrhythmic effect. Most β-blockers have comparable antiarrhythmic properties in adequate dosage; choice is, therefore, based on tolerance to adverse effect. Sotalol has been shown to exhibit type III antiarrhythmic activity (see Chapter 13) and may have a more specific action in treatment of cardiac arrhythmias, in particular supraventricular tachy-cardia.

Negative inotropism. The action of catecholamine agonists on the force of contraction of cardiac muscle is antagonised by β-blockade. The resulting negative inotropic effect is of little significance in normal hearts but may be disastrous in situations where increased sympathetic tone is supporting the 'failing' heart. In theory, compounds with ISA have less negative inotropism by virtue of their partial agonist activity. This putative benefit is, however, of no practical use in cardiac failure when higher than normal sympathetic drive is present.

Antianginal activity. Angina pectoris occurs when oxygen demand exceeds supply. The oxygen demand of the left ventricle depends on contractility, heart rate and the pressure within the ventricle during systole. The reduction in heart rate caused by β-blockade results in a decrease in cardiac work which reduces oxygen demand. A slower heart rate also permits longer diastolic filling time and this allows greater coronary perfusion. β-blockade also reduces exercise induced increases in arterial pressure, velocity of cardiac contraction and oxygen consumption at any work load.

All β-blockers, irrespective of other pharmacological properties, produce some degree of increased capacity for cardiac work in angina patients. They all limit the increase in heart rate during exercise but they differ in their effects on the heart at rest. Those with ISA have less effect on the resting heart rate, which is of particular benefit in patients with an existing low heart rate as it reduces the risk of atrioventricular conduction disturbance. On the other hand, ISA may theoretically increase the metabolic demand of the myocardium. In practice, drugs without ISA may be more effective in patients with angina at rest or very low levels of exercise.

Antihypertensive effect. β-blockers are effective in controlling the arterial pressure of many hypertensive patients. The mechanism of action has not been elucidated fully but it is probable that some of the following are involved:

1. *A direct effect on the cardiovascular system.* This includes a reduction in cardiac output which correlates with a reduction in heart rate and some decrease in myocardial contractility. The significance of the reduction in heart rate is unclear, since in paced hearts, β-blockers reduce cardiac output at rest and during exercise. After long-term oral treatment with β-blockers, cardiac output tends to return to pretreatment values.

2. *A reduction in sympathetic nervous activity.* This may be mediated by an action of β-blockers in the hypothalamus, altering central control of sympathetic tone. However, different drugs may vary widely in their lipophilicity and consequent central nervous system penetration, but have similar effects on arterial pressure control. The significance of the central action of these drugs is, therefore, uncertain.

3. *An effect on plasma renin levels.* β-blockers have variable effects on resting and orthostatic release of renin. The nonselective drugs propranolol and timolol cause the greatest reduction, while drugs with ISA (oxprenolol, pindolol) or β_1-selectivity are less effective. In addition, no correlation has been found between renin lowering effect and antihypertensive activity of these drugs or with dosage of β-blocker used.

4. *An effect on peripheral resistance.* β-blockade does not reduce peripheral resistance directly but may even cause an increase by allowing unopposed α stimulation. Since the vasodilating effect of catecholamines on skeletal muscle is β_2 mediated, unopposed α stimulation would be expected to be less with cardioselective drugs or with those having ISA. However, cardioselectivity decreases with dosage and since hypertensive patients often require large dose of β-blocker, little real advantage is offered. Drugs with ISA may not raise peripheral resistance as much as those without.

5. *The membrane stabilising effect.* This was considered of possible importance when early studies indicated that the antihypertensive effect of propranolol resembled that of quinidine. However, all β-blockers appear to reduce arterial pressure regardless of the presence of membrane stabilising effect.

The full hypotensive effect of β-blockers is not achieved until about two weeks after start of treatment, indicating the involvement of several mechanisms. Possibly, readjustment of cardiovascular reflexes, both central and peripheral, is an important contributory factor to the chronic antihypertensive effect. Arterial pressure reduction begins within an hour of administration of a β-blocker, but several days may elapse before the plateau is reached. During chronic administration, the hypotensive effects of β-blockers last longer than the pharmacological half-life, so that single daily dosage is adequate therapeutically.

In contrast, however, there is a more direct relationship between plasma concentration and cardiac β-blockade so that to achieve adequate antianginal effect, plasma concentrations must be maintained throughout the 24 h. To achieve this in single daily dosage, either the long half-life drugs (e.g. atenolol, nadolol) or slow-release preparations (e.g. oxprenolol-SR, propranolol-LA, metoprolol-SR) are required. Regardless of pharmacological profile, all β-blockers are equally effective as hypotensive drugs at rest and during exercise. Patients unresponsive to one β-blocker are generally unresponsive to all.

Adverse reactions to β-blocking drugs

These can be classified into:

Reactions resulting from β-blockade

1. Induction of bronchospasm in patients relying on sympathetically mediated bronchodilation (β_2), e.g. asthmatics, chronic bronchitics, etc.

2. Precipitation of heart failure in patients with compromised cardiac function. Co-administration with other drugs affecting cardiac contractility (e.g. verapamil, disopyramide, quinidine) is potentially hazardous.

3. Production of cold extremities or worsening symptoms of Raynaud's phenomenon and peripheral vascular disease.

4. Impairment of cardiovascular and metabolic response to insulin-induced hypoglycaemia in diabetics; reduced cardiovascular response (tachycardia — β_1) and hepatic glycogenolysis (β_2).

5. Increased muscle fatigue (perhaps with cramps), possibly resulting from blockade of β_2-mediated vasodilatation in muscles during exercise.

6. A withdrawal phenomenon may occur after abrupt cessation of long-term β-blocker antianginal therapy. This may take the form of rebound tachycardia, worsening angina, or precipitation of myocardial infarction.

Idiosyncratic reactions

1. Central nervous system effects occur with some β-blockers including nightmares, hallucinations, insomnia and depression. These effects are more common with the lipophilic drugs which cross the blood-brain barrier most readily (e.g. propranolol, acebutolol, oxprenolol and metoprolol).

2. Oculomucocutaneous syndrome was recognised in association with practolol therapy. It affects the eye, mucous and serous membranes. There is no firm evidence that any other β-blockers may provoke a similar reaction.

Theoretically, cardioselective (β_1-selective) drugs are less likely to aggravate bronchospasm in asthmatics, but as their selectivity is only relative, high doses still interact with bronchial β_2-adrenoceptors and therefore should not be considered safe. Similarly, β-blockers with ISA are promoted wrongly as safer in patients with mild cardiac failure, since at the higher levels of sympathetic activity seen in these patients, the presence of small amounts of partial agonist activity are of no significance.

α-Adrenoceptor antagonists

α-Adrenoceptor antagonists (α-blockers) are used mainly as vasodilators and as urethral smooth muscle relaxants. Their use has been limited because of the widespread effects of α-adrenoceptor blockade on the sympathetic nervous system which can produce an array of undesirable effects (e.g. postural hypotension, nasal stuffiness, diarrhoea, constipation, abdominal discomfort and inhibition of ejaculation). α-Adrenoceptor blocking drugs still have a role in the preoperative management of phaeochromocytoma although their use in other acute hypertensive situations has been replaced by directly acting vasodilators, e.g. sodium nitroprusside (see Chapter 13). The α-blockers bind selectively to the α subclass of adrenoceptors and, therefore, inhibit catecholamine action at these sites. Drugs in this group may bind covalently (i.e. irreversibly) to the receptor (e.g. phenoxybenzamine) or, as with the β-blockers, in a competitive reversible manner (e.g. phentolamine).

There are differences in the relative abilities of the α blockers to antagonise effects at the two subtypes of α-adrenoceptors, leading to the following classification:

1. Non-selective agents (block equally α_1 and α_2), e.g. phentolamine, tolazoline.

2. α_1-Selective, e.g. prazosin, indoramin, phenoxybenzamine.

3. α_2-Selective, e.g. yohimbine.

Only classes (1) and (2) are relevant presently in clinical practice. α–Blockers produce a decrease in peripheral vascular resistance and an increase in venous capacity resulting from blockade of noradrenergic vaso- and venoconstrictor tone.

The antihypertensive action may be combined synergistically with β-blockade in order to prevent reflex sympathetic tachycardia, consequent upon vasodilatation. *Prazosin* and *indoramin* are the most commonly used agents in this class and in contrast with direct acting vasodilators (hydralazine) and the nonselective α-blockers (phentolamine) reflex tachycardia and postural hypotension are less common. The mechanism of these changes is not completely understood, but may involve a difference in the proportions of α_1 and postsynaptic α_2 adrenoceptors in the arterial and venous smooth muscle. Thus, prazosin and indoramin may produce a more balanced effect on venous and arterial circulations. An alternative explanation is that nonselective α-antagonists block the feedback inhibition of noradrenaline on its own release at presynaptic α_2-adrenoceptors, thus encouraging increased chronotropic action of neuronally released noradrenaline at cardiac β-adrenoceptors. In both instances nonselective α-blockers produce more postural hypotension, more reflex tachycardia and there is a greater tendency for tolerance to develop to their therapeutic effects.

In common with other vasodilators, α-blockers may have indirect positive inotropic actions as a result of reduction in afterload and preload. Prazosin has been used for this effect since it produces balanced vaso- and venodilatation with consequent reduced likelihood of reflex tachycardia. Unfortunately the effects of prazosin in cardiac failure are limited by the development of tachyphylaxis after a few months therapy, and it is being superseded by other agents.

Labetalol is an oral and parenteral antihypertensive agent with both an α_1-blocking and a β-blocking action. In acute use, it may produce a prompt reduction in arterial pressure, suggesting that its α-blocking action predominates. Its β-blocking action may be the more important property during chronic administration. It has been used successfully in the preoperative management of phaeochromocytoma.

DRUG EFFECTS ON THE PARASYMPATHETIC NERVOUS SYSTEM

Stimulation of both the cholinergic synapses in ganglia and, more importantly, the postganglionic muscarinic cholinergic receptors, affects chiefly the following organs.

Cardiovascular system

Acetylcholine has three primary effects on the cardiovascular system — vasodilatation, decrease in cardiac rate (negative chronotropic effect) and a decrease in the force of cardiac contraction (negative inotropic effect). The cardiac effects are characteristic of vagal overactivity and blocked by potganglionic muscarinic antagonists (atropine). These pure effects are often obscured in the whole organism by a number of factors; in particular the release of catecholamines by acetylcholine from cardiac and extracardiac tissues, and the dampening of direct effects by baroreceptor and other reflexes.

Gastrointestinal system

All compounds acting on the parasympathetic nervous system are capable of producing increased tone, amplitude of contractions and peristaltic activity of the alimentary tract in addition to enhanced secretory activity. This may cause nausea, belching, vomiting, cramps and defaecation.

Urinary tract

Drug effects increase ureteral peristalsis, contract the detrusor muscle of the bladder and increase maximal voiding pressure, thus encouraging micturition.

Bronchial tree

Bronchoconstriction is produced in addition to increased mucus secretion. These effects may be a problem in asthmatic and allergic subjects in whom cholinergic drugs should be used with caution. In addition, a significant contribution from reflex cholinergic (vagal) effects inducing bronchospasm in some asthmatics has led to the use of anticholinergics as bronchodilators (see Chapter 13).

Eye

Miosis and spasm of the ciliary muscle occur so that the eye is accommodated for near vision. Intraocular pressure decreases as a result of increased reabsorption of intraocular fluids.

DRUGS ACTING ON THE PARASYMPATHETIC NERVOUS SYSTEM

The major drugs in use which act on the parasympathetic nervous system are parasympathetic agonists (e.g. bethanechol and the anticholinesterases, neostigmine and pyridostigmine) and muscarinic antagonists (e.g. atropine and propantheline).

Parasympathetic agonists

Bethanechol is used as a stimulant of the smooth muscle of the gastro-intestinal tract and bladder. It is given subcutaneously or orally in postoperative abdominal distension and urinary retention.

Bethanechol has mainly muscarinic activity at parasympathetic nerve terminals, an action which lasts several hours, since the drug is not hydrolysed by acetylcholinesterase. Bethanechol has also been used to prevent gastro-oesophageal reflux. Generally it has little effect on the cardiovascular system, although atrial fibrillation can be precipitated in hyperthyroid patients. Bradycardia may also aggravate ischaemic heart disease. Flushing, sweating and excessive salivation are predictable adverse effects which necessitate careful dosage selection. Bethanechol is contraindicated in patients with active peptic ulcer or obstructive airways disease.

Anticholinesterase agents (e.g. neostigmine, pyridostigmine) by decreasing the breakdown of released acetylcholine exert a parasympathomimetic effect in addition to an action on skeletal neuromuscular junctions. Their use in anaesthesia to reverse the neuromuscular blockade of nondepolarizing muscle relaxants is covered in Chapter 11. The action on the autonomic nervous system tends to appear at low doses. Anticholinesterases may be used to increase gastro-intestinal and bladder smooth muscle tone in a similar way to bethanechol. Their other uses include the symptomatic management of myasthenia gravis, where pyridostigmine is a useful, relatively long acting agent. Topical anticholinesterases are also used in ophthalmology as miotic agents.

Physostigmine differs from neostigmine and pyridostigmine in being capable of crossing into the central nervous system, producing excitation. Physostigmine has been used to arouse patients from drug-induced coma, particularly that following poisoning with anticholinergic agents, ketamine, diazepam and tricyclic antidepressants which have anticholinergic effects. This is potentially hazardous since it can induce convulsions and may exacerbate any cardiac bradyarrhythmias associated with direct toxicity of the tricyclic drugs.

Parasympathetic antagonists

Parasympathetic antagonists act by blockade of the muscarinic acetylcholine receptor. They are either tertiary or quaternary amine compounds, which differ in their ability to cross biological membranes. Tertiary amines, e.g. atropine and hyoscine, may affect central acetylcholine receptors and may produce sedative or stimulatory effects. Similar antimuscarinic drugs, e.g. benztropine and procyclidine, are useful anti-Parkinson agents because of their predominant central action.

Many other parasympathetic antagonists which have been developed are quaternary amines, which are less likely to produce central effects but which also tend to be absorbed poorly after oral administration.

Atropine. The muscarinic-blocking action of atropine affects a wide range of parasympathetic autonomic nervous functions, depending upon dosage. Salivary secretion, micturition, heart rate and visual accommodation are impaired (in that order). Central nervous system effects (sedation or excitation) are possible, but uncommon at usual therapeutic doses in medical conditions. In anaesthesia, central effects may be more common, resulting in the 'central cholinergic crisis' described in Chapter 20. Hyoscine crosses into the brain more readily and frequently produces confusion, sedation and ataxia. Hyoscine is also used as an antiemetic.

Atropine is administered subcutaneously or i.v. to counteract bradycardia in the presence of hypotension, or to prevent bradycardia associated with vagal stimulation or the use of anticholinesterase agents. Adverse cardiac effects of atropine include an increase in cardiac work and ventricular arrhythmias. Occasionally after subcutaneous administration, atropine may produce a transient slowing of heart rate, thought to be mediated by a central action. Atropine is also used to block salivary and respiratory secretions in anaesthetic premedication (see Chapter 15, p. 220).

Glycopyrronium bromide. This is a quaternary amine which has similar anticholinergic actions to atropine. It is used for its antisecretory and gastro-intestinal actions. Certain other quaternary amines, e.g. *propantheline* and *dicyclomine* have a mainly peripheral parasympathetic antagonist action and are used as gastro-intestinal and urinary antispasmodics. The extent to which these two agents reduce gastric acidity is limited by their lack of effect on acid secretion and the need to avoid doses which produce undesirable effects such as dry mouth and visual disturbances. Anticholinergic agents also delay gastric emptying, a disadvantage in peptic ulcer disease. *Pirenzepine* is an anticholinergic which has been developed recently to be rather more selective for receptor sites in the gastric mucosa. In general anticholinergic agents have little if any role in the treatment of peptic ulcer disease because of the advent of histamine H_2 antagonists (see Chapter 13, p. 192).

Ipratropium is useful topically as an anticholinergic bronchodilator aerosol.

FURTHER READING

Breckenridge A 1983 Which beta-blocker? British Medical Journal 286: 1085

Goodman-Gilman A, Goodman L S, Gilman A (eds) 1980 The pharmacological basis of therapeutics, 6th edn. Macmillan, New York

Gross F 1982 The place of alpha-adrenoceptor and beta-adrenoceptor blockade in the treatment of hypertension. British Journal of Clinical Pharmacology 13 (suppl): 5S

Heinsimer J A, Lefkowitz R J 1982 Adrenergic receptors: biochemistry, regulation, molecular mechanism and clinical implications. Journal of Laboratory and Clinical Medicine 100: 641

Juan D 1982 Pharmacologic agents in the management of phaeochromocytoma. Southern Medical Journal 75: 211

McDevitt D G 1979 Adrenoceptor blocking drugs: clinical pharmacology and therapeutic use. Drugs 17: 267

Motulsky H J, Insel P A 1982 Adrenergic receptors in man. New England Journal of Medicine 307: 18

Nelson H S 1982 Beta-adrenergic agonists. Chest 82 (suppl): 34S

Opie L H 1980 Drugs and the heart: 5 digitalis and sympathomimetic stimulants. Lancet 1: 912

Prichard B N C 1982 Propranolol and beta-adrenoceptor blocking drugs in the treatment of hypertension. British Journal of Clinical Pharmacology 13: 51

Taylor S H 1981 Vasodilators and alpha-adrenoceptor antagonists in hypertension and heart failure. British Journal of Clinical Pharmacology 12 (suppl 1): 27S

13

Miscellaneous drugs of importance in anaesthesia

DRUGS AFFECTING THE GASTRO-INTESTINAL TRACT

Antacid or histamine H_2 antagonist therapy is used empirically to prevent bleeding from stress ulceration. Cimetidine has been shown to be effective in the prophylaxis against bleeding after severe head injury and erosive bleeding secondary to fulminant liver failure and after renal transplantation. In general, high doses (exceeding 1.2 g daily, i.v.) have been required, with adjustment according to measurement of gastric pH. Cimetidine does not prevent the occurrence of mucosal lesions but affects only the incidence of haemorrhage. Any effect on overall outcome in these patients has yet to be demonstrated. In stress ulcers, cimetidine is less effective in preventing bleeding than hourly, high-dose antacids. Oral or i.v. cimetidine has been advocated $1\frac{1}{2}$–$2\frac{1}{2}$ h preoperatively to prevent pulmonary acid aspiration syndrome in elective Caesarian section. In the treatment of acute upper gastrointestinal haemorrhage histamine H_2 receptor antagonists have not affected the incidence of rebleeding.

Antacids

Antacids raise gastric pH and facilitate ulcer healing only when given in large doses equivalent to around 200 ml daily of a typical magnesium-aluminium preparation. In vitro neutralising capacity varies according to titration technique used and does not correlate with ability to relieve ulcer pain. Antacid mixtures containing local anaesthetics, barbiturates or anticholinergic agents have no proven advantages and are potentially harmful. Calcium-containing antacids should also be avoided since they can cause rebound hyperacidity and hypercalcaemia.

Magnesium compounds can produce diarrhoea whereas aluminium antacids tend to produce constipation. The high sodium content of some antacid mixtures should be taken into account when antacids are used in patients with cardiovascular or renal disease. Antacids may affect the absorption of drugs including tetracyclines, iron, ketoconazole, diflunisal, chlorpromazine, prednisone and (in high doses) cimetidine and ranitidine. Various other drugs may also be affected, so it is advisable to separate all oral medication from high dose antacid therapy by 1–2 h.

Histamine H_2 receptor antagonists

Basal and stimulated gastric acid secretion is mediated by the action of locally secreted histamine on gastric parietal cells. The receptors involved are H_2 receptors which are responsible also for the effect of histamine in increasing heart rate and counteracting uterine contraction. These actions of histamine are unaffected by traditional antihistamines which act on the other elements of the histamine receptor population (H_1 receptors) which are present in bronchi, arteries and gut.

The H_2 receptor antagonists, cimetidine and ranitidine, reduce acid content and volume of gastric secretions. This effect varies with dose and correlates with plasma concentrations of the drugs. Both compounds are effective in healing gastric and duodenal ulcers when given for 4–6 weeks in a twice daily regimen. Their use in single courses of treatment does not affect the high relapse rate of peptic ulcer disease.

Cimetidine and ranitidine do not appear to produce a rebound hypersecretory state after discontinuation and early reports of acute perforation after a course of treatment probably reflect the tendency for peptic ulcers to revert to their former state of activity.

Cimetidine has been used most widely and a variety of adverse effects has been observed. Central nervous system toxicity in elderly and seriously ill patients has led to various, quickly reversible manifestations, e.g. confusion, agitation, psychosis, seizures and decreased consciousness. Pre-existing renal or hepatic impairment have been implicated. Cardiovascular toxicity including bradycardia, hypotension and asystole has been reported after rapid i.v. injection, but no e.c.g. effects have been found during continuous infusions.

Endocrine effects of long-term use include gynaecomastia, oligospermia and impotence. A range of drug interactions are known to occur as a consequence of the effect of cimetidine to inhibit drug metabolism. Of particular importance is the need to monitor drugs including anticonvulsants, amino-phylline/theophylline, warfarin and lignocaine which carry a high risk of toxicity. Dosage of these drugs may need to be reduced by 50% or more. Other drugs which may be affected include benzodiazepines, chlormethiazole, propranolol, morphine and quinidine.

Ranitidine in therapeutic doses seems free of any inhibitory effect on drug metabolism. It may also be free of c.n.s. and endocrine actions, although experience with the drug is much less than with cimetidine.

Antiemetics

Antiemetics are used frequently during the postoperative period since nausea and vomiting result from the use of opioid analgesics and anaesthetic agents. Inhibition of nausea and vomiting may be achieved by drugs which depress the vomiting centre (antihistamines/anticholinergic agents), by drugs which depress the chemoreceptor trigger zone (e.g. phenothiazines and metoclopramide) and by drugs which increase gastrointestinal motility (e.g. metoclopramide, domperidone).

Antihistamines (e.g. cyclizine, promethazine) are most useful in vestibular disorders and are thought to act mainly through an anticholinergic action which blocks stimulation of the vomiting centre from the vestibular nuclei. The anticholinergic agent, hyoscine, is also useful in motion sickness.

Phenothiazines are the most useful antiemetic agents and their action is probably mediated via blockade of dopamine receptors in the chemoreceptor trigger zone. Chlorpromazine, prochlorperazine, thiethyl-perazine and perphenazine are equally effective in nausea and vomiting resulting from infection, uraemia, radiation, neoplastic disease and in anaesthetic or drug-induced vomiting. Sedation (antihistamine and anticholinergic action), hypo-tension (α-adrenoceptor blockade) and dystonic reactions (dopamine-receptor blockade) are the major adverse effects. Sedation and hypotension are most frequent with chlorpromazine but less marked with prochlorperazine and thiethylperazine. Perphenazine is more likely to produce involuntary movements. Acute dystonic reactions involving eyes, head and neck are more likely to occur in children and in the elderly. Phenothiazines may also lower the seizure threshold and therefore should be used with caution in epileptic patients.

Metoclopramide has a central antiemetic action via dopamine blockade (as with the phenothiazines) and a peripheral action which involves increasing the tone of gastro-intestinal smooth muscle. Lower oesophageal sphincter tone, gastric emptying rate and small intestinal transit are increased. The peripheral action of metoclopramide is poorly understood but it seems to mimic the effect of acetylcholine in addition to involving dopamine-receptor blockade. Meto-clopramide may produce drowsiness, dizziness or motor restlessness and, less commonly, acute dystonic reactions. These extrapyramidal reactions are related to dopamine receptor blockade and respond to i.v. diazepam or to an anticholinergic antiparkinsonian agent (e.g. benztropine). Toxic effects of metoclopramide may be mistaken occasionally for idiopathic Parkinsonism. The dosage of metoclopramide should be reduced in moderate/severe renal impairment.

Domperidone is an antiemetic similar to meto-clopramide, but without marked central nervous system actions. Experience is limited at present and extrapyramidal reactions, minor sedation and cardiac arrhythmias have been reported after i.v. bolus so that administration by infusion is preferable.

BRONCHODILATORS

Aminophylline is the most widely used bronchodilator in acute bronchospasm. However, its perioperative use is controversial since individual reports of cardiac arrhythmias during anaesthesia indicate that patients under anaesthesia may be more sensitive to its toxic effects.

Xanthine bronchodilators

Theophylline and its more water soluble ethylene diamine salt, aminophylline, are reliable bronchodilators for acute bronchospasm. Other xanthine derivatives including acepifylline, diprophylline, etamiphylline and proxyphylline have no advantages and are either too short-acting or are poorly absorbed orally.

Xanthines relax smooth muscle producing bronchodilation, a lowering of systemic vascular resistance and a reduction in left ventricular end-diastolic pressure. Venous pooling occurs and this is beneficial in acute pulmonary oedema of cardiac failure. A chronotropic and inotropic effect on the heart in addition to a direct action on renal tubules produces diuresis. The smooth muscle and cardiac effects of xanthines are produced, in part, by inhibition of phosphodiesterase, the enzyme responsible for degradation of cyclic adenosine monophosphate (cAMP) within the muscle cell. Potentiation of the effects of catecholamines and calcium is thought also to be involved. In this way, the pharmacological action of xanthines mimics β-adrenoceptor stimulation (see Chapter 12, p. 177). The therapeutic and toxic effects of xanthines in combination with β-agonists are additive.

Xanthines also cause stimulation of the central nervous system. Stimulation of the respiratory centre is exploited in the treatment of neonatal apnoea and Cheyne-Stokes respiration. C.n.s. stimulation in high doses also produces nausea, vomiting, restlessness, irritability and convulsions. In acute situations, aminophylline should be administered i.v., since the pH (9.4) precludes the i.m. route and rectal administration is too unreliable. Caution should be exercised in the i.v. use of aminophylline because the narrow therapeutic dose range requires attention to selection of dosage and rate of administration. Rapid injection of aminophylline produces high peak blood concentrations exceeding the therapeutic range of 10–20 mg/litre during the first 15 min or so after administration, with the risk of convulsions, tachycardia, nausea and vomiting. Aminophylline should be given i.v. over at least 10–15 min to allow complete distribution of the drug throughout the body during this period.

Variations in dosage requirements arise from variations in metabolism of theophylline, resulting from age, disease and smoking habits. In otherwise healthy adults (nonsmokers) the half-life of theophylline is 7–9 h, whilst the half-life is 4–5 h amongst smokers. In premature infants and patients with severe cirrhosis the half-life is approx. 20–30 h, whereas in children (aged 1–15 yr) the half-life is approx. 3–4 h.

Since aminophylline is normally metabolised rapidly, maintenance treatment is best provided by a continuous i.v. infusion following a standard loading dose of approx. 6 mg/kg. The initial loading dose should be halved if the patient has been taking oral aminophylline/theophylline regularly. The previously recommended adult maintenance infusion rates (0.9 mg/kg/h) have been associated with fatalities from seizures. The initial maintenance dosage should be approx. 0.5–0.6 mg/kg/h and, wherever possible, should be adjusted by measurement of plasma concentration. It is important to appreciate that seizures may not be preceded by other warning symptoms (e.g. nausea). Patients also receiving cimetidine may require up to 50% reduction in maintenance dose (vide supra). Therapeutic benefit can be expected at plasma concentrations of 5–15 mg/litre, with little added benefit above this range and at the cost of greatly increased toxicity above 20 mg/litre. Other drugs (e.g. corticosteroids) should not be added to the infusion fluid. Aminophylline should not be given via a central venous catheter because of its cardiotoxicity.

Theophylline may be given orally in the salt form choline theophyllinate, three times daily, or a slow release preparation, twice daily. In view of the need to adjust dosage individually, oral formulations of combination products of theophylline/aminophylline (with, for example, sympathomimetics) should be avoided.

β-Adrenoceptor agonists

β-Adrenoceptor agonists are based chemically on isoprenaline and structural modification has produced relatively long-acting compounds, many of which are effective orally and most of which are selective to noncardiac (β_2) receptors in therapeutic doses.

The pharmacological profiles of selective β_2-adrenoceptor agonists are identical, differing only in duration of action. β_2-adrenoceptor agonists are popular when administered by self-propelled aerosol. Salbutamol and terbutaline can be given also by injection, by nebuliser and orally. Fenoterol, rimiterol and reproterol are available also for aerosol administration. The majority of β_2-agonists act for 5–7 h after inhalation, except for rimiterol which lasts for only approx. 2 h. Orciprenaline is a nonselective agent. Although these agonists produce less cardiac effects than isoprenaline or orciprenaline, tachycardia may occur after i.v. administration or after high dose nebuliser therapy. The cardiac effects may result partly from reduction in systemic vascular resistance. Other signs of toxicity include tremor, headache and dizziness. These side effects are seen also during oral administration. Measurable tolerance to the therapeutic effects of long term systemic therapy has been demonstrated and is supported by clinical impression.

The relatively small doses used in aerosol inhaler or powder insufflation (100–500 μg per metered dose) do not usually produce systemic effects. Careful attention should be paid to dosage of β_2 agonists administered via nebuliser, since the amounts of drug delivered (2.5–12.5 mg) are markedly greater than those given by aerosol. Drug absorbed by the lung avoids first pass metabolism in the liver and is therefore analogous to parenteral administration. An optimum initial dose of salbutamol or terbutaline by nebuliser is 2.5–5 mg. Apart from convenience of administration, nebuliser therapy is no more effective than aerosol inhalation.

Faulty technique of aerosol administration is a common cause of poor control of chronic obstructive airways disease. Various alternative devices including an automatically triggered aerosol (rimiterol 'Auto-haler'), a powder insufflation (salbutamol 'Rotahaler') and extended aerosol mouth-pieces (terbutaline 'Spacer' and 'Nebuhaler') are available.

Intravenous salbutamol or terbutaline are equally as effective as aminophylline in acute asthma. Intravenous aminophylline offers the advantage of theoretical (but unproven) synergy with inhaled β_2-agonist.

Ipratropium bromide

Ipratropium is an anticholinergic bronchodilator which may be given either by aerosol or nebuliser. It acts by blocking bronchoconstriction via cholinergic receptors and so decreases intracellular ionic calcium and decreases cyclic guanosine monophosphate, an intracellular mediator of bronchoconstriction. Its effects occur within 15 min and slowly peak between 1–2 h. It has been found to be less effective than β_2-adrenoceptor agonists in asthmatic subjects but seems effective in chronic bronchitis. There is no evidence of systemic toxicity with inhaled ipratropium and the drug does not impair clearance of sputum. Ipratropium may have an additive bronchodilator action in combination with β_2-agonists or aminophylline in some patients.

DRUGS ACTING ON THE CARDIOVASCULAR SYSTEM

Diuretics

The management of oedema may require a planned approach to the use of diuretics, demanding an appreciation of the limitations of individual agents and the value of combining diuretics which have different sites and mechanisms of action.

In the renal tubule there are four sites where diuretics affect sodium reabsorption (see Fig. 13.1). Site 1 is the proximal tubule where blockade of active sodium reabsorption is of limited use as a result of development of compensatory mechanisms distally. Site 2 is the ascending loop of Henle. Action at this site produces a brisk, potentially large diuresis even at low glomerular filtration rates. Site 3 is the diluting segment and action at this site produces a moderate diuresis. Site 4 is the distal tubule where blockade of sodium–potassium exchange leads to a mild diuresis and conservation of potassium.

The pharmacological properties of diuretics are indicated in Table 13.1.

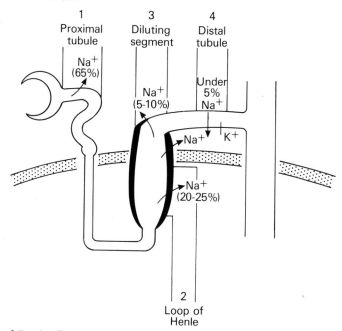

Fig. 13.1 Sites of action of diuretics. Percentages indicate the proportion of intraluminal sodium which is absorbed at different sites in the nephron.

Table 13.1 Commonly used diuretics

Diuretic	Site(s) of action	Route	Onset	Duration (h)	Notes
High potency					
Frusemide	2				Effective at low GFR. Produce hyperuricaemia, hyperglycaemia, hypokalaemia and hypomagnesaemia. Calcium excretion is increased. May cause hearing loss, tinnitus or vertigo after high doses i.v. (especially if too rapid), very high doses orally, in uraemia, or if combined with aminoglycosides
Bumetanide	2	oral & i.v.	30 min	4–6	
Ethacrynic acid	2		5 min	2	
Medium potency					
Thiazides	1 + 3	oral	2 h	6–12 (some longer)	Ineffective at GFR less than 20 ml/min. Maximum diuresis achieved after small increases in dose. Additive effect with high potency diuretics. Produce hyperuricaemia, hyperglycaemia, hypokalaemia and hypomagnesaemia. Calcium excretion is reduced.
Mefruside	1 + 3	oral	2 h	12	
Metolazone	1 + 3	oral	2 h	12–24	Effective at GFR less than 20 ml/min. Synergy with high potency diuretics. Diuresis can be profound, caution with initial dose
Low potency					
Spironolactone	4	oral	12 h	24	Acts by aldosterone inhibition. In absence of loading dose maximum effect takes 3 days
Potassium conrenoate		i.v.	12 h	24	i.v. form is the active metabolite (canrenone). Potassium retaining. Avoid in renal failure
Amiloride	4	oral	2 h	10	Independent of aldosterone. Potentially nephrotoxic. Potassium retaining. Avoid in renal failure
Triamterene	4	oral	2 h	12–16	
Acetazolamide	1	oral i.v./i.m.	2 h	12	Inhibits carbonic anhydrase. Metabolic acidosis during first week leads to tolerance through $Na^+ - H^+$ exchange. Synergy with high potency diuretics

High-potency diuretics are useful in left ventricular failure. After i.v. administration, the immediate beneficial effect of frusemide results partly from an increase in venous capacitance and decrease in preload. In hepatic ascites rapid diuresis may worsen electrolyte imbalance. Spironolactone is particularly beneficial where secondary hyperaldosteronism contributes to the oedema (e.g. hepatic or cardiac failure). Potassium-retaining diuretics are potentially hazardous in the presence of declining renal function or potassium supplementation. When a combination of diuretics is necessary, the objective should be to use maximum tolerable effective doses of each agent.

Cardiac glycosides

Digoxin and other cardiac glycosides improve cardiac output by an inotropic action on myocardial contractility, whilst their ability to suppress atrioventricular conduction is useful in controlling the ventricular rate in supraventricular arrhythmias, particularly atrial fibrillation.

The cardiovascular response to cardiac glycosides is complicated by indirect actions. In the failing heart, a slowing of heart rate occurs, brought about mainly by the reduction in sympathetic tone which results from the increase in cardiac output. In addition there is a direct vagal stimulatory action of cardiac glycosides. Peripheral vasodilatation occurs also as sympathetic tone is diminished but there is no clinically relevant direct effect on peripheral vasculature. Although cardiac glycosides might be expected to increase heart work and therefore oxygen demand, the work of the failing heart is often reduced because of reduced heart rate and cardiac size.

The mechanism of action of cardiac glycosides is incompletely understood but stems from inhibition of the sodium–potassium active exchange at the myocardial cell membrane. There is an associated increase in ionic calcium within the cell, either because of release from intracellular stores or because of increased influx of calcium in lieu of sodium ions. The increased availability of intracellular ionised calcium enhances excitation–contraction coupling within myofibrils.

The ability of cardiac glycosides to suppress conduction in the AV node is the basis for their use in supraventricular arrhythmias. The improvement in cardiac output is therefore most marked in congestive heart failure in the presence of atrial fibrillation. The use of cardiac glycosides in acute left ventricular failure has been superseded gradually by vasodilators and sympathomimetics. The glycosides are of no use in cardiogenic shock and are best avoided after acute myocardial infarction. Any long-term benefit on congestive heart failure in sinus rhythm remains to be demonstrated fully, since in many patients cardiac glycosides can be discontinued without detriment.

There is increased sensitivity to digoxin and similar cardiac glycosides in the presence of hypokalaemia, hypomagnesaemia, hypercalcaemia, renal impairment, chronic pulmonary or heart disease, myxoedema, and hypoxia. There is decreased sensitivity in thyrotoxicosis. Quinidine, and to a lesser extent amiodarone and verapamil, tend to increase plasma digoxin concentrations. β-blockers and verapamil have combined effects on the AV node. Digoxin should be administered cautiously i.v. in situations where AV conduction is already suppressed.

There are various manifestations of cardiac glycoside toxicity. Ventricular arrhythmias (particularly bigeminy and trigeminy) are the commonest. Supraventricular arrhythmias may occur, often with some degree of heart block. Other symptoms are rather unpredictable, and in chronic toxicity, include fatigue, weakness of arms or legs, agitation, nightmares, various visual disturbances, anorexia, and nausea or abdominal pain. These symptoms may not precede cardiac toxicity. Therapeutic and toxic blood concentrations overlap so plasma determinations may be used only to substantiate clinical impressions of digitalis toxicity. Treatment of serious arrhythmias involves careful administration of potassium chloride under e.c.g. control (especially in the presence of heart block or renal impairment). Lignocaine or phenytoin are useful for ventricular arrhythmias, whilst β-blockade is useful in supraventricular arrhythmias. Cardioversion during cardiac glycoside therapy may produce ventricular arrhythmias.

Digoxin has a long half-life (approx. 36 h) which is sensitive to changes in renal function. In the absence of a loading dose, effective plasma concentrations (1–2 μg/litre) occur after approx. 5–7 days. For an acute response, a loading (digitalising) dose is required which should be based approximately on lean body weight. Maintenance doses of digoxin need to take into account the presence of renal impairment. Although the effect of an i.v. injection begins within 30–60 min, distribution into cardiac tissue takes place slowly over the first 6 h following ·oral or i.v. administration. This slow distribution entails that a maximum response occurs 4–6 h after i.v. administration. Blood samples for digoxin measurements taken before this 6-h period cannot be interpreted correctly. Digoxin is absorbed unreliably and i.m. injections are painful.

Other parenteral cardiac glycosides (ouabain and deslanoside) have a marginally shorter onset of effect perhaps as a result of more rapid tissue distribution.

Ouabain has a half-life of 21 h. The effect begins 5–10 min after i.v. administration and reaches a maximum after 1–2 h.

Deslanoside has an onset of action between that of ouabain and digoxin, beginning in 10–30 min after i.v. administration and reaching a maximum after 1–2 h.

Digitoxin is less dependent upon renal function for its elimination. Its long half-life (4–6 days) is a disadvantage, since toxic effects are very persistent.

Vasodilators

Drugs which dilate arteries or veins are now widely used either alone or in conjunction with inotropic agents in the management of acute left ventricular failure. Arterial vasodilators are useful also in the treatment of acute hypertensive episodes and in the selective induction of controlled hypotension to reduce haemorrhage during surgery. Some vasodilators are used investigationally to reduce infarct size after myocardial infarction. The main agents are sodium nitroprusside and the nitrates (isosorbide dinitrate and glyceryl trinitrate). Hydralazine and diazoxide are also important parenteral vasodilators, whereas prazosin, minoxidil and captopril are oral agents which have a place in the chronic management of left ventricular failure and as third line agents in the treatment of hypertension. Calcium slow-channel blocking agents also have a mainly arterial vasodilator action, including an effect on the coronary artery.

The use of vasodilators in left ventricular failure is based on their ability to reduce afterload and preload. In cardiac failure, reflex increase in sympathetic tone creates an increase in systemic vascular resistance in the arterial bed. By lowering this resistance (afterload), the work and oxygen requirements of the heart are reduced. Those vasodilators which are capable of acting on the venous side of the circulation increase venous capacitance, reduce venous return to the heart and so decrease the left ventricular filling pressure (preload). Lowering the filling pressure in the left ventricle decreases the degree of stretch of myocardial fibres and so improves myocardial contractility and cardiac output and reduces myocardial oxygen consumption for the same degree of external cardiac work performed.

Vasodilators may be classified into those which act directly on arterial smooth muscle (nitroprusside, nitrates, hydralazine, diazoxide, minoxidil, calcium slow-channel blocking agents), and those which are neurohumoral antagonists (prazosin and other adrenoceptor antagonists, captopril). This distinction is important since the drugs in the first category have a clear, often sensitive, dose-response relationship which requires haemodynamic monitoring (preferably by invasive techniques), whereas those in the second category have a relatively long duration of action and their intensity of effect is less sensitive to changes in dosage.

Another useful way of comparing vasodilators is to consider on which side of the heart they may act preferentially. Hydralazine and minoxidil act mainly on afterload. Nitroprusside, the α-adrenoceptor antagonists and captopril have a balanced effect on both arteries and veins.

Sodium nitroprusside

Sodium nitroprusside has an immediate, short-lived effect (lasting only for a few minutes) which requires that it be given by continuous infusion. A smooth reduction in arterial pressure can be achieved by adjustment of the infusion rate. The nitroprusside ion is responsible for a direct action on vascular smooth muscle and it is metabolised by red cells to cyanide. Cyanide ions are detoxified by the liver and kidney to thiocyanate (requiring thiosulphate and vitamin B_{12}) which is excreted slowly in the urine.

Sodium nitroprusside produces a balanced reduction in afterload and preload. In larger doses (e.g. when used for hypotensive anaesthesia) its use leads to an increase in heart rate. There is an additive effect with other vasodilators. In medical practice nitroprusside is well tolerated and most symptoms are nonspecific (e.g. drowsiness, perspiration, nausea, dizziness) and are associated with too rapid a decrease in arterial pressure.

The accumulation of cyanide and thiocyanate, with the risk of lactic acidosis, is a possibility but is rare in the absence of impaired renal or hepatic function or if total dosage does not exceed 1.5 mg/kg. Where therapy is high dose or prolonged, plasma bicarbonate monitoring is indicated. Plasma cyanide or thiocyanate concentrations may also be monitored if the drug is used for more than two days. Thiocyanate is potentially neurotoxic and can cause hypothyroidism. Thiosulphate and a specially prepared high dose infusion of hydroxocobalamin have been used to reverse cyanide toxicity. Nitroprusside is photodegraded and infusion solutions should be protected from light.

The use of sodium nitroprusside (SNP), in hypotensive anaesthesia is considered in Chapter 35.

Nitrates

The organic nitrates, glyceryl trinitrate and isosorbide dinitrate, affect mainly preload and are most effective in relieving pulmonary congestion secondary to left ventricular failure. However this selectivity of action decreases with dosage so that a decrease in arterial pressure, tachycardia and headaches may occur. The nitrates have a shortlived effect and may be given i.v. The infusion rate should be carefully controlled according to heart rate and haemodynamic effects. The action of nitrates in left ventricular failure is enhanced by agents, including hydralazine, which preferentially reduce afterload.

The nitrates are absorbed by rubber and plastics (especially PVC infusion bags), so they are best administered from syringe pumps. Intravenous nitrates are used also in unstable angina. The therapeutic effects of nitrates in myocardial ischaemia result not only from preload reduction but also from counteraction of coronary vasospasm and redistribution of blood within the myocardium.

Hydralazine, diazoxide and minoxidil

These drugs are direct-acting arterial vasodilators. Their main action is to reduce afterload, with little or no effect on preload and their main limitation is reflex tachycardia, although this is less prominent in patients with cardiac failure.

In hypertensives, the reduction in arterial pressure is limited by reflex sympathetic discharge which tends to increase cardiac output. Similarly, their antihypertensive action is limited by a tendency to cause sodium and water retention by a direct renal mechanism and by activation of the renin–angiotensin system. These vasodilators therefore often benefit from being combined with a β-adrenoceptor blocker and a diuretic.

Hydralazine is the most widely used direct vasodilator drug. Its half-life is short (less than 5 h) but its antihypertensive effect is relatively prolonged, permitting twice daily dosage.

Diazoxide is of limited use because of its unpredictable duration of action, unrelated to its short plasma half-life. The initial i.v. dose of diazoxide must be given rapidly for maximum effect. A cumulative effect on arterial pressure may make it difficult to control the action of repeated doses.

Minoxidil is available for oral use only and it too has a long duration of action (12–24 h) which is unrelated to its plasma half-life.

Calcium slow-channel blocking agents

Calcium slow-channel blocking agents, such as nifedipine and verapamil, have been used as antianginal and, more recently, as antihypertensive agents. They antagonise coronary artery spasm and relax systemic vascular smooth muscle predominantly on the arterial side of the circulation. Verapamil is also a useful drug for the treatment of supraventricular arrhythmias (vide infra) since it shows some preference for the AV node, through which conduction is dependent upon intracellular calcium (as opposed to sodium) influx. The antihypertensive effects of calcium channel blocking agents have not yet been studied widely but they appear modest and, in the case of nifedipine at least, have been inconsistent.

Intracellular calcium ion availability is important in the conduction of the cardiac action potential and in electromechanical coupling within smooth muscle cells. Drugs which affect the permeability to calcium of the extracellular or intracellular membranes can influence the size of the cytoplasmic pool of calcium ions. This action reduces cardiac contractility (producing a negative inotropic effect) and decreases vascular tone. Calcium slow-channel blocking agents differ in their selectivity for myocardial or arterial tissue, verapamil being rather more selective for cardiac muscle than nifedipine. Nifedipine presents less risk of reducing contractility and has no important effect on conduction through the AV node.

Nifedipine is more potent than verapamil as a systemic and coronary arterial vasodilator, making it the more effective antianginal agent. It is effective in countering coronary artery spasm, which is now thought to be an important component to all forms of angina. The antianginal effect of nifedipine is additive with that of β-adrenergic blocking drugs and nitrates. The marked negative inotropic action of verapamil presents a potential hazard when used in conjunction with β-adrenergic blockers or other cardiodepressant drugs (including disopyramide and the volatile anaesthetic agents) in patients with limited cardiac reserve. However the effects of these agents in individual patients is unpredictable since the failing left ventricle can benefit from reductions in afterload brought about by peripheral vaso-dilatation.

Side effects of nifedipine are related to its vasodilator action and include flushing, headaches, dizziness, tiredness and palpitations. Nifedipine may also cause ankle oedema which arises from peripheral vasodilatation unrelated to any cardiodepressant action of the drug. Reports of nifedipine actually precipitating an anginal attack about half an hour after a dose have received some attention, but more evidence is required in order to clarify their relevance. Nifedipine is available for oral administration only but a swift action in angina can be obtained by advising the patient to bite on the soft gelatin capsule placed in the mouth.

Inhibition of platelet aggregation, protection against bronchospasm, use in Raynaud's syndrome and improvements in lower oesophageal sphincter function are other interesting properties of calcium slow-channel blocking agents which are being investigated currently.

α-Adrenoceptor antagonists

The pharmacology of α-adrenoceptor antagonists (e.g. phentolamine, phenoxybenzamine) has been discussed in Chapter 12, p. 188. These agents have a balanced effect on venous capacitance and systemic arterial resistance. The oral postsynaptic (α_1) blocking agent, prazosin, is a widely used vasodilator in chronic left ventricular failure. It tends to produce little if any increase in heart rate. Initial administration may cause a sudden decrease in arterial pressure and so prazosin should be given as a low first dose, preferably with the patient supine. Syncope is more likely if the patient is receiving nitrates concurrently. There is concern that the short-term benefits of prazosin in left ventricular failure may not be maintained during long-term therapy.

As with many of these drugs, the duration of vasodilator action of prazosin (approx. 12 h) does not correlate with its short half-life in plasma (3–4 h). The short-acting phentolamine and the long-acting phenoxybenzamine are other α-adrenoceptor blocking drugs which are used occasionally by the parenteral route as adjuncts in hypertension or left ventricular failure.

Captopril

Captopril is an oral agent which has a balanced action on preload and afterload. It acts by inhibiting the converting enzyme responsible for the activation of angiotensin from its inactive form in plasma. Captopril also lowers blood volume by blocking the renin–angiotensin–aldosterone sequence. Those patients who have recently been or who are being treated with potent diuretics should be given captopril cautiously to avoid a profound initial response.

Antiarrhythmic agents

The aim of drug treatment of cardiac arrhythmias is either to prevent the emergence of a tachyarrhythmia or to terminate a run of tachycardia. A continuous arrhythmia may be controlled either by slowing the primary mechanism or, in the case of supra-ventricular arrhythmias, by reducing the proportion of impulses transmitted through the AV node and ventricular conducting system.

The emergence of ectopic pacemaker cells may be explained by the phenomenon of re-entry. Re-entrant arrhythmias arise from retrograde conduction along a branch of tissue in which anterograde conduction has been blocked by disease. When retrograde conduction is sufficiently slow it can influence cells which have already discharged and repolarised, triggering a further action potential which is both premature and ectopic. A vicious circle can ensue such that these action potentials become self-sustaining (circus movements) leading to multiple ectopic beats, tachycardia or fibrillation.

The basis for treatment of particular arrhythmias has arisen largely from clinical experience. The known electrophysiological properties of anti-arrhythmics have provided explanations for observed effects and, in particular, it has become clear that any drug with an antiarrhythmic action may itself provoke arrhythmias. Consequently antiarrhythmic agents tend to be used rather more conservatively than in the past.

Antiarrhythmic agents may be classified empirically on the basis of their effectiveness in supraventricular tachycardias (e.g. digoxin, β-blockers and verapamil) or in ventricular arrhythmias (lignocaine, mexiletine, tocainide, phenytoin and bretylium). Many agents (disopyramide, amiodarone, quinidine and procainamide) are effective in both supraventricular and ventricular arrhythmias.

The cardiac action potential

Antiarrhythmic agents are classified conventionally according to their effects on the cardiac action potential (Fig. 13.2) which comprises five phases, each corresponding to a changing state of depolarisation of the myocardial cell.

The action potential is triggered by slow intracellular leak of sodium ions (and calcium ions at the AV node) until a threshold point is reached when sudden rapid influx of sodium ions generates an impulse (phase 0). The action potential starts to reverse (phase 1) but is sustained, whilst there is slower inward movement of calcium ions (phase 2) after which there is gradual termination as efflux of potassium ions brings about repolarisation (phase 3). Thereafter, re-equilibration of sodium and potassium takes place and the resting membrane potential is restored (phase 4).

There are three important components of the cardiac action potential which are amenable to pharmacological intervention.

First, the *automaticity* (tendency to spontaneous discharge) of cells may be reduced. This result can be achieved by reducing the rate of leakage of sodium (reducing the slope of phase 4), by increasing the electronegativity of the resulting membrane potential or by decreasing the electronegativity of the threshold potential.

Second, the speed of *conduction* of the action potential can be suppressed as indicated by a lowering of the height and slope of the phase 0 discharge. A reduction in the electronegativity of the membrane potential at the onset of phase 0 will reduce both the amplitude and the slope of the phase 0 depolarisation. This situation occurs if the cell discharges before it has completely repolarised.

Third, the *rate of repolarisation* can be reduced, which prolongs the refractory period of the discharging cell.

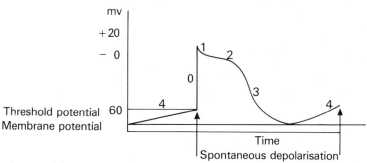

Fig. 13.2 The cardiac action potential.
Phase 0 — rapid depolarisation associated with fast Na^+ influx
    1 — early repolarisation
    2 — maintained depolarisation associated with slow Ca^{++} influx
    3 — repolarisation associated with K^+ efflux
    4 — resting membrane potential; may have upward slope representing slow spontaneous depolarisation in automatic (pacemaker) tissues

On the basis of these pharmacological effects, antiarrhythmic agents can be grouped into four classes (Table 13.2). Those agents in class 1A antagonise primarily the fast influx of sodium ions and so reduce automaticity and conduction velocity,

Table 13.2 Classification of anti-arrhythmic agents

1 Membrane stabilisation	A Quinidine, procainamide, disopyramide
	B Lignocaine, mexiletine, tocainide, phenytoin
2 β-receptor blockade	All β-blockers
3 Prolongation of action potential	Amiodarone, bretylium, sotalol (also class 2)
4 Calcium antagonism	Verapamil

whilst prolonging the refractory period. Those in class 1B also affect automaticity in the same way, but they have much less effect on conduction velocity in usual therapeutic doses and they shorten the refractory period. β-blockers (class 2) depress automaticity but have no other specific effects on the action potential apart from reducing the effect of catecholamines (i.e. the increase in automaticity and conduction velocity in the sinus and AV node). Agents in class 3 lengthen the refractory period by prolonging the action potential. Verapamil (class 4) also prolongs the action potential in addition to depressing automaticity (especially in the AV node).

An appreciation of the general class of action of different antiarrhythmic agents enables the selection of a second agent to be made from a different class, in the event of failure of a primary agent or if there is need for combination therapy.

Quinidine has now been superseded largely by newer agents including disopyramide. Intravenous administration may cause severe hypotension. Toxic effects may be dose related or arise as drug idiosyncrasy. The most serious toxicity is depression of conduction and risk of ventricular fibrillation. Visual and auditory disturbances with vertigo and gastrointestinal symptoms are signs of toxicity. Skin reactions, thrombocytopenia and agranulocytosis may occur also. Quinidine enhances digoxin toxicity by doubling plasma concentrations. It also has an additive effect with hypotensive agents and drugs having cardiodepresssant properties (e.g. disopyramide, β-blockers and calcium antagonists).

Procainamide closely resembles quinidine in its effect on the heart. It may cause hypotension after i.v. administration. Its main application is as an oral antiarrhythmic, although therapy is limited by its short half-life (3 h) requiring frequent administration or the use of a sustained release oral preparation. Procainamide is restricted usually to short-term use because of the risk of drug-induced systemic lupus erythematosus. Other manifestations of hypersensitivity include fever, rash, arthralgia and agranulocytosis.

Disopyramide has properties in common with both quinidine and lignocaine. It is useful in supraventricular tachycardias and as a second line agent to lignocaine in ventricular arrhythmias. Its half-life (8 h) is prolonged in renal impairment and following myocardial infarction, necessitating dosage reduction. Side effects result mainly from the anticholinergic effect of the parent drug and a major metabolite, which can produce urinary retention and blurred vision. Disopyramide is markedly cardiodepressant, especially in combination with β-blockers, quinidine, procainamide or verapamil.

Lignocaine remains the first choice for ventricular arrhythmias. It has a short half-life of less than 2 h, although this is prolonged after myocardial infarction, in liver disease and during cimetidine treatment. The effect of a single loading dose may be brief since lignocaine distributes rapidly after an i.v. dose which may need to be repeated twice. A continuous infusion is used to maintain the effect, with the rate of infusion adjusted according to response. Close adjustment of the infusion rate is required to avoid toxicity (confusion, slurring of speech, numbness, dizziness and convulsions). The presence of heart failure, β-blockade or liver disease should be an indication to reduce maintenance dosage by half. A reduced loading dose is necessary also in heart failure. A common reason for failure of response to lignocaine is the presence of hypokalaemia.

Mexiletine is a longer acting, orally effective, lignocaine analogue which has a half-life of 10 h. It shares lignocaine's low margin of safety, especially after i.v. administration when hypotension and bradycardia have been reported. Most frequent adverse effects involve the central nervous system and include tremors, nystagmus, confusion, speech disturbances, tinnitus, paraesthesiae and convulsions. Gastro-intestinal effects are also common during oral treatment.

Tocainide is another lignocaine analogue which can be given orally and parenterally. It has a half-life of 13

h. Arrhythmias not responding to lignocaine are unlikely to respond to tocainide. Adverse effects resemble those of mexiletine.

Phenytoin is unique in that it accelerates intraventricular conduction and is particularly effective in controlling digitalis-induced ventricular arrhythmias.

β-blockers are used mainly in sinus and supraventricular tachycardias, especially those provoked by emotion or exercise. Their cardio-depressant effects are a disadvantage in the management of arrhythmias after acute myocardial infarction. For further discussion of the pharmacology of β-blockers see Chapter 12 (p. 184).

Amiodarone is a very effective agent against both supraventricular and ventricular arrhythmias. It has a long half-life (over 30 d) so that oral treatment should be commenced with approx. a week of high doses to establish a therapeutic effect. An i.v. form has been used although experience is limited. Intravenous administration may cause bradycardia, hypotension (vasodilatation) and heart block and so it must be diluted in an infusion of dextrose. Long-term accumulation produces reversible microdeposits in the cornea which generally do not interfere with vision. Deposition in the skin produces photosensitivity and blue-grey discolouration. Since amiodarone is an iodinated compound it may disturb thyroid function tests and may produce clinical hyperthyroidism or, less commonly, hypothyroidism. Amiodarone may increase blood concentrations of digoxin.

Bretylium is a quaternary ammonium compound which prevents noradrenaline uptake into sympathetic nerve endings. It has been used in recurrent life-threatening ventricular arrhythmias resistant to lignocaine or DC shock. It has a positive inotropic effect and usually causes an increase in arterial pressure during the first 24 h, followed by a decrease. It may cause bradycardia or asystole and may worsen ventricular arrhythmias transiently.

Verapamil is also a coronary and peripheral vasodilator, useful in angina and hypertension, which is effective both orally and i.v. It is very effective in supraventricular tachycardias, in which it acts by depressing AV conduction and blocking re-entry mechanisms. Similarly, it controls the ventricular rate in atrial fibrillation. Intravenous administration may reduce arterial pressure (by vasodilatation) and

caution is necessary in low output states and in patients treated with negative inotropic agents, e.g. β-blockers, disopyramide, quinidine and procainamide.

DRUGS AFFECTING THE IMMUNE SYSTEM

The major drugs used in acute conditions involving the activation of immunological and inflammatory mechanisms are the corticosteroids and the antihistamines.

Corticosteroids

The corticosteroids have been advocated in a variety of acute life-threatening conditions, although few recommendations are supported by firm evidence of efficacy. Included in these conditions are bacteraemic and anaphylactic shock, adult respiratory distress syndrome, status asthmaticus and cerebral oedema.

Amongst the many complex actions of pharmacological doses of corticosteroids, those affecting the cellular and microvascular components of the inflammatory response are more relevant to any therapeutic benefit achieved in critically ill patients. These pharmacological effects seem to parallel the glucocorticoid properties of individual corticosteroids which are shown in Table 13.3.

The anti-inflammatory action of corticosteroids involves reduction in the permeability of capillaries to intravascular fluid, proteins and chemical mediators of the inflammatory process. The migration and phagocytosis of polymorphonuclear leucocytes is inhibited. In high doses, corticosteroids prevent tissue damage by stabilising lysosomal membranes which reduces the extent of autolysis and hinders the perpetuation of the local inflammatory response. Corticosteroid administration leads to a relative lymphocytopenia which results from redistribution into the reticulo-endothelial system and a cytolytic action affecting preferentially the T lymphocyte population. The action on B lymphocytes is less marked and antibody formation is reduced only by high doses.

High doses of steroids have a cardiac inotropic effect and they also reduce systemic and pulmonary vascular resistance. Capillary flow is increased and there is mobilisation of interstitial fluid and protein.

Table 13.3 Glucocorticoid corticosteroids

	Equivalent dosage (mg)	Mean dose to suppress HPA * (mg/day)	Half-life in plasma (h)	Half-life of pharmacological effect ** (h)
Hydrocortisone	20	15–30	1.5	8–12
Cortisone	25	20–35	1.5	8–12
Prednisolone	5	7.5–10	3+	18–36
Prednisone	5	7.5–10	3+	18–36
Methylprednisolone	4	7.5–10	3+	18–36
Dexamethasone	0.75	1–1.5	5+	36–54
Triamcinolone	4	7.5–10	3+	18–36
Betamethasone	0.6	1–1.5	5+	36–54

* HPA = hypothalamic–pituitary–adrenal axis
** Based on duration of suppression of HPA axis

The use of corticosteroids in septic shock has gained theoretical support from the knowledge that the inflammatory process includes an early phase of vasodilatation and extensive capillary leakage which leads to hypovolaemia. β-Endorphin is probably also involved in vasodilatation and it is derived from the same precursor molecule as ACTH. Early administration of high dose corticosteroids may conceivably affect both ACTH and β-endorphin release. However, the results of clinical studies carried out to date are controversial. There is no evidence for any beneficial effect of corticosteroids in cardiogenic shock.

An effect on pulmonary capillary leakage has formed the theoretical basis for the use of corticosteroids in the adult respiratory distress syndrome. It is likely that the drugs should be given early to be effective and this may be practical when respiratory distress is provoked by a specific event such as pulmonary aspiration. However the evidence for benefit of corticosteroids in adult respiratory distress syndrome is inconclusive and there is likely to be a greater risk of infection if steroids are used routinely. Experimentally, steroids have been demonstrated to be beneficial in animal models of ARDS.

In acute allergic emergencies, including status asthmaticus, the use of corticosteroids is empirical, hydrocortisone being most commonly used. Intensive corticosteroid therapy should be for as short a period as possible (ideally limited to within 48–72 h). In such instances, the dosage need not be tapered or may be tapered quickly over the next 48–72 h except for conditions (such as asthma) in which there may be a relapse unless dosage is reduced carefully. In asthma, a change to oral prednisolone should be undertaken once an adequate response has been obtained. Dosage can be tapered gradually over 1–2 weeks. There is no evidence that very high dose potent steroids are more effective than conventional doses of hydrocortisone in acute allergy.

In cerebral oedema, corticosteroids (most commonly dexamethasone) have been used successfully to reduce raised intracranial pressure of varying aetiology. Steroids tend to be most effective in vasogenic oedema. Symptomatic improvement can be obtained when oedema results from tumour or benign intracranial hypertension. In the case of head injury or stroke any benefits of corticosteroids are uncertain. In cerebral malaria steroid treatment is detrimental.

The potential hazards of corticosteroids argue against their use in indications where their effectiveness is in doubt. The most important risk is infection, as a consequence of the suppressed inflammatory response. Glucose intolerance and gastro-intestinal haemorrhage are also risks to be considered, although an accurate assessment of their clinical importance is lacking. Effective antimicrobial cover is essential whenever corticosteroids are used in the critically ill.

Antihistamines

Although there are two distinct populations of histamine receptors (H_1 and H_2) the term antihistamines is still used to refer to those drugs which block selectively histamine H_1 receptors found in the bronchi, arteries and gut. There are no compounds currently in therapeutic use which influence both H_1 and H_2 receptors.

Histamine is only one of many mediators which may be involved in acute allergic reactions. Some consequences of these substances (e.g. hypotension and bronchospasm) may be counteracted most effectively by adrenaline and the β-adrenoceptor agonists. Antihistamines (e.g. chlorpheniramine, promethazine) tend to have only a secondary role in the management of acute allergy. They are most effective against symptoms including itch, oedema and urticaria. They are less effective against hypotension, and ineffective against bronchospasm, fever and arthralgia.

The most important adverse effect of antihistamines is sedation, although occasionally they may produce central nervous system stimulation (e.g. agitation or convulsions) especially in children. A new generation of antihistamines, e.g. terfenadine, has been developed which is relatively less sedative.

All antihistamines have anticholinergic effects which tend to dry mucosal secretions and may cause tachycardia.

FURTHER READING

Bowman W C, Rand M J 1980 Textbook of pharmacology, 2nd edn. Blackwell Scientific Publications, Oxford

Goodman-Gilman A, Goodman L S, Gilman A (eds) 1980 The pharmacological basis of therapeutics, 6th edn. Macmillan, New York

Vickers M D, Schneiden H, Ward-Smith F G 1984 Drugs in anaesthetic practice, 6th edn. Butterworths, London

14

Local anaesthetic agents

Local anaesthetic drugs act by producing a reversible block to the transmission of peripheral nerve impulses. A reversible block may be produced also by physical factors including pressure and cold. Although nerve compression is of purely historical interest, cold (produced by the evaporation of ethyl chloride, the application of ice packs or use of the cryoprobe) still has a limited use.

Many types of drug have local anaesthetic actions (e.g. β-blockers and antihistamines), but all those known and used as local anaesthetics have originated from cocaine, the alkaloid found in the leaves of the South American bush *Erythroxylon coca*. Its local anaesthetic action was demonstrated first by Koller, an ophthalmic surgeon working in Vienna. Although most of the major local anaesthetic techniques were described within a few years of that discovery, the drug was not used widely other than as a topical agent because of its systemic toxicity, central nervous stimulant and addictive properties and tendency to produce allergic reactions.

The demonstration of the physical structure of cocaine as an ester of benzoic acid permitted the production of safer agents, all with the same general structure of an aromatic group joined to an amine by an intermediate chain (Fig. 14.1). Procaine, synthesised in 1904, was the first significant advance

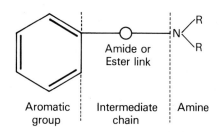

Fig. 14.1 General formula for local anaesthetic drugs.

and it allowed wider use of local anaesthetic techniques. Many other drugs were introduced, but none displaced procaine as the standard until the synthesis of lignocaine in the 1940s. The intermediate chain in lignocaine contains an amide bond and this obviated many of the problems associated with the ester group present in the older drugs. The subsequent production of other amide agents with varying clinical profiles has greatly extended the scope of modern local anaesthesia.

The mode of action of local anaesthetics is by blocking membrane depolarisation in all excitable tissues. Since local anaesthetics are injected at their site of action, only peripheral nerve is usually exposed to concentrations high enough to have a significant effect. However, if sufficient drug reaches other organs via the circulation, more widespread effects occur.

MODE OF ACTION

Neural Transmission (Fig. 14.2)

During the resting phase the interior of a peripheral nerve fibre has a potential difference of about -70 mV relative to the outside. When the nerve is stimulated there is a rapid increase in the membrane potential to approx. $+20$ mV, followed by an immediate restoration to the resting level. This depolarisation/repolarisation sequence lasts 1–2 ms and produces the familiar action potential associated with the passage of a nerve impulse.

The resting potential is the net result of several factors affecting the distribution of ions across the cell membrane. Electrochemical and concentration gradients modify ionic diffusion which is adjusted further by the semipermeable nature of the membrane and the action of the sodium/potassium pump.

Depolarisation of the fibre is the result of a sudden increase in membrane permeability to sodium which can thus diffuse down both electrochemical and concentration gradients. Sodium ions enter the cell through large protein molecules in the membrane (known as channels), which are closed during the resting phase. Stimulation of the nerve changes the configuration of these protein molecules so that the channels open and allow positively charged sodium ions to enter the cell. This increases the membrane potential to approx. +20 mV, when the electrochemical and concentration gradients for sodium balance each other and the channels close. Both concentration and electrochemical gradients then favour movement of potassium out through the membrane until the resting potential is restored. Relative to the total amounts present, only small numbers of ions take part in this exchange and the sodium/potassium pump restores their distribution during the resting phase.

At sensory nerve endings the initial opening of sodium channels is produced by the appropriate physiological stimulus, which may be chemically mediated in some instances. The impulse is transmitted along the axon because a local current flows between the depolarised segment of nerve (which has a positive charge) and the next segment (which has a negative charge). The voltage change associated with this current causes the configurational change in the sodium channels in the next segment, so that the action potential is propagated along the nerve.

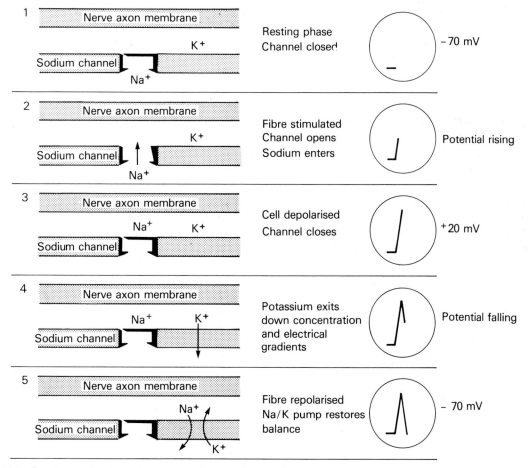

Fig. 14.2 Events occurring during transmission of a nerve impulse along an axon.

Effect of local anaesthetic drugs (Fig. 14.3)

Local anaesthetics are usually injected in an acid solution as the hydrochloride salt (pH approx. 5). The tertiary amine group becomes quaternary and they are thus soluble in water and suitable for injection. Following injection, the pH increases as a result of buffering in the tissues and a portion of the drug dissociates to release free base, the amount dependent on the pK of the drug. Being lipid soluble, the free base is able to pass through the lipid cell membrane to the interior of the axon where reionisation takes place. The reionised portion enters the sodium channels, and may be thought of simply as plugging them so that sodium ions cannot enter the cell. As a result, no action potential is generated or transmitted, and conduction blockade has occurred. Because it is the ionised form of drug that is active and reionisation has to take place intracellularly, individual drug pK has little effect on rate of onset of blockade.

In addition to diffusing into nerves at the site of injection the drug also enters capillaries and is removed by the circulation. Eventually, tissue concentration decreases below that in the nerves and the drug diffuses out, so allowing restoration of normal function.

Systemic toxicity

If significant amounts of local anaesthetic drug reach the tissues of heart and brain they have exactly the same 'membrane stabilising' effect as they have on peripheral nerve, resulting in a progressive depression of function. The earliest feature of systemic toxicity is numbness or tingling of the tongue and circumoral area — a result of a rich blood supply depositing enough drug to have an effect on the nerve endings. The patient may become lightheaded, anxious, drowsy and/or complain of tinnitus. If concentrations continue to rise, consciousness is lost and this may be preceded or followed by convulsions.

Coma and apnoea may develop subsequently. Cardiovascular collapse may result from direct myocardial depression and vasodilatation, but more commonly, it is a result of hypoxia secondary to apnoea.

Factors affecting toxicity

The most common cause of life-threatening systemic toxicity is an inadvertent intravascular injection, but it may result also from absolute overdosage. The changes in plasma concentration of drug following injection (Fig. 14.4) are dependent on the total dose administered, the rate of absorption, the pattern of distribution to other tissues and the rate of metabolism.

Absorption. Absorption from the site of injection depends on the blood flow — the higher the blood flow, the more rapid is the increase in plasma concentration, and the greater the resultant peak. Of the common sites of injection of large doses, the intercostal space has the highest blood supply, followed in turn by the extradural space, the brachial plexus and the sites of major lower limb nerve block. Absorption is slowest after infiltration anaesthesia.

Intravenous regional anaesthesia is a special case. If the tourniquet deflates immediately after drug injection, a large dose enters the circulation very rapidly. Following 20 min of tourniquet application sufficient drug has diffused out of the vessels into the tissues to result in the increase in systemic

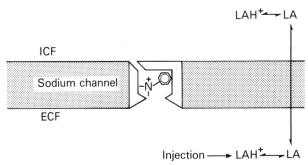

Fig. 14.3 Mode of action of a local anaesthetic drug. In order to penetrate the lipid cell membrane, the drug must be in free base form, while to effect a block reionisation must occur.

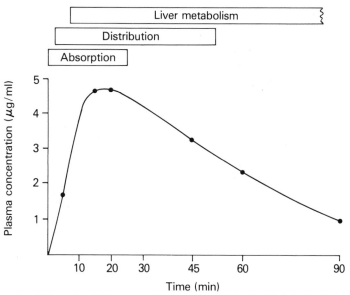

Fig. 14.4 Plasma concentration of lignocaine. The concentrations are shown following the injection into the lumbar extradural space of 400 mg of lignocaine without adrenaline. The injection was made at zero time and the phases of absorption, distribution, and metabolism are indicated.

concentration being smaller than that following brachial plexus block.

Blood supply may be modified by the inherent vaso-active properties of the particular drug and by the addition of vasoconstrictors to the solution. Use of the latter permits the safe dose to be increased by 50–100%.

Distribution. (Fig. 14.5) Following absorption, local anaesthetic drugs are distributed rapidly to, and taken up by, organs with a large blood supply and high affinity, e.g. brain, heart, liver and lungs. Muscle and fat, with low blood supplies, equilibrate more slowly, but the high affinity of fat for these drugs ensures that a large amount is taken up into adipose tissues. The lungs sequester (and possibly metabolise) local anaesthetic drugs, thereby preventing a large portion of the injected dose from reaching the coronary and cerebral circulations.

Metabolism. In general, ester drugs are broken down so rapidly by plasma cholinesterase that systemic toxicity is unusual. Toxicity may occur with some of the slowly hydrolysed drugs or in patients with abnormal enzymes (cf. suxamethonium). The amides are metabolised by amidases located predominantly in the liver. Hepatocellular disease has to be severe before the rate of metabolism is slowed

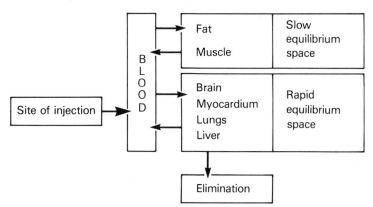

Fig. 14.5 Distribution of local anaesthetic drug following absorption from the site of injection.

significantly, and in general the rate of disappearance of drug is dependent more upon liver blood flow. This has practical relevance in the use of lignocaine as an antiarrhythmic in cardiogenic shock, where liver blood flow is diminished.

Protein binding. Local anaesthetics are bound to plasma proteins in varying degrees. It is assumed sometimes that drugs with the greatest degrees of protein binding are less toxic because only a small fraction of the plasma level is free to diffuse into the tissues and produce toxic effects. However, values for protein binding are obtained under laboratory conditions and probably bear little relationship to the dynamic situation existing during the phase of rapid absorption. Furthermore, even if a drug is bound to protein, it is still available to diffuse into the tissues down a concentration gradient since the bound portion is in equilibrium with that in solution. Thus, values for protein binding do not relate to acute toxicity of a drug.

Placental transfer. Much theoretical concern has been expressed about the mechanisms and effects of placental transfer of local anaesthetics administered to the mother during labour. Local anaesthetics cross the placenta as readily as other membranes, but their effects are of minimal significance when compared with those of conventional methods of analgesia and anaesthesia.

Fetal plasma protein may bind some drugs to a lesser extent than maternal protein so that *total* plasma concentration may be lower in the baby. It is claimed that such drugs are safer for the fetus. However, the concentration of *free* drug on each side of the placental membrane is the same and as a result tissue concentrations are more similar in mother and fetus than total plasma concentrations. The neonatal liver metabolises drugs slowly, but provided that delivery does not occur immediately after a toxic reaction, there should be little concern about effects on the baby.

Prevention of toxicity

The single most important factor in the prevention of toxicity is the avoidance of accidental intravascular injection. Careful aspiration tests are vital and should be repeated each time the needle is moved. However, a negative test is not an absolute guarantee, especially when catheter techniques are used. The initial injection of 2–3 ml of solution containing adrenaline (1:200 000) has been advocated — an increase in heart rate during the succeeding 1–2 min should indicate an intravascular injection. However, adrenaline is not the safest of drugs and this method is no guarantee against subsequent migration of needle or cannula into a vessel.

An alternative is to repeat the aspiration test after each 5–10 ml of solution, and to inject slowly. The patient should be watched for early signs of toxicity so that the injection may be stopped before there are major sequelae. Particular care should be taken when performing head and neck blocks because a very small dose may produce a major reaction if injected into a carotid or vertebral artery.

Overdosage may be avoided by consideration of the behaviour of the various drugs following injection at the particular site. Most practical manuals indicate the appropriate drug and dosage for each block, and these recommendations should be followed. Maximum safe dosages (for use in any situation) are often quoted for local anaesthetics with and without vasoconstrictor, but such recommendations are not really helpful since they ignore variations by factors including the site of injection, the patient's general condition and the concomitant use of a general anaesthetic. Assuming that the same dose is used, variations in drug concentration have no effect on toxicity. In adults, body weight correlates poorly with the risk of toxicity and it is better to modify the dose to be used in the light of an informed assessment of the patient's general condition.

Treatment of toxicity

No matter how careful the anaesthetist is in regard to prevention, facilities for treatment must always be available. The airway is maintained and oxygen administered by facemask, using artificial ventilation if apnoea occurs. Convulsions may be controlled with small increments of either diazepam (2.5 mg) or thiopentone (50 mg). The latter is usually more readily available and acts more rapidly. Excessive doses should not be given to control convulsions, since cardiorespiratory depression may be exacerbated. If cardiovascular collapse occurs despite adequate oxygenation (and this is *rare*), it should be treated with an adrenergic drug with α and β properties, e.g. ephedrine in 5 mg increments.

Additional side effects

Local anaesthetics are remarkably free from side effects other than systemic toxicity which is an extension of pharmacological action. Complications of specific drugs are discussed later, but there are two general features.

Allergic reactions

Allergy to the esters was relatively common, particularly with procaine, and was caused by para-aminobenzoic acid produced on hydrolysis. Most reactions were dermal in personnel handling the drugs, but fatal anaphylaxis has been recorded. Allergy to the amides is extremely rare and most 'reactions' result from systemic toxicity, overdosage with vasoconstrictors, or are manifestations of anxiety. The occasional genuine allergic reaction is usually to a preservative in the solution rather than the drug itself.

Drug interactions

Interactions with other drugs are possible theoretically, but rarely give rise to clinical problems. For instance, therapy with anticholinesterases for myasthenia, or the concomitant administration of other drugs hydrolysed by plasma cholinesterase, increases the toxicity of the ester drugs, and competition for plasma protein binding sites may occur with the amides. Of more practical importance is that heavy sedation with anti-convulsants (e.g. benzodiazepines) may mask the early signs of toxicity. These drugs may even prevent convulsions so that if a severe reaction does occur, the patient may suddenly become deeply unconscious.

PHARMACOLOGY OF INDIVIDUAL DRUGS

The local anaesthetic drugs in current use vary in their clinical profile (stability, potency, duration, toxicity, etc.). These differences may be related to variations in physicochemical properties.

Local anaesthetic drug chemistry

As indicated above (Fig. 14.1) all the local anaesthetic drugs have a three-part structure, with either an ester or amide bond at the centre. The important effects of the nature of this linkage on the route of metabolism and allergenicity have been discussed. The ester drugs also have short shelf lives because they tend to hydrolyse spontaneously, especially on warming. The amides may be stored for long periods without loss of potency and are not heat sensitive unless mixed with dextrose to produce hyperbaric spinal solutions. As a general rule solutions of amides in dextrose and of any ester may be heat sterilised once, and should be used soon after autoclaving.

The aromatic end of the molecule determines fat solubility and the amine affects its water solubility. Addition of other organic groups increases lipid solubility, and therefore potency, since ability to penetrate the lipid cell membrane is increased. Duration of action increases in proportion to the extent of protein binding, which is also a property of the aromatic group. Sodium channels are formed from large protein molecules to which are bound for longer periods the drugs with longer durations of action.

The effects of a local anaesthetic drug on blood vessels also modify its profile. Cocaine is a vasoconstrictor, but most of the other agents produce some degree of vasodilatation, which tends to shorten duration of action and increase toxicity.

The effects of differences in molecular structure often interact in complex ways, but a simple example of a structure-activity relationship is the addition of a butyl group to mepivacaine to produce bupivacaine, which is four times as potent and significantly longer acting. Alterations in structure also affect the rate, and the products, of metabolism.

Clinical factors affecting drug profile

Increasing the dose of a drug shortens its onset time and increases the duration of block. Dose may be increased by using either a higher concentration or a larger volume, but with the same total dose a large volume of a dilute solution is usually more effective than the converse.

The site of injection also affects onset time and duration (in addition to potential toxicity). Onset is almost immediate after infiltration and is progressively delayed with spinal, peripheral nerve and extradural blocks respectively. The slowest onsets follow brachial plexus block. The dose required and the likely duration of action tend to increase in much the same order as with onset.

Pregnancy and age have been shown to increase segmental spread of extradurals. For many blocks, younger, fitter, taller patients seem to require more drug, as do obese, alcoholic or anxious patients, the last perhaps because they react to any sensation from the operative area.

Individual drug properties

Only when all the above factors are taken into account may the properties of various drugs be compared. It is doubtful if, at *equipotent* concentrations, there are any real differences in speed of onset, but there are certainly variations in potency, duration and toxicity. The features of individual drugs are described below and in Table 14.1.

Cocaine. Cocaine has little place in modern anaesthetic practice, although it is used in ENT surgery for its vasoconstrictor action. Because of its use as a drug of addiction, it is increasingly difficult to obtain cocaine legitimately at a reasonable price.

Benzocaine. This is an excellent topical agent of low toxicity. It does not ionise and therefore its use is limited to topical application. In addition its mode of action cannot be explained according to the theory outlined above. Instead, it is thought that benzocaine diffuses into the cell membrane, but not into the cytoplasm, and either causes the membrane to expand in the same way as is suggested for general anaesthetics (see Chapter 5) or enters the sodium channel from the lipid phase of the membrane. Whichever is the case, the mechanism may also be relevant to the action of the other agents.

Procaine. The incidence of allergic problems, short shelf life and brief duration of action of procaine result in its infrequent use at the present time.

Chloroprocaine is a relatively new ester which is widely used in the U.S.A. Its profile is very similar to procaine from which it differs only by the addition of a chlorine atom (Table 14.1). As a result it is hydrolysed four times as quickly by cholinesterase and seems to be less allergenic. It is claimed to be more rapidly acting than any other agent, but this may relate to its very low toxicity, permitting use of relatively larger doses.

Amethocaine is relatively toxic for an ester because it is hydrolysed very slowly by cholinesterase. It is also very potent and is the standard drug in North America for spinal anaesthesia.

Lignocaine. Having been used safely and effectively for every possible type of local anaesthetic procedure, lignocaine is currently the standard agent. It has no unusual features and is also a standard anti-arrhythmic.

Mepivacaine is very similar and seems to have neither advantages nor disadvantages.

Prilocaine. This is an under-rated agent. It is equipotent to lignocaine, but has virtually no vasodilator action, is either metabolised or sequestered to a greater degree by the lungs, and is more rapidly metabolised by the liver. As a result it is slightly longer acting, considerably less toxic and is the drug of choice when the risk of toxicity is high. Metabolism produces *o*-toluidine which reduces haemoglobin, so methaemoglobinaemia is a theoretical possibility (but only with a dose considerably in excess of 600 mg). However, methaemoglobinaemia is of minimal significance since cyanosis appears only when 1.5 g/dl of haemoglobin are reduced, and treatment with methylene blue (1 mg/kg) is effective immediately. Fetal haemoglobin is more sensitive, and prilocaine should not be used during labour.

Cinchocaine. Cinchocaine was the first amide agent to be produced (two decades before lignocaine). It is very potent and toxic so, like amethocaine, it is used mainly for spinal anaesthesia.

Bupivacaine. The introduction of bupivacaine represented a significant advance in anaesthesia. Relative to potency, its acute toxicity is only slightly less than that of lignocaine, but its longer duration of action obviates repeated dosage leading to cumulative toxicity.

An interesting point is that some reports of toxic reactions have described ventricular fibrillation — a surprising effect for a membrane stabilising drug. It is difficult to judge the extent to which hypoxia may have contributed.

Etidocaine. The newest of the amide drugs is a derivative of lignocaine. Possibly it is even longer acting than bupivacaine and is of particular interest as it seems to have a more profound effect on motor than sensory nerves. With the other drugs, the converse is true.

Table 14.1   Features of individual local anaesthetics

Proper name / formula	% Equivalent concentration*	Relative duration*	Toxicity	pK	Partition coefficient	% protein bound	Main use by anaesthetists in the UK
COCAINE	1	0.50	V. high	8.7	?	?	Nil
BENZOCAINE	N/A	2	Low	2.9	?	?	Topical
PROCAINE	2	0.75	Low	8.9	0.6	5.8	Nil
CHLOROPROCAINE	1	0.75	Low	9.1	1	?	Not available
AMETHOCAINE	0.25	2	High	8.5	80	76	Topical
LIGNOCAINE	1	1	Medium	7.7	3	64	Infiltration Nerve block Extradural
MEPIVACAINE	1	1.	Medium	7.6	1	77	Not available
PRILOCAINE	1	1.50	Low	7.7	1	55	Infiltration Nerve block IVRA
CINCHOCAINE	0.25	2	High	7.9	?	?	Spinal
BUPIVACAINE	0.25	2-4	Medium	8.1	28	95	Extradural Spinal Nerve block
ETIDOCAINE	0.5	2-4	Medium	7.7	141	94	Not available

*Lignocaine = 1; N/A = not applicable — not used in solution;
? = information not available.
NB. All figures are approximations as there is some variation in published values.

Additives

Many substances are added to local anaesthetics for pharmaceutical purposes. Sodium hydroxide and hydrochloric acid are used to adjust the pH, sodium chloride the toxicity, and dextrose and water the baricity of solutions. Preservatives, e.g. methyl hydroxybenzoate are added to multidose bottles and manufacturers recommend that these should not be used for spinal or extradural blocks. Other additions are made for pharmacological reasons.

Vasoconstrictors

By slowing the rate of absorption, vasoconstrictors reduce toxicity, prolong duration and perhaps result in more profound blocks. These are all desirable effects, but vasoconstrictors are not used universally for several reasons. Because of the risk of ischaemia they are absolutely contraindicated for injection close to end-arteries (ring blocks of digits and penis) and in intravenous regional anaesthesia.

Adrenaline is the most potent agent, has its own systemic toxicity, and should be used with particular care, if at all, in patients with cardiac disease. Even in healthy patients concentrations greater than 1:200 000 should not be used, and the maximum dose administered should not exceed 0.5 mg. Interactions with other sympathomimetic drugs, including tricyclic antidepressants, may occur especially when adrenergic drugs are used systemically to treat hypotension.

Felypressin is a safer drug although it causes pallor and may constrict the coronary circulation. It is available usually only for dental use.

There is also a theoretical risk that the use of vasoconstrictors may increase the risk of permanent neurological deficit by rendering nerve tissue ischaemic. While evidence is inconclusive, many anaesthetists feel that vasoconstrictors should not be used unless there is no alternative method of prolonging duration or reducing toxicity in the particular clinical situation.

Carbon dioxide

In order to speed the onset of blockade, some local anaesthetics have been produced as the carbonated salt, with carbon dioxide dissolved in the solution under pressure. It is theorised that, following injection, the carbon dioxide lowers intracellular pH and favours formation of more of the ionised active form of the drug. With blocks of slower onset there is good evidence that a significant improvement is obtained.

Dextrans

There have been many attempts to prolong duration of action, by mixing local anaesthetics with high molecular weight dextrans. The results are inconclusive, but it has been suggested that the very large dextrans may be effective, especially in combination with adrenaline. It is postulated that 'macromolecules' are formed between dextran and local anaesthetic so that the latter is held in the tissues for longer periods.

Hyaluronidase

For many years the enzyme hyaluronidase was added to local anaesthetics to aid spread by breaking down tissue barriers. There was little evidence that it had a significant effect and this practice has been abandoned.

CHOICE OF LOCAL ANAESTHETIC AGENT

When using a local technique the anaesthetist has to decide upon the concentration, volume and nature of the agent to be used. For lignocaine (the relative potencies of other agents are shown in Table 14.1) concentrations required are:

skin infiltration } i.v. regional	0.5%
minor nerve block	1.0%
brachial plexus } sciatic/femoral	1.0–1.5%
extradural	1.5–2.0%
spinal	2.0–5.0%

Greater concentrations than these may be used to produce more profound blocks of faster onset. The volumes required for particular techniques are described in Chapter 22 and the inter-relationships that exist between patient status and the required amount of drug have been discussed above.

Ideally, several drugs of different potency, duration and toxicity should be available to permit a rational choice based upon the required dose, the particular risk of toxicity in that block and patient, and the likely duration of surgery. Often this is not possible, mainly for commercial reasons. For example, in the UK, lignocaine and bupivacaine are marketed in a full range of concentrations, but little else is available apart from the more dilute solutions of prilocaine. The availability of spinal anaesthetic solutions is particularly poor. For more peripheral blocks, lignocaine and bupivacaine may be used safely unless the risk of toxicity is relatively high (e.g. i.v. regional) when prilocaine is preferred. When large volumes of more concentrated solutions are needed and the higher concentrations of prilocaine are not available, then one of the other agents should be used in combination with adrenaline.

FURTHER READING

Covino B G 1980 The mechanisms of local anaesthesia. In: Norman J, Whitwam J G (eds) Topical reviews in anaesthesia. John Wright & Sons, Bristol

Covino B G, Vassallo H G 1976 Local anesthetics: mechanisms of action and clinical use. Grune and Stratton, New York

Henderson J J, Nimmo W S 1983 Practical regional anaesthesia. Blackwell Scientific Publications, Oxford

Stanton-Hicks M d'A (ed) 1978 Regional anesthesia: advances and selected topics. International Anesthesiology Clinic 16(4)

Wade A (ed) 1977 Martindale: the extra pharmacopoeia. The Pharmaceutical Press, London

15

Preoperative assessment and premedication

It is essential that the anaesthetist visits every patient in the ward prior to surgery, partly in order to assess 'fitness for anaesthesia', but also to allay fear and anxiety by careful explanation and reassurance (psychotherapy) and to prescribe drugs for administration prior to induction of anaesthesia (premedication).

Since 'fitness for anaesthesia' is determined largely by the presence and severity of coexisting medical disease, this chapter should be read in conjunction with Chapter 36 on intercurrent disease and anaesthesia.

Since the majority of patients are seen by the anaesthetist only after planned admission to hospital for elective surgery, it is occasionally necessary for the anaesthetist to postpone the planned operation date for the patient. This may be avoided by the provision of anaesthetic assessment outpatient clinics to which patients may be referred directly before a definitive admission date is given.

Preoperative assessment of patients should embrace two broad questions:

1. Is the patient in optimum physical condition for anaesthesia? If there is any medical condition which may be improved (e.g. hypertension, cardiac failure, chronic bronchitis, etc) surgery should be postponed and appropriate therapy instituted.

2. If an increased anaesthetic and surgical risk produced by concurrent medical disease is present, is it offset by the anticipated benefits of surgery? It is difficult to quantify the morbidity and mortality for an individual patient and frequently a decision can be made only by discussion between surgeon and anaesthetist.

There has been considerable interest recently amongst academic anaesthetists in defining prognostic criteria which correlate with postoperative complications (e.g. development of postoperative myocardial infarction). Nonetheless, despite its apparent simplicity the most useful method of classifying a patient's physical condition pre-operatively is still that established by the American Society of Anesthesiologists (ASA) (Table 15.1). The ASA classification should be applied to all patients prior to anaesthesia.

Table 15.1 ASA classification

Class*	Physical status
1	Normal, healthy
2	Mild systemic disease
3	Severe systemic disease that limits activity but is not incapacitating
4	Incapacitating systemic disease that is a constant threat to life
5	Moribund; not expected to survive 24 h with or without operation

*In the event of an emergency operation, precede the class number with an E

Common causes for postponing surgery

1. Acute upper respiratory tract infection ('common cold'). Although many patients may admit to the presence of a cold, clarification of such an admission should be made. In general, the presence of nasal secretions or a pyrexia, or the unexpected presence of physical signs on clinical examination of the chest suggest that surgery should be postponed for a few weeks until the patient has recovered.

2. Existing medical disease (cardiac, respiratory, endocrine) which is not under optimum control (see Chapter 36).

3. Emergency surgery where the patient has not been resuscitated adequately. Postponement may be necessary for only one or two hours to permit

restoration of circulating blood volume. This important principle may be breached if haemorrhage is extensive and continuous.

4. Recent ingestion of food. In general, anaesthesia for elective surgery should not be undertaken within four to six hours of ingestion of food or liquids.

5. Failure to obtain informed consent. Informed consent for surgery should be obtained from all patients, but it should be noted that such consent is invalid if obtained after the patient has received premedicant drugs. Consent from a parent or guardian is required if the patient is under 16 yr of age in England and Wales or under 14 yr of age in Scotland. When parents or guardians cannot be contacted, consent may be obtained from a Court of Law, or in the case of emergency surgery from a District Medical Officer.

6. Drug therapy. It is unwise to proceed to anaesthesia if the patient is receiving some form of drug therapy (vide infra) which is not under optimal control.

THE PREOPERATIVE VISIT

Preoperative assessment of a patient should be similar to any full medical examination. Normally, the patient has been clerked and examined by a house physician or surgeon and the anaesthetist may confine himself to systems of particular anaesthetic relevance (especially the cardiovascular and respiratory systems). Nonetheless, the anaesthetist should ensure that all systems have been examined correctly prior to anaesthesia.

The preoperative visit comprises:

History
Physical examination
Special investigations
Premedication
Special instructions

History

Aspects of the presenting complaint require scrutiny by the anaesthetist. Since the most important symptom relevant to fitness for anaesthesia is exertional dyspnoea, it may be necessary to enquire closely when exercise is limited by intermittent claudication, arthritis, etc.

Previous medical history is of great importance and direct questions should be asked in respect of cardiac and respiratory disease. This is described in greater detail in Chapter 36.

Enquiries should be made in respect of drug allergies, any previous anaesthetic history of postoperative nausea and vomiting, and more serious complications including deep vein thrombosis or respiratory problems.

A familial history of hereditary conditions associated with anaesthetic problems, e.g. malignant hyperpyrexia, dystrophia myotonica, porphyria, or cholinesterase abnormalities may indicate the necessity for appropriate investigation.

If previous anaesthetic records are available, they should be inspected to ascertain the type and efficacy of premedication, the size and type of endotracheal tube, the presence of difficulty with tracheal intubation, and the anaesthetic agents used. It is generally recommended that halothane anaesthesia should not be repeated within three months of a previous halothane anaesthetic.

Alcohol

A moderate alcohol intake is associated frequently with tolerance to anaesthetic drugs, and excessive alcohol intake may cause both liver and cardiac damage. In alcoholics, delirium tremens may occur during the postoperative recovery phase as a result of withdrawal of the drug.

Smoking

History of cigarette smoking is associated with the development of chronic bronchitis and coronary artery disease, both of which increase substantially the risks during anaesthesia. However, in the absence of these diseases, cigarette smoking provokes mucus secretion by irritation of the tracheobronchial tree which may render induction of anaesthesia less smooth than anticipated.

Drug History

Cardiac glycosides. Digoxin should be continued up to and including the morning of operation (with the possible exception of cardiac surgery).

There are several anaesthetic implications:

1. Suxamethonium may cause serious ventricular arrhythmias in the fully digitalised patient and care should be taken to avoid precipitating factors, including hypoxia.

2. Potentiation of the vagotonic effects of digitalis by halothane and neostigmine may lead to excessive bradycardia.

3. Digitalis toxicity may be precipitated by hypercalcaemia or hypokalaemia.

Antihypertensive drugs. These should also be continued up to and including the morning of operation. The anaesthetic implications are that interactions may occur between these drugs and anaesthetic agents, and also that hypertensive patients tend to exhibit a more labile cardiovascular response to surgical stress (see p. 466).

β-Adrenergic blocking agents. These should be continued up to and including the morning of operation. There may be additive effects with the myocardial depressant actions of volatile anaesthetic agents.

Diuretics. These drugs may produce hypokalaemia which can precipitate digitalis toxicity. In addition, the action of neuromuscular blocking drugs may be enhanced and prolonged. Hypokalaemia also affects myocardial conduction leading to arrhythmias.

Anticoagulants. Anticoagulant therapy must be controlled carefully prior to surgery as described on page 497. Usually, regional anaesthetic techniques are contraindicated unless clotting times are near normal.

Steroids. Patients who are receiving steroid drugs, or who have received steroids within six months before surgery, may suffer from induced adrenocortical insufficiency. Steroid cover should therefore be given over the perioperative period. An appropriate regimen is described on page 485.

Antibiotics. Many antibiotics exhibit neuromuscular blocking activity and may therefore potentiate the effects of competitive muscle relaxant drugs. These drugs include:

1. Streptomycin and related compounds neomycin and kanamycin.
2. Polymyxins.
3. Tetracyclines.

These antibiotics are excreted primarily via the kidney and therefore patients with renal disease are particularly susceptible to synergistic effects with competitive relaxants.

Oral contraceptive agents. These drugs cause a small but definite increase in the incidence of DVT, an effect which persists for three months after discontinuing the drugs. It is common practice either to discontinue these drugs for three months prior to surgery or to treat the patient with low dose subcutaneous heparin for prophylaxis against development of DVT.

Monoamine oxidase inhibitors (MAOI).

(a) Phenelzine	(d) Pargyline
(b) Nialamide	(e) Iproniazid
(c) Isocarboxazid	(f) Tranylcypromine

These drugs permit accumulation of noradrenaline; the action of indirectly acting vasopressor drugs (amphetamines, phenylephrine and ephedrine) are potentiated. Reactions occur also with narcotic analgesics especially pethidine, leading to hyper- or hypotension.

The MAOI drugs should be withdrawn at least three weeks prior to surgery. Psychiatric advice may be required for prescription of alternative antidepressant drugs.

Tricyclic antidepressant drugs (imipramine, amitriptyline). These drugs act by blocking the reuptake of noradrenaline and therefore enhance the action of adrenaline and noradrenaline. They also exert prominent anticholinergic effects causing tachycardia, arrhythmias and hypotension.

Levodopa. This is the Levo isomer of dihydroxyphenylalanine and is used in the therapy of Parkinson's disease. Side effects include ectopic beats with palpitations, dyspnoea and angina. Care should be taken when using anaesthetic agents which sensitise the myocardium to the effects of catecholamines.

Ophthalmic drugs. Ecothiopate iodide is an anticholinesterase drug used in the treatment of glaucoma. It may cause increased sensitivity to, and prolonged duration of the action of drugs metabolised by cholinesterase, e.g. suxamethonium.

Sedatives and tranquillisers. These drugs usually present few problems during anaesthesia, but in combination with premedicant drugs and anaesthetic agents may lead to prolonged recovery from anaesthesia. There may be a greater predisposition to development of hypotension in patients receiving phenothiazines.

Antidiabetic drugs. The management of diabetes mellitus is described on page 488.

Physical examination

A full physical examination should be undertaken and documented in the patient's records prior to anaesthesia. Examination must include cardiovascular system, respiratory system, alimentary tract, musculoskeletal system and central nervous system. Usually this full examination will have been undertaken by the house surgeon and the anaesthetist may confine himself to examination of the essential details in the cardiovascular and respiratory systems. In addition, the anaesthetist pays particular attention to ascertaining whether or not tracheal intubation may prove difficult. Thus the teeth are examined carefully for the presence of dentures, loose teeth, and protrusion, particularly of upper incisors. Full opening of the mouth and extension of the cervical spine is confirmed. Features associated with difficulty in intubation are discussed more fully on page 278.

Although it may seem irrelevant to undertake a full neurological examination of a healthy patient presented for minor surgery, documentation that the nervous system is normal is essential since neurological complications occur, albeit extremely rarely, following both general anaesthetic techniques and regional blocks.

Special investigations

The following investigations are required in every patient:

1. Urinalysis — occasionally unsuspected diabetes mellitus may be diagnosed.

2. Haemoglobin estimation. This reveals previously undiagnosed anaemia and also provides an indication of the quantity of blood which should be requested from the Transfusion Service prior to major surgery. Patients with previously unsuspected anaemia should be investigated and the cause of the condition elicited before proceeding to surgery. If the anaemia is associated with the surgical condition, preoperative transfusion of blood is not necessary unless the haemoglobin is less than 10 g/dl.

In addition, the following investigations should be undertaken where indicated:

3. Serum electrolytes and urea — in patients receiving drug therapy with diuretics, antihypertensives, or digoxin and patients with metabolic diseases or a history of diarrhoea, vomiting, or abstention from food or liquids.

4. Chest X-ray — radiography of the chest is expensive and should be undertaken only if there are particular indications, e.g. cardiac or respiratory disease. However, because of the frequency of chest infections after abdominal surgery, it is customary to obtain a chest radiograph in patients undergoing upper abdominal surgery and in patients over the age of 40 yr undergoing any major surgery.

5. E.c.g. should be obtained where special indications exist and in all patients over the age of 40 yr.

6. Respiratory function tests should be undertaken in all patients who have severe dyspnoea on mild to moderate exertion.

7. Blood gas analysis is required in all patients with dyspnoea at rest.

8. Cervical X-rays should be obtained in some situations where difficulty in endotracheal intubation may be anticipated, e.g. in patients with a large goitre (together with thoracic inlet X-rays) and patients with severe limitation of movement of the cervical spine.

Premedication

Premedication developed in the early part of the twentieth century predominantly for two purposes: firstly, to allay fear and anxiety prior to anaesthesia — this was particularly important with chloroform which is a potent agent in sensitising the heart to circulating catecholamines. Secondly, to reduce secretions from the oropharynx and tracheobronchial tree as these may impair smooth induction and maintenance of anaesthesia with ether.

With the advent of newer nonirritant anaesthetic agents, this second reason now assumes only minor importance whilst the overall improvement in safety of anaesthesia and surgery combined with greater sophistication and greater emphasis on explanation and reassurance has also reduced the necessity for anxiolytic drugs.

Nonetheless, it is still customary to prescribe

premedication, which should be regarded as part of the overall balanced anaesthetic technique. Currently, the purposes of administering premedicant drugs are:

1. To allay anxiety and fear before anaesthesia and operation. It may seem surprising that the most frequent fear expressed by patients is not related to surgery per se, but is fear of loss of, and recovery from, consciousness, which is conceptually difficult for the nonbiologist to understand. Reassurance and explanation is undoubtedly of more importance than drug therapy in allaying these fears.

2. To reduce secretions. Although ether and cyclopropane are rarely used, some 60% of anaesthetists in the United Kingdom still prescribe anticholinergic drugs to reduce secretions produced by the presence of an airway or endotracheal tube in the mouth and larynx.

3. To enhance the hypnotic effect of general anaesthetic agents, i.e. as part of the overall anaesthetic technique. This is particularly important when opioid analgesic drugs are given as premedication for an anaesthetic technique which comprises spontaneous ventilation with nitrous oxide, oxygen and a volatile agent. The opioid helps to reduce tachypnoea associated with use of the volatile agent and also provides analgesia in the immediate postoperative period.

4. To reduce postoperative nausea and vomiting.

5. To produce amnesia.

6. To reduce the volume and raise the pH of gastric contents in patients in whom the risk of vomiting or regurgitation (followed by aspiration) are known to be high.

7. To reduce vagal reflexes which may occur on induction of anaesthesia in response to suxamethonium and/or tracheal intubation.

It may be seen from the above list that some of the objectives of premedication can be achieved by administration of drugs at the time of induction or during maintenance of anaesthesia and this accounts for the very wide variation in prescribing habits for premedicant drugs. The only real essential of premedication is that a patient arrives in the operating theatre in a calm and happy frame of mind.

A wide variety of drugs may be used for premedication (Table 15.2) either alone or in combinations. The commonest regimens are shown in Table 15.3.

Table 15.2 Drugs used for premedication

Opioid analgesics	Benzodiazepines	Butyrophenones	Phenothiazines	Anticholinergics	Antiemetics
Morphine	Diazepam	Haloperidol	Promethazine	Atropine	Metoclopramide
Papaveretum	Nitrazepam	Droperidol	Promazine	Hyoscine	*Butyrophenones*
Pethidine	Flurazepam		Trimeprazine	Glycopyrrolate	*Phenothiazines*
Phenoperidine	Lorazepam		Chlorpromazine		
Fentanyl	Flunitrazepam				
Pentazocine	Temazepam				
Buprenorphine					

Table 15.3 Common premedication regimens (doses are suitable only for healthy adult male)

Drug (combination)	Dose (mg)	Route of administration	Comments
Papaveretum	20	i.m.	Profound sedation 'Omnopon & Scopolamine' still very
Hyoscine	0.4	i.m.	commonly used combination.
Diazepam	10–15	Oral	Good anxiolysis but effect variable
Lorazepam	2–3	Oral	Marked anterograde amnesia. Prolonged action
Diazepam	10	Oral	Metoclopramide increases the tone of the lower
Metoclopramide	10	Oral	oesophageal sphincter and possesses antiemetic effect
Morphine	10	i.m.	Frequently used when less profound sedation is required
Atropine	0.6	i.m.	than 'Omnopon & Scopolamine'
Promethazine	50	i.m.	Frequently prescribed for asthmatic patients
Atropine	0.6	i.m.	

Opioid analgesics

These drugs are used particularly when a patient has pain preoperatively; in combination with hyoscine they provide very effective sedation and relief of anxiety. Tachypnoea occurring with the volatile agents (halothane, enflurane, and particularly trichloroethylene) is reduced, and a lower concentration of anaesthetic agent is required for maintenance of anaesthesia. In addition, the incidence of awareness is reduced during a N_2O/O_2 relaxant technique.

The disadvantage of these drugs is that they may produce respiratory depression and delay resumption of spontaneous ventilation at the end of a N_2O/O_2/relaxant technique. All these drugs are associated with a high incidence of postoperative nausea and vomiting which may be reduced by combination with hyoscine or a phenothiazine.

These drugs should be used cautiously in the very young or elderly patient, those with asthma or respiratory disease, and in the presence of MAOI drugs.

Benzodiazepines

The most commonly used drugs in this group are diazepam and lorazepam. The advantage of diazepam over the opioid analgesic drugs is that it may be given orally. Indeed its gastro-intestinal absorption is more reliable than that following i.m. administration. The i.v. route should be avoided because of the high incidence of thrombophlebitis. The benzodiazepines are particularly useful, producing relief from anxiety with little soporific or respiratory depressant effect unless given in very large doses. They may also be usefully employed as hypnotics on the night before operation. Unfortunately, there is a very wide variability in the response of patients to these drugs and the effects may be unpredictable.

Butyrophenones

These drugs possess neuroleptic effects and are prescribed commonly as part of the neuroleptanalgesic technique or for their antiemetic properties (see Chapter 10, page 162). They possess a very long duration of action and this may delay recovery from anaesthesia particularly in elderly patients. Relatively modest doses should be employed since extrapyramidal effects are not uncommon.

Phenothiazines

Useful properties of these drugs for premedication include antisialagogue, antiemetic, sedative and tranquillising effects. Disadvantages include extrapyramidal side effects (restlessness, muscle tremor and rigidity), synergism with opioids to delay postoperative recovery, and potentiation of the hypotensive effects of other anaesthetic agents. Postoperatively the patient may exhibit pallor with mild tachycardia and hypotension which mimic the signs of surgically induced bleeding.

Anticholinergic agents

Atropine. The advantages of atropine for premedication are that it blocks secretions when irritant anaesthetic gases are used and reduces excessive secretion and bradycardia associated with suxamethonium given either repeatedly or in the form of an infusion. Atropine is used very commonly as premedication in ophthalmic surgery to block the oculocardiac reflex in patients undergoing squint surgery. It is useful in small children to reduce the bradycardia which may occur in association with halothane anaesthesia.

The disadvantages of atropine are that administration by i.m. injection is extremely painful and the excessive drying of the oropharynx is very uncomfortable. Tachycardia should be avoided in cardiac conditions (obstructive cardiomyopathies, valvular stenosis, and ischaemic heart disease) and when a hypotensive anaesthetic technique is planned. The drug should also be avoided in pyrexial children.

Hyoscine. In standard clinical doses hyoscine 0.4 mg differs from atropine 0.6 mg in that there is a greater antisialagogue effect and little action on cardiac vagal receptors. It possesses marked sedative and amnesic actions and, in contrast with atropine, does not cause stimulation of higher centres. Hyoscine should be avoided in the elderly (over 60 yr of age) as it produces dysphoria and restlessness.

Glycopyrrolate. Unlike atropine and hyoscine, this drug does not cross the blood-brain barrier and therefore central actions are avoided. In addition the drug has a much longer duration of action.

All the anticholinergic drugs cause reduction in

lower oesophageal sphincter pressure tone, thereby enhancing the likelihood of gastro-oesophageal regurgitation.

Special instructions

In addition to premedication drugs other forms of therapy may require prescription depending upon the patient's medical condition.

Chest physiotherapy should be commenced preoperatively in patients with severe respiratory disease and sputum should be obtained for bacteriological examination and culture to determine optimum antibiotic therapy in the event of postoperative chest infection.

Prophylactic antibiotics are required in patients with cardiac lesions who are at risk of developing subacute bacterial endocarditis (see page 471).

Bronchodilators and/or physiotherapy are required in patients with asthma, or severe chronic bronchitis.

FURTHER READING

Miller R D (ed) 1981 Anesthesia, vol 1 & 2. Churchill Livingstone, Edinburgh

16

Anaesthetic apparatus

It is essential that every anaesthetist has a thorough knowledge of the functioning of all anaesthetic equipment at his disposal, and that he checks it conscientiously every time before use. In some respects, the routine of testing that anaesthetic equipment is functional is akin to the airline pilot's check list which is an essential preliminary to aircraft flight. The purpose of this chapter is to describe briefly equipment with which the junior anaesthetist must be familiar.

THE ANAESTHETIC MACHINE

The anaesthetic machine (Fig. 16.1) comprises:

1. A supply of compressed gases.
2. A means of releasing and metering the gases.
3. A method of vaporising volatile anaesthetic agents.
4. Apparatus for delivery of gases and vapours to the patient.
5. A mechanism for scavenging anaesthetic gases in order to reduce environmental pollution.

Additional apparatus of various kinds is stored on the flat surface of the machine.

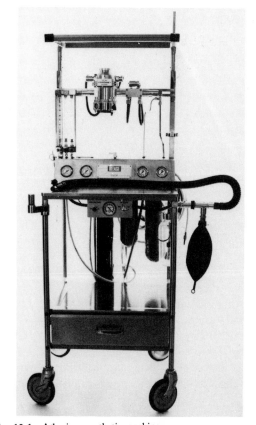

Fig. 16.1 A basic anaesthetic machine.

Anaesthetic gases

Oxygen may be obtained in hospital either from a pipeline source or as compressed gas in cylinders of various sizes. In larger hospitals, pipeline oxygen originates from a liquid oxygen store. Liquid oxygen is stored at a temperature of approx. $-165°$ C at 10.5 bar in a giant thermos flask — a Vacuum Insulated Evaporator (VIE). Some heat passes through the insulating layer between the two shells of the flask, increasing the tendency to evaporation and elevation of pressure. Pressure is usually maintained constant by transfer of gaseous oxygen into the pipeline system (via a warming device). However, if the pressure increases above 17 bar, a safety valve opens and oxygen runs to waste. When the supply of oxygen resulting from slow evaporation from the surface in the VIE is inadequate, the pressure decreases, and a valve opens to allow liquid oxygen to pass into an evaporator, from which gas passes into the pipeline system.

In smaller hospitals, where it is uneconomical to site a liquid oxygen store, the hospital pipeline is supplied by a double bank of large cylinders. Pipeline systems ensure continuity of supply and are more reliable in this respect than small cylinders which are the sole oxygen supply to an anaesthetic machine. Emptying of cylinders has been responsible for patient fatalities in the past despite the presence of warning devices.

In addition to oxygen, nitrous oxide, compressed air, and Entonox are sometimes piped, and very occasionally carbon dioxide. Thus a gas other than oxygen might be obtained from the 'oxygen outlet'. A designated member of the pharmacy staff should test the gas obtained from the sockets using an oxygen analyser when a new system is installed or servicing of an existing pipeline system has been undertaken.

Malfunction of an oxygen-air mixing device may result in entry of compressed air into the oxygen pipeline, rendering an anaesthetic mixture hypoxic. Because of this possibility it has been advocated that oxygen analysers be used routinely during anaesthesia.

Oxygen in a cylinder (Table 16.1) is stored at a pressure of 137 bar (1987 lbf/in^2) and is in the form of compressed gas. Thus a pressure gauge provides a reliable indication of the proportion of the original contents still remaining (by Boyle's law). Oxygen cylinders are constructed of molybdenum steel, and are much lighter in comparison with the earlier cast variety. After manufacture, each cylinder is tested to ensure that it can withstand enormous hydraulic pressure. One cylinder in every hundred is cut into strips to test the metal for tensile strength. The sealant between valve and cylinder melts at high temperatures, thereby allowing the gas to escape slowly, and reducing the possibility of an explosion in the event of fire.

Nitrous oxide cylinders are colour-coded blue. Nitrous oxide is liquid at room temperature when compressed, and exerts a pressure of 44 bar (638 lbf/in^2) at 15°C. When nitrous oxide gas escapes from the cylinder, some of the liquid nitrous oxide evaporates into the gaseous phase. This process absorbs heat, causing a reduction in temperature of the contents and cylinder and consequently a decrease in pressure which is restored as the cylinder warms up towards room temperature again. Only when all the liquid has evaporated does the nitrous oxide pressure gauge start to indicate a decrease, signalling imminent emptying of the cylinder.

When a nitrous oxide cylinder in use is almost empty, water vapour condenses as ice on the lower part of the cylinder. This tendency is less with a full cylinder because of the larger thermal capacity of the liquid nitrous oxide which is in contact with a larger area of metal.

Entonox is a 50:50 mixture of oxygen and nitrous oxide supplied in cylinders (colour-coded blue with white segments on the shoulders) at a pressure of 137 bar (1987 lbf/in^2) at 15°C. The constituent gases in a full cylinder separate at −7°C, the nitrous oxide liquefying. Such a cylinder delivers initially a mixture rich in oxygen, and as the cylinder empties, a mixture deficient in oxygen. Prior to use, cylinders of Entonox should be stored horizontally at a temperature exceeding 10°C for 24 h. If required urgently, the cylinders should be stored at a temperature exceeding 10°C for 2 h then inverted

Table 16.1 Medical gas cylinders

	Colour		Pressure at 15°C	
	Body	Shoulder	lbf/in^2	bar
Oxygen	Black	White	1987	137
Nitrous oxide	Blue	Blue	638	44
Cyclopropane	Orange	Orange	73	5
CO$_2$	Grey	Grey	725	50
Helium	Brown	Brown	1987	137
Air	Grey	White/black quarters	1987	137
O$_2$/helium	Black	White/brown quarters	1987	137
O$_2$/CO$_2$	Black	White/grey quarters	1987	137
N$_2$O/O$_2$ (Entonox)	Blue	White/blue quarters	1987	137

three times. Alternatively, a cylinder may be placed in a bath of water at body temperature for 5 min and inverted three times to promote thorough mixing of the contents.

Types of cylinder

There are six sizes (Table 16.2) of oxygen cylinder (sizes C, D, E, F, G and J) and five sizes of nitrous oxide (sizes C, D, E, F, and G). The larger oxygen cylinders are fitted with a bull-nose valve, which may be connected to the pipeline manifold, or oxygen therapy apparatus. The larger nitrous oxide cylinders, F and G, are fitted with a handwheel valve.

Pin-index valves are provided for the smaller cylinders of oxygen and nitrous oxide (and also carbon dioxide and cyclopropane) which may be attached to anaesthetic machines. The pegs on the inlet connection (Fig. 16.2) slot into corresponding holes on the cylinder valve and obstruct any attempt to fit a cylinder on to an inappropriate inlet connection. However, if a pin has been broken it may be possible to attach a cylinder inappropriately.

When fitting a cylinder to a machine, the yoke is positioned and tightened with the handle of the yoke spindle. Before this joint is tightened fully the valve spindle should be opened until gas is heard leaking. The yoke spindle is then tightened to eliminate the leak.

Whenever a cylinder is to be fitted to an anaesthetic machine the anaesthetist must check that it is full and that there are no leaks at the gland nut or the pin-index junction caused by absence of, or damage to the washer (Bodok seal) (Fig. 16.2).

In the essential preliminary checking of the anaesthetic machine before each operating session, the anaesthetist must ensure that all oxygen and

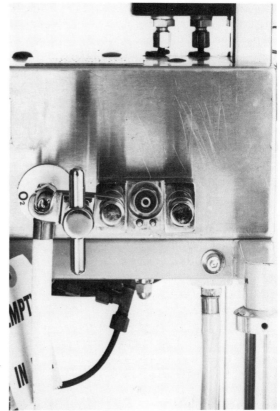

Fig. 16.2 An oxygen inlet connection for a cylinder. Note the black Bodok seal around the oxygen inlet, and the two pegs of the pin index system which slot into corresponding holes in the cylinder valve.

nitrous oxide cylinders are usable even if the machine is supplied by pipeline gases.

Pressure regulators

The pressure in the gas lines of a modern anaesthetic machine is 4 bar (60 lbf/in^2) and therefore the

Table 16.2 Medical gas cylinder sizes and capacities

Cylinder size	A	B	C	D	E	F	G	J
Height (in)	10	10	14	18	31	34	49	57
Capacities (litre)								
Oxygen			170	340	680	1360	3400	6800
Nitrous oxide			450	900	1800	3600	9000	
Cyclopropane	90	180						
CO$_2$			450	900	1800			
Helium				300		1200		
Air							3200	6400
O$_2$/Helium					600	1200		
O$_2$/CO$_2$						1360	3400	
Entonox							3200	6400

pressure in a cylinder is modified by a 'reducing valve', described more accurately as a pressure regulator (Fig. 16.3). The gas is conducted into the chamber of the reducing valve where it distorts a diaphragm to which a toggle mechanism is connected, which in turn causes the entry orifice to be occluded,

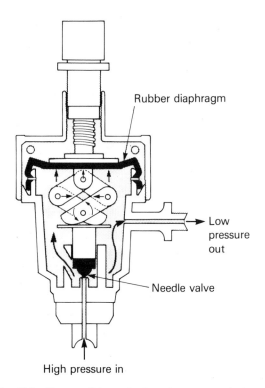

Rubber diaphragm

Low pressure out

Needle valve

High pressure in

Fig. 16.3 Diagram of the mechanism of a pressure reducing valve. The spring above the diaphragm exerts a force limiting the escape of gas through the needle valve.

thus limiting the flow of gas into the chamber. This prevents the pressure from increasing above a predetermined limit. When gas flows out of the chamber of the reducing valve, the ensuing decrease in pressure causes opening of the entry port. As the gas expands on entering the chamber of the reducing valve, heat is absorbed, and the valve cools. Condensation may therefore form on the outside of the valve. Precautions are taken during manufacture to ensure that the contents of cylinders are free from water, so that ice does not form *inside* the reducing valve. The earlier reducing valve possessed 'fins' designed to augment acquisition of heat from the environment.

Flowmeters

Gas issues from the reducing valve at a pressure of 4 bar (60 lbf/in^2), and is conducted to the needle valve of the appropriate flowmeter (Fig. 16.4). The needle valve permits fine adjustment of the quantity of gas flow. Modern flowmeters may be of either the 'ball'

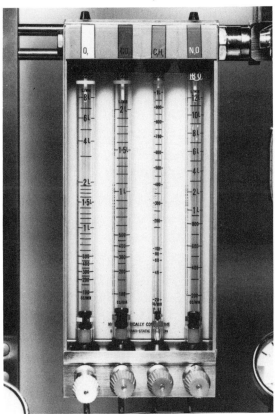

Fig. 16.4 A flowmeter bank, showing needle valves and bobbin flowmeters for (from left) oxygen, carbon dioxide, cyclopropane and nitrous oxide.

or 'bobbin' type. In the former the glass tube is of uniform diameter and gas flow between the ball and glass wall is 'orificial' in physical terms, resulting in turbulent flow. For turbulent flow;

$$\text{gas flow} \propto \frac{1}{d} \text{, where } d \text{ is gas density}$$

In the bobbin type of flowmeter the glass tube is tapered, being narrower at the bottom. At high gas flow rates, flow is turbulent, but at low flows, gas passes through a cylinder annulus, resulting in laminar flow which may be quantified using the Hagen-Poiseuille equation;

$$\text{gas flow} = \frac{P \, r^4 \pi}{8\eta l}$$

where P = pressure decrease at each end of the cylinder, r = radius of cylinder, l = length of cylinder and η = gas viscosity.

Thus with the bobbin type of flowmeter, the physical property determining flow is gas viscosity at low flow rates, and gas density at high flow rates. Hence each flowmeter is calibrated for a specific gas.

When gas is flowing, and the bobbin is suspended, downthrust from the weight of the bobbin balances exactly the upthrust, which corresponds to the gas pressure difference above and below the bobbin. The pressure difference above and below the bobbin is therefore constant, and this necessitates an increase in the size of the aperture as the flow increases.

The glass tube is calibrated to an accuracy of $\pm 2\%$. The top of the bobbin denotes the flow rate. The bobbin rotates because of flow of gas past spirally cut grooves, designed to prevent sticking of the bobbin to the glass tube — a white dot provides clear indication that the bobbin is rotating freely.

The needle valves associated with the flow meters must be handled gently. Excessive force on closure may lead to damage of the spindle or seating of the valve. It must be ensured that pipes, hoses and other pieces of apparatus do not accidentally rotate the flowmeter controls.

Anticonfusion test

When checking the anaesthetic machine, it is important to verify that the gas which issues from the oxygen pipeline or cylinder is the same as that which passes through the oxygen flowmeter. Fatalities have occurred because pipes on the machine were connected incorrectly. To test for this error in plumbing, all pipelines are disconnected and cylinders turned off. The needle valves of *all* flowmeters are opened. An oxygen cylinder is turned on. This should cause *only* the bobbin of the oxygen flowmeter to rise. The cylinder is then turned off, and the oxygen pipeline, if present, is attached. The flowmeters are observed again.

After turning on all cylinders required, all the bobbins should be inspected carefully. The carbon dioxide flowmeter may be fully opened, and the bobbin unnoticed at the very top of the tube.

Miscellaneous problems

In the U.K. it is customary for the oxygen flowmeter to be on the left, and the nitrous oxide on the right (of

the observer) with carbon dioxide and sometimes cyclopropane between (Fig. 16.4). As mixed gas leaves the flowmeter unit to the right, a leak from a faulty carbon dioxide or cyclopropane flowmeter causes a preferential loss of oxygen, resulting in delivery of a hypoxic mixture to the patient. In the U.S.A. the oxygen flowmeter is situated on the right of the flowmeter bank to avoid this hazard.

On older machines, an emergency oxygen flush lever was positioned near the needle valve so that all the oxygen passed through the flowmeter and also, incidentally, through the vaporiser. On modern machines, the oxygen flush button or lever is situated downstream from the vaporisers. This leads to dilution of the anaesthetic mixture with excess oxygen if the emergency oxygen tap is opened by mistake.

On some anaesthetic machines there is a knob or lever, often quite inconspicuous, which channels gas either to the outlet for an 'open circuit' or to the circle-absorber/ventilator circuit. Death from asphyxia has been caused by failure to recognise that no gas was issuing from the 'open circuit' port. Reports of consciousness during supposed anaesthesia have resulted from the use of an electrically powered ventilator in which the anaesthetic mixture was flowing directly into the atmosphere through the 'open circuit' outlet, while the curarised patient was receiving air.

Oxygen failure warning device

Many anaesthetic machines are equipped with an oxygen failure warning device. This may take the form of a battery-powered buzzer which is activated by a decrease in oxygen pressure. Some devices rely on the pressure of nitrous oxide to operate a whistle, the valve to which is opened if the oxygen pressure decreases. Both these types of device rely on sources of power which may also fail. Perhaps the best device is a whistle activated by compressed oxygen in a reservoir tank which is charged automatically through a nonreturn valve when the oxygen supply is connected initially. When the oxygen pressure decreases below a preset level (16–26 lbf/in^2) a pneumatic valve allows this reservoir to discharge through a whistle which sounds for approx. 10 s. A second valve may turn off the nitrous oxide supply, which is a desirable feature since total cessation of gas supply is noticed more quickly than a situation in which nitrous oxide alone continues to flow. However, it should be a matter of pride with every anaesthetist that the oxygen supply must never fail, even momentarily.

Quantiflex

The Quantiflex Mixer flowmeter (Fig. 16.5) eliminates the possibility of reducing the oxygen supply inadvertently. One dial is set to the desired percentage of oxygen and nitrous oxide, and the total flow-rate adjusted independently. The percentage of oxygen may be varied from 20% or 30% to 100%. Each gas passes through a flowmeter prior to mixture, providing evidence of correct functioning of the dual needle valves. Both gases arrive via linked pressure reducing regulators. The Quantiflex is useful in particular for varying the volume of fresh gas flow from moment to moment, whilst keeping the proportions constant.

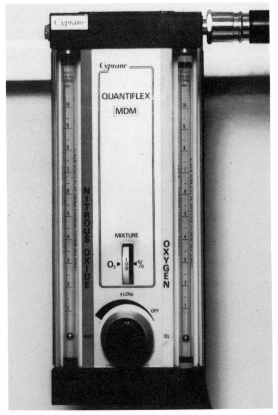

Fig. 16.5 A Quantiflex flowmeter. The required oxygen percentage is selected using the dial, and total flow of the required mixture adjusted using the black knob.

Vaporisers

Originally, anaesthetic agents were vaporised from liquid dripped on to a piece of absorbent material held over the patient's mouth and nose, but kept slightly away from the patient's skin by a small frame, e.g. Schimmelbusch mask.

More economical and convenient ways evolved, which provide a known concentration of vapour. If a carrier gas, e.g. oxygen, is mixed intimately with liquid ether at 20°C (room temperature) by causing tiny bubbles to pass through the liquid, the resulting mixture becomes fully saturated with ether. At this temperature, the saturated vapour pressure (SVP) exerted by ether is 425 mmHg. As the volume of the gas present is proportional to its partial pressure, then, assuming an atmospheric pressure of 760 mmHg, the partial pressure of oxygen in the mixture will be 760−425 = 335 mmHg. Thus for each 335 ml of oxygen, there are 425 ml of ether vapour, i.e. 1 ml of oxygen to 1.27 ml of ether vapour.

Thus, a flow of 400 ml of oxygen picks up approx. 500 ml of ether vapour. If this total of 900 ml is added to 4 litre of an oxygen/nitrous oxide mixture, the resultant 4.9 litre contain approx. 10% ether vapour. The percentage of vapour presented to the patient may be varied by adjusting the proportion of gas passing through the vaporiser.

Evaporation is accompanied by cooling. During use, the vaporiser cools. SVP, which is determined for a particular agent solely by temperature, is reduced and therefore concentration of vapour in the final gas mixture decreases. Cooling of the vaporiser may be minimised by a construction of copper (a highly conductive metal) and provision of a large surface area for the absorption of heat from the atmosphere. This system is known as the Copper Kettle and although popular in the U.S.A. has never enjoyed widespread use in the U.K. or Europe.

Modern vaporisers may be classified as either:

1. *Plenum vaporisers.* These are intended for unidirectional gas flow, have a relatively high resistance to gas flow and are unsuitable for use as either draw-over vaporisers or in circle systems. Examples include the Fluotec (Fig. 16.6) for halothane, Pentec for methoxyflurane, Tritec for trichloroethylene and Enfluratec for enflurane.

2. *Draw-over vaporisers.* These have a very low resistance to gas flow and may be used for obstetric

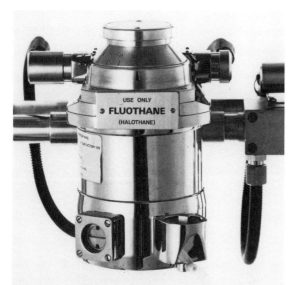

Fig. 16.6 The Fluotec flow and temperature compensated halothane vaporiser.

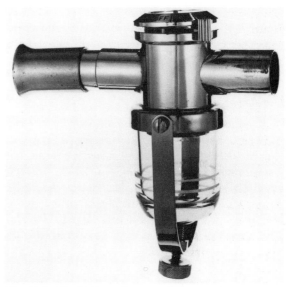

Fig. 16.8 The Goldman draw-over vaporiser.

analgesia (Emotril or Tecota, Fig. 16.7), dental anaesthesia (Goldman vaporiser, Fig. 16.8) or for emergency use in the field (e.g. EMO vaporiser, Fig. 16.9).

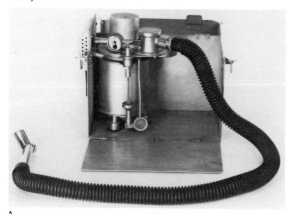

A

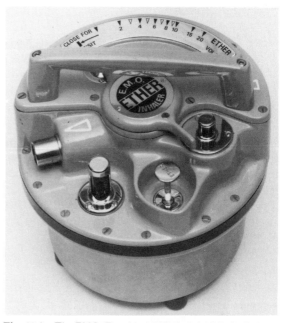

Fig. 16.9 The EMO (Epstein and Macintosh of Oxford) draw-over ether vaporiser.

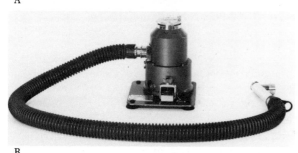

B

Fig. 16.7 The Emotril (**a**) and Tecota (**b**) draw-over vaporisers for delivery of 0.35% or 0.5% trichloroethylene in air.

The concentration of anaesthetic gas delivered by these vaporisers is dependent upon:

(a) The SVP of the agent.

(b) The temperature of the liquid anaesthetic. Modern vaporisers (e.g. Fluotec) are temperature compensated by means of a bimetallic strip which varies gas flow through the vaporising chamber. In the EMO a metallic bellows filled with ether vapour changes the operation of an outlet port. The Blease Universal Vaporiser also carries a bellows for thermal regulation. The most accurate vaporiser is the Drager 'Vapor' in which there is manual compensation for temperature changes. In addition changes in temperature may be reduced by increasing the thermal capacity of the vaporiser, e.g. Copper Kettle described above, water jacket in an EMO.

(c) The surface area of liquid exposed to the carrier gas. In order to ensure complete saturation of vapour in the Fluotec, a large surface area for evaporation is provided by a wick embracing an annular spiral of copper.

When there are two vaporisers in series on an anaesthetic machine it is undesirable to allow one vapour to enter the other vaporiser, as this will cause contamination which, in some circumstances, may be harmful.

Anaesthetic-specific connections are now available to link the supply bottle (container of liquid anaesthetic agent) to the appropriate vaporiser. These connections reduce the extent of spillage (and thus atmospheric pollution) and also the likelihood of filling the vaporiser with an inappropriate liquid. Some of these liquids contain nonvolatile additives, e.g. waxoline blue added to trichloroethylene for colouring, and thymol to halothane to increase stability. These additives may accumulate in the vaporiser and impair evaporation. Each vaporiser should therefore be emptied periodically and recharged with fresh liquid.

Breathing systems

The delivery system which conducts the anaesthetic mixture from the machine to the patient is termed colloquially a 'circuit' but is described more accurately as a breathing system since this does not imply that gas returns to the site of entry. Circuits are variously classified as 'open circuits', 'semiopen circuits' or 'semiclosed circuits' but these terms should be avoided.

Some breathing systems incorporate a spill valve, which is designed to vent gas if positive pressure is exerted upon it from within the system. During spontaneous respiration, the valve opens when the

patient generates a small positive pressure within the system, and it permits gas to be vented with minimal resistance to flow. During positive pressure ventilation, the valve is adjusted to restrict the leak of gases from the system while permitting an appropriate pressure to develop within the system for inflation of the patient's lungs.

In 1954 Mapleson classified anaesthetic breathing systems into five types: A, B, C, D and E (Fig. 16.10).

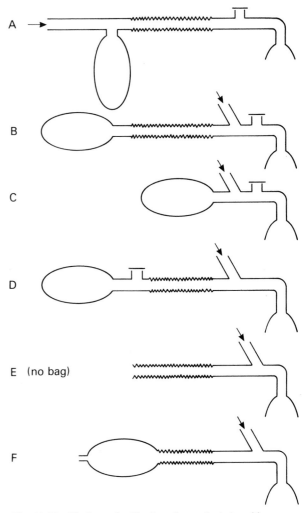

Fig. 16.10 Mapleson classification of anaesthetic breathing systems. The arrow indicates entry of fresh gas to the system.

Mapleson A

The most commonly used version of this is the Magill attachment (Fig. 16.11). At the end of inspiration, the reservoir bag is relatively empty and the pressure in

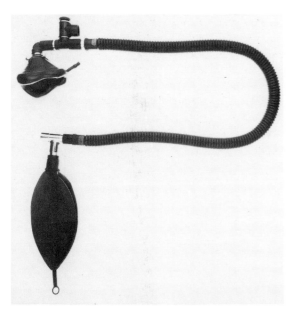

Fig. 16.11   The Magill attachment.

the system low, allowing the spring-loaded expiratory valve to remain closed. When expiration starts, the first part of the exhaled breath — the dead space gas — travels back into the corrugated tubing, causing the bag to fill. At the same time, fresh gas enters the bag from the machine. When the bag is distended, pressure in the system increases sufficiently to open the valve. As the patient continues exhaling, alveolar gas passes out through the expiratory valve.

If the circuit is used in the most economical way possible, only alveolar gas is voided through the valve (assuming no linear mixing). Therefore the fresh gas flow rate should equal the minute alveolar ventilation.

At the end of expiration, the cavity of the mask is filled with alveolar gas which is reinspired. This 'apparatus dead space' may be approx. 100 ml. This renders the Magill system in its usual form unsuitable for babies and small children.

During operations on the head and neck, it is inconvenient to have the expiratory valve underneath the surgical drapes, especially if a gas-scavenging device is in use. Lack has devised a modification in which a long tube is interposed between the patient-end of the corrugated tube and the expiratory valve. This long tube is housed inside the wide-bore corrugated tube in a coaxial arrangement (Fig. 16.12b). The inner expiratory tube should be of

adequate diameter to allow rapid escape of gas during expiration. The outer tube must therefore be of larger diameter than that of a Magill attachment. A fresh gas flow rate equivalent to the patient's total minute volume is required to eliminate rebreathing in the Lack circuit.

The Mapleson A circuits are not ideal for controlled or assisted ventilation. When inflating the patient's lungs, the valve should be fairly tightly closed. When the bag is squeezed, the patient's lungs are inflated, whilst some fresh gas spills from the valve. During expiration, the corrugated tube fills mainly with expired gas, the valve stays shut, and the reservoir bag fills with fresh gas and, if the fresh gas flow rate is low, with expired gas. Thus rebreathing occurs and the circuit is unsuitable for IPPV unless a large fresh gas flow is used.

Mapleson B and C

These systems are more efficient than the Mapleson A during IPPV but less efficient during spontaneous ventilation. They are not used commonly.

Mapleson D

The Bain coaxial system (Fig. 16.12a) is the most commonly used version of the Mapleson D. The inflow tube of the Bain is housed conveniently inside the corrugated tube.

During spontaneous ventilation, the fresh gas flow for a Mapleson D system should be at least 2.5 times the minute volume, in order to obviate significant rebreathing. For an adult this is approx. 15 litre/min, which is uneconomical of gases and vapours. In some patients a fresh gas flow of 250 ml/kg/min may be required to prevent rebreathing.

If the stream of fresh gas is directed into the cavity of the mask (without an angle piece) the dead space of the mask is greatly reduced. This makes the system more suitable for use in young children than the Magill.

It is important to check that gas is being delivered through the end of the inner tube. If this tube has developed a leak at the machine end, or become occluded by twisting, the patient will be asphyxiated. The end of the little finger, or the plunger of a 2 ml syringe, should be used to occlude the spout of the inner tube momentarily, while gas is flowing through

(a)

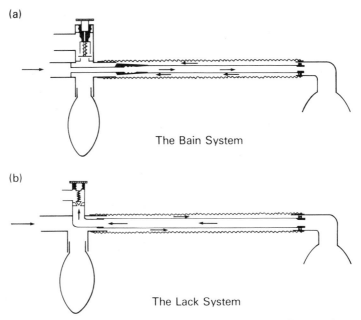

The Bain System

(b)

The Lack System

Fig. 16.12   Coaxial anaesthetic breathing systems. (**a**) The Bain System (Mapleson D). (**b**) The Lack System (Mapleson A).

the tube. Sound effects indicate if this manoeuvre causes a build-up of pressure, and confirm that the inner tube is intact. Movement of the reservoir bag with respiration does *not* indicate that fresh gas is being delivered to the patient.

The Bain circuit is more efficient than the Magill for IPPV and a fresh gas flow of 80 ml/kg/min provides moderate hypocapnia.

Mapleson E

This is commonly known as the Ayre's T-piece without a reservoir bag. Traditionally, this circuit has been used for babies and small children. Before the advantages of PEEP and CPAP in infants were recognised, it was commended for its low resistance to expiration. With a high fresh gas flow, the stream of gas tends to drive away expired gas from the cavity of the mask during the pause before inspiration, thereby reducing apparatus dead-space.

The fresh gas inflow should be 2.5 to 3 times the minute volume, and at least 4 litre/min. Some anaesthetists attach a visual indicator such as a piece of paper or a feather to the end of the reservoir tube to serve as an indication that gas is flowing.

If the volume inspired by the patient is greater than

the combined volume of the reservoir tube plus the fresh gas arriving during inspiration, some air is entrained during the latter part of inspiration, leading to lightening of anaesthesia.

The Ayre's T-piece may be used for IPPV by intermittent occlusion of the end of the reservoir tube with the thumb. Unfortunately, it is not possible to assess the pressure generated in the circuit with this technique.

Mapleson F

The F category was added as a postscript to describe the Ayre's T-piece with the Jackson-Rees modification (an open-ended bag on the end of the reservoir limb). It has several advantages over the Ayre's T-piece:

1. It provides visual evidence that the child is breathing.

2. By occluding the open end of the bag temporarily, it is possible to confirm that fresh gas is still entering the system.

3. It provides a degree of continuous positive airway pressure (CPAP) or positive end-expiratory pressure (PEEP) instead of allowing the patient to breathe out to atmospheric pressure.

4. It provides a convenient method of assisting or controlling ventilation. The open end of the reservoir bag is occluded between finger and thumb, and the bag squeezed. Some expired gas is directed back into the patient, but with IPPV this may be desirable, inasmuch as it permits large tidal volumes without producing hypocapnia. Large tidal volumes during IPPV may reduce the extent of atelectasis.

5. It is possible to assess (approximately) the inspiratory pressure during manual ventilation of the lungs, and to detect changes in lung or chest compliance.

The Waters 'To and Fro' system

Introduced by Ralph Waters in 1924, this system is similar to the Mapleson C except that a canister of soda-lime is interposed between the bag and the junction of the inflow tube (Fig. 16.13). As the patient exhales, carbon dioxide is absorbed by the more proximal granules in the canister, which are exhausted first, causing the apparatus dead-space to increase progressively. If the canister is not well

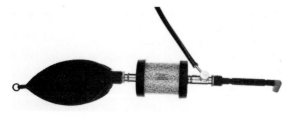

Fig. 16.13 The Waters' anaesthetic breathing system, incorporating a canister of soda lime.

filled, expired gas shunts to and fro in the channel above the granules, taking the course of least resistance and thereby increasing apparatus dead-space. Even in a properly filled can, channelling of gas tends to occur in the periphery.

The distance between the face-piece or endotracheal tube and the canister must be kept small to minimise dead-space and this renders the system rather inconvenient to use.

The minimum requirements for fresh gas flow depend on several factors which are not usually measured; the rates of uptake of oxygen and anaesthetic gases, and the concentration of nitrogen in the system. Most anaesthetists do not use it as a closed system, but employ a relatively high fresh gas flow rate, so that the concentrations of oxygen, anaesthetic gas and vapour in the system are similar to the input concentrations. A generous input is necessary at the outset of anaesthesia for the removal of nitrogen and to allow for the uptake of anaesthetic.

This system also helps to maintain humidity in the inspired gas mixture.

The Circle system

This system comprises an inspiratory hose, an expiratory hose, a soda-lime canister, two uni-directional valves, a reservoir bag usually on the end of a third hose, pressure relief valves and an inflow tube (Fig. 16.14).

Although the apparatus is more bulky and complex than the Waters', it is more convenient to use, as the

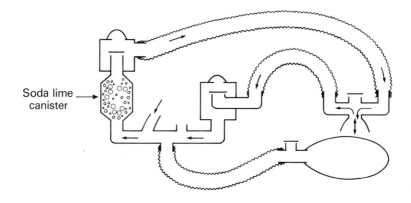

Circle System : Closed or semi-closed circuit

Fig. 16.14 The circle system: closed or semiclosed circuit.

Soda lime canister

heavy parts are carried by the anaesthetic machine, and the endotracheal tube is not disturbed when the reservoir bag is squeezed. The anaesthetist may also use an expiratory valve distant from the patient, and this is convenient during head and neck surgery.

The soda-lime canister is positioned vertically, which reduces the possibility of channelling through unfilled areas. The volume of the canister should be at least as large as the patient's tidal volume, so that the expired gas has adequate time for contact with the granules.

The Circle is seldom used as a totally closed system because of uncertainty regarding gas concentrations. During use, the fresh gas supply is diluted by mixing with the patient's expired gas. This applies particularly during induction, when the expired gas contains appreciably less anaesthetic gas and vapour than the inspired. Thus, with a modest fresh gas flow, the concentration of vapour in the circle is much smaller than that delivered by a vaporiser outside the circle (VOC). Later, as the rate of uptake of anaesthetic gases declines, the difference between inspired and expired concentrations decreases.

A vaporiser may also be used within the circle system (VIC). It should have low resistance to flow, e.g. the Goldman vaporiser (Fig. 16.8). The gas input may then be limited to the basal requirements for oxygen (approx. 250 ml/min) to keep the reservoir bag adequately filled. The depth of anaesthesia must be assessed continually, and the vaporiser tap opened or closed accordingly. During spontaneous ventilation, deepening of anaesthesia results in diminished alveolar ventilation, and thus diminished uptake of vapour, which permits anaesthesia to lighten. Conversely lightness of anaesthesia results in increased ventilation and uptake increases. To a certain extent there is therefore a protective feedback system. However, during IPPV this safety factor is not present, and it is dangerously easy to produce very high vapour concentrations in the inspired gas mixture.

With low fresh gas flows, e.g. less than 1.5 litre/min, into a circle system, nitrous oxide should *not* be used unless an oxygen analyser is employed to monitor inspired oxygen concentration. Preferably, all gas concentrations should be monitored during low flow anaesthesia (O_2, CO_2, volatile agents). Using oxygen alone at a fresh gas flow rate of approx. 300–500 ml/min into a circle system, the inspired nitrogen concentration rarely diminishes below 10%.

Soda Lime has the following approximate composition:

$Ca(OH)_2$	94%
NaOH	5%
KOH	1%
Silica	0.2%
Moisture content	14–19%
Indicators,	e.g. 'Durasorb' changes from pink to white

Absorption of CO_2 occurs by the following chemical reactions:

$$CO_2 + 2NaOH \rightarrow Na_2CO_3 + H_2O + heat$$
$$Na_2CO_3 + Ca(OH)_2 \rightarrow 2NaOH + CaCO_3$$

Trichloroethylene must not be used in any system involving soda-lime granules, as toxic substances, viz. dichloracetylene, phosgene and carbon monoxide, are produced if the vapour comes into contact with granules which have become hot by reacting with carbon dioxide.

Testing the anaesthetic machine for leaks

A significant high pressure leak is usually audible but leaks from the lower pressure side of the apparatus may be inaudible, difficult to detect and potentially more dangerous.

To test for leaks, the vaporisers should be turned on and the oxygen needle valve regulated to provide a flow of 500 ml/min. Occlusion of the 'open circuit' port with the thumb for 10 s should cause a small fall in the oxygen flowmeter bobbin and sudden removal of the thumb should be accompanied by a 'pop' as pressurised gas escapes.

The anaesthetic breathing circuit should be tested by filling the reservoir bag, closing the expiratory valve, blocking the patient connection port, turning off the inflow, and squeezing the reservoir bag. This manoeuvre does not diagnose leaks in the flowmeters and vaporisers, as there is usually a one-way valve at the right-hand end of the back bar on the anaesthetic machine.

VENTILATORS

The concept of artificial ventilation dates back to antiquity. In the early nineteenth century, the eccentric explorer Charles Waterton described the technique as 'a difficult and tedious mode of cure' for the effects of the deadly curare poison. A century later, attempts to make this mode of cure less tedious resulted in the invention of machines for mechanical ventilation. The polio epidemic of the 1950s increased interest in mechanical ventilation, and coincided with the increased use of relaxants during anaesthesia, improved understanding of respiratory physiology, and the more frequent use of endotracheal intubation.

An enormous selection of ventilators exists, and this brief section can attempt only to draw the reader's attention to some principles involved in their use and to stress that it is *absolutely essential* that the trainee understands the functioning of a mechanical ventilator before utilising it during anaesthesia. Even in recent times tragedies have occurred because of failure to understand the functioning of a machine despite apparently adequate ventilation of the patient. In addition, accidental disconnection, sticking valves, and incorrect adjustment of taps have all caused problems.

Each ventilator should be examined thoroughly prior to use. It is often helpful to use a 'dummy lung', i.e. a rubber bag on the patient connection, and to discuss with a senior colleague the particular capabilities and limitations of the machine.

With simple ventilators, observation of the patient is the only means of assessing the adequacy of ventilation, and with all machines continuous clinical observation is essential even in the presence of sophisticated monitoring and warning devices. Minimum monitoring should include the use of a spirometer on the expiratory limb to measure expiratory tidal volume and most machines possess a manometer for airway pressure. Continuous monitoring of oxygen, carbon dioxide and anaesthetic vapour concentrations are desirable but not always available.

Additional features of more complicated ventilators include ventilation failure alarms and humidifiers and warning devices which are important for children and longer procedures. The patient circuit should be either disposable or autoclavable. Alternatively, bacterial filters may be used.

The principle of operation of ventilators is best described by considering how they operate during each phase of the respiratory cycle:

1. Inspiration
2. Changeover from inspiration to expiration (cycling)
3. Expiration
4. Changeover from expiration to inspiration

Inspiration

Simplistically, ventilators may be regarded as producing inspiration by exerting either a predetermined flow of gas (*flow generators*) or a predetermined pressure (*pressure generators*). The effects of constant flow and constant pressure generators on airway pressures and lung volume are shown in Figure 16.15. Flow generators do not necessarily produce constant flow; flow may be sinusoidal if the mechanism is via a crank, e.g. Cape-Waine ventilator. With pressure generators, the pressure exerted is generally constant.

To a certain extent, pressure generators compensate for leaks in the circuit but not for change in pulmonary compliance. In contrast, flow generators, to a certain extent, compensate for changes in airway resistance or compliance but not for leaks in the circuit.

Pressure generator. Because the machine is producing a constant pressure, increased resistance to flow in the machine, tubes or patient may reduce the volume of gas received by the patient. With a Blease Manley ventilator a preset tidal volume is selected by the anaesthetist and this may not be achieved if:

(i) resistance increases (e.g. bronchospasm or constriction of anaesthetic tubing)

(ii) compliance decreases (e.g. increased muscle tone, the surgeon leaning on the chest, or the peritoneal cavity filled with CO_2)

(iii) leaks develop anywhere in the system.

Constant flow generator. The flow may be initiated by a piston compressing a bellows. Changes in resistance and compliance make little difference to the delivered volume unless a predetermined pressure is exceeded. Tidal volume and the frequency can be varied independently. The Bird ventilators, and the Cyclator, generate a flow by the Venturi effect. The Sheffield ventilator operates by intermittently occluding the outflow from an Ayre's T-piece.

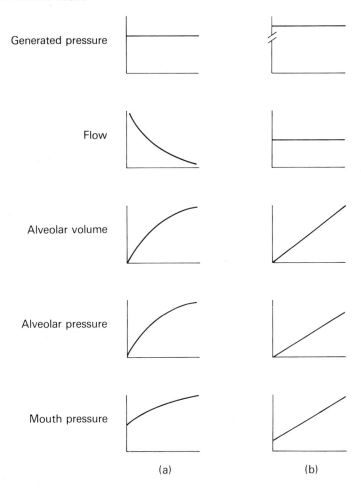

Fig. 16.15 Diagrammatic relationships between pressures, flow and volume using (**a**) a constant pressure generator and (**b**) a constant flow generator to inflate the lungs.

(**a**) A constant pressure generator exerts a low (e.g. 15 cmH$_2$O) pressure. At the start of inspiration, the pressure in the alveoli is zero. Gas flows rapidly into the alveoli, resulting in a rapid increase in alveolar volume. The pressure generated at the mouth (or endotracheal tube) is determined by the internal resistance of the ventilator and its connections. The initial rate of flow of gas into the alveoli depends both on that resistance, and the resistance of the endotracheal tube and tracheobronchial tree. As the alveolar pressure increases, the pressure gradient between ventilator and alveoli decreases, and flow rate diminishes. The pressure differences between ventilator and mouth, and mouth and alveoli, decrease because resistance diminishes with decreasing flow rate. When the alveolar pressure equals ventilator pressure, flow ceases.

(**b**) A constant flow generator generates a very high internal pressure (e.g. 4000 cmH$_2$O), but has a very high internal resistance to limit the flow rate. Because the pressure gradient between ventilator and alveoli is reduced by a negligible amount during an inspiratory cycle (e.g. 4000 to 3985 cmH$_2$O), flow rate is effectively constant. Thus, the increase in alveolar volume is linear, and, assuming constant lung/chest wall compliance, alveolar pressure also increases linearly. Because flow rate is constant, resistance is constant, as is the pressure gradient between mouth and alveoli.

Changeover from inspiration to expiration (cycling)

Volume cycled ventilators. When the predetermined volume has been delivered through the inspiratory limb, valves operate to allow expiration. Within limits, increases of resistance and decreases of compliance do not diminish the volume delivered.

Such changes in the airway and lungs increase the pressure required for delivery of the preset tidal volume.

Pressure cycled ventilators, e.g. Bird and Cyclator. These compensate for leaks by maintaining the inspiratory phase for a longer period and delivering a larger volume until a predetermined pressure has been achieved. If confronted with increased resistance or decreased compliance, the cycling pressure is reached earlier, and the tidal volume decreases. If airway resistance decreases, hyperventilation occurs unless the cycling pressure is reduced.

Time cycled ventilators. The duration of inspiration and of expiration may be predetermined on this type of ventilator. The maximum flow rate and/or the tidal volume should also be preselected.

Expiration

Usually the patient is allowed to exhale to atmospheric pressure. Subatmospheric ('negative') pressure is seldom used as it may cause bronchospasm and air trapping. Some ventilators may provide PEEP which helps to reduce pulmonary collapse, and minimise airway closure.

The expiratory port of the ventilator should be connected to an antipollution system. If malfunctioning, this may cause obstruction or suction.

On some machines, the expired air is passed through soda-lime as in the circle system. Such machines (e.g. East-Radcliffe and Cape-Waine) may be used with minimal gas inflow.

Changeover from expiration to inspiration

This may be triggered by a subatmospheric pressure created by the patient, but is usually brought about according to a predetermined time pattern or when the ventilator bellows have filled with a set volume of gas.

SCAVENGING

Because of the possible adverse effects of pollution of the operating theatre environment on anaesthetic, nursing, and surgical staff (see Chapter 41, p. 540), measures should be taken to reduce the extent of contamination of the atmosphere to a minimum. In the United Kingdom no target levels have been set by the DHSS but in the United States, it has been recommended by the National Institute of Occupational Safety and Hygiene that the level of contamination should be maintained below 2 parts per million (ppm) of a halogenated anaesthetic agent

or 25 ppm of nitrous oxide in combination with 0.5 ppm of a halogenated agent.

Pollution of the atmosphere with anaesthetic gases and vapours takes place in the operating theatre, the anaesthetic room, the recovery room, dental anaesthetic theatre, and obstetric delivery suites (where Entonox is used widely).

Sources of pollution include;

1. Gas discharge from ventilators.
2. Expired gas vented from the expiratory valve of anaesthetic breathing systems (Fig. 16.16).
3. Leaks from equipment, e.g. under the skirting of face masks.
4. Expired air from the patient in the recovery period.
5. Spillage arising from filling of anaesthetic vaporisers.

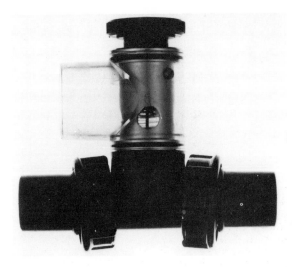

Fig. 16.16   An expiratory spill valve with scavenging attachment.

Although most attention has concentrated on removing gas from expiratory valves in anaesthetic breathing systems and ventilators, close attention should also be paid to the following;

1. Reduced usage of anaesthetics. In recent times there has been increased interest in the use of closed and low-flow semiclosed breathing systems. In addition, use of anaesthetic gases and volatile agents may be obviated totally by the use of total i.v.

anaesthesia (see Chapter 9, p. 151) or local anaesthetic techniques.

2. Air conditioning. Normal standards exist for operating theatre departments but particular problems arise in dental surgeries, recovery rooms and obstetric delivery suites.

3. Care in the filling of anaesthetic vaporisers. Great care should be taken to ensure nonspillage of volatile anaesthetic agents when recharging anaesthetic vaporisers. In some countries portable fume cupboards exist for this purpose.

Scavenging of anaesthetic breathing systems

(a) *Passive systems* (Fig. 16.17)

Passive systems permit the venting of patient expired gas from the anaesthetic system either to the outside atmosphere or to a ventilation extract duct. Long lengths of pipework must be avoided since the resistance to gas flow should not exceed 50 pascal (0.5 cmH$_2$O) at 30 litre/min.

(b) *Active systems* (Fig. 16.18)

An active system implies that active suction is applied near to the expiratory port of the anaesthetic breathing system to remove waste gases. The exhaust should be capable of accommodating 75 litre/min

continuous flow with a peak of 130 litre/min. Since the application of mains suction pressure (usually −54 kPa) would produce severe lung damage, it is essential that a suction pressure limiting device is included in the scavenging system.

There is a large number of different scavenging systems on the market as manufacturers of anaesthetic equipment produce their own devices. As with all items of equipment, it is essential that the anaesthetist understands the functioning of the apparatus before he utilises it. In addition, great care is necessary to avoid exposing the patient to increased resistance to expiration by compression of the expired ducting system (e.g. by allowing tubing to trail on the floor where it may be subjected to compression by items of equipment).

LARYNGOSCOPES (Fig. 16.19)

Straight-bladed (e.g. Magill)

When using a straight-bladed laryngoscope, it is usual to 'pick up' the epiglottis. The tip of the laryngoscope presses it upwards on to the root of the tongue so that it is not visible during tracheal intubation. The laryngoscope may be inserted initially deep into the pharynx, and withdrawn slowly, until the arytenoids and cords drop into view. This technique is useful for

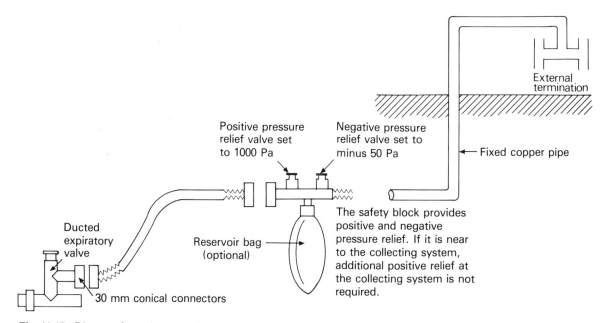

Fig. 16.17 Diagram of a passive scavenging system.

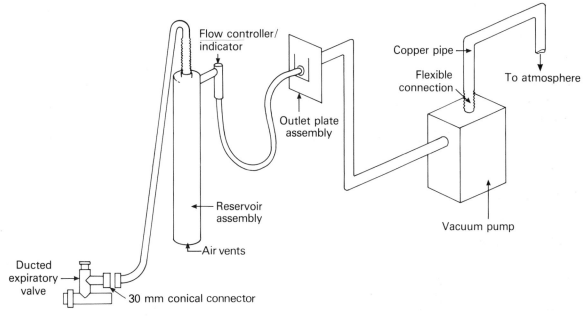

Fig. 16.18 Diagram of an active scavenging system.

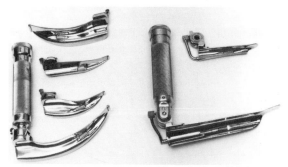

Fig. 16.19 Two laryngoscopes with a selection of blades. Right: Magill infant blade (above) and Magill adult blade (below). Left (from above downwards): Macintosh left-handed blade, Robertshaw blade, Macintosh infant blade and Macintosh adult blade.

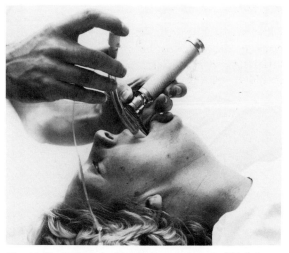

Fig. 16.20 Endotracheal intubation using a curved-bladed laryngoscope.

babies, as the epiglottis is rather floppy, and obscures the view of the cords if not elevated.

Curved-bladed (e.g. Macintosh)

The handle is held firmly in the left hand (Fig. 16.20). The mouth may be opened using left thumb and right forefinger. The right thumb is used for retracting the upper lip, and the right middle finger keeps the lower lip away to obviate its entrapment between teeth and blade. The tip of the laryngoscope is advanced carefully over the surface of the tongue until it reaches the vallecula. The tip is rotated upwards to lift the larynx, but without using the incisor teeth (or gum margin) as a fulcrum. When the arytenoids and posterior ends of the cords are seen, gentle pressure on the larynx using the right thumb and forefinger may help to provide a good view. The epiglottis is less likely to be bruised when a curved-bladed laryngoscope is used.

Laryngoscopes are usually constructed in such a way that the bulb is illuminated when the blade is opened. With this construction the electrical contact points are subject to corrosion and sometimes, when stress is placed on the hinge of the laryngoscope, the light goes out unexpectedly. Thus two functional laryngoscopes should always be available when embarking on tracheal intubation.

ENDOTRACHEAL TUBES (Figs 16.21–16.24)

Plain tubes

Noncuffed tubes are available in red rubber, latex rubber (armoured) and in PVC. There may be a leak unless the tube fits snugly. Fluids appearing in the pharynx may be aspirated into the trachea during inspiration. The incidence of sore throat after tracheal intubation is 40% and this is not reduced significantly by the use of a plain as opposed to a cuffed tube.

Cuffed tubes

When IPPV is planned, it is usual to use a cuffed tube. IPPV is employed usually in abdominal,

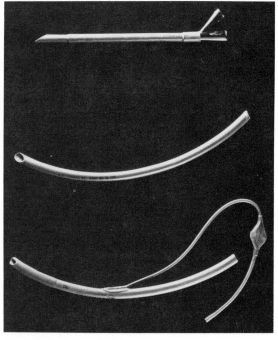

Fig. 16.21   Red rubber endotracheal tubes. Top to bottom: flexometallic, uncuffed nasal, and cuffed oral tubes.

thoracic, and neuro-surgery. It is also indicated when intra- and postoperative safety is improved by using a technique involving relaxants and analgesics in doses which would prevent adequate spontaneous ventilation.

A cuffed tube is indicated if there is a danger of aspiration of oesophageal, gastric or intestinal contents, or if blood, pus, saliva or irrigation fluids may enter the pharynx.

Cuff volume

A tube with a low volume cuff may require inflation to a high pressure to produce a good seal. A high-pressure cuff may exert little or no pressure on the tracheal mucosa unless it has been overinflated or because nitrous oxide diffuses into a cuff filled with air, thereby leading to an increase in pressure. It has been advocated that either cuff pressure be monitored continuously or the cuff be filled with an oxygen/nitrous oxide mixture. Alternatively the cuff volume may be readjusted after 10–15 min of anaesthesia.

High volume, low pressure 'floppy' cuffed tubes may fit an irregularly shaped trachea better, but may be more difficult and traumatic to insert. The cuff is in intimate contact with the mucosa over a larger area, and may cause ridges and furrows if the large cuff is puckered in a relatively small trachea.

Size of tube

In adults there is little to be gained in the way of reduction of resistance by choosing a tube larger than 8.0 mm. There is no compelling reason to find the largest possible tube for each adult, and it is most convenient to use a cuffed tube when an airtight seal is required. However it is usual to use an 8.5 mm tube for females and a 9.5 mm tube for males. Appropriate sizes of endotracheal tube for use in children are shown in Appendix V, p. 554

Red rubber cuffed tubes

These are satisfactory for most purposes. They have a suitable curve and are relatively easy to insert. They have a limited life (approx. 3 yr) and should be destroyed when signs of deterioration are seen. As with other cuffed tubes, the cuff should always be left inflated for several minutes before use to check for leaks.

Armoured latex cuffed tubes (Fig. 16.22)

These are particularly useful when there is a special danger of kinking, as the nylon spiral prevents obliteration of the lumen. However, if the cuff is overinflated it may 'herniate' downwards and obstruct airflow, especially during expiration. The pilot tube may develop a dilatation inside the main lumen of the tube causing obstruction. A wire or stilette, bent to the appropriate curve, is used when inserting this type of tube.

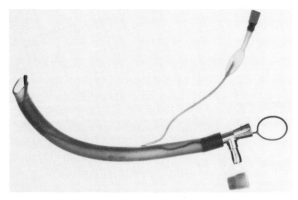

Fig. 16.22 Armoured latex cuffed endotracheal tube, with stilette for introduction.

Disposable plastic tubes (Figs 16.23 & 16.24)

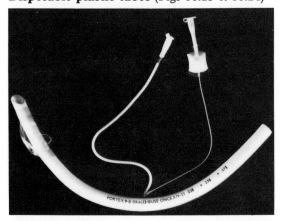

Fig. 16.23 A disposable plastic endotracheal tube. This type has an additional narrow side-lumen for sampling gas from the distal part of the tube.

These are becoming increasingly popular, and eliminate the problems of collecting, cleaning, checking and sterilising reusable tubes. Most anaesthetists prefer to shorten the tube before attaching the 15 mm tapered connection provided (Fig. 16.25). The tube is presented in a sterile package and care should be exercised to maintain the sterility of the distal end.

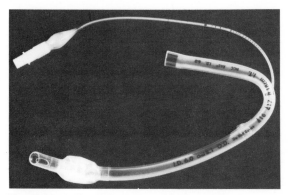

Fig. 16.24 A disposable plastic endotracheal tube.

Connections

British Standard connections with a 22 mm diameter are used in breathing circuits. Endotracheal connectors normally have a diameter of 15 mm.

Endotracheal tube connections (Fig. 16.25)

15 mm disposable. These are provided with plastic disposable tracheal tubes and are normally used with these tubes unless there is an indication for a different connector.

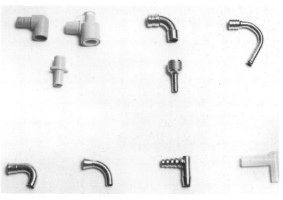

Fig. 16.25 A variety of endotracheal connectors. From top left in clockwise rotation: Portex and Portex swivel with 15 mm endotracheal tube connector, Nosworthy, Worcester, Cobbs, Rowbotham, Magill (oral), Magill (nasal).

Magill's connections are frequently used, especially with reusable tubes, during head/neck surgery.

Cobb's suction union is a modification of a Rowbotham connector. It was designed to permit the passage of a suction catheter down the tube. This may also be undertaken, of course, with the 15 mm disposable connector.

OTHER APPARATUS

Intubating forceps

The most commonly used intubating forceps is that designed by Magill (Fig. 16.26). The instrument is employed to manipulate a nasotracheal or nasogastric tube through the oropharynx and into the correct position.

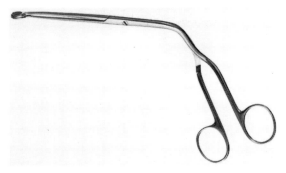

Fig. 16.26   The Magill intubating forceps.

Laryngeal spray

A laryngeal spray (Fig. 16.27) is used to deposite a fine mist of local anaesthetic solution (usually lignocaine 4%) on the mucosa of the larynx and upper

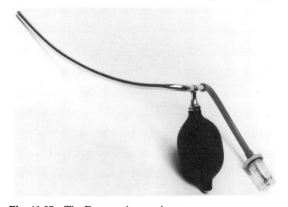

Fig. 16.27   The Forrester laryngeal spray.

trachea in order to minimise the autonomic reflexes and circulatory changes associated with endotracheal intubation.

Mouth gag

A mouth gag (Fig. 16.28) is employed during dental anaesthesia; it is also required occasionally to open the mouth in patients with trismus or in those who develop masseter spasm. It is positioned between the molar teeth, and must be used with care if damage to the teeth is to be avoided.

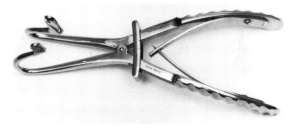

Fig. 16.28   The Fergusson mouth gag.

The gum elastic bougie (Fig. 16.29)

When the patient's upper and lower teeth are so close that the larynx cannot be visualised or the tube cannot be manoeuvred into the larynx, the easiest solution may be to insert a gum-elastic bougie into the trachea, remove the laryngoscope and gently slide the lubricated tube down over the bougie (also lubricated) with the tube rotated a quarter-turn anticlockwise so that its tip lies anteriorly in close contact with the bougie.

Bending plastic tubes

The curvature of a plastic tube may be increased easily when necessary. If the plastic has been held in the required position for several seconds it regains its original shape slowly. This requires no additional apparatus and does not involve touching the sterile end of the tube. One type of disposable cuffed tube can have its curvature increased during insertion by pulling on a ring loop.

Stilettes

Any type of tube can have its curvature altered by using a malleable wire or stilette which should be lubricated before use.

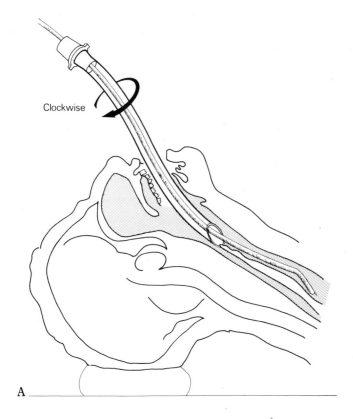

Clockwise

A

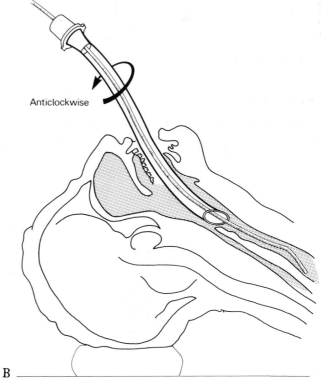

Anticlockwise

B

Fig. 16.29   A gum elastic bougie passed into the trachea. After insertion of the endotracheal tube, clockwise rotation of the tube (A) may cause it to lodge against the ary-epiglottic fold whilst anti-clockwise rotation (B) permits the tube to slide past the fold into the trachea.

Airways

An oropharyngeal airway (Guedel airway, Fig. 16.30) is frequently required to maintain a patent airway during spontaneous ventilation with a mask or if a patient's lungs cannot be ventilated prior to tracheal intubation because of obstruction in the oropharynx.

A nasopharyngeal airway (Fig. 16.31) is particularly useful for maintaining an airway during dental anaesthesia or in situations in which it is difficult to insert an oral airway (e.g. because of trismus or during recovery from anaesthesia because of increased muscle tone).

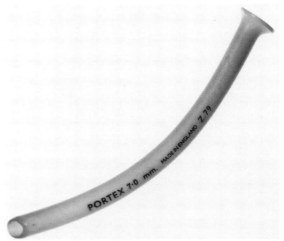

Fig. 16.31 A nasopharyngeal airway.

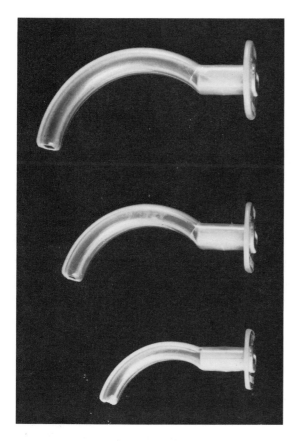

Fig. 16.30 Small, medium and large Guedel airways. Smaller sizes are available for use in infants and children.

FURTHER READING

Aldrete J A, Lowe H J, Virtue R W 1980 Low flow and closed system anaesthesia. Grune and Stratton, New York

Mushin W W, Rendell-Baker L, Thompson P W, Mapleson W W 1980 Automatic ventilation of the lungs, 3rd edn. Blackwell Scientific Publications, Oxford

Scurr C, Feldman S 1983 Scientific Foundations of Anaesthesia, 3rd edn. Heinemann, London

Sykes M K, Hull C J, Vickers M D 1981 Principles of clinical measurement. Blackwell Scientific Publications, Oxford

Ward C S 1975 Anaesthetic equipment: physical principles and maintenance. Baillière Tindall, London

17

The practical conduct of anaesthesia

Planning the conduct of anaesthesia normally commences after details concerning the surgical procedure and the medical condition of the patient have been ascertained at the preoperative visit. Preoperative assessment and selection of appropriate premedication are discussed in Chapter 15.

PREPARATION FOR ANAESTHESIA

Before embarking on the anaesthetic, consideration should be given to the induction and maintenance of anaesthesia, the position of the patient on the operating table, equipment necessary for monitoring, the use of intravenous fluids or blood for infusion, and the postoperative care and recovery facilities which will be required. The availability and function of all anaesthetic equipment should be checked before commencing (see Table 17.1). After the patient's arrival in the anaesthetic room the anaesthetist should be satisfied that the correct operation is being performed upon the correct patient, and that consent

Table 17.1 Equipment required for endotracheal intubation

Correct size laryngoscope and spare (in case of light failure)
Endotracheal tube of correct size + an alternative small size
Endotracheal tube connector
Wire stilette
Gum elastic bougies
Magill forceps
Cuff inflating syringe
Artery forceps
Securing tape or bandage
Catheter mount(s)
Local anaesthetic spray — 4% lignocaine
Cocaine spray/gel for nasal intubation
Endotracheal tube lubricant
Throat packs
Anaesthetic breathing circuit and face masks — tested with O_2 to
  ensure no leaks present

has been given. The patient must be on a tilting bed or trolley and the anaesthetist should have a competent assistant.

INDUCTION OF ANAESTHESIA

Anaesthesia is induced using one of the following techniques.

Inhalational induction

The most common indications for induction of anaesthesia by an inhalational technique are listed in Table 17.2.

Table 17.2 Indications for inhalational induction

Young or unco-operative children
Upper airway obstruction, e.g. epiglottitis
Lower airway obstruction with foreign body
Bronchopleural fistula or empyema
Poor risk patient unsuitable for i.v. induction

The proposed procedure should be explained to the patient. A 'no mask' technique using a cupped hand around the fresh gas delivery tube may be preferred for young children. Some anaesthetists favour allowing a child to play with the mask before connecting the anaesthetic tubing. The mask or hand is introduced *gradually* to the face from the side since the sight of a black mask descending to the face may be disturbing. While talking to the patient the anaesthetist selects the gas mixture and observes the patient's reactions. Initially 70% nitrous oxide in oxygen is used and anaesthesia deepened by the gradual introduction of increments of a volatile agent, e.g. halothane 1–3%; enflurane 1–3%. Maintenance levels of halothane (1–1.5%) or enflurane (1–2%) are used when anaesthesia has been established. Cyclopropane 50% in oxygen provides a rapid induction and anaesthesia may be maintained with a concentration of 5–10% in oxygen using a closed circuit.

If spontaneous ventilation is to be maintained throughout the procedure, the mask is applied more firmly as consciousness is lost and the airway is supported by the anaesthetist. Observation of the pattern of respiration and the patient's colour, together with palpation of a pulse, measurement of arterial pressure and monitoring of e.c.g. are important in the conduct of induction. Insertion of an oropharyngeal or endotracheal airway may be considered when anaesthesia has been established.

Difficulties and complications. Slow induction of anaesthesia (but cyclopropane is more rapid).

Problems particularly during stage 2 (vide infra).

Salivation — especially with cyclopropane and ether, therefore atropine premedication is required.

Airway obstruction, bronchospasm

Laryngeal spasm, hiccups

Environmental pollution.

Intravenous induction

Induction of anaesthesia using an i.v. anaesthetic agent is suitable for most routine purposes and avoids many of the complications associated with an inhalational induction. In addition, it is normally the most appropriate method of induction in the patient undergoing emergency surgery, where there is a risk of regurgitation of gastric contents.

All the drugs which may be required at induction should be prepared and i.v. access established. If an existing i.v. cannula is to be used, its function must be checked. 'Butterfly' type needles or cannulae with a side injection port ('Venflon' type) are useful; large cannulae (e.g. 16G, 14G) are necessary for transfusion of fluids or blood. A vein in the forearm or back of the hand is preferable; veins in the antecubital fossae are best avoided because of the risks of intra-arterial injection. After selection of a suitable vein, skin preparation is performed using iodine or alcohol. Subcutaneous local anaesthetic may be used where a large cannula is to be employed. Intravenous entry is confirmed with blood aspiration and the device secured firmly with tape. 'Opsite' dressing

may be used when long term use is anticipated. Arterial pressure should be measured, and e.c.g. monitoring may be attached to the patient at this stage. Preoxygenation is carried out, if appropriate, by administration of 100% oxygen by face-mask.

Doses of the common i.v. agents are shown in Table 17.3; induction dose varies with the patient's weight, age, state of nutrition, state of circulation, premedication and concurrent medications. A small

Table 17.3 Intravenous induction agents

Agent	Induction dose
Thiopentone	3–5 mg/kg
Methohexitone	1–1.5 mg/kg
Etomidate	0.3 mg/kg
Ketamine	2 mg/kg

test dose should be administered and its effect observed; slow injection is recommended in the aged, and patients with slow circulation time (e.g. shock, hypovolaemia, cardiac disease). Monitoring the effects of the drug on the cardiovascular system and on respiration is important. Rapid induction of anaesthesia through to stage 3 is achieved and this is maintained by the rapid introduction of inhalation agents, by repeated bolus injection, or by a continuous i.v. infusion of anaesthetic agent.

For patients undergoing emergency surgery and those in whom vomiting and/or regurgitation is a potential problem, rapid induction of anaesthesia using a 'crash' i.v. induction is indicated. The problems associated with emergency anaesthesia are discussed in Chapter 30.

Complications and difficulties

1. *Regurgitation and vomiting.* If regurgitation occurs, the patient should be placed immediately into a Trendelenburg position and material aspirated with suction apparatus. Should inhalation of gastric contents occur, treatment with 100% oxygen, bronchodilators, endotracheal suction and toilet, steroids, and antibiotics should be commenced immediately. Continued IPPV may be required if the resultant pneumonitis is severe.

2. *Intra-arterial injection of thiopentone.* This causes pain and blanching in hand and fingers as a result of crystal formation in the capillaries. The needle should

be left in the artery and 5 ml 0.5% procaine and 40 mg papaverine injected. Further treatment includes stellate ganglion block, brachial plexus block or i.v. guanethidine sympathetic block.

3. *Perivenous injection.* This causes blanching and pain and may lead to a small degree of tissue necrosis. Methohexitone is said to produce less tissue damage than thiopentone. Hyaluronidase may be used to speed dispersal of the drug.

4. *Cardiovascular depression.* This is particularly likely to occur in the hypovolaemic or the untreated hypertensive patient. Infusion of i.v. fluid (e.g. 500 ml compound sodium lactate) is usually adequate to restore arterial pressure toward normal.

5. *Respiratory depression.* Slow injection of induction agents may reduce the degree of respiratory depression. Respiratory adequacy must be assessed carefully, and the anaesthetist should be ready to assist ventilation if necessary.

6. *Histamine release.* Thiopentone, methohexitone, Althesin and propanidid may all cause release of histamine with subsequent formation of typical wheals.

7. *Reaction to individual i.v. agents.* Appropriate drugs and fluids should be available in the anaesthetic room to cope with this eventuality.

8. *Porphyria.* An acute porphyric episode may be precipitated in susceptible individuals by barbiturates.

9. *Other complications.* Hiccup, muscular movement, pain on injection, especially with methohexitone or etomidate.

POSITION OF PATIENT FOR SURGERY

Following induction, the patient is placed on the operating table in a position appropriate for the proposed surgery. When positioning the patient, the anaesthetist should take into account surgical access, patient safety, anaesthetic technique, monitoring and position of i.v. lines, etc.

Some commonly used positions are shown in Figure 17.1. Each may have adverse effects in terms of skeletal, neurological, ventilatory and circulatory effects.

The *Trendelenburg* position may produce increased pressure on the diaphragm or damage to the brachial plexus with arm abduction. *Lithotomy* position may result in nerve damage on the medial or lateral side of the leg by pressure from stirrups. Great care must be taken to elevate the legs simultaneously to avoid pelvic asymmetry and resulting backache. The *prone* position may cause abdominal compression, which may result in respiratory and circulatory embarrassment. To prevent this, support must be provided beneath shoulders and iliac crests. Extension of the shoulder should be avoided. The *lateral* position results in asymmetrical lung ventilation, and care is required with arm position and i.v. infusions. The *sitting* position requires careful head support. In addition, venous pooling with resultant cardiovascular instability can be a problem. The *supine* position carries the risk of inhalation, and the supine hypotensive syndrome during pregnancy.

MAINTENANCE OF ANAESTHESIA

Anaesthesia may be continued using inhalational agents, i.v. anaesthetic agents, or i.v. opioids either alone or in combination. Endotracheal intubation with or without muscle relaxants may be employed. Regional anaesthesia may be used to supplement any of these techniques.

Inhalational anaesthesia with spontaneous ventilation

This is an appropriate form of maintenance for superficial operations, minor procedures producing little reflex or painful stimulation, and operations for which profound muscle relaxation is not required.

Conduct

Following induction, gaseous and/or volatile agents may be used for the spontaneously ventilating patient. Halothane in 70% nitrous oxide/30% oxygen may be employed at a maintenance level of 1–2%, depending upon the nature of the surgery, the provision of analgesia in the premedication, and the patient's response in terms of respiration, circulation, heart rate and rhythm. Enflurane 1.5–2.5% is an alternative agent. Trichloroethylene is more soluble and thus slower in onset and must be administered at a relatively high concentration (1–1.5%) initially, although this may be reduced to 0.4–0.6% after

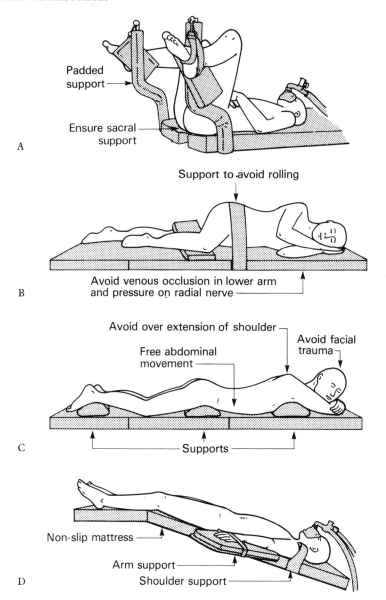

Fig. 17.1 Positions on the operating table **(a)** lithotomy, **(b)** lateral, **(c)** prone, **(d)** Trendelenburg.

10–15 min. Cyclopropane is used occasionally for maintenance of anaesthesia, but because of its explosive property, it must be administered in a closed system, usually in a concentration of 5–10% in oxygen.

Minimum alveolar concentration (MAC)

The MAC is the alveolar concentration of an inhaled anaesthetic agent which prevents reflex movement in response to surgical incision in 50% of subjects.

MAC values of commonly used inhalational agents are shown in the Appendix (p. 548).

MAC varies little with metabolic factors, but is reduced by opioid premedication and when mixtures of anaesthetic agents (e.g. volatile agent + N_2O/O_2) are used. MAC is higher in neonates and reduced in the aged. It is reduced by hypothermia.

The rate at which MAC is attained can be increased by raising the inspired concentration and preventing airway obstruction.

Increasing ventilation at a constant inspired concentration produces more rapid equilibration. The time taken for equilibration increases with the solubility coefficient of the agent in blood. Thus, anaesthetic agents of moderate or high solubility do not reach equilibrium for several hours (see Chapter 7, p. 117). It follows that, when using such agents, the inspired concentration should be higher than MAC, in order to produce an adequate alveolar concentration.

Control of depth by varying the inspired concentration of volatile agent requires constant assessment of the patient's reaction to anaesthesia and surgery to produce adequate anaesthesia while avoiding overdosage and excessively 'deep' anaesthesia. This rapid control is one of the main advantages of inhalational anaesthesia. The signs of an inadequate depth of anaesthesia include tachypnoea, tachycardia, hypertension and sweating.

Signs of Anaesthesia (Fig. 17.2)

Guedel's classical signs of anaesthesia are those seen in patients premedicated with morphine and atropine, and breathing ether in air. The clinical signs associated with anaesthesia produced by other inhalational agents follow a similar course, but the divisions between the stages and planes are less precise.

Stage 1: the stage of analgesia. This is the stage attained when using nitrous oxide 50% in oxygen, as employed in the technique of relative analgesia (see Chapter 33).

Stage 2: stage of excitement. This is seen with inhalational induction, but rapidly passed during i.v. induction. Respiration is erratic, breath-holding may occur, laryngeal and pharyngeal reflexes are active and stimulation of pharynx or larynx can produce laryngeal spasm. The eyelash reflex (used as a sign of unconsciousness with i.v. induction) is abolished in stage 2, but the eyelid reflex (resistance to elevation of eyelid) remains present.

Stage 3: surgical anaesthesia. This deepens through 4 planes (in practice 3 — light, medium, deep) with increasing concentration of anaesthetic drug.

STAGE	RESPIRATION	PUPILS	EYE REFLEXES	URT & RESPIRATORY REFLEXES
1 Analgesia	Regular Small volume	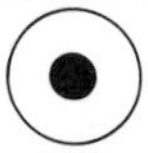 ◉		
2 Excitement	Irregular	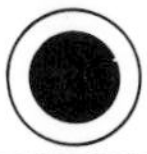 ⬤	Eyelash absent	
3 Anaesthesia Plane I	Regular Large volume	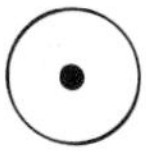 ⊙	Eyelid absent Conjunctival depressed	Pharyngeal & vomiting depressed
Plane II	Regular Large volume	⊙	Corneal depressed	
Plane III	Regular Becoming diaphragmatic Small volume	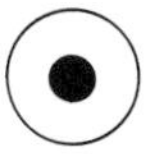 ⬤		Laryngeal depressed
Plane IV	Irregular Diaphragmatic Small volume	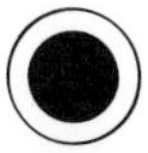 ⬤		Carinal depressed
4 Overdose	Apnoea	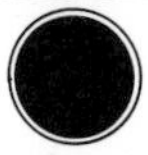 ⬤		

Fig. 17.2 Stages of anaesthesia, modified from Guedel.

Respiration assumes a rhythmic pattern and the thoracic component diminishes with depth of anaesthesia. Respiratory reflexes become suppressed but the carinal reflex is abolished only at plane IV (therefore an endotracheal tube which is too long may produce carinal stimulation at an otherwise adequate depth). Pupils are central and gradually enlarge with depth. Lacrimation is active in light planes but absent in planes III and IV — a useful sign in a patient not premedicated with an anticholinergic.

Stage 4: stage of impending respiratory and circulatory failure. Brainstem reflexes are depressed by the high anaesthetic concentration. Pupils are enlarged and unreactive. The patient should not be permitted to reach this stage. Withdrawal of the anaesthetic agents and administration of 100% oxygen lightens anaesthesia.

Observation of other reflexes provides a guide to depth of anaesthesia. Swallowing occurs in the light plane of stage 3. The gag reflex is abolished in upper stage 3. Stretching of the anal sphincter produces reflex laryngospasm even at plane III of stage 3.

Complications/difficulties during inhalational anaesthesia

Airway obstruction. Relieved with appropriate positioning and equipment (vide infra).

Laryngeal spasm. This may occur as a result of stimulation above light-medium stage 3. Treatment is to stop the stimulation and gently deepen anaesthesia. If spasm is severe, 100% oxygen is applied with the face mask held tightly, maintaining the airway by hand and applying pressure to the reservoir bag. Attempts to ventilate the patient's lungs usually result only in gastric inflation. However, as the larynx partially opens, 100% oxygen flows through under pressure. Further gentle deepening of anaesthesia may then take place. In severe laryngeal spasm, suxamethonium may be required and after the patient has been oxygenated it is advisable to intubate the trachea.

Bronchospasm. This may occur if volatile anaesthetic agents are introduced rapidly, particularly in smokers with excessive bronchial secretions. Humidification and warming of gases may minimise the problem. Bronchospasm may accompany laryngospasm. Administration of bronchodilators may be required. These respiratory reflexes are induced more readily in the presence of an upper respiratory tract infection.

Malignant hyperpyrexia. Volatile agents in addition to suxamethonium and amide-type local anaesthetic agents may trigger this syndrome in susceptible individuals (see Chapter 19).

Raised intracranial pressure (ICP). All volatile agents may produce an increase in ICP, and this is accentuated by retention of CO_2 which accompanies the use of volatile agents in the spontaneously breathing patient. A spontaneous ventilation technique is therefore contraindicated in patients with an intracranial space occupying lesion or cerebral oedema.

Atmospheric pollution. The use of the appropriate scavenging apparatus helps to reduce levels of theatre pollution by volatile and gaseous agents (see Chapter 16).

Airway maintenance during inhalational anaesthesia

Airway maintenance is one of the most important aspects of the anaesthetist's task. Inhalational anaesthesia usually involves the use of the face mask; these take many forms and selection of one of the correct size to provide a gas tight seal is important. For children, a mask with excessive dead space should be avoided. Nasal masks are required during chairside dental anaesthesia. The patient's head position during mask anaesthesia is important; the mandible is held 'into' the mask by the anaesthetist with his fingers holding the mandible itself rather than pressing into the soft tissues, which may result in airway obstruction (especially in children). The mandible is held forward, helping to prevent posterior movement of the tongue obstructing the airway.

The importance of observation of the airway during mask anaesthesia should be stressed. Indrawing of the suprasternal and supraclavicular areas is evidence of upper airway obstruction. Noisy respiration or inspiratory stridor is further evidence that airway obstruction is present and requires correction. An oropharyngeal (Guedel) airway may be used to assist in preventing obstruction. The patient must be anaesthetised adequately before insertion of the airway since stimulation of the pharynx may produce coughing, breath-holding or laryngeal spasm. Nasopharyngeal airways may be tolerated better. Once the airway is established and the patient's respiratory pattern has settled, the use of a Clausen harness frees the anaesthetist's hands; the straps should be applied carefully and symmetrically for success. Support of the mandible may be achieved with a well-padded tongue spatula or an oropharyngeal airway inserted between the straps.

Endotracheal anaesthesia

Indications for endotracheal anaesthesia

1. Provision of a clear airway, e.g. difficulty anticipated in using mask anaesthesia in the edentulous patient.

2. Where the patient is in an 'unusual' position, e.g. prone or sitting. A reinforced nonkinking tube may be necessary.

3. Operations on the head and neck, e.g. ENT, dental. A nasal endotracheal tube may be required.

4. Protection of the respiratory tract, e.g. from blood during upper respiratory tract or oral surgery and from inhalation of gastric contents in emergency surgery or patients with oesophageal obstruction. The use of a cuffed tube for adults is mandatory in these circumstances.

5. During anaesthesia using IPPV and muscle relaxants.

6. To facilitate suction of the respiratory tract and during thoracic operations.

Contraindications

There are few contraindications. In emergency situations, hypoxia must be relieved if at all possible before insertion of an endotracheal tube.

Preparations for endotracheal intubation

Before commencing, the anaesthetist must check the availability and function of the necessary equipment. He should have a 'dedicated' and experienced assistant present. Laryngoscopes of the correct size are chosen and the function of bulb and batteries checked, the patency of the endotracheal tube is checked and the integrity of the cuff ensured. Various aids to intubation must also be present (see Table 17.1).

Choice of equipment

Laryngoscopes. Laryngoscopes abound in many shapes and sizes. There are two basic types of blade — straight and curved. Straight blade laryngoscopes (e.g. Magill) are favoured for children, in whom the epiglottis is floppy, and are designed to pass posterior to the epiglottis and lift it anteriorly, exposing the larynx (Fig. 17.3). The curved blade (e.g. Macintosh) is designed so that the tip lies anterior to the epiglottis in the vallecula, pressing on the hyo-epiglottic ligament and moving it anteriorly to expose the larynx and vocal cords (Fig. 17.3).

Endotracheal tubes. Most endotracheal tubes are made either of rubber or plastic. The latter are disposable and less irritant to the tracheal mucosa. In certain circumstances, e.g. head and neck or throat surgery, the endotracheal tube may be subjected to direct or indirect pressure, and standard tubes may kink or become compressed. It may be appropriate to use a tube which is reinforced with nylon or steel in such cases. Endotracheal tubes are normally

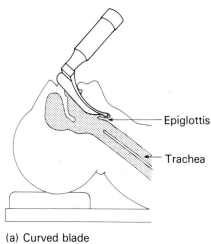

(a) Curved blade

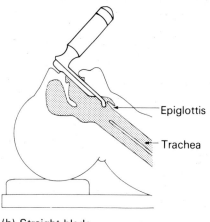

(b) Straight blade

Fig. 17.3 Use of the laryngoscope.

introduced through the mouth, although it may be preferable to pass the tube through the nose, particularly for oral surgery. The length of disposable endotracheal tubes exceeds that normally required for oral intubation, and the tube should be cut to the appropriate length before use. During thoracic surgery, it may be necessary to ventilate the lungs independently, and endobronchial or double-lumen tubes are required (see Chapter 28).

In order to seal the airway, most endotracheal tubes are manufactured with an inflatable cuff at the distal end. The cuff may be of low or high volume; low volume cuffs produce a seal over a smaller area of tracheal mucosa, and tend to exert a high pressure on the mucosal cells, reducing their capillary blood supply and rendering them potentially ischaemic. High volume cuffs cover a wide area of mucosa; the pressure exerted varies during the respiratory cycle, but is on average lower than that produced by a low volume cuff.

Endotracheal tubes of different sizes are required. The size usually quoted is the internal diameter (ID). Adult males normally require a tube of 9–10 mm ID, and females 8–8.5 mm. For oral intubation, the tube should be 20–23 cm long. The appropriate internal diameter of tube for paediatric use can be calculated from the formula $(\frac{Age}{4} + 4)$ mm. This is an approximation, and a tube 0.5 mm smaller and 0.5 mm larger should also be prepared. The length of tube required for oral intubation is approximately equal to $(\frac{Age}{2} + 12)$ cm. A tube of slightly smaller internal diameter may be required for nasal intubation, and its length may be calculated from the formula $(\frac{Age}{2} + 15)$ cm.

An appropriate connector is required between the endotracheal tube and the anaesthetic circuit, e.g. curved connector for nasal tube, lightweight plastic with low deadspace for children, or a connector with a suction port for thoracic surgery.

Anaesthesia for endotracheal intubation

Endotracheal intubation may be performed with the patient awake (e.g. neonates), under local anaesthesia using topical spray, transtracheal spray and superior laryngeal nerve block, or under general anaesthesia, either i.v. or inhalational with or without the use of muscle relaxation. The usual approach is to provide general anaesthesia and muscle relaxation, perform laryngoscopy and direct vision intubation, and then to maintain anaesthesia via the endotracheal tube with spontaneous or controlled ventilation. Adequate anaesthesia and muscle relaxation must be provided for laryngoscopy.

Inhalational technique for intubation. Adequate depth of anaesthesia is necessary to depress the laryngeal reflexes and provide a degree of relaxation of the laryngeal and pharyngeal muscles. Halothane in concentrations up to 4% may provide rapid attainment of necessary depth, which can be judged from a pattern of respiration with predominance of diaphragmatic breathing (a useful sign in children is the 'dissociation' of the thoracic and abdominal excursion). The mask is removed and laryngoscopy and intubation performed. The anaesthetic circuit is then connected to the endotracheal tube and anaesthesia maintained at a depth appropriate for surgery.

Relaxant anaesthesia for intubation. Following i.v. or inhalational induction of anaesthesia, the short-acting depolarising muscle relaxant suxamethonium may be used to provide ideal relaxation for endotracheal intubation. Following loss of consciousness, the patient breathes 100% oxygen or 50% nitrous oxide/oxygen and suxamethonium is administered in a dose of 1mg/kg. Ventilation is maintained via the mask until muscle relaxation occurs (except in emergency patients and those likely to regurgitate) and laryngoscopy and intubation are carried out. Inhalational anaesthesia is continued with manual ventilation until the effects of suxamethonium have ceased. Anaesthesia may be continued via the endotracheal tube with spontaneous ventilation, or, if appropriate, neuromuscular blockade continued, and ventilation controlled.

Conduct of laryngoscopy

The position of the patient's head and neck is important. The neck is flexed and the head extended with support of a pillow to achieve this. Thus the oral, pharyngeal and tracheal axes are brought towards alignment (Fig. 17.4). The laryngoscope is designed for left hand use and is introduced into the right side of the mouth while the right hand opens the mouth, parting the lips to avoid interposing them between laryngoscope and teeth. The teeth may be protected from blade trauma with the fingers or the

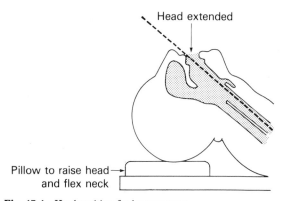

Head extended

Pillow to raise head →
and flex neck

Fig. 17.4 Head position for laryngoscopy.

use of a plastic 'guard'. The laryngoscope blade deflects the tongue to the left and the length of the blade is passed over the contour of the tongue. The laryngoscope is lifted upwards and forwards, avoiding a levering movement which can damage the upper teeth. Using a straight blade, the tip is passed posterior to the epiglottis, which is lifted anteriorly and the vocal cords visualised. With a curved blade, the tip is inserted into the vallecula and pressure on the hyo-epiglottic ligament moves the epiglottis to expose the vocal cords. External pressure on the thyroid cartilage by an assistant may help laryngeal visualisation at this stage.

Conduct of intubation

After laryngeal visualisation the supraglottic area and cords may be sprayed with local anaesthetic spray (4% lignocaine) if desired. The endotracheal tube is passed from the right side of the mouth (which may be held open by the assistant's finger if necessary) permitting a clear view of the midline. The tip is passed between the vocal cords and into the trachea until the cuff is below the vocal cords.

A semirigid stilette may be used during intubation to provide the correct degree of curvature of the endotracheal tube to permit intubation. The tube cuff is inflated sufficiently to abolish the audible gas leak on inflation; the position of the tube is confirmed by auscultation, ensuring that bronchial intubation has been avoided.

Tube fixation. The tube is secured in position using either cotton tape or bandage, or sticking plaster strips. Tube fixation is important if the head is inaccessible during the operation, e.g. patient in a prone position.

Nasal intubation

Nasal intubation may be employed for dental operations, ENT operations, etc., and may be preferred for long-term intubation by providing easier tube fixation, easier oral toilet and greater patient comfort.

A slightly smaller tube is used, and is introduced preferentially to the right nostril since the left-facing bevel of the tube favours this approach. The tube is passed along the floor of the nose and advanced *gently* into the pharynx, avoiding excessive force. Laryngoscopy then takes place, and the tube is advanced into the trachea by manipulation of the proximal end or by grasping the tip with Magill's intubating forceps to pass it between the cords.

Throat packing may be employed after intubation especially for oropharyngeal operations. The moist gauze pack is introduced using the laryngoscope and Magill forceps. The pharynx should be packed on each side of the endotracheal tube. The pack should be applied gently to avoid abrasion of the mucosa. A 'tail' of the pack is left protruding from the mouth and the anaesthetist must accept responsibility for removal of the pack before extubation. A latex 'foam' pack may be used as an alternative to cotton gauze.

Difficult intubation

Difficult intubation may be anticipated or unanticipated. Difficulty may be expected from evidence sought at the preoperative visit. The unexpected case should be acknowledged as such at the time of intubation and the anaesthetist should have contingency plans to overcome the situation. This subject is discussed in Chapter 19.

Complications of endotracheal intubation

Complications may be mechanical, respiratory, or cardiovascular and may occur early or late.

Early complications. Trauma may occur to lips and teeth or dental crowns. Jaw dislocation and dislocation of arytenoids may be produced. Trauma during intubation may result in damage to larynx and vocal cords. Nasal intubation may produce epistaxis, trauma to the pharyngeal wall or dislodgement of adenoid tissue. Obstruction or kinking of the tube can occur and carinal stimulation or endobronchial intubation may take place if the tube is too long. Laryngeal trauma may produce postoperative croup, bronchospasm or laryngospasm, especially in children. Mechanical complications may be avoided with careful technique. Broken teeth, etc., must be retrieved and the event documented. Respiratory complications immediately postoperatively may be minimised by humidification of inspired gases. Cardiovascular complications of intubation include arrhythmias and hypertension, especially in untreated hypertensive patients.

Late complications. These are more common after long-term intubation. Tracheal stenosis is rare, but damage to tracheal mucosa from a cuffed tube may be related to its design; high volume-low pressure cuffs may be preferred for long-term intubation. Trauma to vocal cords may result in ulceration or granulomata which may require surgical removal. Cord trauma may be more likely in the presence of an upper respiratory tract infection.

Relaxant anaesthesia

Indications for relaxant anaesthesia

As an alternative to deep anaesthesia with spontaneous ventilation and volatile agents leading to multisystem depression, the triad of sleep, analgesia and muscle relaxation may be provided separately with specific agents. Relaxation anaesthesia provides muscle relaxation, permitting lighter anaesthesia with preservation of autonomic reflexes. Thus the technique is appropriate for major abdominal operations, intraperitoneal operations, thoracic operations, intracranial operations, prolonged operations where spontaneous ventilation would lead to respiratory depression, and operations in a position in which respiration is impaired mechanically.

Conduct of relaxant anaesthesia

Induction of anaesthesia is followed by endotracheal intubation after administration of a depolarising muscle relaxant. When its action has worn off, relaxation is provided by a longer-acting nondepolarising relaxant (Table 11.1). The choice of agent depends upon operative indications (e.g. tubocurarine may be preferred when induced hypotension is proposed) or the patient's condition (e.g. pancuronium does not produce cardiovascular depression).

Controlled ventilation is instituted, first manually, by compression of the reservoir bag, and then by a mechanical ventilator delivering the appropriate tidal and minute volume (see Appendix VII, p. 557). Anaesthesia and analgesia are usually provided by nitrous oxide/oxygen, together with a volatile agent and/or i.v. analgesic. Analgesia may be provided by opioid premedication. Volatile agents are used in an inspired concentration less than MAC when ventilation is controlled. Intravenous agents, e.g. morphine, papaveretum, phenoperidine, fentanyl or buprenorphine may be employed in small doses.

Assessment of relaxant anaesthesia

Light anaesthesia with preservation of reflexes permits the use of physical signs for the continued assessment of the adequacy of anaesthesia.

Adequacy of anaesthesia. Autonomic reflex activity with lacrimation, sweating, tachycardia, hypertension, or reflex movement in response to surgery, indicate 'light' anaesthesia and response to surgical stimulation and warn that the depth of anaesthesia should be increased or further increments of i.v. analgesic given.

'Awareness' during relaxant anaesthesia. The possibility of awareness or inadequate anaesthesia exists in a patient paralysed with muscle relaxant drugs and therefore unable to move in response to stimulation. The anaesthetist should ensure that this possibility is avoided. The clinical signs of inadequate anaesthesia should be sought and appropriate action taken.

Adequacy of muscle relaxation. Signs of returning muscle tone include retraction of wound edges during abdominal operations, and abdominal muscle, diaphragmatic or facial movement. An increase in inflation pressure (with a volume-cycled ventilator) may indicate increase in muscle tone (or bronchospasm). Small increments (e.g. $\frac{1}{4} - \frac{1}{3}$ of the original dose) of muscle relaxant may be given to maintain relaxation. Quantitative estimation of muscle paralysis may be performed with a peripheral nerve stimulator (see Chapter 11). The duration of action of muscle relaxants (Table 11.1) may be prolonged in the presence of volatile agents.

Adequacy of ventilation. Clinical signs of inadequate ventilation and an increase in Pa_{CO_2} include venous dilatation, wound oozing, tachycardia, hypertension and attempts at spontaneous respiration by the patient.

Measurement of arterial $P\text{CO}_2$, end-expired $P\text{CO}_2$ or minute volume provide more objective information upon which mechanical ventilation may be adjusted.

Reversal of relaxation

At the end of operation, residual neuromuscular blockade is antagonised and spontaneous respiration established before the tracheal tube is removed and the patient awakened. Neuromuscular block is antagonised with neostigmine 2.5–5 mg (0.08 mg/kg in children). Atropine (0.6–1.2 mg) counteracts the nicotinic side effects of the anticholinesterase and is given before or with neostigmine. Care is required with atropine in the presence of an existing tachycardia or CO_2 retention.

Resumption of spontaneous ventilation is aided by adding 5% CO_2 to the inspired gas mixture to restore normocapnia when hyperventilation has been employed. Tracheobronchial suction (vide infra) has the beneficial side-effect of stimulating respiration.

Extubation

This may take place with the patient supine if the anaesthetist is satisfied that airway patency can be maintained by the patient in this position and there is no risk of regurgitation. In patients at risk of regurgitation and potential aspiration, the lateral position is preferred. However, it is safer to employ the lateral recovery position after extubation (Fig. 17.5). Return of respiratory reflexes is signified by coughing and resistance to the presence of the endotracheal tube.

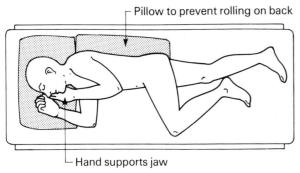

Pillow to prevent rolling on back

Hand supports jaw

Fig. 17.5   Recovery position.

Tracheobronchial suction via the endotracheal tube is carried out using a soft sterile suction catheter whose external diameter is less than half the internal diameter of the tube. Preoxygenation precedes suctioning since the oxygen stores may be depleted by suctioning. The catheter is occluded during insertion and suction applied during withdrawal.

Pharyngeal suction is best performed under direct vision, avoiding trauma to the pharyngeal mucosa, uvula or epiglottis.

Extubation is performed preferably during an inspiration when the larynx dilates; the cuff is deflated and the tube withdrawn along its curved axis. Some anaesthetists generate a positive pressure in the trachea during this manoeuvre by 'squeezing the bag' in order to propel secretions into the pharynx.

Following extubation, the patient's ability to maintain the airway is ensured, the ability to cough and clear secretions is assessed and an oropharyngeal airway employed if required. 100% oxygen replaces the anaesthetic mixture at this stage to counteract the effect of diffusion hypoxia (Chapter 20). Preparations are made for recovery.

Precautions and complications associated with extubation

Laryngeal spasm. This may follow stimulation during extubation. Extubation during deep anaesthesia and subsequent maintenance with a mask may be used. Local anaesthetic spray to the larynx may block the reflex, and pharyngeal suction before extubation removes secretions causing stimulation.

Regurgitation/inhalation. Aspiration of a nasogastric tube (if present) should be performed before extubation to remove gastric liquid. Extubation with the patient 'awake' is practised in emergency patients so that airway control is continuous. Some laryngeal incompetence may occur in the immediate post-extubation period, especially if local anaesthetic spray has been employed. Recovery should take place in the lateral head-down position with facilities for suction, reintubation and oxygenation at hand.

EMERGENCE AND RECOVERY

Following extubation and at the end of mask anaesthesia, the anaesthetic agents are withdrawn and

100% oxygen is delivered via the facemask. The patient's airway is supported until the respiratory reflexes are intact. The patient's muscle power and co-ordination are assessed by testing hand grip, tongue protrusion or lifting the head from the pillow in response to command. Return of adequate muscle power must be ensured before the patient leaves theatre (Chapter 11, Table 11.3).

The patient is then ready for transfer from operating table to bed or trolley and further recovery takes place in a recovery area of theatre or recovery ward (Chapter 20).

The lateral coma position (Fig. 17.5) is adopted for recovery unless the anaesthetist is satisfied that this is unnecessary. The patient is turned on one side, upper leg flexed and lower extended; the head is on one side and the tongue falls forward under gravity, thus avoiding airway obstruction.

FURTHER READING

Adams A P, Henville J D 1979 Anaesthetic circuits and flexible pipelines for medical gases. In: Langton Hewer C, Atkinson R S (eds) Recent advances in anaesthesia and analgesia, no. 13. Churchill Livingstone, Edinburgh
Brit B 1979 Malignant hyperthermia. International Anesthesiology Clinics 17. Little, Brown, Boston
Crawford J S 1978 Principles and practice of obstetric anaesthesia. Blackwell Scientific Publications, Oxford
Dundee J W, Wyant G M 1977 Intravenous anaesthesia. Churchill Livingstone, Edinburgh, Ch 6
Harrison G G 1978 Death attributable to anaesthesia. British Journal of Anaesthesia 50: 1041

Prys-Roberts C 1977 Hypertension and systemic arterial disease. In: Vickers M D (ed) Medicine for anaesthetists. Blackwell Scientific Publications, Oxford
Strunin L 1979 Liver dysfunction and repeat anaesthesia. British Journal of Anaesthesia 51: 1097
Stenquist O, Nilsson K 1982 Postoperative sore throat related to tracheal cuff design. Canadian Anaesthetists Society Journal 29: 384
Utting J E 1982 In: Atkinson R S, Langton Hewer C (eds) Recent advances in anaesthesia and analgesia, no. 14. Churchill Livingstone, Edinburgh
Watkins J, Milford-Ward A 1978 Adverse response to intravenous drugs. Academic Press, London

18

Monitoring during anaesthesia

The word 'monitor' is derived from the Latin verb *'monere'*— to warn. The purpose of a monitoring device is to measure a physiological variable and to indicate trends of change, thus enabling appropriate therapeutic action to be taken.

A monitor, as the derivation suggests, can only warn. No mechanical or electrical device can replace simple, conscientious observation of the patient. Information from monitoring equipment requires clinical interpretation.

It is essential to ensure that all monitoring equipment is maintained properly and that it functions accurately, so that the information it provides is reliable. The user should understand the basic principles on which monitoring equipment is based and be able to interpret the information provided.

The anaesthetic record

Varying levels of complexity of patient monitoring during anaesthesia are appropriate in different clinical situations; major cardiovascular surgery and dilatation and curettage, for instance, represent opposite ends of the monitoring spectrum.

The importance of meticulous record keeping for all patients undergoing anaesthesia cannot be stressed too highly. Detailed, accurate charts provide not only a valuable record of trends occurring during anaesthesia, but are also useful for reference purposes, should further anaesthetic administrations be necessary. In addition, they may be required for medicolegal purposes. Cases of litigation may be brought many years following the event.

A suitable chart is shown in Figure 18.1.

The basic requirements of such a chart are that it should provide space to record cardiovascular parameters (pulse, arterial pressure, central venous pressure, and urine output), respiratory parameters (including ventilator settings), dosages of all drugs used, details of all i.v. fluids, the apparatus employed, sites of i.v. and intra-arterial cannulation, volume of blood lost and any problems or difficulties encountered. In addition, it is essential that details of the preoperative anaesthetic assessment should be recorded.

THE CARDIOVASCULAR SYSTEM

Electrocardiography

Valuble information concerning cardiac rhythm may be obtained by the use of the e.c.g. Most e.c.g. machines calculate ventricular rate. This should not distract the anaesthetist from monitoring the peripheral pulse rate.

E.c.g. monitors have become increasingly reliable electrically and less subject to interference. As the technique is noninvasive, simple and accurate, many anaesthetists now regard it as mandatory that the electrocardiogram should be monitored in all patients undergoing anaesthesia, no matter how minor the surgical procedure.

Standard lead II monitoring is used widely. However, the CM_5 lead configuration (Fig. 18.2) has been advocated for routine intraoperative monitoring because it reveals more readily ST segment changes produced by left ventricular ischaemia.

It is important to appreciate that the e.c.g. is an index only of electrical activity. It is possible to have a normal electrical waveform with negligible cardiac output to the tissues. Information from the e.c.g. should therefore be used in conjunction with data acquired from monitoring of perfusion.

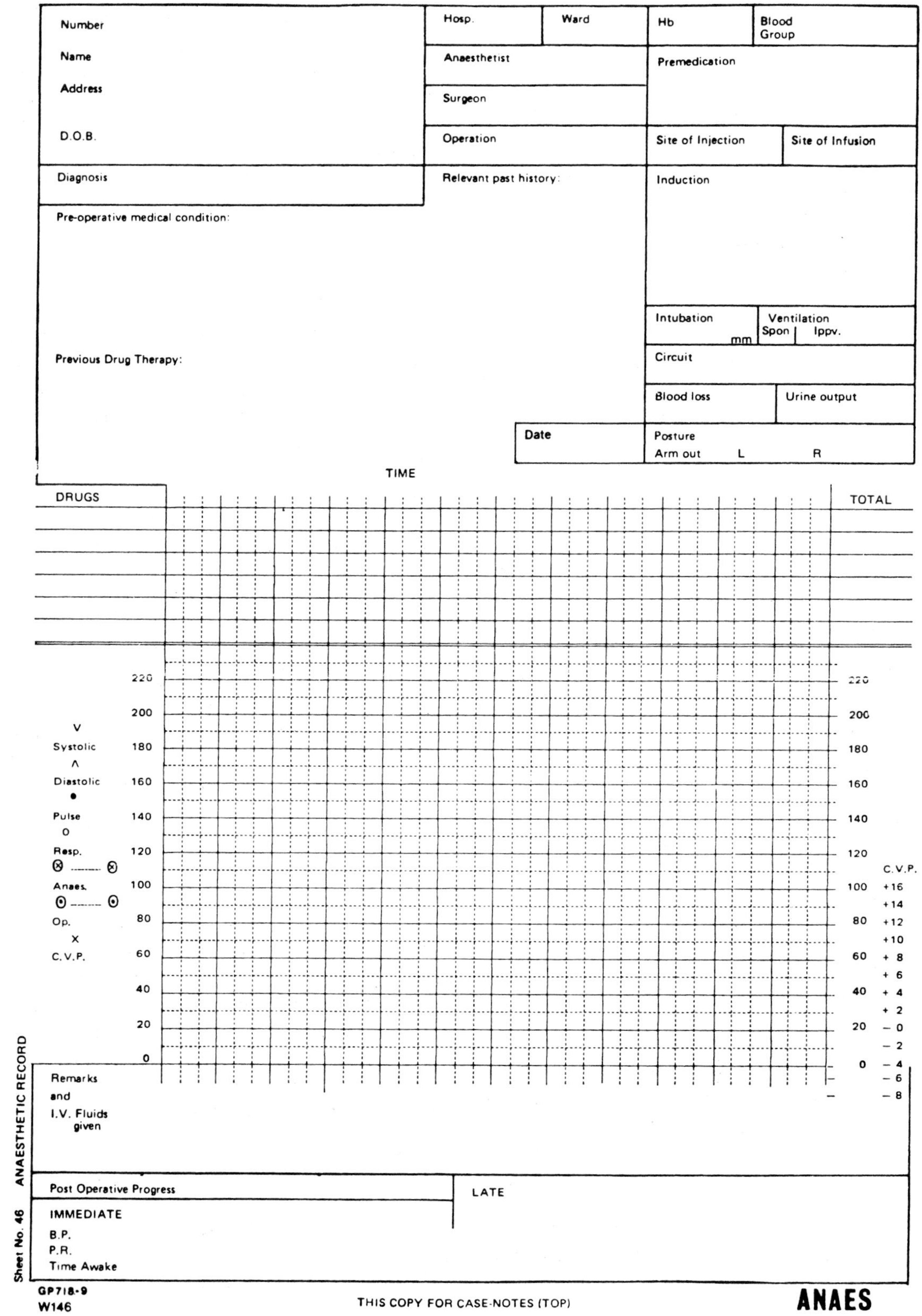

Number		Hosp.	Ward	Hb	Blood Group
Name		Anaesthetist		Premedication	
Address		Surgeon			
D.O.B.		Operation		Site of Injection	Site of Infusion
Diagnosis		Relevant past history:		Induction	

Pre-operative medical condition:

Intubation	Ventilation	
	Spon	Ippv.
mm		

Circuit

Blood loss | Urine output

| Date | Posture |
| | Arm out   L   R |

Previous Drug Therapy:

TIME

| DRUGS | | TOTAL |

V
Systolic   180
Λ
Diastolic   160
●
Pulse   140
O
Resp.   120
⊗ ----- ⊗
Anaes.   100
⊙ ----- ⊙
Op.   80
X
C.V.P.   60
             40
             20
              0

220
200
180
160
140
120
100
80
60
40
20
0

C.V.P.
+16
+14
+12
+10
+ 8
+ 6
+ 4
+ 2
− 0
− 2
− 4
− 6
− 8

Remarks
and
I.V. Fluids
   given

ANAESTHETIC RECORD

Sheet No. 46

Post Operative Progress	LATE
IMMEDIATE	
B.P.	
P.R.	
Time Awake	

GP718-9
W146

THIS COPY FOR CASE-NOTES (TOP)

ANAES

Fig. 18.1 Anaesthetic record.

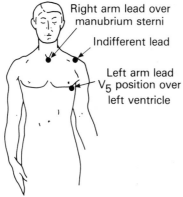

Right arm lead over
manubrium sterni

Indifferent lead

Left arm lead
V$_5$ position over
left ventricle

Fig. 18.2 CM$_5$ lead configuration for e.c.g. monitoring.

Monitoring the circulation

Maintenance of perfusion of vital organs is one of the principal tasks of the anaesthetist during surgery. Adequate perfusion is dependent largely on cardiac output, arterial pressure and venous return to the heart.

Direct measurement of cardiac output and blood volume during anaesthesia are difficult and require invasive procedures which are inappropriate in many situations. Alternatively, adequacy of cardiac output and circulating blood volume may be inferred indirectly from observation of the following variables:

1. Peripheral pulse.
2. Peripheral perfusion.
3. Urine production.
4. Arterial pressure

The peripheral pulse

Regular palpation of the peripheral pulse is one of the simplest and most useful methods of monitoring during anaesthesia and is mandatory for even the most minor surgery. Information may be obtained by observation of the rate, volume and rhythm of the pulse.

Automated devices are available for monitoring peripheral pulsation. They are based on the principle of photoplethysmography. The skin of a suitable digit, or of the pinna of the ear, is illuminated by a weak source of light. The intensity of light transmitted through or reflected by the digit waxes and wanes with each capillary pulsation, and this is detected by a photoelectric cell, the signal of which is transduced to display a wave form on an oscilloscope.

When a finger is used, inflation of an arterial pressure recording cuff causes the wave form from the pulse meter to flatten. Oscillations reappear when the cuff is deflated below systolic arterial pressure. The pulse monitor provides a guide to the pulse pressure. Thus an increased signal may be seen in peripheral vasodilatation or increased cardiac output and a low pulse pressure is seen during vasoconstriction or low cardiac output states.

Peripheral perfusion

Peripheral perfusion is gauged most usefully by observation of the patient's extremities. Warm, dry, pink skin indicates adequate peripheral perfusion. Cold, white peripheries imply the converse. This is particularly useful in children where cool peripheries usually indicate a degree of hypovolaemia. Other methods exist for estimating peripheral blood flow including ultrasound and venous occlusion plethysmography, but these are not useful for routine monitoring.

The core to peripheral temperature gradient is a useful index of adequacy of peripheral perfusion. One temperature probe is placed centrally (e.g. in the nasopharynx) and the other peripherally (e.g. on the great toe). The temperature gradient increases with vasoconstriction and low cardiac output, and decreases gradually as vasodilatation occurs with increasing limb blood flow consequent upon increasing cardiac output.

Urine output

Adequacy of renal perfusion may be inferred from the volume of urine produced. The kidney is the only organ whose function may be monitored directly in this way. Adequate urine production implies that perfusion of the other vital organs is likely to be adequate. Accurate measurement of urine volumes with, for example, a urimeter, is particularly indicated in the following situations:

1. Major vascular surgery
2. Massive fluid or blood loss.
3. Major trauma.
4. Critically ill/shocked patients.
5. Cardiac surgery
6. Surgery in the jaundiced patient.

The aim is to achieve a urine production of 0.5–1 ml/kg/h.

Systemic arterial pressure

Measurement of arterial pressure may be classified into indirect or direct methods.

Indirect	Direct
1. Palpation	1. Intra-arterial pressure manometry
2. Auscultation	
3. Oscillotonometry	
4. Doppler ultrasound	

Measurement of arterial pressure is mandatory during anaesthesia in all patients. It is an indirect method of estimating adequacy of cardiac output since:

Cardiac output = arterial pressure ÷ peripheral resistance

Taken in conjunction with estimation of the peripheral perfusion, it is an invaluable measurement.

Indirect, noninvasive methods are appropriate for most types of surgery.

Palpation. Palpation of the radial pulse as the

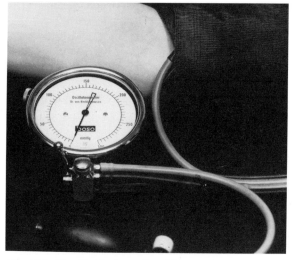

Fig. 18.3   Von Recklinghausen's oscillotonometer.

sphygmomanometer cuff is deflated is the commonest method of measuring arterial pressure. This method, although simple, is inaccurate at low pressures or when vasoconstriction is present.

Auscultation. Auscultation of the Korotkoff sounds is too cumbersome for routine use during anaesthesia.

Oscillotonometry. Von Recklinghausen's oscillotonometer (Figs 18.3 and 18.4), as used widely in

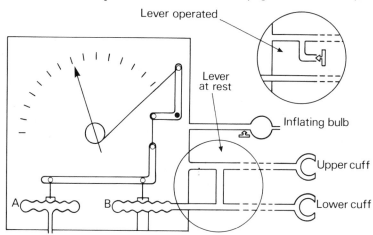

Fig. 18.4   Principle of oscillotonometer.
With the control lever at rest, air is pumped into the cuffs and the airtight case of the instrument using the inflating bulb to a pressure exceeding the patient's systolic arterial pressure. By operating the lever, the lower cuff is isolated, and the pressure in the upper cuff and instrument case allowed to decrease slowly through an adjustable leak. As systolic pressure is reached, pulsation of the artery under the lower cuff results in an increase in pressure within the cuff and an anaeroid capsule B. The pressure changes are transmitted by a mechanical amplification system to the pointer, which swings with each pulsation. As the pressure in the upper cuff decreases below diastolic pressure, the pulsation ceases. Anaeroid manometer A is connected to atmosphere, and changes in pressure inside the instrument case (and upper cuff) result in deflection of the pointer. Although systolic and diastolic pressures are detected when the lever is operated, the true pressure in the upper cuff is recorded with the lever at rest. The lever is therefore operated intermittently, and readings made on detection of pulsatile movement of the pointer.

anaesthetic practice, exemplifies the principles of oscillotonometry.

A double cuff, consisting of an upper small occluding cuff which overlaps a lower and longer sensing cuff, is connected to the oscillotonometer. The cuffs are inflated above the anticipated systolic pressure and a slow leak from both cuffs is obtained by unscrewing the case valve and depressing the lever. A complex mechanical amplification system enables the pressure waves arriving at the lower cuff to be displayed as oscillations of the needle. When the needle begins to oscillate, the lever is released and the pressure recorded on the gauge approximates to the systolic pressure. The significance of the maximum oscillation point which occurs as the cuffs are deflated is uncertain, and the diastolic pressure cannot be measured accurately with this device. However, systolic pressure corresponds more accurately to changes in cardiac output during anaesthesia.

This device is reliable at low pressures and no stethoscope is necessary. However, it is prone to artefact, e.g. as a result of patient movement or pressure from a surgeon's arm. It is also delicate, and must be serviced regularly.

The Dinamap (Fig. 18.5) provides an automated method of oscillotonometry. This machine automatically inflates the cuff at preset time intervals. It measures heart rate and systolic and diastolic pressures as the cuff deflates. A model suitable for infants is also available.

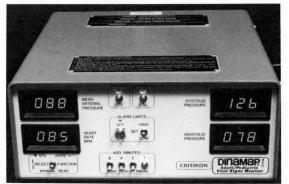

Fig. 18.5 Dinamap automated oscillotonometer.

Doppler ultrasound. The Doppler principle is utilised in the Arteriosonde. An ultrasound emitter and receiver are placed over the brachial artery and surrounded by an inflatable cuff. As the cuff deflates from just above systolic pressure, the vessel walls

begin to move apart during systole. Each movement generates a signal detected by the machine. As the pressure in the cuff decreases further, the vessel walls remain open for longer during each pulsation and when the cuff pressure equals diastolic pressure, movement ceases. Two mercury columns display systolic and diastolic pressures. The main advantages of the method are that it is accurate at low pressures, and that it is suitable for use in children. Disadvantages include its expense and size.

Direct measurement of arterial pressure. This is achieved by attaching a transducer to an intra-arterial cannula inserted percutaneously into a peripheral artery. This is an invasive procedure which carries potential morbidity. Therefore the method is justified only when rapid changes in arterial pressure are anticipated during anaesthesia. Some indications for arterial cannulation are shown in Table 18.1.

Table 18.1 Common indications for arterial cannulation

(1) Major vascular surgery
(2) Cardiothoracic surgery
(3) Induced hypotension
(4) Critically ill and shocked patients
(5) Phaeochromocytoma surgery
(6) Neurosurgery
(7) Frequent blood gas analysis necessary

The radial or dorsalis pedis arteries are selected most frequently. When using the radial artery, the adequacy of the collateral ulnar circulation should first be assessed by using Allen's test, and the nondominant hand used preferentially. Complications of short-term cannulation (up to 48 h) are relatively minor and infrequent.

Long-term cannulation carries risks of morbidity (Table 18.2). Most of these may be minimised by meticulous attention to antisepsis, continuous slow flushing of the cannula with heparinised saline, the use of Teflon, parallel sided cannulae of small diameter (20G or 22G), and the use of Luer-Lok connections.

Table 18.2 Morbidity associated with long-term arterial cannulation

Arterial wall damage and thrombosis
Embolisation
Disconnection and haemorrhage
Sepsis
Tissue necrosis

The availability of accurate, low volume displacement, miniature strain-gauge transducers has helped to simplify recording of arterial pressure. The transducer should be zeroed, i.e. placed at the same level as the left ventricle, and the system should be calibrated. The transducer is connected to the arterial cannula via a short length of stiff saline-filled manometer tubing. The pressure signal is usually displayed as a waveform on an oscilloscope screen (Fig. 18.6), and systolic, diastolic and mean arterial pressures displayed digitally.

Damping of the system should be adjusted carefully in order to reproduce pressures accurately.

The commonest causes of a 'damped' trace are:

1. Air bubbles/blood in the system.
2. Kinking of the cannula.
3. Arterial spasm.

Other techniques

There are two other monitoring techniques which may be employed to provide further information on the volaemic status and function of the myocardium.

Central venous pressure

The placement of a central venous catheter with its tip in the lower superior vena cava or right atrium provides valuable information concerning the volume status of the patient during anaesthesia.

Measurement of the central venous pressure is useful in situations similar to those warranting direct arterial pressure measurement.

Catheters are usually inserted percutaneously via one of the following routes:

1. *Peripheral arm vein.* This route is the least likely to provide correct placement of the catheter (approx. 40%). However, it avoids most of the serious complications of other routes of insertion. Thrombophlebitis and sepsis are common when a peripheral arm vein is used, particularly if the catheter is left in place for more than 48 h.

2. *Internal jugular vein* (Fig. 1.8). This route is associated with the highest incidence of correct placement of the catheter (approx. 90%). Numerous techniques have been described for insertion of a catheter into the internal jugular vein. Common complications are listed in Table 18.3.

Table 18.3 Complications of internal jugular cannulation

Air embolism
Carotid artery puncture
Brachial plexus/phrenic nerve damage
Ectopic placement (numerous sites)
Sepsis
Pneumothorax

Secure fixation of internal jugular catheters is difficult.

3. *Subclavian vein.* This approach is more hazardous than the internal jugular, and less likely to provide correct catheter placement. However, it is the most suitable route if long-term cannulation is contemplated, e.g. to facilitate parenteral feeding. The main complications of insertion at this site are shown in Table 18.4.

Table 18.4 Complications of subclavian vein cannulation

Pneumothorax
Subclavian artery puncture
Air embolism
Thoracic duct damage (left side)

Whichever route is chosen, meticulous attention to antisepsis is necessary. Backflow of blood should always be confirmed before commencing infusion of fluid. Numerous complications have been docu-

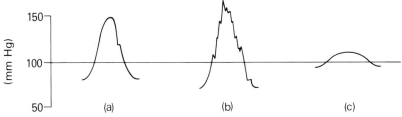

Fig. 18.6 Arterial pressure waveform.
(a) Correct, optimally damped waveform.
(b) Underdamped waveform, resulting in overestimation of systolic and underestimation of diastolic pressure.
(c) Overdamped waveform, resulting in underestimation of systolic and overestimation of diastolic pressure.

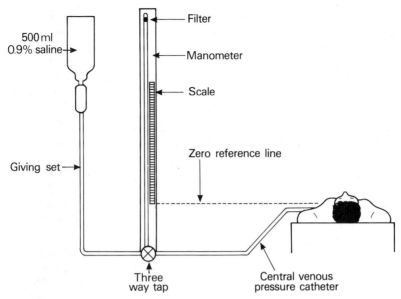

Fig. 18.7 Measurement of CVP using a manometer. The manometer tubing is filled from the infusion bag, and the tap turned to connect the manometer to the central venous catheter. The fluid level in the manometer falls until the height of the fluid column above the zero reference point is equal to the central venous pressure.

mented, particularly associated with routes of insertion in the neck, and these approaches are unsuitable for the unskilled unless properly supervised.

Measurement of CVP. Once in situ, the catheter is connected to a fluid-filled water manometer column via a three-way stopcock (Fig. 18.7). Alternatively, the catheter may be connected to a transducer, as with arterial pressure monitoring, and the wave form displayed on a screen. The position of any central venous catheter should be checked by chest X-ray as soon as possible following insertion.

Definite swings of pressure should be observed with respiration. Excessive pulsation may be indicative of placement in the right ventricle, and the catheter should be withdrawn accordingly.

The surface markings of the right atrium, the true zero reference point, are shown in Figure 18.8. The normal range of values is 0–6 cmH$_2$O. It is sometimes simpler to use the manubriosternal junction as the reference point, in which case the value obtained for central venous pressure is 5–10 cm lower than the true right atrial measurement at the midaxillary line.

Trends   in   measured   observations   are   more

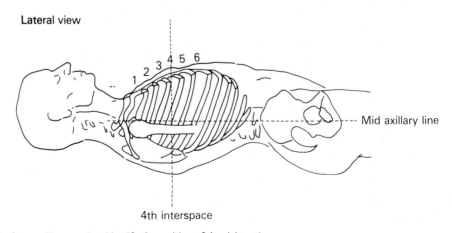

Fig. 18.8 Surface markings used to identify the position of the right atrium.

important than absolute values. For example, in a patient undergoing major arterial surgery, a decrease in CVP from +5 to +1 may indicate considerable fluid loss, and warrants therapeutic intervention, even though the lower value is still within the normal range.

Measurement of CVP is a valuable aid to blood and fluid replacement. If the central venous pressure increases above normal and remains high with no improvement in arterial pressure, it is likely that myocardial failure has occurred and inotropic support may be required.

Pulmonary artery pressure monitoring

In the normal individual, CVP measurement provides a reasonably accurate estimate of the pressures in both right and left atria. In certain clinical situations, however, the central venous or right atrial pressure does not correlate with pressure in the left atrium, and infusion of fluids or inotropic agents titrated against CVP may not result in optimum cardiac function.

Dissociation between left atrial and central venous (right atrial) pressures occurs in:

1. Left ventricular failure with pulmonary oedema.
2. Interstitial pulmonary oedema — of any aetiology.
3. Chronic pulmonary disease.
4. Valvular heart disease

If such patients are about to undergo major surgery, it may be desirable to monitor pressures in the pulmonary circulation and left side of the heart.

The introduction of the flow-directed balloon-tipped pulmonary artery catheter (Figs 18.9–18.10) into clinical practice, has made these measurements possible.

The simplest form of catheter has two channels, one for inflation of the balloon, and one for

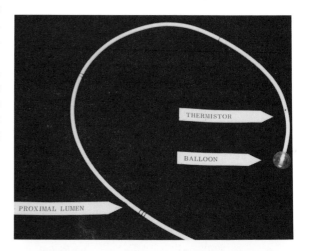

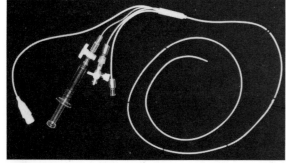

Fig. 18.9   Pulmonary artery catheter.

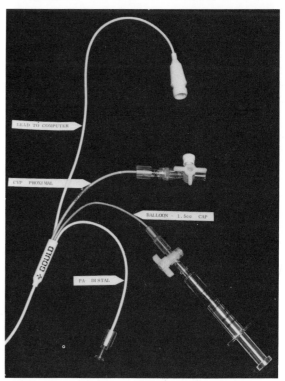

Fig. 18.10   **(a)** Distal end of pulmonary artery catheter, showing inflated balloon, thermistor, and position of end of proximal lumen.
(b) Proximal end of pulmonary artery catheter. The proximal lumen may be used for measurement of CVP, and the distal lumen for measurement of pulmonary artery pressure. The connection from the thermistor is used in conjunction with a cardiac output computer. The balloon capacity is normally 1–1.5 ml.

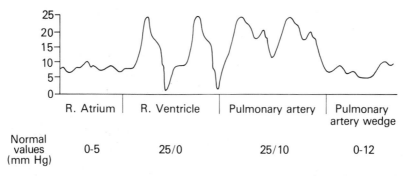

Normal values (mm Hg)	R. Atrium	R. Ventricle	Pulmonary artery	Pulmonary artery wedge
	0-5	25/0	25/10	0-12

Fig. 18.11 Diagrammatic representation of pressure waveforms seen on an oscilloscope as the tip of a pulmonary artery catheter is advanced through the right atrium and right ventricle to lie in the pulmonary artery. The 'pulmonary artery wedge' waveform is seen when the balloon is inflated with the tip of the catheter in a branch of the pulmonary artery. Normal values shown represent pressures in a spontaneously breathing patient.

measurement of pressure at the tip. In order to ease placement it is marked at 10 cm intervals.

The most sophisticated version of this device has four lumina:

1. *The proximal lumen.* This is situated approx. 25 cm from the tip and should lie in the right atrium following final placement of the catheter. Central venous pressure may be measured using this lumen.

2. *The distal lumen.* Situated at the tip of the catheter, this lumen lies in a major branch of the pulmonary artery following final placement of the catheter and may be used to measure pulmonary artery pressure when connected to a suitable transducer.

3. *The balloon lumen.* This lumen permits the introduction of approx. 1 ml of air into the balloon which surrounds the distal tip of the catheter.

4. *Thermistor lumen.* A bead thermistor is situated 4 cm from the tip of the catheter and measures the temperature of blood at this site. This is used in measurement of cardiac output (vide infra).

The pulmonary artery catheter is inserted via a central vein, usually the internal jugular or subclavian. A vein dilator is necessary to facilitate its introduction. When the catheter reaches the right atrium (indicated by a venous pressure wave form on the screen; Fig. 18.11) the balloon is inflated and the catheter advanced slowly and gently. The balloon helps to 'float' the catheter through the right ventricle, where the typical ventricular waveform replaces that of the atrium. The catheter then passes into the pulmonary artery when the waveform again

alters (Fig. 18.11). Further advancement of the catheter into a branch of the pulmonary artery should show typical 'wedging' of the waveform. At this stage a continuous column of fluid connects the left atrium via the pulmonary veins and capillaries to the catheter. Hence the pressure measured reflects left atrial pressure. As soon as this pressure is obtained, the balloon is deflated. Constant inflation may cause pulmonary arterial infarction.

Occasionally arrhythmias may be encountered during insertion, and suitable therapeutic agents should be available.

Uses of the pulmonary artery catheter include:

1. The assessment of the volume status of the patient in conditions where CVP is unreliable (vide supra).

2. Sampling of true mixed venous blood in order to calculate shunt fraction (see Chapter 3).

3. Measurement of cardiac output using the thermodilution method.

Measurement of cardiac output. The thermistor lead is connected to a cardiac output computer (Fig. 18.12). Ten ml of dextrose 5% at room temperature are injected as quickly as possible through the

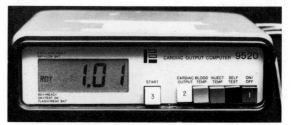

Fig. 18.12 A cardiac output computer.

proximal lumen, preferably at a fixed part of the respiratory cycle. The temperature of the blood arriving at the thermistor near the tip of the catheter is measured. The computer calculates the degree of dilution of the relatively cold injectate, and from this extrapolates the cardiac output. This method has been shown to correlate well with the Fick method of measuring cardiac output.

Complications of pulmonary artery catheterisation are not negligible and include:

1. Arrhythmias on insertion.
2. Knotting of the catheter in the right ventricle.
3. Balloon rupture.
4. Pulmonary infarction.
5. Infection.

This device should be used for as short a period of time as necessary and only in exceptional circumstances for longer than 48 h.

Measurement of blood loss

Losses of up to 10% of blood volume (approx. 70 ml/kg in the adult) are tolerated well and may be replaced by an appropriate volume of crystalloid solution. Blood loss in excess of 20% of blood volume during surgery should be replaced as whole blood.

It is prudent to weigh wet swabs when losses appear to be mounting and then subtract the weight of an equivalent number of dry swabs in order to obtain an estimate of blood lost. This is particularly important in children. However, the method is notoriously inaccurate; it ignores blood lost on drapes, gowns, etc., and unless weighing is carried out promptly, weight is lost because of evaporation of liquid. A more accurate method is that which employs colorimetry. Swabs, gowns, and drapes are 'washed' with a known volume of fluid, and the haemoglobin content measured colorimetrically. Clearly, this can be performed only at the end of the procedure.

THE RESPIRATORY SYSTEM

Clinical monitoring of ventilation

Continuous observation should be made of the following: the patient's colour, respiratory rate, adequacy of chest movement and the movement of the reservoir bag or ventilator bellows. Auscultation of both lung fields should also be performed frequently in order to detect equality of air entry, intubation of a bronchus, the presence of secretions or the occurrence of a pneumothorax. In addition the anaesthetist must check regularly for signs of respiratory obstruction as evidenced by tracheal tug, parodoxical abdominal movement and absence of bag deflation. Some ventilators make a regular noise during part of the ventilatory cycle and this is a valuable audible monitor.

Measurement of airway pressure

A simple manometer which measures the pressure of the gases delivered to the airway is incorporated into most mechanical ventilators. Observation of changes in this pressure is vital. It reflects changes in lung and chest wall compliance if the ventilator is of the volume-cycled or time-cycled volume preset variety. Chest wall compliance may be influenced by the degree of muscle paralysis, surgical manipulation and the position of the patient, and lung compliance by accumulation of secretions, or the development of a pneumothorax. Increased resistance to airflow caused by bronchospasm or obstruction of the endotracheal tube is reflected by an increased peak airway pressure.

Trouble shooting check if airway pressure becomes excessively raised

1. Kinking of ventilator tubing or endotracheal tube (e.t.t.).
2. Overinflation of e.t.t. cuff with consequent obstruction of the lumen of the tube.
3. Increased secretions.
4. Pneumothorax.
5. Bronchospasm.
6. Is another dose of relaxant needed?

Ensuring an uninterrupted breathing system

The continuity of the anaesthetic circuit and hence gas delivery to the patient may be monitored using a disconnection alarm. This may be incorporated into a mechanical ventilator and is activated if the airway pressure decreases below a preset limit, indicating a large leak or disconnection. This does not obviate the necessity for visual surveillance of the continuity of the circuit, particularly when the patient is breathing spontaneously.

Measurement of inspired and expired volumes

A device for measuring inspired and expired lung volumes should always be incorporated into the breathing system when a patient receives intermittent positive pressure ventilation (IPPV). A Wright respirometer (Fig. 18.13) is used commonly and is mounted usually in the expiratory limb of the circuit,

so that leaks which develop during delivery of gases are eliminated from the evaluation of expired minute volume. It should be sited as near to the endotracheal tube as possible to minimise the effects of circuit compliance on its function.

The Wright respirometer is a vane anemometer. The vane rotates within a small cylinder, the walls of which are perforated with a number of tangential slits, so that the air stream causes the vane to rotate. Rotation of the vane drives the pointer around the dial and gas volume is recorded. It tends to over-read at high tidal volumes and under-read at low volumes as a result of its inertia. Its function is affected by moisture, which causes the pointer to stick. Thus, it should be switched off when not in use. In the electronic version (Fig. 18.14) rotation of the vane is detected electronically; this reduces the inaccuracies caused by water condensation. The pneumotachograph (Fig. 18.15) measures gas flow rate and integrates this signal with time to produce a calculated gas volume. The flow rate is derived from the pressure decrease across a resistance. Laminar

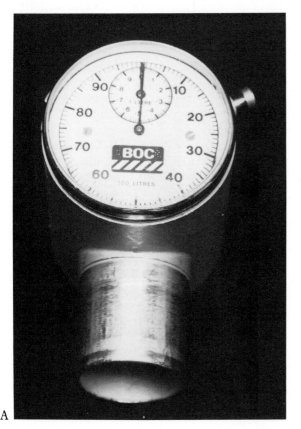

A

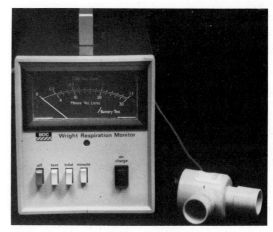

Fig. 18.14 Electronic Wright respirometer.

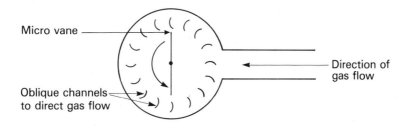

B

Fig. 18.13 (a) Wright respirometer.
(b) Diagrammatic representation of mechanism (see text for details).

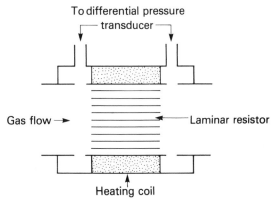

To differential pressure
transducer

Gas flow →　←— Laminar resistor

Heating coil

Fig. 18.15 Diagrammatic representation of pneumotachograph (see text for details).

flow is produced by using multiple small tubes. The head may be heated electrically to avoid water condensation which increases resistance to flow.

However, this instrument is expensive and requires expert calibration and maintenance. Consequently it is not used routinely, although pneumotachographs are incorporated into some ventilators used in intensive care units.

MONITORING GAS DELIVERY AND EXCRETION

1. Oxygen delivery

a. *To the patient*

Before using an anaesthetic machine, the anaesthetist should check that it is functioning correctly, particularly with regard to delivery of oxygen (see Chapter 16). All anaesthetic machines should be

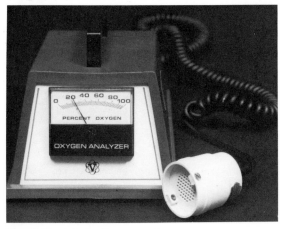

Fig. 18.16 A fuel cell oxygen analyser.

fitted with an oxygen failure alarm which provides an audible and/or visual warning should the oxygen pressure decrease. A full spare cylinder of oxygen should always be available on the anaesthetic machine when piped gases are in use.

Oxygen analysers may be used in an anaesthetic circuit to ensure that the required percentage concentration of oxygen is delivered to the patient. Fuel cell oxygen analysers (Fig. 18.16) generate a current proportional to the oxygen concentration. These instruments may be placed in the inspiratory limb of the circuit and have a 90% response time of approx. 20 s. They are accurate to within ±3%, are calibrated using air, are not affected by humidity and require no external power source.

These analysers are particularly valuable when circle systems are employed using low fresh gas flows.

b. *To the tissues*

Transcutaneous PO_2 measurement — $TcPO_2$. The instrument used to measure this parameter is a modified Clark electrode (Fig. 18.17) applied to the skin surface. However, to ensure that $TcPO_2$ approximates to Pa_{O_2}, the skin must be rendered hyperaemic by heating to 45°C. The transcutaneous PO_2 electrode provides a continuous, noninvasive estimate of arterial oxygen tension.

The instrument requires a warm-up period of 15 min, calibration, and subsequently a 5 min equilibration period. There is good correlation at least in infants between $TcPO_2$ and Pa_{O_2}. The response time is 10–15 s when the skin is thin, and the device is reliable in following trends. However, the equipment is cumbersome and expensive. In adults with a thicker skin, correlation is less good and decreases with increasing age.

2. Carbon dioxide excretion

a. *In expired gas*

It is important to ensure adequate carbon dioxide elimination during anaesthesia, because of the deleterious effects of raised arterial carbon dioxide tension (Pa_{CO_2}).

Capnography. End-tidal CO_2 (PE'_{CO_2}) correlates with Pa_{CO_2} in patients without significant pulmonary disease. It may be measured using the principle of

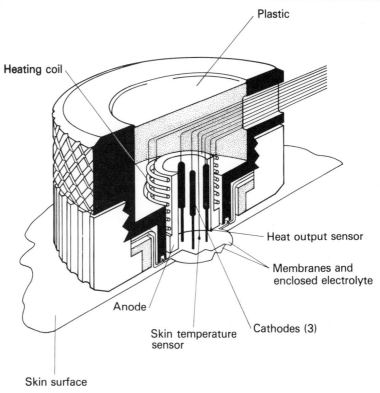

Fig. 18.17 Diagram of a transcutaneous P_{O_2} electrode.

infrared absorption spectrophotometry. A number of machines are marketed for this purpose, an example of which is shown in Figure 18.18.

The sampling probe is inserted usually into the catheter mount of the gas delivery system. E.t. tubes which have a pilot tube specifically for sampling end tidal gas are available. $P_{E'_{CO_2}}$ may be displayed

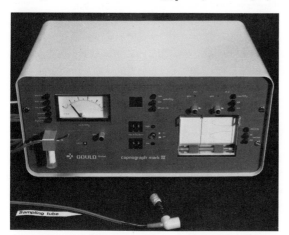

Fig. 18.18 A capnograph for measurement of CO_2 concentration in a gas mixture.

digitally, or a permanant trace of CO_2 concentration obtained (Fig. 18.19). This form of monitoring may be useful in the following clinical situations:

1. Detection of air/fat/pulmonary embolism — sudden decrease in $P_{E'_{CO_2}}$ occurs as a result of an increase in dead space.

2. Patients at risk of malignant hyperpyrexia — progressive increase in $P_{E'_{CO_2}}$ occurs as a result of raised muscle metabolism.

3. Monitoring of elderly patients to ensure normocapnia and assist in preserving adequate cerebral perfusion.

4. Carotid artery surgery — to ensure normal $P_{a_{CO_2}}$ and consequently maintain cerebral perfusion.

5. Routine intraoperative monitoring of the adequacy of ventilation.

b. *Tissue level*

Transcutaneous P_{CO_2} monitoring TcP_{CO_2}. Devices for measurement of TcP_{CO_2} are at present undergoing clinical trials and have already proved useful in the management of acutely ill neonates. In adults there are numerous technical problems.

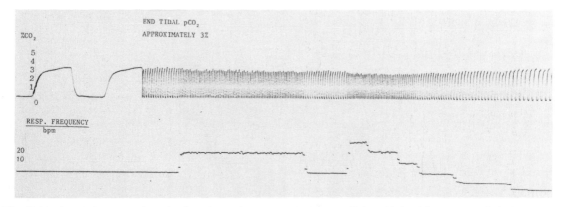

Fig. 18.19 A typical capnograph tracing from the respiratory tract during controlled ventilation. The upper graph shows two initial calibration traces followed by a record of tidal CO_2 concentration.

Pa_{CO_2} changes much less rapidly than Pa_{O_2} following apnoea, making TcP_{CO_2} less useful as an emergency warning device. In addition the instrument has a slow response time; 5 min to 90% response.

TcP_{CO_2} consistently reads higher than arterial P_{CO_2}, but there is a good correlation over a wide range of values up to 8 kPa. The skin must be heated to increase blood flow and reduce arterial to capillary P_{CO_2} gradient. This device may prove to be a useful addition to respiratory monitoring in the future, possibly in combination with the TcP_{O_2} electrode.

Oesophageal stethoscope

This method of monitoring the cardiovascular and respiratory systems is in common use in the U.S.A., but is seldom employed in the UK. When fitted with a moulded earpiece (Fig. 18.20) it permits the anaesthetist to monitor heart and breath sounds continuously. Alterations in heart sounds, air entry to the tracheobronchial tree, and the development of abnormal breath sounds, e.g. crepitations or rhonchi, may be detected readily. In procedures subject to the risk of air embolism, e.g. hip joint replacement and certain neurosurgical operations, air entering the great veins or cardiac chambers is audible.

The oesophageal stethoscope is simple, cheap, safe, noninvasive and free from electrical interference. Its routine use in intraoperative monitoring is recommended.

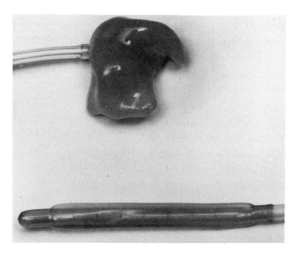

Fig. 18.20 An oesophageal stethoscope.

MONITORING ANAESTHETIC VAPOUR DELIVERY

'Emma' analyser

It is now possible to measure the concentration of a particular vapour delivered to the patient. The 'Emma' multigas analyser (Fig. 18.21) monitors the concentration of halothane, enflurane and isoflurane on a breath-to-breath basis.

The principle of this device is based on the resonant frequency of a highly stable quartz crystal oscillator which changes as a result of interaction between the coating of the crystal and the surrounding gas,

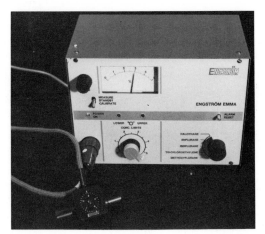

Fig. 18.21 'Emma' multigas analyser.

producing an electrical signal which is proportional to the gas concentration. The crystal is mounted in a compact measuring head which is positioned in the anaesthetic circuit. It is said to be sensitive to a concentration of as little as 0.02% halothane. Water vapour produces some artefact.

This monitor may prove to be particularly valuable during closed-circuit anaesthesia.

Mass spectrometer

This versatile but bulky and expensive instrument is used mainly as a research tool, but it provides rapid accurate measurements of a number of gases simultaneously. Gas concentrations in the airway may be measured.

THE NERVOUS SYSTEM

Central nervous system

Monitoring the central nervous system during anaesthesia is concerned primarily with estimation of depth of unconsciousness, in order to avoid awareness or vivid unpleasant dreams.

Clinical monitoring

Observation of the signs of sympathetic overactivity (lacrimation, sweating, increase in pupil size, increase in heart rate or arterial pressure) and reflex movements indicate that anaesthesia is too 'light'.

However, numerous investigations have shown these signs are unreliable indicators of inadequate narcosis.

A more sophisticated attempt to detect the occurrence of awareness comprises isolation of one arm from the rest of the circulation by inflation of a tourniquet on the upper arm prior to injection of relaxant into the systemic circulation. It is suggested that in this way contact may be maintained with the patient, who indicates when he or she is aware by responding to the anaesthetist's questions with a squeeze of the isolated hand. However, many anaesthetists regard this technique as unsatisfactory.

The cerebral function monitor (c.f.m.)

Since the conventional electroencephalograph (e.e.g.) is too cumbersome for routine theatre use, a device has been designed which integrates the total electrical activity in the brain.

Two parietal needle electrodes record the electrical signal for display on an X-Y plotter. The height of the signal against the axis is proportional to the frequency of cerebral electrical rhythms. Changes in the height and width of the trace correspond to changes in cerebral electrical function (Fig. 18.22). This device appears to be capable of detecting changes in depth of total i.v. anaesthesia, but is unreliable when volatile agents are used. It is used principally in situations where cerebral ischaemia may occur (e.g. carotid artery surgery, cardiac surgery).

A more recent model, the cerebral function analysing monitor (c.f.a.m.) provides the facility to display both the amplitude and frequency of cerebral activity separately, again indicating trends in cerebral activity. Separate electrodes enable the function of each hemisphere to be monitored. The data provided are amenable to statistical analysis by computer. This device is also capable of computing evoked potentials (see Chapter 5) and of measuring the spontaneous scalp electromyogram (e.m.g.). Increasing amplitude of the e.m.g. reflects an increase in patient activity. Facial and scalp muscles are less sensitive to muscle relaxants than peripheral muscles and this may be a promising way of detecting pain and awareness during relaxant anaesthesia.

This machine, with the aid of a nerve stimulator, may also assess and display the response to train of four stimulation (see Chapter 11).

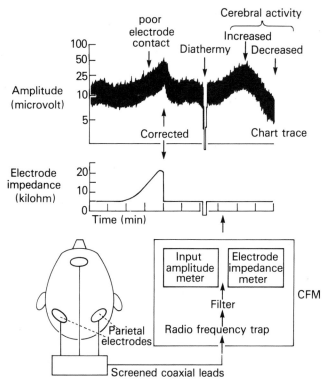

Fig. 18.22 The integrated cerebral function monitor. Screened electrical signals displayed on upper trace depict cerebral activity. Allowance must be made for alterations in electrode impedance, and interference from extraneous electrical sources.

Situations where c.f.m. may be useful
1. Cardiac surgery.
2. Carotid artery surgery.
3. Neurosurgery.
4. Total i.v. anaesthesia.
5. Status epilepticus — when neuromuscular blockers are used.
6. Hypotensive anaesthesia.
7. Drug overdose.

Cerebral blood flow (c.b.f.)

The measurement of c.b.f. using a gamma camera and radioactive isotope injection provides the most accurate measurement of cerebral perfusion. However, this method is too cumbersome and complicated for routine application.

MONITORING THE NEUROMUSCULAR JUNCTION (See Chapter 11)

MONITORING OF METABOLISM

Homeostasis of the main metabolic processes of the body must be assured during anaesthesia. Monitoring of the following functions should be considered for all but minor surgery: (a) temperature regulation, (b) fluid and electrolyte balance, (c) blood gas and acid–base status, (d) hormonal status, especially in relation to blood sugar control and (e) assessment of the coagulation system.

a. Temperature regulation

General anaesthesia inhibits the patient's ability to maintain his or her body temperature by depressing the thermoregulatory centre in the hypothalamus. Heat loss during anaesthesia is potentiated by surgery of long duration and exposure of large surface areas of tissue, e.g. the abdominal contents during gastrointestinal operations. The use of wet packs and dry inspired gases potentiate the problem. These sources of heat loss assume even more importance in children, especially small babies, whose surface area is much larger in proportion to body weight, than in the adult.

During operations where these factors are important, core temperature must be monitored and efforts made to minimise heat loss. Measures to minimise heat loss include the following:

1. An operating room temperature as high as is comfortable for the theatre staff.
2. A warming mattress placed beneath the patient.
3. Swaddling of exposed surfaces with warm gauze or foil, especially in neonates.
4. Warming of all i.v. fluids.
5. Warming and humidifying inspired gases.

The most commonly used type of temperature measuring device is the thermistor probe. This consists of a bead of a mixture of nonmetal oxides which is thermally sensitive and the resistance of which varies nonlinearly with temperature.

The probe may be placed in the following positions in order to measure core temperature:

a. in the nasopharynx — approximates to brain temperature,
b. in the oesophagus — approximates to cardiac temperature,
c. on the tympanic membrane — best for core temperature, but the membrane is delicate and easily damaged,
d. in the rectum — reads 1°C higher than core.

It is also useful to measure the temperature of the inspired gases when an efficient humidifier is employed in order to avoid thermal burns to the respiratory tract.

If core temperature decreases during anaesthesia, the heat debt has to be repaid during recovery, and this may result in intense shivering. This in turn results in increased oxygen consumption (5–10 times normal), disturbances of blood gas homeostasis, increased demands on the cardiovascular system, and discomfort to the patient.

Rarely, a rapid increase in temperature occurs during anaesthesia. This is associated usually with the rare inherited disorder of malignant hyperpyrexia. The rapid increase in muscle metabolism and temperature result in profound metabolic acidosis, hypercapnia and hyperkalaemia. Prompt therapeutic action is required to prevent a fatal outcome (see Chapter 19).

b. Fluid and electrolyte status

Blood and fluid loss may be considerable during surgery and empirical calculations of electrolyte losses may be erroneous. Estimation of fluid losses includes measurement of blood loss on swabs and drapes (vide supra), fluid collection in suction jars, and an allowance for evaporative loss. Fluid input and output must be measured as accurately as possible in babies and young children.

Measurement of serum sodium and potassium concentrations in the laboratory is relatively simple and this provides guidance on replacement with appropriate i.v. fluids. However, there may be some delay in obtaining laboratory results. Bedside flame photometers and ion-specific electrodes are now available for measurement of serum and urine electrolytes.

c. Blood gas and acid-base status

Monitoring of oxygen delivery to the tissues and of adequate carbon dioxide elimination is assessed most accurately by the measurement of arterial blood gases. This is facilitated by the presence of an arterial cannula and the availability of an automated blood gas analyser. Modern blood gas analysers use micro-electrode systems and require very small quantities (approx. 0.2 ml) of heparinised blood. These machines provide results within 2–3 min and there is no doubt that they have helped improve the management of patients undergoing major surgery.

Indications for measurement of blood gases/acid-base status

1. Major vascular surgery.
2. One-lung anaesthesia.
3. Hypotensive anaesthesia.
4. Critically ill patients.
5. Neurosurgical anaesthesia.

d. Monitoring of hormonal status

The metabolic response to anaesthesia and surgery consists of an elevation of the plasma levels of all the catabolic hormones; cortisol, catecholamines, growth hormone, and depression of the secretion of insulin. The magnitude of this response is proportional to the extent and duration of surgery.

The consequent elevation of blood sugar levels may be detrimental, particularly to the diabetic patient and to patients who are critically ill and already in a catabolic phase. Therefore in such patients, blood sugar concentrations should be monitored at appropriate intervals and an insulin infusion administered as appropriate. The introduction of 'BM stix' strips has made blood sugar estimation from a thumb prick rapid and accurate.

e. Assessment of clotting status

Assessment of the adequacy of blood coagulation is of obvious importance during surgery. However, in particular situations, e.g. patients with inherent disorders of clotting, those receiving massive transfusions, those on anticoagulant therapy, or those suspected of developing disseminated intravascular coagulation (DIC) it is mandatory to monitor clotting status.

Massive transfusion

Storage of blood induces the following changes:

1. Decrease in platelet count.
2. Decrease in labile clotting factors, mainly V and VIII.
3. Decrease in 2,3-DPG.
4. Increase in extracellular K^+
5. Decrease in Ca^{++}
6. Decrease in pH (6.6–7.1)

When large quantities of stored blood are transfused, coagulation may be affected adversely. The following tests my be helpful in assessing the necessity for platelet transfusion, transfusion of fresh frozen plasma, or calcium therapy.

1. Platelet count (n. range 150–400 × 10^9/litre).
2. Prothombin time (n. range 12–14 s) — tests extrinsic system.
3. K.C.C.T. (n. range 35–45 s) — tests intrinsic system.

If K.C.C.T. is prolonged more than 10 s above the upper limit of normal, infusion of fresh frozen plasma is indicated. Spontaneous bleeding may not occur until the platelet count is less than 10 × 10^9/litre but platelet transfusion should be considered if the platelet count is less than 50 × 10^9/litre and the patient is bleeding actively. If DIC is suspected the fibrinogen level (n. range 2–4 g/litre) and fibrin degradation product titre (n. range < 1/40) should also be measured.

Anticoagulant therapy

Patients receiving oral anticoagulants should not be considered for surgery until the British Corrected Ratio (BCR) is less than twice normal. If emergency surgery is necessary, fresh frozen plasma should be available.

Peroperative heparin therapy may be monitored by measuring the activated clotting time. A commercially available kit (Haemochron) may be used in the operating theatre. It consists of a test tube which contains a magnet and some diatomaceous earth. The blood sample is injected into the test tube which is placed in the machine. The test tube is rotated slowly and when clot forms it enmeshes the magnet which then rotates along with the tube and activates a detector. The activated clotting time is kept at two to three times normal (approx. 120 s) for adequate heparin anticoagulation.

THE FUTURE

A number of new methods of patient monitoring are being investigated, for example, the use of evoked potentials to assess the function of brain-stem pathways and possibly depth of anaesthesia, the application of aortovelography to measure cardiac output noninvasively and the use of computers to analyse arterial waveforms in order to monitor alterations in cardiac output.

However, the level of monitoring appropriate for the individual patient depends on his pathological lesion, the general level of fitness and the type of surgery contemplated. There is no substitute for simple monitoring — palpation of the peripheral pulse, observation of the patient's colour and peripheral perfusion, measurement of arterial pressure, auscultation of air entry to the chest and monitoring of the e.c.g. More sophisticated monitoring requires justification. Invasive monitoring needs skilled interpretation and may possess complications. Time spent in making complex machinery function properly may detract from routine but vital patient observation.

FURTHER READING

Franklin C B Monitoring 1979 In: Atkinson R S, Langton Hewer C (eds) Recent advances in anaesthesia and analgesia No 13. Churchill Livingstone, Edinburgh

Gerson G R (ed) 1981 Monitoring during anaesthesia. International Anesthesiology Clinics, vol 19. Little, Brown, Boston

Henville J D 1982 Recent developments in Anaesthetic Apparatus and Ventilators. In: Kaufman L (ed) Anaesthesia review I. Churchill Livingstone, Edinburgh

Saidman L J, Smith N T 1978 Monitoring in anesthesia. Wiley, New York

Spence A A 1982 Respiratory monitoring in intensive care. Churchill Livingstone, Edinburgh

19

Complications during anaesthesia

RESPIRATORY OBSTRUCTION

Respiratory obstruction is a very common and potentially hazardous complication in the anaesthetised patient. If allowed to persist it may lead to coughing, straining and regurgitation or vomiting, resulting in hypoxaemia. In addition, the depth of anaesthesia may be reduced. Airway obstruction should be suspected when there is snoring, inadequate movement of the reservoir bag associated with respiration, or an obstructed respiratory pattern (paradoxical chest and abdominal movements which result in little or no gas exchange). In the artificially ventilated patient, an excessive inflation pressure is required to deliver the preset tidal volume. It may be difficult to inflate the lungs manually and, in extreme cases, the duration of expiration may be prolonged.

Airway causes

The lips may close tightly together in the edentulous patient as the mandible is supported in order to maintain the airway.

The tongue

As consciousness is lost, the tongue falls back into the oropharynx. In the overweight, short-necked individual, it may be difficult to pull the tongue and floor of the mouth forward sufficiently to maintain a clear airway.

Supraglottic structures

Swelling, oedema, tumours of the supraglottic area, or strictures may render maintenance of the airway difficult. Irradiation may result in rigidity and irritability of the structures of the floor of the mouth,

so that the airway cannot be maintained when consciousness is lost. In epiglottitis, airway obstruction may be so severe that it is difficult to deepen anaesthesia sufficiently to permit intubation of the trachea.

A tumour of the larynx may act as a flap valve in the anaesthetised patient and cause intermittent obstruction. Alternatively, the laryngeal narrowing may result in turbulent flow which decreases the rate of induction of anaesthesia. In laryngo-tracheobronchitis, inflammation and oedema narrow the airway at both glottic and subglottic levels.

Large goitres may cause tracheal compression or deviation, and malignant thyroid tumours may infiltrate the trachea.

Mechanical obstruction

This usually occurs when the trachea has been intubated. The catheter mount may twist and obstruct. The endotracheal tube itself may kink. This is most likely to occur close to the connector, particularly when PVC endotracheal tubes of small diameter are used. These become more pliable when they reach body temperature. Armoured latex tubes contain an unreinforced area at the proximal end and if the connector is not inserted fully to reach the nylon reinforcement spiral, the soft latex may kink.

A Boyle Davis gag or palatal gag used in plastic surgery may obstruct the endotracheal tube near the lips.

Red rubber tubes and to a lesser extent PVC tubes may kink in the oropharynx. While the degree of narrowing of the airway is likely to be small, the resulting obstruction may be sufficient to increase alveolar P_{CO_2}.

Overinflation of the cuff of the tube may cause

herniation of the cuff over the distal end of the tube with resulting obstruction; in nylon latex tubes herniation may obstruct the internal diameter of the tube. On occasions, the distal orifice of the tube may lie against the wall of the trachea.

ENDOBRONCHIAL INTUBATION

Unintentional endobronchial intubation leads to hypoxaemia, may precipitate bronchospasm, and increases the risk of postoperative pulmonary collapse and infection. At induction of anaesthesia with volatile agents, rate of induction may be slowed considerably in comparison with the anticipated rate.

When the endotracheal tube has not been cut to the appropriate length, inadvertent endobronchial intubation is more likely to occur. This seems to be most common when intubation has been performed as an emergency by nonanaesthetic personnel.

To avoid endobronchial ventilation, it is important to cut the endotracheal tube to the appropriate length for each patient, and to listen to both lung fields with a stethoscope before securing the tube and after any change of posture. Usually, the endotracheal tube passes into the right main bronchus.

BRONCHOSPASM

Bronchospasm during anaesthesia is an undesirable, sometimes severe complication. It may be so intense that oxygenation of the patient is impossible and death may ensue.

Preoperative assessment and adequate preparation of the asthmatic or wheezy bronchitic patient diminishes intraoperative problems and allows an appropriate anaesthetic technique to be selected. Bronchodilator therapy should be continued until immediately before anaesthesia. Respiratory function tests may demonstrate a reversible element in the respiratory obstruction of a bronchitic which should be treated by bronchodilator agents. Physiotherapy is required when chest secretions are present.

Bronchospasm may be triggered by chemical, mechanical or neurogenic factors.

Inhalational agents, e.g. halothane or enflurane, are relatively nonirritant to the bronchial tree compared with ether or trichloroethylene. Bronchial secretions tend to increase during anaesthesia and may trigger an already irritable bronchial tree. The presence of an endotracheal tube near the carina often initiates bronchospasm. Surgical stimulation may act as a trigger, either when the incision is made in a patient who is too lightly anaesthetised or during upper abdominal operations. Pneumothorax may mimic bronchospasm and should always be excluded. Unsuspected aspiration of stomach contents on induction or during the course of anaesthesia may precipitate bronchospasm, as may drugs, either as a side effect or as part of an adverse reaction.

The presence of bronchospasm should be suspected when there is an audible wheeze and prolonged expiratory phase, or an increased inflation pressure is required to deliver a preset tidal volume. The diagnosis is made only after the position and patency of the endotracheal tube have been checked, secretions aspirated and the possibility of a pneumothorax eliminated.

Intravenous aminophylline 250 mg (50 mg/min) or salbutamol 25 mg (5 mg/min) are the drugs of first choice and both may be continued in an infusion. Hydrocortisone 100 mg i.v. may be useful. Intractable bronchospasm sometimes responds to halothane, enflurane or ether.

It is important to achieve adequate oxygenation while treating bronchospasm.

Anaesthesia and the wheezy patient

A preoperative visit helps to allay anxiety, and premedication should be designed to aid bronchodilation. Most recently introduced induction agents have been both recommended and deemed to be unsuitable for the patient with bronchospasm. It is accepted generally that an inhalational induction is more likely to increase anxiety and therefore to trigger bronchospasm. If surgery is essential in the presence of severe bronchospasm, etomidate or ketamine together with pancuronium is an appropriate combination. Alternatively, a regional technique with adequate sedation may be employed.

LARYNGEAL SPASM

Partial laryngeal spasm is manifest as a crowing inspiratory noise and may progress to complete spasm resulting in hypoxaemia. Laryngeal spasm occurs most commonly during induction and although i.v.

barbiturates are not primary stimulants, they enhance respiratory reflexes during light anaesthesia. The stimulus may be premature insertion of an airway or laryngoscope, or pharyngeal secretions or vomit irritating the larynx; or surgical incision when anaesthesia is too light.

Certain surgical operations, particularly anal stretch, breast surgery or dilatation of the cervix often produce a degree of laryngeal spasm in the apparently well-anaesthetised patient.

At the end of surgery, laryngeal spasm may be encountered after extubation. Rarely, trauma to the recurrent laryngeal nerves at the time of thyroid surgery produces adduction of the vocal cords and stridor.

Minor degrees of laryngeal spasm are treated with 100% oxygen with respiratory assistance. The operation should be stopped until control is regained if surgical stimulation is the cause. On rare occasions it may be necessary to administer suxamethonium to allow intubation of the larynx.

Recently doxapram has been shown to be effective when laryngeal spasm occurs after tracheal extubation.

HICCUPS

Hiccups result from inco-ordinated diaphragmatic movements, often as a result of vagal stimulation. Their incidence is increased when muscle relaxants are used. Patients undergoing subarachnoid or extradural techniques may also suffer this complication. Hiccups occur less commonly when atropine or hyoscine are used for premedication. Induction agents including methohexitone or Althesin are more likely to produce hiccup than thiopentone.

Hiccup is most commonly encountered during upper abdominal surgery and has been ascribed to hypocapnia, unduly light anaesthesia and insufficient dosage of nondepolarising muscle relaxants. The suggested remedies reflect these views; hand ventilate, administer more muscle relaxant, or deepen anaesthesia. Stimulation of the postnasal space with a suction catheter may be successful when other methods have failed.

Hiccup may be remarkably difficult to treat during anaesthesia. The trainee should beware of the temptation to administer excessive quantities of muscle relaxant. If hiccup is not inconveniencing the surgeon, the best course of action may be to ignore this problem.

PNEUMOTHORAX

The presence of pneumothorax may cause serious problems during anaesthesia. As nitrous oxide diffuses into the pleural space, a pneumothorax enlarges, producing haemodynamic disturbances. Positive pressure ventilation augments the problem and a tension pneumothorax may result as additional gas enters the pleural space.

The common causes of pneumothorax during anaesthesia are listed in Table 19.1. Iatrogenic pneumothorax is the most common cause of problems during anaesthesia, especially when a subclavian catheter has been inserted to monitor a hypovolaemic patient. The anaesthetist should inspect the chest X-ray before inducing anaesthesia.

Table 19.1 Common causes of pneumothorax during anaesthesia

Traumatic	chest injury	
	rib fracture	
Iatrogenic	sublavian cannulae	cervical surgery
	internal jugular cannulae	thoracic surgery
	brachial plexus block	
	inadvertent barotrauma	
Spontaneous	localised disorder, e.g. congenital bullae, Marfan's syndrome	
	generalised emphysema	
	secondary to lung disease abscess	
	spontaneous mediastinal emphysema	
	asthma	
	rapid decompression of divers	

A chest drain should be inserted prior to inducing anaesthesia in the presence of a known pneumothorax or recent rib fractures, particularly if IPPV is to be employed. On rare occasions this rule may be ignored and ketamine or a continuous inhalational technique avoiding nitrous oxide may be used if spontaneous respiration is maintained.

Detection of pneumothorax

Pneumothorax may present during anaesthesia as unexplained tachycardia, hypotension, broncho-spasm, altered pattern of breathing, cyanosis and surgical emphysema. Diagnosis is made by clinical examination of the chest, surgery being suspended if necessary to allow the anaesthetist adequate access.

Action

Nitrous oxide should be discontinued immediately, and oxygen 100% administered while the diagnosis is confirmed by percussion of the chest and by needle aspiration of the suspected side via the 2nd intercostal space in the mid clavicular line. A tension pneumothorax may be relieved by inserting an i.v. cannula at this site temporarily while the underwater seal and intercostal drain are prepared.

Pneumomediastinum

Air in the mediastinum may result from trauma or barotrauma. In barotrauma, it usually precedes the development of a pneumothorax. Pneumo-mediastinum is common after tracheostomy.

DIFFICULT INTUBATION

Relative ease of endotracheal intubation reflects the experience and skill of the individual anaesthetist. During the preoperative visit, common anatomical causes of difficulty in intubation should be detected. However, from time to time every anaesthetist encounters a patient in whom endotracheal intubation is either extremely difficult or impossible.

There are two problems; firstly recognising the potentially difficult intubation and planning how to overcome the problem, and secondly ensuring the safety of the patient when planned intubation has failed. Approx. 1 in 65 patients is likely to present difficulties in tracheal intubation.

Causes

Congenital

Pierre Robin syndrome
Cystic hygroma
Treacher-Collins syndrome
Gargoylism
Achondroplasia
Marfan's syndrome

Anatomical

Eight anatomical features associated with difficult intubation have been identified:

1. A short muscular neck and full set of teeth.
2. Receding lower jaw with obtuse mandibular angles.
3. Protruding incisors, with relative overgrowth of the premaxilla.
4. Long high arched palate with a long narrow mouth.
5. Increased alveolar-mental distance requiring wide opening of the mandible for laryngoscopy.
6. Poor mobility of the mandible.
7. Increase in posterior depth of the mandible hindering displacement of the mandible.
8. Decreased distance between the occiput and the spinous process of Cl.

Recent work suggests that this last cause is the most important factor.

Acquired

Restricted jaw opening. Trismus is caused by spasm of the medial pterygoid and masseter muscles and is often secondary to an infective cause, e.g. dental abscess. Fibrosis may follow infection, and restrict temporomandibular joint (TMJ) movement. Rheumatoid or osteo-arthritis affecting the TMJ also restrict mouth opening. Mandibular fractures may impede TMJ movement and also produce trismus.

Restricted neck movement. Osteo-arthritis commonly affects the cervical spine, and undue neck movement during anaesthesia may worsen the patient's symptoms. Ankylosing spondylitis is less common, but may result in total rigidity of the cervical spine. This may be encountered also in patients who have undergone fusion of the cervical spine.

Neck instability. Intubation may be made difficult if neck movement (especially the flexion required for endotracheal intubation) is prohibited because it may cause cord damage, e.g. in the presence of a cervical spine injury or severe rheumatoid arthritis.

Soft tissue swelling. Facial swelling occurs with dental infections, trauma and immediately after burns. There may be associated intra-oral swelling which distorts the upper airway and makes it difficult to see the larynx.

Bleeding after thyroidectomy or other neck operations produces both compression of neck structures and oedema of the oropharynx and larynx making intubation hazardous.

Scarring. Skin and soft tissue contractures develop after burns, making the floor of the mouth rigid. Radiotherapy also produces a 'wooden' mouth floor which cannot be displaced easily to allow laryngoscopy.

Other causes. Laryngeal and tracheal causes are discussed above.

In the morbidly obese individual, direct laryngoscopy may be physically difficult to perform. Excessive weight gain in pregnancy may limit the range of movements necessary for easy laryngoscopy as the laryngoscope handle infringes on the anterior chest wall.

Management

There are three questions the trainee should ask himself on approaching a patient in whom intubation may prove difficult;

1. Is the patient likely to regurgitate as a result of a full stomach following recent ingestion of food or liquid, or because of pregnancy or gastrointestinal pathology, e.g. pharyngeal pouch, hiatus hernia, pyloric stenosis, paralytic ileus?

2. Is intubation likely to prove difficult because of respiratory tract obstruction?

3. Is intubation likely to be difficult because of difficulty in laryngoscopy, e.g. inability to open the mouth or extend the atlanto-occipital joint?

The trainee should never attempt to perform endotracheal intubation using an i.v. induction agent and long acting muscle relaxant in any of the above situations.

Endotracheal intubation and a failed intubation drill in obstetric anaesthesia is described in detail in Chapter 31 (p. 418), whilst difficult intubation in emergency anaesthesia is described in Chapter 30 (p. 399).

The following manoeuvres are used in non-emergency anaesthesia and items 1 to 5 represent progressive anticipated difficulty in laryngoscopy and/or tracheal intubation.

1. Where there is minimal difficulty anticipated in either laryngoscopy or intubation, the following may be attempted. After setting up an i.v. infusion and following preoxygenation for 3 min, a small dose of induction agent is administered i.v. and manual ventilation of the lungs via a face mask is attempted. If satisfactory ventilation of the lungs is achieved, then suxamethonium may be given prior to laryngoscopy. If laryngoscopy is difficult, anaesthesia should be maintained with nitrous oxide, oxygen and halothane. In most instances a bougie may be passed into the trachea and an endotracheal tube 'railroaded' over it. If this fails, blind nasal intubation should be considered with the patient breathing spontaneously a volatile agent, e.g. halothane, or, for those who are experienced, ether. Alternatively, if visualisation of the larynx is impossible, it may be possible to thread an endotracheal tube over an extradural catheter passed through the cricothyroid membrane via an extradural needle and passed up through the oropharynx.

2. In the presence of respiratory tract obstruction severe enough to cause dyspnoea on exercise, i.v. agents should not be used and anaesthesia should be induced with a volatile agent with 50% nitrous oxide in oxygen. The reason for this is that minor degrees of respiratory tract obstruction may progress to complete obstruction when muscle tone decreases following loss of consciousness. The use of a gas induction is beneficial since muscle tone diminishes gradually with progressive loss of consciousness, and if ventilation ceases because of total respiratory tract obstruction the patient wakes up rapidly. For this reason, experienced anaesthetists would consider cyclopropane as the gas induction of choice in these situations as the rate of induction and recovery is more rapid than with the volatile agents.

3. Following sedation with i.v. benzodiazepines, local anaesthetic solution may be applied to the nose, pharynx and trachea to enable an endotracheal tube to be passed blindly in the awake patient before anaesthesia is induced. This is an appropriate technique in patients when laryngoscopy is impossible, e.g. severe trismus.

4. A fibre-optic laryngoscope may be used under local anaesthesia and an endotracheal tube threaded over the laryngoscope prior to use. However, the anaesthetist requires considerable practice with this instrument in order to be able to acquire familiarity with the normal anatomical landmarks.

5. Tracheostomy may be performed surgically under local anaesthesia and the airway maintained safely via the tracheostomy tube.

In respiratory tract obstruction which is severe enough to cause dyspnoea at rest, only manoeuvres 3–5 should be contemplated.

If it is anticipated that the level of difficulty in intubation warrants manoeuvres 2–5, surgery should be undertaken under local anaesthesia if appropriate.

Failed intubation drill

If intubation fails when neither experienced help nor alternative aids to intubation are available, it is essential to have a contingency plan. The failed intubation drill was devised for obstetric patients undergoing general anaesthesia, but deserves to be applied more widely. In emergency anaesthesia, from the moment of loss of consciousness, cricoid pressure must be maintained, and the patient positioned head down on the left side. Manual ventilation is continued via the face mask and pharyngeal secretions aspirated if necessary. Surgical anaesthesia is established using nitrous oxide, oxygen and a volatile agent until spontaneous respiration returns, or if oxygenation is difficult, the patient is allowed to wake up and the situation reassessed.

It is essential to record in the patient's notes that intubation has proved to be difficult.

A failed intubation drill for obstetric patients is described on page 418.

HYPOTENSION

Hypotension during anaesthesia may be defined as a decrease in systolic arterial pressure below 70 mmHg.

Causes (see Table 19.2)

Preoperative resuscitation of a patient for emergency anaesthesia may have been inadequate. This is most likely to occur when the magnitude of fluid loss has been underestimated, e.g. in the patient with intestinal obstruction, intra-abdominal haemorrhage or multiple fractures of long bones or pelvis. Induction of anaesthesia produces vasodilatation and abolishes compensatory vasoconstriction, resulting in hypotension.

Table 19.2 Common causes of hypotension during anaesthesia

Hypovolaemia	preoperative hypovolaemia surgical haemorrhage
Induction agents	relative overdosage in very young, very old, very ill, or patients with cardiovascular disease absolute overdosage
Volatile agents	halothane, enflurane, isoflurane
Muscle relaxants	d-tubocurarine
SAB and extradural	hypotension proportional to height of block
Cardiovascular disease	myocardial infarction arrhythmias pulmonary embolus
Respiratory disease	pneumothorax
Hypersensitivity reactions	induction agent muscle relaxants blood or colloid infusions

When given in equipotent doses, all induction agents, with the exception of ketamine and possibly etomidate, produce similar cardiovascular effects, viz. an increase in heart rate and a decrease in systolic and diastolic arterial pressures, central venous pressure and cardiac output.

Excessive dosage is likely to lead to a decrease in arterial pressure, particularly in the elderly. Those who have coexisting myocardial disease or inadequately treated hypertension often show a greater arteriolar dilatation and are much more susceptible to the hypotensive effects of induction agents.

Volatile anaesthetic agents, particularly halothane, enflurane and isoflurane, produce myocardial depression, and may result in hypotension. This is more likely to occur if large concentrations are used or IPPV is employed. The concurrent use of d-tubocurarine with its ganglion blocking properties may compound the hypotensive effect. IPPV may result in decrease in arterial pressure resulting from a decrease in cardiac output caused by increased intrathoracic pressure. This responds usually to infusion of i.v. fluids.

Spinal or extradural anaesthesia produces vasodilatation because of sympathetic blockade. Hypotension and bradycardia may require correction with i.v. fluids and ephedrine. Hypotension during anaesthesia may be caused also by surgical manoeuvres (e.g. haemorrhage, pressure on great veins), anaphylactic reactions to drugs or blood transfusion, pneumothorax, myocardial infarction, or cardiac arrhythmias.

HYPERTENSION

Hypertension during anaesthesia is an undesirable complication because of the risk of myocardial ischaemia or infarction, or vascular damage. Some causes are listed in Table 19.3.

Table 19.3 Common causes of hypertension during anaesthesia

Light anaesthesia	inadequate analgesia
	inadequate hypnosis
	coughing, straining on e.t.t.
Coexisting hypertension	untreated
	treated
	undiagnosed phaeochromocytoma
Aortic cross-clamping	
Hypercapnia	
Drugs	
adrenaline	
ergometrine	
ketamine	
Pre-eclampsia	

There is no doubt that poorly controlled hypertension intra- and postoperatively leads to an increased mortality and morbidity. However, moderate hypertension with a diastolic arterial pressure < 110 mmHg is not a risk provided it is controlled during surgery and the early postoperative period.

In patients with a phaeochromocytoma, coarctation of the aorta or renal artery stenosis, particular attention should be paid to preoperative treatment if intraoperative fluctuations are to be avoided.

A hypertensive response commonly occurs to laryngoscopy. β-Blockers given at induction may partly attenuate this. Coughing and straining on the endotracheal tube may be diminished by topical analgesia of the larynx with lignocaine.

Surgical stimulation results in hypertension if the depth of anaesthesia is inadequate.

Ketamine should be avoided in patients with ischaemic heart disease or hypertension. Ergometrine is contraindicated in the obstetric patient with pre-eclampsia.

Cross-clamping the aorta greatly increases peripheral resistance and afterload. Increased myocardial

work may result in hypertension and subendocardial ischaemia. Halothane or sodium nitroprusside may be used to control arterial pressure at a level normal for that patient.

Hypercapnia may lead to hypertension, tachycardia or ventricular arrhythmias. In the absence of end-tidal CO_2 monitoring, it is essential to ensure that the carbon dioxide cylinder on the anaesthetic machine is not accidentally in operation and that fresh gas flows are appropriate for the anaesthetic breathing system in use.

CARDIAC ARRHYTHMIAS (see also Chapter 36, p. 469)

As perioperative disturbances of cardiac rhythm are common, all anaesthetised patients warrant continuous e.c.g. monitoring in conjunction with the other standard aspects of monitoring including capillary refill, arterial pressure and pulse. Electrocardiographic evidence of sinus rhythm implies normal cardiac impulse generation and conduction, and is not indicative of adequate cardiac output or tissue perfusion.

The e.c.g. allows early and accurate detection and analysis of abnormal rhythms, some of which may go unnoticed clinically. For example, ventricular bigeminy may exist in the presence of a normal radial pulse.

Whilst arrhythmias which compromise cardiac function, e.g. ventricular tachycardia, always require immediate treatment, some arrhythmias do not. Treatment is required in the following situations:

1. When they interfere significantly with cardiac output and tissue perfusion, i.e. in the presence of hypotension.
2. When they predispose to ventricular fibrillation or asystole (which are associated with circulatory standstill and may be difficult to treat).
3. When they are associated with significant myocardial ischaemia.

Treatment

Supraventricular tachyarrhythmias, (see Appendix IVc for doses of drugs), e.g. atrial fibrillation, flutter or supraventricular tachycardia may result in heart rates sufficiently fast to embarrass cardiac function and these should probably not be allowed to persist untreated. It should be remembered that anti-arrhythmic drugs are potent depressants of cardiac conduction and contractility and should not be used unless there is a good indication. In this context any underlying factors which may precipitate or perpetuate arrhythmias (hypoxia, hypercapnia, electrolyte disturbances, light anaesthesia) should be corrected before resorting to drug therapy.

Perioperative arrhythmias are rarely primary cardiac events and often may be attributed to extracardiac factors. Sinus tachycardia may result from hypovolaemia, sepsis, pain or light anaesthesia and treatment should be directed at the underlying cause. Atrial premature contractions do not usually warrant specific treatment but on occasion herald atrial fibrillation which may be associated with haemodynamic deterioration.

Ventricular tachycardia and fibrillation should be treated immediately with DC shock if cardiac function is compromised. Premature ventricular contractions and ventricular tachycardia with a well preserved cardiac output should be treated with lignocaine.

Aetiology

There are many potential causes of arrhythmias during anaesthesia (Table 19.4). Most can be avoided by adequate preoperative assessment and skilful intraoperative management. However, there are some arrhythmias that occur despite good anaesthesia.

Table 19.4 Common causes of arrhythmia during anaesthesia

Surgical	ophthalmic ⎫
	nasal ⎬ surgery
	dental ⎭
	mesenteric traction
	anal stretch
Metabolic	hyperthyroidism
	hypercapnia
	hypokalaemia
Disease	congenital heart disease
	ischaemic heart disease
Drugs	atropine
	adrenaline
	halothane
	cyclopropane

Ischaemic heart disease is by far the commonest cardiac disorder encountered in the surgical population. In these patients, any change in circulatory status that adversely affects the myocardial oxygen supply:demand ratio (e.g. hypertension, hypotension, bradycardia, tachycardia) may precipitate ventricular arrhythmias. Pharmacological suppression of any ectopic focus should be accompanied by attempts to improve myocardial metabolism.

Patients with inadequately treated hypertension are also prone to perioperative arrhythmias, as are patients with chronic rheumatic heart disease associated with valvular stenosis or regurgitation. The pre-excitation syndromes, e.g. the Wolff-Parkinson-White syndrome, which are not as uncommon as once supposed, may present with a supraventricular tachycardia during anaesthesia. Similarly, sino-atrial dysfunction is being increasingly recognised and may result in sinus bradycardia and sinus arrest which predispose to junctional escape rhythms. Paroxysmal tachycardia followed by a prolonged period of sinus arrest may also be a prominent feature of this syndrome.

Patients with undiagnosed hyperthyroidism may develop atrial fibrillation in the perioperative period, whereas unheralded hypertensive crises together with malignant ventricular arrhythmias are the hallmarks of an unsuspected phaeochromocytoma.

Apart from pre-existing cardiac or endocrine disease, the two commonest causes of perioperative rhythm disturbances are arterial hypoxaemia and hypercapnia. Hypercapnia provokes the release of endogenous catecholamines which may trigger ventricular arrhythmias especially in the presence of halothane, cyclopropane or trichloroethylene in a spontaneously breathing patient. This interaction between adrenaline and halothane is also important in the context of exogenous adrenaline injected to reduce blood loss. From the practical viewpoint, in the presence of halothane the maximum dose of adrenaline for infiltration should not exceed 100 μg (i.e. 10 ml of 1:100 000) during any 10-min period. Enflurane is much safer in this respect and problems are unlikely if oxygenation and ventilation are guaranteed.

Halothane, and to a lesser extent enflurane, cause a dose-dependent depression of sinus node automaticity. This suppression of the dominant pacemaker may encourage the emergence of a secondary pacemaker in AV junctional tissue. The resulting junctional escape rhythm is a common occurrence in patients anaesthetised with these agents. Treatment is only necessary if the junctional focus is very slow (less than 50 beat/min), or if the concomitant loss of 'atrial kick' causes hypotension. Small doses of atropine (0.3 mg) usually restore sinus rhythm.

Hyperventilation and hypocapnia are associated with transcellular potassium shifts resulting in relative extracellular hypokalaemia. Serum potassium may decrease 0.5 mmol/litre for every 1.3 kPa decrease in $P\text{CO}_2$ and the resulting hypokalaemia increases the resting membrane potential of excitable tissues, causing hyperpolarisation of cell membranes. The overall effect is an irritable, excitable myocardium that is more prone to arrhythmias. This situation exists in hypokalaemia of any aetiology including that commonly seen in the surgical population.

Hyperkalaemia decreases the resting membrane potential and the resulting membrane hypo-polarisation predisposes to arrhythmias. An increased serum potassium is typically seen in renal insufficiency when excretion of potassium is limited, but can also occur with ionic redistribution. In patients with burns, or extensive denervation of skeletal muscle (paraplegia), or certain neuromuscular or myopathic diseases, large amounts of potassium are released from muscle in response to suxamethonium. This may result in acute hyperkalaemia and cardiac arrest.

Many nonanaesthetic drugs predispose to arrhythmias — digoxin, tricyclic antidepressants, aminophylline and some sympathomimetic inotropes. In each instance toxicity should be excluded prior to anaesthesia.

If anaesthesia is too light, surgical stimulation may result in extreme reflex sympathetic and para-sympathetic activity, and this may be associated with arrhythmias. However, more extreme rhythm abnormalities occur in the form of traction reflexes presenting during certain surgical manipulations. Traction on hollow viscera during laparotomy, or on the external ocular muscles during squint surgery, may produce extreme bradycardia which, although usually transient, can result in asystole. Atropine may be used to both prevent and treat these disturbances.

In neuro-anaesthetic practice, severe rhythm abnormalities are seen when the brain stem and/or cranial nerves are encroached upon in posterior fossa explorations. More importantly to general anaesthetists, stimulation and traction on the pharynx and larynx is commonly associated with transient ventricular arrhythmias. These are seen during tracheal intubation and are reflected in the high incidence of arrhythmias during ENT, oral and dental surgery.

EMBOLISM

Venous

Venous embolism during anaesthesia is uncommon. However, prophylactic measures should be used to decrease the incidence of postoperative venous thrombosis and embolism. Preoperatively, sub-cutaneous heparin is used most frequently. Intra-operatively, the venous return may be improved by squeezing the calves mechanically or stimulating the calf muscles electrically.

The choice of anaesthetic technique influences the incidence of DVT. DVT may be more common when IPPV and a muscle relaxant is used than when a regional or spontaneously breathing technique is employed.

Arterial

The most common source of arterial emboli during anaesthesia is an indwelling cannula, and is often associated with excessive flushing of an arterial line with either a 2 ml syringe or an automatic flushing device. More than 15 drops may flush clots retrogradely from the radial artery into the arterial tree.

Air

The possibility of an air embolism exists in many types of surgical operation (Table 19.5), whenever atmospheric pressure is greater than intravascular pressure. In many situations, careful positioning of the patient so that the heart is higher than, or at the same level as, the operating site prevents this complication.

Table 19.5 Surgical and other causes of air embolism

Neurosurgery:	posterior fossa operations in sitting position
Abdominal surgery:	laparoscopy hysterectomy D & C and insufflation
Orthopaedic surgery:	arthrography hip surgery
Chest:	open heart surgery breast operations
Miscellaneous:	middle ear surgery neck surgery blood transfusion CVP lines pressure at depth arterial monitoring extradural injection

Pathophysiology

Symptoms of venous air embolism are produced if air enters a vessel at a rate of 0.5 ml/kg/min or greater. A hissing sound may be heard in the wound. As the air enters the right side of the heart, mechanical distension is produced, cardiac output and arterial pressure decrease, heart rate increases and a 'millwheel' murmur is heard. The air passes into the pulmonary vein producing coughing, gasping and cyanosis. End-tidal CO_2 decreases, and pulmonary artery pressure and central venous pressure increase. Asphyxia results from obstruction to the pulmonary circulation. Paradoxical air embolism may occur via a 'probe patent' foramen ovale, or air may cross the pulmonary capillary bed, to enter the coronary or cerebral circulations causing myocardial ischaemia or convulsions.

Detection

Precordial or oesophageal stethoscope; end-tidal CO_2 monitoring; Doppler studies — chest wall, oesophageal; echocardiography.

Treatment

Haemostasis is achieved by compression, or the operative field may be flooded by the surgeon. The patient is tipped head down on the left side so that air may be aspirated from the right atrium via a central venous line. In extreme situations, a cannula may be inserted percutaneously into the right ventricle for aspiration of air. Neurosurgical air embolism may be obviated almost completely if the patient is placed prone and not in the sitting position.

HYPOVOLAEMIA

Prior to anaesthesia, it is essential to assess the extent of fluid deficit and to correct hypovolaemia. Thirst, apathy, a dry tongue, inelastic tissue and a decreased urine output indicate fluid depletion which may be confirmed biochemically and haematologically. Poor peripheral perfusion, decreased urine production (<0.5 ml/kg/min) in the presence of a raised heart rate, hypotension and low central venous pressure confirm the diagnosis. β-Blocking drugs may prevent a compensatory tachycardia and obscure the diagnosis.

Induction of anaesthesia in a hypovolaemic patient may result in cardiovascular collapse as peripheral vasodilatation occurs and as the adrenergic vasoconstrictor response is depressed by barbiturates. Therefore, fluid losses should be replaced preoperatively, if necessary measuring CVP when large volumes are required.

Table 19.6 indicates some common causes of fluid loss in the perioperative period.

Table 19.6 Causes of fluid loss

Pre-existing deficit	
Haemorrhage	trauma gastro-intestinal obstetric major vessel rupture
Gastro-intestinal	vomiting obstruction fistula diarrhoea
Other causes	diuretics
Continuing physiological loss Evaporation Sequestration of fluids	
Continuing current abnormal losses Haemorrhage Drainage of ascites Decompression of obstructed bowel Burns	

Haemorrhage

In children a blood loss greater than 10% of circulating blood volume (wt in kg × 80 ml) should be replaced with blood. In adults, blood losses up to

1 litre may be replaced by crystalloid or plasma substitutes, but larger losses should be replaced with warmed filtered blood.

Allowance must be made for additional fluid loss by sequestration as interstitial fluid when increased vascular permeability in damaged areas is likely to occur, e.g. crush injuries, intestinal obstruction. 5 ml/kg/h of a balanced electrolyte solution is usually sufficient to cover these losses.

Evaporation

Insensible loss from skin and lungs forms part of normal body fluid losses and 0.5–2 litre of water per day may be lost. Electrolyte loss is increased significantly by sweating. Evaporative losses are increased during anaesthesia and surgery. The patient loses fluid and latent heat of vaporisation in humidifying dry inspired gas and from exposed abdominal contents. Humidification of inspired gas decreases respiratory heat and water loss and helps to maintain body temperature. Condenser humidifiers are suitable, but they achieve only 70% relative humidity and an airway temperature of 32°C. They may also increase airway resistance on becoming blocked, and represent an additional site of potential disconnection.

HYPERVOLAEMIA (Table 19.7)

Table 19.7   Factors resulting in hypervolaemia

1. Myocardial failure
2. Overenthusiastic replacement in response to:
    drug-induced hypotension
    caval compression
3. Inability to excrete a fluid load
4. Misleading monitoring, CVP not indicating left ventricular function
5. Pregnancy — circulatory changes at delivery
6. Hypoproteinaemia
7. Water intoxication following transurethral resection of prostrate

Fluid should be administered according to the requirements of the individual patient. Overenthusiastic administration of crystalloid may lead to pulmonary oedema if the interstitial fluid volume is expanded by more than 30%. Special care should be taken when crystalloid is used to correct hypotension produced by anaesthetic drugs. Myocardial failure may occur, particularly in the elderly patient with ischaemic heart disease.

During anaesthesia hypervolaemia may be suspected if there is an elevated CVP, tachycardia and low arterial pressure after rapid fluid infusion. Distended neck veins, a third heart sound, pulmonary crepitations and a raised inflation pressure confirm the diagnosis. During longer procedures, facial oedema may develop.

Inotropic support should be provided with dopamine and digoxin, and loop diuretics used to excrete the excess fluid. If CVP monitoring is misleading and does not reflect left heart function, pulmonary artery and pulmonary capillary wedge pressure measurement should be considered.

HYPOTHERMIA

Induced hypothermia is used to reduce metabolic rate and oxygen consumption to increase the ability of the brain to withstand hypoxia without producing irreversible damage, e.g. in cardiac surgery, neurosurgery and intensive therapy. Surface cooling is used in small children before induction of profound hypothermia (15–20°C) and circulatory arrest to allow repair of congenital heart defects. Non-depolarising muscle relaxants are used to prevent shivering, and carbon dioxide added to inspired gases to shift the oxygen dissociation curve to the right, thereby allowing greater oxygen release in the tissues.

Inadvertent hypothermia

During surgery a patient loses heat to the cooler theatre environment. This heat loss may be increased by evaporative loss from exposed viscera, the use of dry anaesthetic gases, and replacement of fluid loss with cold i.v. solutions.

The temperature may decrease to 33–34°C during prolonged surgery. Drugs are metabolised more slowly and their duration of action is prolonged. At the end of surgery, a cold patient has to expend energy to regain body temperature, and may shiver. Shivering increases oxygen consumption significantly and may compromise myocardial oxygen supply since cardiac output is depressed by the residual effects of anaesthesia. Measures which may be employed to reduce heat loss during anaesthesia and surgery are shown in Table 19.8.

Table 19.8 Prevention of heat loss

Swaddling of small children
Warming mattress
Space blanket
Humidification
    Swedish nose
    heated water bath
Enclose exposed viscera in plastic bags
Warm surgical preparation fluids
Warm irrigation fluids
Warm i.v. solutions
Increase ambient temperature and humidity

MALIGNANT HYPERPYREXIA

This is a potentially fatal condition in which, as a result of an inherited abnormality in skeletal muscle cells, exposure to certain anaesthetic agents may precipitate a rapid increase in body temperature of at least 2°C/h.

Aetiology

Susceptible individuals inherit a defect in calcium binding in the sarcoplasmic reticulum of skeletal and possibly cardiac muscle cells. In the presence of certain trigger agents, calcium is released into the cytoplasm, producing myofibrillar contraction, accelerated lactic acid and carbon dioxide production, increased oxygen consumption, a profound metabolic acidosis, and the production of heat. Membrane stability is lost, and potassium leaks from the cells into the extracellular fluid causing hyperkalaemia.

Susceptibility is inherited as an autosomal dominant. Susceptible individuals frequently have muscular disorders or myopathies, or may be normal on clinical examination.

Trigger agents

Most drugs used in anaesthesia have been incriminated in the precipitation of malignant hyperpyrexia. Halothane and suxamethonium are the two agents most likely to produce the condition, although all volatile anaesthetic agents should be avoided in an individual who is known to be susceptible. Lignocaine is probably unsafe.

Clinical signs

There may be increased muscle tone following the injection of suxamethonium, particularly in young patients. In other patients, hyperpyrexia with or without rigidity appear later during the anaesthetic, or in the early postoperative period, and are accompanied by tachycardia, hyperpnoea, cyanosis, hypoxaemia, metabolic acidosis, hyperkalaemia, hypocalcaemia, tetany, myoglobinuria, acute renal failure, and cardiac failure. Arrhythmias may occur at any time. Until the introduction of dantrolene (vide infra) the mortality associated with malignant hyperpyrexia was 64%.

Treatment

Volatile agents should be discontinued. 100% oxygen should be administered, if necessary by IPPV. Attempts should be made to reduce body temperature using ice or ice-packs, and sodium bicarbonate should be infused to treat the metabolic acidosis. Insulin may be required to treat hyperkalaemia.

Dantrolene is the only drug available for the specific treatment of malignant hyperpyrexia. It should be administered i.v. in a dose of 1–2 mg/kg and repeated every 5–10 min up to a maximum dose of 10 mg/kg in total until control of the condition has been obtained.

Investigation of susceptible individuals

Although measurement of serum creatine phosphokinase has been recommended as a screening test for susceptible individuals, its results are unreliable. Susceptible individuals, and members of their family, require muscle biopsy for histological evidence of the condition and for in vitro exposure to trigger agents. These investigations are highly specialised, and the patient and his family should be referred to a malignant hyperpyrexia investigation centre.

Anaesthesia in the susceptible individual

In a patient known to be susceptible to the condition, or a relative of such a patient, all attempts should be made to prevent triggering of malignant hyperpyrexia. It is probably advisable to avoid premedication, and anticholinergic agents should not be administered. Induction with a barbiturate, muscle relaxation using pancuronium, and maintenance of anaesthesia with nitrous oxide supplemented by an opioid agent, appears to be the safest technique available. Although regional anaesthesia may have advantages, malignant hyperpyrexia has been reported in patients undergoing spinal nerve block. Throughout the course of the anaesthetic, temperature should be monitored using needle probes inserted into muscle, and an oesophageal or nasopharyngeal temperature probe. Dantrolene and all necessary resuscitation equipment should be immediately available.

HYPERSENSITIVITY

Hypersensitivity reactions refer to uncommon, unpredictable drug toxicity, in most cases involving the release of histamine, and not exaggerated normal pharmacological actions resulting from relative or absolute overdosage. Reactions occur most commonly to induction agents and muscle relaxant drugs.

Anaphylactic or type I hypersensitivity

Type I hypersensitivity to a drug, e.g. thiopentone, involves production of specific IgE antibodies as a result of previous exposure. Occasionally a primary IgG mediated response is seen.

Anaphylactoid

This is a descriptive term used for responses which are clinically similar to a type I response but which involve pharmacological as opposed to immunological release of histamine.

Althesin commonly produces histamine release by immediate chemical activation of complement C_3 via the alternate pathway.

Recognition

Reactions are more likely to occur in the female patient in her mid-thirties. Allergies (particularly to cosmetics) atopy and asthma are more common in reactors than in the general population. Most reactions present within the first 5 min of anaesthesia, but in 10% the onset is delayed. The first apparent feature is variable, but flushing over the upper half of the body, absent peripheral pulses, bronchospasm or transient difficulty in lung inflation are the most common (Table 19.9).

Table 19.9 Manifestations of hypersensitivity

Cutaneous	flushing
	large urticarial weals
	rash
Oedema	early (within minutes)
	head, eyelids, upper airway
	significant loss of fluid
	late (slow to resolve)
	generalised
Cardiovascular collapse	
	Vasodilatation — absent peripheral pulses
	e.c.g. — tachycardia
	asystole
	VF
Bronchospasm	mild — transient difficulty in ventilation
	severe — likely to be asthmatic
Gastro-intestinal symptoms	
	cramping abdominal pain
	nausea, vomiting
	diarrhoea
Haematological abnormalities	
	present in 10–15%
	? should surgery proceed

Treatment

This is designed to prevent hypoxaemia and restore the circulation. In many reactions, spontaneous recovery occurs but a severe reaction comprising hypotension and bronchospasm may be fatal. When a severe reaction occurs, the following steps should be followed:

1. Administer 100% oxygen.
2. Intermittent positive pressure ventilation and external cardiac massage if necessary.
3. 500–1500 ml HPPF i.v. — crystalloid escapes via leaky capillaries.
4. Consider administering adrenaline 0.3–0.5 ml 1:1000 i.v. or i.m. to counter vasodilatation.
5. Steroids
   Aminophylline   } may be required
   Sympathomimetic drugs } for bronchospasm.
6. Surgery should not commence after treatment of a severe reaction because there is increased risk of abnormal coagulation. In one series, the average length of treatment was 143 min.

Investigation

The mechanism of the reaction may be elucidated by detecting complement conversion or formation of IgE antibodies in sequential blood samples taken into

EDTA bottles at time 0, 3 h, 6 h and 24 h after the reaction.

Some anaesthetists advocate intradermal testing on the basis that it is safe, highly sensitive, and a ready source of antigen is provided. Others query the safety and particularly the reliability for drugs which have the capacity to release histamine. Intradermal testing is performed one month after the reaction when all drugs which might modify the result have been discontinued.

Prevention

The patient should be advised to wear a warning bracelet describing sensitivity to drugs. Prophylaxis with antihistamines and steroids is not usually successful. The evidence for the use of H_2 receptor antagonists is ill defined. It has been suggested that disodium cromoglycate may have a role.

Blood transfusion reactions

Most transfusion reactions are febrile or urticarial in nature and are induced by leucocyte or platelet antigens. Microfiltration of blood recovers 90% of the granulocytes and decreases the incidence of reactions.

Pretreatment with chlorpheniramine or other antihistamines may be indicated in a patient who has had a previous reaction.

Anaesthesia masks the signs of incompatible transfusion but tachycardia, hypotension, cyanosis or unexplained oozing from the wound shortly after a transfusion has commenced, may be indicative of mismatched blood. At times of stress, the wrong blood may be given to a patient and surveys have shown that this is most likely to occur in the operating theatre or ITU.

Plasma substitutes

Haemaccel (mol. wt 35 000) and Dextran 70 (av. mol. wt 70 000) are most likely to produce hypersensitivity, urticaria, tachycardia and hypotension when they are infused rapidly. The incidence of these reactions varies according to different surveys but the most commonly quoted figures are:

0.008% for Dextrans
0.038% for Haemaccel
0.003% for plasma protein solutions.

Haemaccel has been reformulated and a lower incidence of reactions is now claimed by its manufacturers.

FURTHER READING

Albin M S 1983 Editorial: The sights and sounds of air. Anesthesiology 58: 113
Cass N M, James N R, Lines V 1956 Difficult direct laryngoscopy complicating intubation for anaesthesia. British Medical Journal 1: 488
Clarke R S J 1982 Hypersensitivity reactions to intravenous anaesthetic drugs. In: Atkinson R S, Langton Hewer C (eds) Recent advances in anaesthesia and analgesia, 14. Churchill Livingstone
Ellis F R 1982 Malignant hyperpyrexia. In: Vickers M D (ed) Medicine for anaesthetists, part II, 2nd edn. Blackwell Scientific Publications, Oxford
Hirsham C A 1983 Airway reactivity in humans. Anesthetic implications. Anesthesiology 58: 170

Hooper G 1981 Malignant hyperpyrexia: a review. Eaton Laboratories, Woking
Horsey P J 1982 Blood transfusion. In: Atkinson R S, Langton Hewer C (eds) Recent advances in anaesthesia and analgesia, 14. Churchill Livingstone, Edinburgh
Prys-Roberts C (ed) 1980 The circulation in anaesthesia. Blackwell, Edinburgh
Tunstall M E 1976 Failed intubation drill. Anaesthesia 31: 850
Watkins J 1982 Hypersensitivity responses to drugs and plasma substitutes used in anaesthesia and surgery. In: Watkins J, Salo M (eds) Trauma stress immunity in anaesthesia and surgery. Butterworths, London
White A, Kauder P L 1975 Anatomical factors in difficult direct laryngoscopy. British Journal of Anaesthesia 47: 468
Willatts S M 1982 Lecture notes on fluid and electrolyte balance. Blackwell, Edinburgh

20

Recovery from anaesthesia

The patient arriving in the recovery ward after a general anaesthetic has usually received agents by injection and/or inhalation, which have interfered with the vital functions of consciousness, respiration and circulation. During recovery, these functions should be monitored and if necessary supported. The patient should not leave the recovery area until:

(a) consciousness has returned and he can maintain his airway,

(b) ventilation is adequate and

(c) circulation is stable, (unless he is transferred to the ITU or CCU).

The recovery period is also useful for close inspection of surgical wounds and drains for bleeding, and frequently analgesic therapy is administered in the recovery area.

The recovery area (Fig. 20.1) should be equipped adequately and staffed by specially trained nurses. However, the anaesthetist remains responsible for his patient in the recovery area and he (or another anaesthetist) must be immediately available.

The patient is nursed on either a bed (if a prolonged stay is anticipated) or on a trolley, either of which may be tilted quickly to a head-down position, should vomiting occur. Within reach of each trolley should be suction apparatus, catheters, an oxygen supply and facilities for arterial pressure measurements. Full resuscitation equipment must be stationed within the recovery area. This includes an anaesthetic bag and

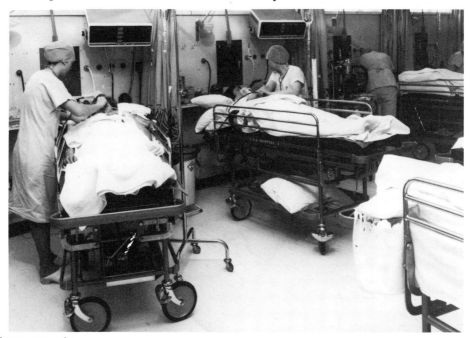

Fig. 20.1 A recovery ward.

Table 20.1 Drugs available in the recovery room

Adrenaline	Insulin
Aminophylline	Isoprenaline
Atropine	Lignocaine
Bupivacaine	Mannitol
Calcium	Morphine
Chlorpromazine	Naloxone
Dextrose 50%	Neostigmine
Diazepam	Pancuronium
Digoxin	Pethidine
Dopamine	Practolol
Doxapram	Propranolol
Ephedrine	Saline 0.9%
Frusemide	Sodium bicarbonate
Hydrocortisone	Sodium nitroprusside
	Suxamethonium

mask, airways, laryngoscopes, selection of endotracheal tubes with bougies, i.v. cannulae, fluids, emergency drugs (Table 20.1), facilities for e.c.g. monitoring and a defibrillator. Equipment for emergency tracheostomy including wide-bore needles and tracheostomy tubes should be available.

Problems occurring during the recovery period concern ventilation, circulation and the level of consciousness. The minimal extent of monitoring in recovery therefore comprises clinical assessment of breathing and conscious level, pulse (providing information on heart rate, pulse pressure and the presence of arrhythmias), arterial pressure and assessment of the peripheral circulation from colour, temperature and the presence of sweating.

Urine output provides information on renal perfusion and fluid balance and inspection of wounds and drains reveals any continuous bleeding. Depending on the magnitude of surgery and the state of the patient, monitoring may be extended to include e.c.g., central venous pressure, intra-arterial pressure,

pulmonary artery and wedge pressures, expiratory carbon dioxide concentration, etc.

The management of postoperative pain is described in detail in Chapter 22; in the recovery room, pain must be differentiated from hypercapnia or hypovolaemia (see Table 20.2), and the appropriate therapy instituted.

COMMON PROBLEMS IN RECOVERY

Hypoventilation (Fig. 20.2)

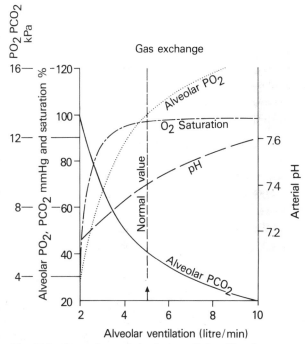

Fig. 20.2 Gas exchange during hypoventilation. Note the relatively rapid increase in P_{CO_2} compared with the slow decrease in arterial O_2 saturation.

Table 20.2 Common problems in the recovery room: symptoms and signs

	Pain	Hypercapnia	Hypovolaemia
Conscious level	May be restless May be quiescent if severe pain	Comatose	Restlessness or quiescent depending on extent of analgesia and residual anaesthesia
Periphery	Vasoconstriction: pallor ±sweating	Warm, flushed with bounding pulse (if normovolaemic)	Vasoconstriction: pallor ±sweating
H.R.	Tachycardia	Tachycardia	Tachycardia
B.P.	s.a.p. ↑ d.a.p. ↑ Pulse pressure normal	s.a.p. ↑ d.a.p. ↑↓ Pulse pressure ↑	s.a.p. and d.a.p. may be normal until marked fall in stroke volume then ↓ Pulse pressure ↓

Airway

Some problems which may occur are listed in Table 20.3. The patient should be kept in the lateral position until he is awake and can protect his own airway. This position helps to maintain a free airway by preventing the tongue from falling against the back of the pharynx. In addition, it decreases the risk of aspiration of gastric contents should regurgitation or vomiting occur. Similarly this position is important after ENT or dental surgery where bleeding from the nose or oral cavity may be expected.

The sign of incomplete *upper airway obstruction* (usually caused by the tongue) is noisy respiration. As the obstruction increases, tracheal tug and indrawing of the supraclavicular area occur on inspiration; stridor may occur also. With complete upper airway obstruction, respiratory sounds are absent and paradoxical movement occurs between the abdomen and thorax. An initial tachycardia and hypertension is followed by bradycardia, hypotension, cyanosis, arrhythmias and ultimately cardiac arrest unless a clear airway is re-established.

If the lateral position per se does not ensure the patency of a patient's airway, the mandible must be displaced anteriorly. In addition, an oral airway may be used although this can stimulate gagging, vomiting and even laryngeal spasm. Often a nasal airway is tolerated better. If a clear airway cannot be obtained by these simple methods, tracheal intubation must be considered and if this fails (an exceedingly rare event), tracheostomy undertaken.

Upper airway obstruction may be caused also by a foreign body. Dentures should have been removed before the operation. There have been some fatalities following failure to remove throat packs. Tumour is another cause of obstruction.

Laryngeal spasm, usually partial, is not uncommon after general anaesthesia. It is caused usually by irritation of the cords from secretions, vomiting, blood or an artificial airway. Painful peripheral stimuli during a light plane of anaesthesia may cause spasm, as may extubation after inhalation anaesthesia during a light level of unconsciousness. Treatment comprises firstly the administration of 100% oxygen followed by removal of any stimulating factors, e.g. removal of artificial airway, aspiration of pharyngeal secretions, treatment of pain with analgesia. Oxygen administration using positive pressure with a bag and mask usually forces oxygen between the cords and maintains oxygenation until the spasm has subsided. If attempts to ventilate in this way are unsuccessful, muscle relaxation with suxamethonium may be necessary to break the spasm and enable the lungs to be ventilated. After suxamethonium has been administered, tracheal intubation may or may not be performed depending on the situation, but it is probably advisable since oxygen may have been blown into the stomach, thereby increasing the risk of regurgitation.

Laryngeal oedema may occur occasionally after tracheal intubation and may cause severe obstruction, particularly in a child. Depending on severity, treatment is either immediate reintubation or in a milder case, the use of humidified oxygen-enriched air in a tent under close observation, and dexamethasone i.v.

Bronchospasm may be the result of airway stimulation by inhaled material, secretions, blood, airways etc. It may result also from intrinsic asthma, or be part of an anaphylactic reaction. Several drugs in anaesthetic practice predispose to broncho-constriction including d-tubocurarine, Althesin,

Table 20.3 Causes of postoperative hypoventilation

Factors affecting airway	Factors affecting respiratory drive	Peripheral factors

Upper airway obstruction:
  tongue
  laryngospasm
  oedema
  foreign body
  tumour
Bronchospasm
	Respiratory depressant drugs
	Preoperative c.n.s. pathology
	Intra- or postoperative
	  cerebrovascular accident
	Hypothermia
	Recent hyperventilation (Pa_{CO_2} low)
		Muscle weakness
		  residual neuromuscular block
		  preoperative neuromuscular disease
		  electrolyte abnormalities
		Pain
		Abdominal distension
		Obesity
		Tight dressings
		Pneumo/haemothorax

morphine, neostigmine and barbiturates. Treatment comprises removal of any stimuli, and the administration of oxygen and bronchodilators.

Respiratory drive

There are several possible causes of reduced respiratory drive (see Table 20.3) but the most common is the residual effect of drugs administered by the anaesthetist in the operating theatre or recovery room.

Often, it is obvious that ventilation is inadequate from the low respiratory rate or inadequate tidal volume, or the patient may complain of inability to breathe adequately. However, hypoventilation may be mild and difficult to detect by casual inspection; the signs of moderate hypercapnia (tachycardia and hypertension) may be masked by the residual effects of volatile anaesthetic drugs, or misdiagnosed as pain (Table 20.2).

Undiagnosed hypercapnia may lead to the development of arrhythmias and eventually apnoea.

All opioid analgesics produce a dose-dependent depression of respiration. A sufficiently high dose stops involuntary breathing completely, but it is important to remember that the patient may still take deep breaths on command. That a patient is awake is therefore no guarantee of adequate ventilation. The elderly are particularly sensitive to respiratory depressant effects of opioid drugs.

The pure opioid antagonist, naloxone, dramatically reverses the effect on respiration. The recommended dose is 1–2 μg/kg i.v. which may be repeated every 2–3 min until the desired effect is achieved. There have been reports of severe hypertension after naloxone when higher doses have been given quickly. An unnecessarily high dose may reverse some of the analgesic effect of the opioid. Very rapid reversal may cause tremor, nausea, vomiting, sweating and tachycardia.

The effect of naloxone i.v. lasts only 30 to 40 min although the opioid administered originally may have a considerably longer duration of effect. Thus respiratory depression may occur suddenly and at a time when patient monitoring has diminished. To prevent this, it has been recommended that half the initial i.v. dose of naloxone should also be administered i.m.

Peripheral factors

Often, insufficient reversal of neuromuscular block may be recognised from inco-ordinated muscle activity. However, when the patient is very sedated, inco-ordinated muscle activity is seen. It is possible for a patient to maintain an adequate tidal volume with 80% of the motor end-plate receptors blocked, but without the ability to cough effectively (which is necessary for protection of the airway in the event of regurgitation). If a patient can maintain a head lift above the trolley for several seconds and if he can maintain good hand-grip strength, there is sufficient reversal of neuromuscular block for maintenance of a safe airway and adequate ventilation. Further subjective tests are described in Table 11.3. The disadvantage of this assessment is that it requires patient co-operation. A more objective test of neuromuscular transmission is the use of the nerve stimulator and the use of these instruments is described in detail in Chapter 11.

If residual neuromuscular blockade of a competitive type is diagnosed, further doses of neostigmine may be administered (with atropine) to a total of 5 mg. If this dose fails to antagonise the block, artificial ventilation should be maintained and the cause sought.

Factors responsible for difficulty in reversing a nondepolarising block include overdosage with muscle relaxant, hypokalaemia, respiratory acidosis, certain antibiotics, local anaesthetic agents, quinidine, diseases affecting neuromuscular transmission (e.g. myasthenia gravis) or muscle disease (Table 20.3).

If the excretion of a nondepolarising drug is impaired (e.g. by renal or hepatic failure) a risk of recurarisation exists since the duration of action of neostigmine is approx. $\frac{1}{2}$–1 h. Development of respiratory acidosis or an increase in temperature after hypothermia may also lead to a degree of recurarisation.

Prolonged neuromuscular blockade following suxamethonium occurs in the presence of atypical pseudocholinesterase or a low plasma concentration of normal pseudocholinesterase. When a patient is homozygous for the atypical enzyme, the duration of block is usually only of the order of 2 h. It is necessary for the patient's lungs to be ventilated artificially for the duration of the block.

Other factors which may interfere with respiratory movements and contribute to inadequate respiration include abdominal distension, obesity, tight dressings and pain.

Pneumothorax may occur after IPPV (following trauma or spontaneously) and careful clinical examination of the respiratory system is an essential element of the assessment of the patient with inadequate postoperative ventilation. Pneumothorax is also a complication of intercostal block and central venous cannulation, and surgery on the kidney or in the neck.

When hypothermia or hyperventilation has been utilised, a patient may hypoventilate either because of low CO_2 production or depletion of CO_2 stores respectively.

Hypoxia

The classical causes of hypoxia are shown in Table 20.4. Ventilation-perfusion abnormalities initially and a degree of true shunting subsequently are the main causes of reduction in arterial oxygenation seen after surgery, particularly thoracic and abdominal.

Table 20.4 Classical causes of hypoxaemia

Reduced inspired oxygen concentration
Ventilation-perfusion abnormalities
Anatomical shunt
Hypoventilation
Diffusion impairment

Ventilation-perfusion abnormalities

Ventilation-perfusion abnormalities result from variations in cardiac output and a reduction in FRC with encroachment of closing volume into the tidal breathing range. When extreme, this may be apparent as a true shunt but in addition, diffuse airway collapse occurs which may not be visible as miliary atelectasis on chest radiography.

Diffusion hypoxia

At the termination of an anaesthetic when the patient's inspired gas mixture is changed from O_2/N_2O to O_2/N_2, the condition termed diffusion hypoxia occurs. The mechanism of this phenomenon is dependent upon the different blood solubilities of N_2O and N_2. The former, being 40 times more soluble than N_2, passes out into the alveoli from mixed venous blood in much greater volumes than the volume of N_2 taken up from the alveoli. In consequence, the alveolar concentration of O_2 is diluted, resulting in arterial hypoxaemia. The effect is also equivalent to increased alveolar ventilation and this is manifest as a small and temporary elevation of Pa_{CO_2}. In healthy patients, diffusion hypoxia has a short duration of only some 5 min and the extent of reduction in Pa_{O_2} is only of the order of 0.5–1.5 kPa. However, in patients with significant respiratory dysfunction, diffusion hypoxia may be significant.

Correction of diffusion hypoxia is achieved easily by the administration of 40% O_2 for the first 5–10 min after termination of anaesthesia. However, administration of oxygen is utilised frequently for longer periods because of continuing depression of cardiac output, and/or persistence of $\dot{V}/\dot{Q}$ abnormalities.

Temporary depression of ventilation

This is usually secondary to the various pharmacological agents used prior to and during anaesthesia. It is usually self-limiting and the use of oxygen in concentrations between 30% and 40% is sufficient to correct the reduced arterial oxygen tension.

Oxygen delivery to the tissues is dependent not only on arterial oxygenation, but also upon haemoglobin concentration, P_{50} of haemoglobin, and cardiac output.

Increased oxygen utilisation

Tissue hypoxia may result also from increased oxygen consumption caused by fever, shivering, restlessness or seizures. Many anaesthetists advocate elective ventilation for some hours after extensive surgery (e.g. following resection of aortic aneurysm). This ensures that the patient is well ventilated and oxygenated during the warming-up period when there are increased demands on the cardiorespiratory systems resulting from raised oxygen consumption and carbon dioxide production.

Shivering and increased muscle activity (seen commonly after halothane anaesthesia) is partly a result of diminished temperature (augmented by vasodilatation produced by the drug) and an effect on temperature-regulating centres.

Shivering in the postoperative period must be distinguished carefully from restlessness, which is a common sign of hypoxia or pain. Less commonly, it may result from distension of stomach or bladder. Restlessness may also be drug-induced. Ketamine may cause confusion and hallucinations. Patients who have received ketamine should be allowed to recover with as little disturbance and stimulation as possible. Atropine crosses the blood-brain barrier and may cause the 'central cholinergic syndrome', characterised by restlessness and confusion in addition to obvious peripheral antimuscarinic effects. This condition is not uncommon in the recovery room as a result of the concomitant use of atropine with neostigmine to reverse the residual effects of competitive muscle relaxant drugs. Glycopyrrolate does not cross the blood-brain barrier and it has been suggested that it is preferable to atropine at the end of an IPPV/relaxant/opioid anaesthetic technique. An additional advantage of glycopyrrolate is its longer duration of action.

Oxygen therapy

Following anaesthesia and surgery, for reasons discussed above, there is often a period of hypoxia. Thus it is advisable to administer oxygen to all patients in the recovery room. Clearly, any avoidable cause of hypoxaemia, e.g. drug-induced respiratory depression, should be treated appropriately.

Certain individuals are more vulnerable to the effects of a reduction in arterial oxygen content, in particular those suffering from ischaemic heart disease, abnormal liver function and those who are anaemic. It is prudent to use oxygen for a more prolonged period in circumstances such as these.

As with most forms of therapy, oxygen may have undesirable side-effects (Chapter 8, p. 125). Both its therapeutic effects and its complications are dose-related. It is therefore important to administer oxygen in a known concentration.

Patients receiving oxygen therapy may be classified into two main groups:

1. Those with normal ventilatory control
2. Those with abnormal ventilatory control.

The latter group lose their sensitivity to carbon dioxide and the main stimulus to ventilation is reduced Pa_{O_2}. The administration of oxygen to this group of patients may lead to the abolition of the hypoxic drive. This results in respiratory depression, further elevation of Pa_{CO_2} and not infrequently, apnoea. If it is thought that a patient has abnormal ventilatory control, then controlled oxygen therapy is indicated.

Controlled oxygen therapy

This implies that the amount given is known and the response to it monitored. In the first instance 24% oxygen is usually administered (see Fig. 20.3). If the Pa_{O_2} increases as a result, and the Pa_{CO_2} rises by no

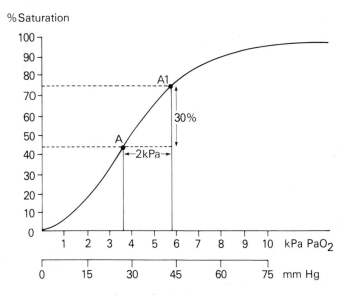

Fig. 20.3 Theory of controlled oxygen therapy. (See text for details.)

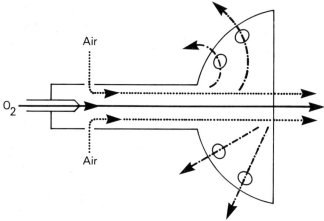

Fig. 20.4 Diagram of Venturi mask.

more than 1.3–1.5 kPa, then if the patient remains conscious and is able to cough, the inspired concentration of oxygen may be increased to 28% if a further increase in Pa_{O_2} is desirable. Arterial blood gases are then rechecked, and in a step-wise fashion the inspired oxygen concentration is adjusted until both Pa_{O_2} and Pa_{CO_2} are optimal.

Oxygen therapy devices

Fixed peformance devices. These provide an inspired gas mixture of known composition. The oxygen concentration delivered does not vary in response to alterations in the patient's pattern of respiration.

Accurate control of inspired gas concentration is possible only if air and oxygen are premixed and delivered to the patient without further dilution.

Premixing may be achieved by the use of:

1. Metered flows of compressed air and oxygen. Dilution of oxygen may be avoided only by use of a tightly fitting mask and a reservoir system (e.g. a Mapleson type A system).

2. An oxygen driven injector entraining a fixed proportion of room air. A high flow rate of premixed gas prevents dilution. The flow rate required must be in excess of the patient's peak inspiratory flow rate (PIFR). This is normally between 20–30 litre/min. Provided the premixed gas is supplied at a rate above this, dilution of oxygen does not occur. This method is often referred to as High Airflow Oxygen Enrichment (HAFOE).

This is the principle used in the Venturi masks (Fig. 20.4). By using injectors of different sizes at the oxygen flow rates recommended by the manufacturers, a range of predictable oxygen concentrations may be administered as appropriate.

Variable performance devices. Most of the other commonly used devices for postoperative oxygen delivery are included in this category. Oxygen is supplied at a flow rate which is less than the patient's minute volume. The actual inspired oxygen concentration is determined by the relationship of these two factors. As respiration is rarely completely regular postoperatively, the tidal volume and thus the inspired oxygen concentration vary from breath to breath. Thus, accurate prediction of inspired oxygen concentration is not possible. In addition, the volume of the mask increases the patient's dead space, and rebreathing is possible. The degree of rebreathing varies with the volume of the mask, the oxygen flow rate and the length of the expiratory pause.

Although these masks are relatively inaccurate, they are adequate for the needs of the majority of patients immediately after anaesthesia. Table 20.5 shows the approximate oxygen concentrations achieved at different oxygen flow rates for some of the more commonly used variable performance devices.

Nasal catheters and speculae also function as variable performance devices, although rebreathing is not a problem.

Figure 20.5 shows a selection of fixed and variable performance oxygen therapy devices.

Normally, an inspired oxygen concentration of 35–40% is sufficient to prevent hypoxia resulting from the causes described above. Thus, oxygen may

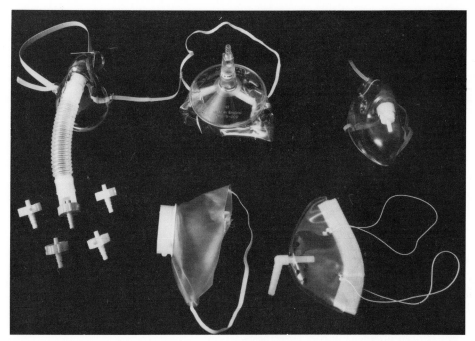

Fig. 20.5 Various types of oxygen mask. In clockwise rotation from top left: Accurox with various Venturi attachments for obtaining different but fixed inspired O$_2$ concentrations; Ventimask; Hudson mask; M.C. mask; Edinburgh mask.

Table 20.5 Oxygen masks, flow rates and approx. O$_2$ concentrations delivered

Type of mask	Oxygen flow (litre/min)	Oxygen concentration (approx. %)
Edinburgh	1	24–29
	2	29–36
	4	33–39
Nasal cannulae	1	25–29
	2	29–35
	4	32–39
Hudson	2	24–38
	4	35–45
	6	51–61
	8	57–67
	10	61–73
M.C.	2	28–50
	4	41–70
	6	53–74
	8	60–77
	10	67–81

be administered postoperatively by a variable performance face mask (e.g. M.C., Hudson).

In severe lung dysfunction caused by large degrees of intrapulmonary shunting, e.g. following aspiration, very high inspired O$_2$ concentrations are required (Fig. 20.6).

Hypotension

Hypovolaemia

This may result from inadequately replaced fluid or blood losses (before or during surgery) or continued postoperative bleeding. The latter may be obvious if

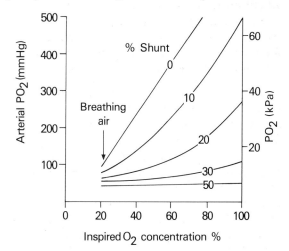

Fig. 20.6 Response of arterial P_{O_2} to increased inspired oxygen concentrations in a lung with various amounts of shunt. Note that the P_{O_2} remains well below the normal level for 100% oxygen. Nevertheless, useful increases in oxygenation occur even with severe degrees of shunting.

there is bleeding into drains or swelling around the wound, which should be inspected carefully. However, intra-abdominal or retroperitoneal bleeding may remain concealed. Diagnosis is dependent on the presence of impaired circulation with hypotension and failure of a sustained response to transfusion.

The usual cause of postoperative bleeding is inadequate surgical haemostasis. However, there may be coagulation disorders particularly after massive transfusions of bank blood in which clotting factors and platelets are reduced. Disseminated intravascular coagulation (DIC), pre-existing bleeding disorders and treatment with anticoagulants are additional causes. Clotting abnormalities may be suspected if there is a general tendency to bleed at venepuncture sites, petechiae, bruising, and oozing from the wound. Coagulation tests must be performed and fresh frozen plasma, platelets, etc given as discussed in Chapter 37.

Hypovolaemia may also be relative, e.g. if vasodilatation has been produced during anaesthesia by anaesthetic agents, specific vasodilators or a sympathetic block caused by subarachnoid or extradural anaesthesia. Lowering of the legs from lithotomy position may also unmask hypovolaemia.

Hypovolaemia is diagnosed by hypotension, tachycardia (although this may be masked in the presence of β-blockers or following the administration of neostigmine), a low CVP as judged from neck vein filling or measured with a central venous catheter, cold, clammy periphery and low urine output (less than 30 ml/h). Treatment comprises elevation of the legs to increase preload, i.v. crystalloids, plasma expanders or blood, and oxygen.

Cardiac failure

Failure of the left ventricle causing hypotension results most frequently from perioperative myocardial infarction or overtransfusion.

Diagnosis is made from the presence of hypotension and poor peripheral circulation. The CVP is usually elevated and pulmonary oedema may be present.

Treatment comprises oxygen therapy, fluid restriction, diuretics and if necessary inotropic support. The e.c.g. should be monitored and cardiac enzymes estimated to confirm or exclude myocardial infarction.

Differentiation between hypovolaemia and cardiac failure may not be easy since both conditions may coexist and the CVP may not reflect left atrial pressure in the presence of pulmonary hypertension. If hypovolaemia is the predominant cause of hypotension, a beneficial effect on arterial pressure would be expected following the rapid infusion of 200 ml of fluid, but this challenge must be undertaken cautiously with close observation of the CVP. Where diagnosis is in doubt, a pulmonary artery catheter may be required.

Septic shock

In septic shock, the patient usually has a high cardiac output and low peripheral resistance. Large volumes of i.v. fluids are required to replace losses from capillary leakage and inotropic support is often needed. Appropriate antibiotic therapy is required, and steroids (e.g. methylprednisolone 30 mg/kg) are usually administered.

Hypertension

Postoperative hypertension is common. Causes include inadequately treated preoperative hypertension, hypoxia, hypercapnia, overtransfusion and the use of vasopressor drugs. However, the commonest cause is pain. As with hypotension the cause should be sought and if possible treated. It is essential to elicit and remedy the cause rapidly since hypertension leads to increased cardiac work and myocardial oxygen consumption and may result in postoperative myocardial infarction or cardiac failure.

Treatment comprises:

1. Oxygen therapy.
2. Positioning the patient head-up (if conscious).
3. If hypoxia, hypercapnia and pain have been eliminated, treatment with an antihypertensive agent, e.g. hydralazine, diazoxide, SNP or trimetaphan.

Cardiac arrhythmias

Arrhythmias are frequently seen intra- and post-operatively. They are often benign, requiring no treatment, but their nature, cause and effects on the circulation should be investigated.

The causes of arrhythmias are legion but the following require exclusion:

Pain

Hypercapnia

Hypoxia

Volatile anaesthetic agents, e.g. trichloroethylene, cyclopropane, halothane, enflurane

Electrolyte and acid/base disturbance

Stimulation of the trachea by an endotracheal tube

Laryngeal or pharyngeal suction

Myocardial ischaemia or infarction

Cardiac failure

Sinus tachycardia is common in the recovery room. It may be a reflex response to hypovolaemia and therefore be responsive to adequate fluid replacement. Hypoxia, hypercapnia, anaemia, raised oxygen consumption in the presence of fever, shivering, increased work of breathing and restlessness are also possible causes. However, the commonest cause is pain. IF no treatable cause can be found for persistent tachycardia, a β-blocker should be given (particularly if the patient has myocardial ischaemia) slowly and carefully (e.g. practolol 2–4 mg) under e.c.g. observation. Treatment of tachycardia is important since a rapid ventricular rate decreases coronary perfusion whilst increasing myocardial oxygen demand. A combination of tachycardia and hypertension is particularly undesirable. The rate pressure product (heart rate × systolic arterial pressure) is an approximate correlate with myocardial oxygen demand, and values below 12–15 000 are desirable in the ischaemic heart.

Sinus bradycardia is very common immediately on arrival in the recovery ward and usually is a result of inadequate antagonism by atropine of the cardiac effect of neostigmine. Additional atropine may be given if the heart rate is less than 50 beat/min. Atropine should also be given if there is a persistent slow rhythm associated with ventricular escape beats or hypotension.

Sinus bradycardia may be caused also by drugs (e.g. β-blockers, digitalis), hypoxia (especially in babies), and raised intracranial pressure.

Ventricular bradycardia may be seen in myocardial infarct or heart block.

Atrial fibrillation, flutter or supraventricular tachyarrhythmias are treated as in other circumstances. Atrial fibrillation with normal ventricular rate and arterial pressure may be left untreated during the recovery period. Digitalisation is commenced if ventricular rate is rapid in fibrillation or flutter, unless hypotension is present in which case cardioversion should be undertaken. Carotid massage, verapamil or digitalis is usually successful in treating supraventricular tachycardia.

Premature ventricular contractions that are frequent (1 in 15 or less), multifocal, occur in runs, or commence on the preceding T-wave (R on T) require *immediate* treatment with lignocaine i.v. (1–2 mg/kg) in a bolus dose followed if necessary by infusion. Treatment of ventricular fibrillation and cardiac arrest is described in Chapter 38.

Conscious level

It is easy to ascribe postoperative unconsciousness to the effect of agents given pre- or intraoperatively. This is true in most instances, but it must not be forgotten that there may be other causes of unexpectedly prolonged or deep unconsciousness and it is important to recognise these situations early if the cause is to be treated.

Hypoglycaemia

It is important to measure blood sugar pre-, intra- and postoperatively in diabetic patients receiving oral hypoglycaemic drugs or insulin (see Chapter 36). The normal stress response to surgery produces elevation of blood sugar and hypoglycaemia usually results from residual effects of oral hypoglycaemic drugs, or the injudicious use of insulin. Hyperglycaemia developing in a previously undiagnosed diabetic rarely produces a prolonged postoperative coma, but the onset of diabetes may present occasionally as symptoms of an acute abdomen.

Cerebral causes

1. Brain damage from episodes of hypoxia or hypotension during anaesthesia.

2. Intracranial bleeding, cerebral thrombosis or embolism (including air embolism).

3. Pre-existing brain tumour.

4. Epilepsy.

Other causes

1. Existing hypoxia.
2. Hypercapnia. A Pa_{CO_2} in excess of 9–10 kPa produces unconsciousness.
3. Hypotension.
4. Hypothermia.
5. Hypo-osmolar syndrome especially after TURP — the diagnosis is confirmed by demonstration of a low serum Na^+.
6. Hypothyroidism previously unrecognised.
7. Rarely in liver and renal failure.

FURTHER READING

Churchill-Davidson H C 1979 A practice of anaesthesia, 4th edn. Lloyd-Luke, London

Gray T C, Nunn J F, Utting J E (eds) 1980 General anaesthesia, 4th edn. Butterworths, London

Miller R D (ed) 1981 Anaesthesia, vol 2. Churchill Livingstone, London

West J B 1979 Pulmonary pathophysiology. Blackwell, London

21

Postoperative sequelae

Anaesthesia and surgery are not without side-effects. This chapter describes some of the commoner complications in the postoperative period, ranging from severe and life-threatening conditions to 'minor' causes of morbidity.

CARDIOVASCULAR SEQUELAE

Myocardial infarction

The incidence of myocardial infarction (MI) after operation in patients over the age of 50 with no pre-existing evidence of ischaemic heart disease is 0.66%. However, the incidence is increased to an average of 6.6% in patients with a history of previous MI.

In addition, mortality among patients suffering a postoperative MI is 70% if there has been one previous infarct, compared with 26.5% in those with no history of ischaemic heart disease. The most important factor related to reinfarction is the time interval between surgery and the previous infarct:

Time interval	Reinfarction rate
< 3 months	37%
> 3 months < 6 months	16%
> 6 months	4.5%

Other factors which increase the risk of reinfarction include untreated preoperative hypertension, intra-operative hypotension and abdominal and noncardiac thoracic procedures lasting longer than three hours.

One extensive study into risk factors showed that there are nine preoperative factors which correlate strongly with the development of serious cardiac complications postoperatively:

1. A 3rd heart sound or elevated venous pressure.
2. MI within the previous 6 months.
3. The presence of an abnormal rhythm on the preoperative e.c.g.

4. More than 5 premature ventricular contractions per minute.
5. Intrathoracic and upper abdominal procedures.
6. Age > 70 y.
7. Significant aortic stenosis.
8. Emergency surgery.
9. Poor general medical condition.

If several of the above features are present concurrently, elective surgery should be postponed until those factors amenable to treatment are managed appropriately.

Patients who have undergone coronary artery bypass surgery for ischaemic heart disease are at no increased risk.

The choice of anaesthetic or anaesthetic technique appears to play no significant role in affecting the incidence of MI postoperatively. However, the anaesthetic management of patients at risk should involve a thorough preoperative assessment and the correction of any treatable risk factors (see Chapter 36, p. 467).

Although the actual anaesthetic technique employed is not of great significance, it would seem prudent to preoxygenate all patients at risk and avoid hypoxia, tachycardia, hypotension and hypertension.

The e.c.g. should be monitored continuously in all patients. The most useful electrode position is the so-called CM_5 position (see Chapter 18).

Postoperatively oxygen should be administered for an appropriate time period, which is dependent on the type of surgery performed.

Diagnosis. MI or reinfarction may be difficult to diagnose in the postoperative period. It occurs most frequently on the third postoperative day. The classical distribution of pain is present in only 25% of patients.

The diagnosis should be considered in any patient at risk who develops an arrhythmia or becomes hypotensive in the postoperative period. Premature ventricular extrasystoles occur in 90% of patients who experience an MI. Sinus bradycardia and varying degrees of atrioventricular heart block frequently accompany MI. There is often a pyrexia of up to 39°C.

The diagnosis is confirmed most frequently by changes in serial e.c.g. recordings and cardiac enzymes. The most useful enzymes for establishing the diagnosis postoperatively are the myocardial specific iso-enzymes for creatinine phosphokinase (CPK) and lactate dehydrogenase (LDH). CPK levels are raised at 3 h, peak at 12 h and return to normal within 36 h. LDH levels rise at 2 days, peak at 4–5 days and return to normal by 10 days.

Thrombo-embolism: (1) deep venous thrombosis (DVT)

The main factors postulated by Virchow as contributing to the formation of venous thrombi are:

1. Changes in the composition of blood.
2. Damage to blood vessel walls.
3. Decreased blood flow.

However, the exact 'trigger' mechanism which initiates thrombosis remains unknown.

Risk factors

A higher incidence of DVT has been reported in patients with:

Extensive trauma
Infection
Heart failure
Blood dyscrasias
Malignancy
Metabolic disorders

DVT is commoner following hip, pelvic and abdominal surgery than other types of surgery. Although the association between spontaneous DVT and the oral contraceptive is well established, the number of women developing this complication is small. However, the incidence increases if surgery is performed while the patient is currently taking the drug.

Diagnosis

Approximately 70% of patients with a DVT have neither symptoms nor signs. Ankle oedema is a more reliable sign than calf pain. Fifty per cent of patients with calf pain and tenderness on dorsiflexion of the foot do not have a DVT. Often there is mild pyrexia.

Investigations

Venography. With modern X-ray equipment this is now established as an effective method for demonstrating most thrombi of clinical importance.

Radioactive fibrinogen uptake. Iodine-labelled fibrinogen is used because this is taken up preferentially by a growing thrombus. The investigation is quick to perform and can detect small thrombi in the calf vessels. Its main disadvantage is that it cannot be used to detect iliac and pelvic vein thrombi. It does not correlate well with pulmonary embolism.

Ultrasonography. This is noninvasive and simple to perform. However, it is insensitive and is useful only for confirming the diagnosis of a major thrombus.

Impedance plethysmography. Like ultrasonography, this investigation is noninvasive but can be used only for confirming major thrombi.

Prophylaxis

Elimination of stasis. The efficacy of early ambulation after operation in reducing the incidence of DVT is not clear. Attempts directed at preventing stasis, including physiotherapy, elastic stockings or elevation of the feet have resulted in only a small reduction in the occurrence of DVT.

Two methods are in use currently for increasing venous return from the lower limbs during surgery:

1. Electrical stimulation of the calf muscles: A low voltage current is applied across the calf to contract the muscles every 2–4 s.
2. Pneumatic compression of the calves: The legs are encased in an envelope of plastic material, which is rhythmically inflated and deflated, thus squeezing the calves intermittently. This technique can be continued postoperatively.

Alteration of blood coagulability

Platelet aggregation. Various drugs which interfere with different aspects of platelet function have been investigated. These include Dextran 70, dipyridamole, aspirin and chloroquine. There is no evidence to suggest that dipyridamole or aspirin prevent DVT. Dextran infusion during and after surgery reduces the incidence of fatal pulmonary embolism. Its role in the prevention of peripheral venous thrombosis is undetermined.

The coagulation mechanism. Oral anticoagulant therapy instituted before operation is the most effective method of preventing venous thrombosis. The risk of severe haemorrhage is high and may exceed the dangers of thromboembolism. Low-dose heparin, 5000 units s.c. 2 h before operation and subsequently at 12-hrly intervals for a week, is the most promising regimen for prevention of DVT and carries little risk of major haemorrhage.

(2) Pulmonary embolism (PE)

This term covers a range of events from sudden circulatory collapse and death, through minor episodes of pleurisy and haemoptysis, to the long-standing disability of patients with chronic thromboembolic pulmonary hypertension. Following anaesthesia and surgery, the acute forms of PE are encountered.

The common sites of origin for pulmonary embolus are the veins of the pelvis and lower extremities. The most common time for a postoperative PE to present is during the second week. In certain patients, predisposing factors may have existed for a period of time preoperatively, and the whole time scale of events may be shifted. The embolus may then occur at the time of, or shortly after surgery.

Diagnosis

Presenting features. The principal features are circulatory collapse and sudden dyspnoea, often associated with chest pain. If the embolus is large enough then the pulmonary artery outflow is blocked and sudden death results. If the embolus involves more than 50% of the main pulmonary arteries it is termed 'massive'.

Physical signs. A low cardiac output state is found. Tachypnoea and central cyanosis are usual. There is arterial hypotension, sinus tachycardia and a constricted peripheral circulation. The jugular venous pressure is elevated. On auscultation a fourth heart sound is usually present.

Investigations

E.c.g. (Fig. 21.1). This reflects acute right ventricular strain, with features which often include right axis deviation, T wave inversion in leads V1–V4 and sometimes right bundle branch block. The classical $S_1Q_3T_3$ pattern is less common.

Chest X-ray. This is often unremarkable. It may show areas of oligaemia reflecting pulmonary vascular obstruction.

Arterial blood gases. There is usually hypoxaemia due to ventilation-perfusion imbalance, and hypocapnia resulting from hyperventilation.

Pulmonary embolus

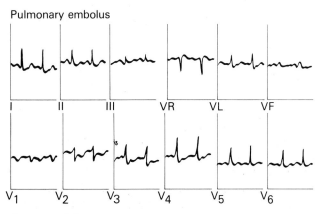

Fig. 21.1 E.c.g. changes in pulmonary embolus.

Perfusion and ventilation lung scans. The perfusion scan shows uneven circulation with perfusion defects delineating the emboli. A simultaneous ventilation scan is usually normal.

Pulmonary angiography. This gives a definitive diagnosis of major obstruction in the pulmonary circulation. This investigation is particularly useful if the patient is critically ill and the diagnosis is in doubt, and is essential if pulmonary embolectomy is planned. However, it is invasive and normally requires transfer of the patient to the X-ray department.

Treatment

DVT. The mainstay of therapy is anticoagulation. Initially, i.v. heparin is infused in a dose of 40 000 units per day. At the same time oral anticoagulants are commenced. Warfarin is used most commonly. Heparin may be discontinued after 48 h. Oral anticoagulants are continued for at least 3 months.

Pulmonary embolism. The immediate treatment consists of the administration of oxygen in a high concentration and i.v. heparin. Digoxin is often useful. Sometimes it is necessary to use additional inotropic support for the circulation. Heparin is continued for 5–6 days. Oral anticoagulants are commenced as soon as possible and are continued for at least 6 months.

Massive pulmonary embolus which does not respond to the above measures may warrant the use of thrombolytic agents, e.g. streptokinase. The chance of haemorrhage with these agents is considerably higher than with heparin. If the cardiovascular effects of the embolism are life-threatening, open pulmonary embolectomy under cardiopulmonary bypass may be considered.

LOCAL VASCULAR COMPLICATIONS

Haematoma formation is probably the commonest complication following i.v. injection. This results usually from inadequate pressure at the injection site following removal of the needle. Phlebitis, thrombosis or thrombophlebitis may result after the use of certain i.v. induction agents. Etomidate, propanidid and methohexitone are probably the most troublesome in this respect, although some studies have shown little difference between the various induction agents. Intravenous diazepam is a potent cause of phlebitis, although a new formulation of diazepam in a fat emulsion (Diazemuls) has overcome the problem. Intravenous infusions commonly cause thrombophlebitis. The incidence is related to the duration of infusion. This is far more important than the type of cannula used. If the infusion is changed every 12 h thrombophlebitis is rare. If it is changed every 72 h, the incidence of thrombophlebitis is 70%. Of the cannulae available, those made of polytetrafluorethylene (Teflon) appear to be least thrombogenic.

Arterial cannulation is performed commonly to permit continuous monitoring of blood pressure during major surgery. Unfortunately it is not without sequelae. Intimal damage may lead to thrombosis and occasionally aneurysm formation. Even if complete occlusion occurs, recannulation of the vessel may be possible. Nevertheless, gangrene of the extremities is an occasional complication. This is particularly likely to occur if there is inadequate collateral circulation. If cannulation of a radial artery is considered, it is important to perform Allen's test to establish the adequacy of the collateral supply from the ulnar artery. In clinical practice a modified Allen's test is performed:

The patient is asked to clench his fist, and radial and ulnar arteries are compressed by the examiner. The patient is then instructed to unclench his fist. The examiner releases the ulnar artery and observes the palm of the hand. If there is adequate collateral flow a prompt return of colour to the palm is seen. If there is little or no return of colour within 15 s Allen's test is said to be negative and it is unwise to cannulate the radial artery of that hand.

The incidence of arterial thrombosis has been reduced by the use of cannulae made of Teflon and by selection of a cannula whose diameter is small relative to the size of the artery.

POSTOPERATIVE PULMONARY SEQUELAE

Impaired oxygenation

In all but the shortest of procedures on healthy young patients, there is a significant decrease in the arterial oxygen tension (Pa_{O_2}). The mechanism of this defect is not understood fully. It is assumed to be a continuation of the factors which cause an increase in the alveolar-arterial O_2 partial pressure difference (A–a PO_2) following the induction of anaesthesia. In most instances the Pa_{O_2} may be restored to its original value by the administration of 30–35% O_2.

Following abdominal surgery

Patients with previously normal lungs suffer impairment of oxygenation for at least 48 h. The extent of this impairment is related to the site of operation. It is less marked following lower abdominal surgery and worst after upper abdominal midline or paramedian incisions.

In these circumstances the differences between pre- and postoperative Pa_{O_2} may be as much as 4 kPa. Factors implicated in impaired oxygenation in the postoperative period include:

Reduction in functional residual capacity (FRC). This also is related to the site of surgical incision. The greatest reduction in FRC follows upper abdominal surgery. The exact cause of the decrease in FRC is not known. There is an initial decrease following induction of anaesthesia. Postoperatively this decrease is compounded by wound pain, causing spasm of the expiratory muscles, and abdominal distension leading to diaphragmatic splinting. The supine position also reduces FRC. The relationship between changes in FRC and Pa_{O_2} postoperatively is shown in Figure 21.2.

Relationship of FRC to closing volume (CV). Postoperatively, there is an increase in CV. This together with the reduced FRC, may lead to CV impinging upon the tidal volume range. This results in small airways closure during normal tidal respiration. Gas trapping occurs in the affected airways and subsequent absorption of air may lead to areas of atelectasis. This occurs mainly in the dependent parts of the lung.

The end result is an increase in the number of areas of low ventilation/perfusion (V/Q) ratios within the lungs.

In most patients these abnormalities return towards normal by the fifth or sixth postoperative day. However, if the changes have been marked, the areas of atelectasis may become a focus for infection. This is particularly so in the presence of retained secretions. Factors which contribute to the retention of secretions postoperatively are:

1. Inability to cough. This is mostly a direct result of wound pain. However, excessive sedation produces a similar situation. Postoperative electrolyte imbalance, especially hypokalaemia and hypo-

.... Minor non-abdominal surgery

------- Lower abdominal surgery

——— Upper abdominal surgery

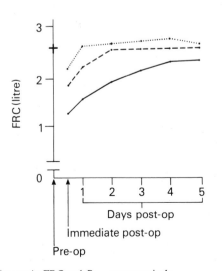

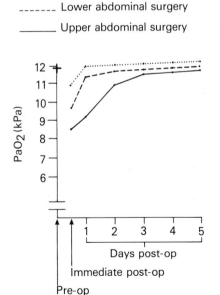

Fig. 21.2 Changes in FRC and Pa_{O_2} postoperatively.

phosphataemia, may compound the situation by interfering with muscle function.

2. Suppression of bronchial mucosal ciliary activity. This is primarily a result of the use of unhumidified anaesthetic gases.

3. Antisialagogue drugs. When antisialagogue premedicants have been used the secretions become more viscid. The dry mucosa itself is more prone to inflammatory reaction. If this occurs, the exudate produced increases the problem still further.

4. Infection. If pulmonary infection supervenes, impairment of oxygenation may contribute to a lack of co-operation in clearing secretions. A combination of these factors may result in retention of secretions, leading to further areas of pulmonary collapse, and an increase in the work of breathing. Ultimately, oxygenation of the blood may become inadequate despite oxygen therapy, or carbon dioxide retention may occur. The sequence of events culminating in ventilatory failure is shown in Figure 21.3.

Predisposing factors

Site of surgery. The total incidence of pulmonary complications reaches 40% following upper abdominal surgery, compared with 10–20% after lower abdominal operations.

Pre-existing respiratory disease increases the complication rate. This is particularly so if excessive secretions or infection are present at the time of operation.

Smokers have an increased incidence of pulmonary complications compared with nonsmokers.

Obesity is associated with a high incidence of pulmonary complications. Obese patients have low FRC and increased work of breathing preoperatively.

The anaesthetic technique used has little effect on pulmonary complications.

Clinical features

Atelectasis. The first signs of atelectasis may be seen within 24 h of operation. The triad of pyrexia, tachycardia and tachypnoea is often present. The temperature is usually in the range of 38–39°C. There is often a productive cough. If atelectasis is extensive, the patient is cyanosed. On physical examination, localising signs are uncommon unless

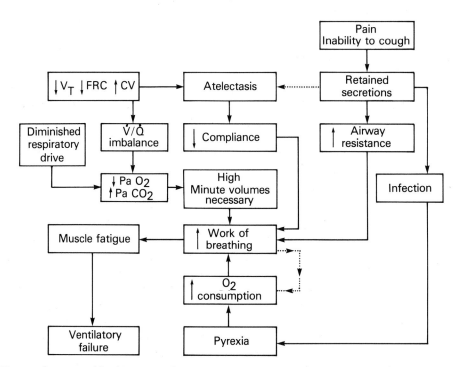

Fig. 21.3 Diagram of events resulting in postoperative ventilatory failure.

the area of involvement is large. A chest X-ray reveals patchy areas of atelectasis.

Pneumonia. Lobar pneumonia is rarely seen postoperatively. Bronchopneumonia is more common. This is especially so in the elderly. The onset of symptoms is not as rapid as in atelectasis. There is usually a fever and associated tachycardia with an increase in the respiratory rate. Physical examination usually reveals areas of consolidation, predominantly at the lung bases. This should be confirmed radiologically.

Treatment

Pulmonary complications are seen usually within the first three days postoperatively. Pyrexia and an increase in respiratory rate are often the presenting signs. If a pulmonary complication is suspected, a sputum sample should be sent to the laboratory for bacteriological analysis. Appropriate antibiotic therapy may then be commenced.

Intensive physiotherapy should be prescribed in an attempt to remove secretions and re-expand atelectatic areas of the lung.

Patients with pulmonary collapse are usually hypoxic, but the Pa_{CO_2} remains normal or may be low as a result of tachypnoea, at least in the early stages. Oxygen in moderate concentrations (30–40%) is usually sufficient to correct the hypoxia, but this should be confirmed by blood gas analysis. If the patient fails to respond to these measures, signs of respiratory distress develop. The patient becomes drowsy and respiration is laboured, with rapid shallow breathing using the accessory muscles. The Pa_{CO_2} increases and arterial oxygenation deteriorates despite oxygen therapy. The presence of continued deterioration in blood gases is an indication for ventilatory support.

Reducing postoperative morbidity

It should be remembered that prevention of pulmonary complications begins preoperatively. Upper and lower respiratory tract infections should be treated prior to surgery. Dental sepsis and sinus infections should be eradicated. Pre-existing chronic respiratory disorders should be treated so that the patient is in optimal condition before the operation. Spirometry is useful to monitor such treatment. Smoking should be discouraged and weight loss

encouraged where indicated. In patients with increased risk factors, heavy premedication is best avoided to ensure minimal respiratory depression at the end of the procedure.

During surgery. At induction care should be taken not to introduce infection by way of contaminated equipment. All equipment should be checked to see that it is clean prior to use. During prolonged procedures, the anaesthetic gases should be humidified.

If neuromuscular blocking agents are used, particular care should be taken to ensure that reversal is adequate.

Postoperatively. Analgesia should be optimal to ensure adequate coughing and co-operation during physiotherapy, which should be commenced as soon as possible postoperatively.

POSTOPERATIVE RENAL DYSFUNCTION

The kidney is vulnerable to a wide range of drugs and chemicals. It is particularly susceptible to toxic substances for the following reasons:

Large blood flow per unit mass.
High oxygen consumption.
Non-resorbable substances concentrated by tubules.
Permeability of tubular cells.

All anaesthetic techniques depress renal haemodynamics and, secondary to this, interfere with renal function. Provided prolonged hypotension is avoided the effects are temporary. There is, however, one exception.

Methoxyflurane

The administration of this volatile anaesthetic agent is associated with a high incidence of renal dysfunction. Clinically, the defect is characterised by a failure in the concentrating ability of the kidney. In certain cases this may progress to high-output renal failure. The nephrotoxicity of methoxyflurane is a dose-related phenomenon. During the metabolism of methoxyflurane, inorganic fluoride ions are produced which interfere with renal tubular function. It has been suggested that fluoride levels of greater than 40 μmol/litre are nephrotoxic. Toxicity may result from lower fluoride levels. Although the toxicity is dose-related, tubular damage may result from only a relatively small amount of methoxyflurane if patients are taking drugs which cause enzyme induction. Methoxyflurane administration in combination with other nephrotoxic drugs, e.g. aminoglycosides or tetracyclines, is particularly hazardous.

Enflurane is also metabolised to fluoride ions, but to a much lesser extent. Only 2.4% of enflurance undergoes biodegradation compared with 45% of methoxyflurane. As yet, there is no evidence to suggest that enflurane causes serious renal dysfunction.

POSTOPERATIVE HEPATIC DYSFUNCTION

There are many causes of postoperative hepatic dysfunction. They are summarised in Table 21.1.

Most patients who have undergone anaesthesia and surgery present no clinical signs of hepatic damage. If hepatic dysfunction does occur, it is usually attributable to one or more of the causes listed in Table 21.1. When hepatic dysfunction occurs without apparent explanation after anaesthesia, consideration must be given to the possible hepatotoxicity of the anaesthetic agents used.

Chloroform

Although rarely used nowadays, this was the first volatile agent suspected of causing liver damage. It is thought that the damage caused by chloroform is a result of products of its metabolism. A hepatitis syndrome results, centrilobular hepatic necrosis being the histological picture.

Methoxyflurane

There have been reports of severe hepatic dysfunction and death in which methoxyflurane was named as the causative agent. Whereas renal damage is dose-related and due to fluoride ion production, hepatic damage is not. The clinical picture is very similar to viral hepatitis. The mechanism of damage is not understood. It is thought that an immune-mediated response is involved and that cross-sensitivity with halothane may contribute. Methoxyflurane-associated hepatitis is rarer than that associated with halothane.

Halothane

Attention was first focused on halothane-associated hepatitis in the early 1960s. Numerous reports prompted the largest retrospective study ever undertaken (United States National Halothane Study) in 1969. It reviewed the incidence of fatal hepatic necrosis occurring within six days of anaesthesia. The incidence of fatal hepatic necrosis was found to be 1 in 10 000. The incidence following halothane administration was 1 in 35 000. This was not significantly greater than that associated with any other anaesthetic agent. However, although an issue surrounded by controversy, the most widely held current view is that there is a small number of patients who develop postanaesthetic jaundice in which the aetiological agent is probably halothane.

The histological picture is very similar to that seen in type-A viral hepatitis and other forms of drug-associated hepatitis. Clinically there is hepatocellular jaundice with elevation of the aminotransferase enzymes. The exact mechanism involved is not yet known. At present there are two main hypotheses:

1. Metabolites of reductive halothane metabolism are capable of bonding covalently to hepatocyte macromolecules, leading to hepatocellular damage.

2. Halothane or any of its metabolites react with hepatocyte proteins to form antigenic compounds, against which the body mounts an immune response and hepatocellular damage results.

Table 21.1 Causes of postoperative hepatic dysfunction

Increased bilirubin load	Hepatocellular damage	Extrahepatic biliary obstruction
Blood transfusion	Pre-existing liver disease	Gallstones
Haemolysis and haemolytic diseases	Viral hepatitis	Ascending cholangitis
Abnormalities of bilirubin metabolism	Sepsis	Pancreatitis
	Hypotension/hypoxia	Surgical misadventure
	Drug induced hepatitis	
	Congestive heart failure	

From the extensive work relating to this subject some practical points have arisen:

Following a general anaesthetic involving halothane, unexplained jaundice, especially if connected with an unexplained pyrexia, should contraindicate a further halothane anaesthetic.

The following groups of patients are more likely to develop hepatitis following the administration of halothane: patients subjected to repeated anaesthesia at short intervals of time (less than 3 months); obese, middle-aged women, especially those with evidence of organ specific autoimmunity.

MINOR SEQUELAE TO ANAESTHESIA

Nausea and vomiting

These may cause only mild discomfort to the patient. However, in severe cases, much distress and even fluid and electrolyte imbalance may result. In some circumstances, notably ophthalmic surgery, the result of the operation may be put at risk by persistent postoperative vomiting.

Many studies have been undertaken to investigate nausea and vomiting after anaesthesia and surgery. The incidence varies from 14.7%–82%. The wide range results largely from differences in the design of studies. There are several factors to be considered in the aetiology of postoperative nausea and vomiting.

Patient. Some people are prone to sickness even after the most minor events. Those individuals who are prone to motion sickness are more likely to vomit postoperatively. Women are more likely to vomit than men, and children more so than adults.

Pre- and postoperative medication. All of the commonly used opioid preparations have marked emetic properties. This is most noticeable if they are given alone. The use of antisialagogues for premedication, especially hyoscine, reduces the incidence of postoperative vomiting.

Anaesthetic agent used. Ether produces a high incidence of postoperative vomiting. Both cyclopropane and trichloroethylene cause vomiting postoperatively in a large proportion of patients. When compared to the above agents, a barbiturate/relaxant technique has been shown to reduce the incidence of vomiting. However, there appears to be little difference between this technique and a halothane anaesthetic.

Site of operation. Abdominal procedures are more likely to lead to vomiting than operations in other areas. Because of the proximity of the vestibular apparatus, middle-ear operations are associated with a high incidence of vomiting. Dilatation of the cervix, especially if combined with the administration of ergometrine, produces vomiting in a high proportion of women.

Other factors. The duration of surgery is related directly to the incidence of postoperative vomiting. Both operative and postoperative hypoxia cause vomiting, as may the premature resumption of oral fluids.

Prevention and treatment

Prevention of sickness requires a careful choice of drugs before, during and after surgery. Numerous antiemetics are available for use. This fact alone highlights the lack of efficacy of any one particular agent.

Metoclopramide is a very popular drug, but it has yet to be shown as a useful agent for this purpose in clinical trials. Other drugs which enjoy popularity at the present time are prochlorperazine and perphenazine. Probably the most effective drugs are those derived from the phenothiazines and butyrophenones (see Chapter 13).

Headache

The reported incidence of postoperative headache (12–35%) varies greatly from one study to another, methodology accounting for most of the variation.

Factors

Personality of the patient. This appears to be an important factor. Those individuals prone to suffer from headaches under stress and other similar circumstances are more likely to report a headache postoperatively.

Duration of surgery. The incidence of postoperative headache is related inversely to the duration of surgery.

Agent used. Many investigations have failed to single out any particular anaesthetic technique as being more likely to produce headache. However, halothane is often regarded as being an important causative factor. There is very little evidence to substantiate this. In fact, much of the work relating to postoperative headache suggests that general anaesthesia *per se* has very little effect.

Sore throat

Investigations into postoperative morbidity reveal a high incidence of sore throat. Some of the common causes include:

Trauma during intubation. Damage to the pharynx and tonsillar fauces may be caused by the laryngoscope blade.

Irritation of the larynx by an endotracheal tube is a more common cause of sore throat. It is more likely to occur following the use of an endotracheal tube made from red rubber than the less irritant plastic tubes. A poorly fixed endotracheal tube causes more frictional damage to the vocal cords than one which is fixed securely.

Trauma to the pharynx. This may result from the passage of a nasogastric tube, an endotracheal tube, or the insertion of a throat pack.

Other factors. It should not be forgotten that sore throat may occur in the absence of endotracheal intubation. The mucous membrane of the upper airways is very sensitive to the effects of unhumidified anaesthetic gases. The drying effect of the gases, often combined with a preoperative antisialogogue, is a potent cause of sore throat.

The use of topical local anaesthetics does not reduce the incidence of postoperative sore throat.

Postoperative sore throat is usually of short duration, patients being symptom-free within 48 h.

Hoarseness

This should not be confused with sore throat. It is nearly always associated with endotracheal intubation. Implicated factors are prolonged abduction of, and pressure on, the vocal cords.

Laryngeal granulomata

This is an unusual complication of endotracheal intubation. The granulomata arise from areas of ulceration, usually on the posterior aspect of the vocal cords. The ulcers are caused by pressure and subsequent ischaemia, the vocal processes of the arytenoid cartilage being the sites most frequently involved. Granulomata are reported most often following thyroidectomy.

If hoarseness persists for greater than one week postoperatively, indirect laryngoscopy should be performed. If ulceration is present, complete voice rest is indicated. If a granuloma is present, it should be excised. Untreated granulomata may grow to such a size as to obstruct the airway.

Trauma to teeth

Damage to teeth during the administration of a general anaesthetic is upsetting to the patient, and may have medicolegal consequences. Damage usually occurs during laryngoscopy, particularly if endotracheal intubation is proving difficult. Loose teeth, crowns, caps and bridges are particularly prone to damage. Preoperative enquiry and examination should alert the anaesthetist to the possibility of damage.

Ocular complications

Carelessness is the commonest cause of damage to the eyes, corneal abrasions being the most frequent type of damage. The eyes are often allowed to remain partially open during anaesthesia. The cornea is thus exposed and vulnerable to the irritant effects of skin preparations, dust and even surgical drapes. This type of damage is prevented easily by suitable covering of the eyes.

Much less likely is retinal infarction, which may result from excess pressure on the eyeball from a face mask.

Suxamethonium pains

Muscle pain following the administration of suxamethonium was reported shortly after its introduction into clinical practice. The muscles involved most frequently are those of the shoulder girdle, neck and thorax.

The factors affecting the incidence of muscle pain can be summarised as follows:

Age. Unusual in young children and old age.

Sex. Women are more susceptible than men. The incidence is reduced during pregnancy.

Type of surgery. There is an increased incidence following minor procedures where early ambulation is likely.

Physical fitness. The incidence is higher in individuals who are physically fit.

Repeated doses. If further doses of suxamethonium are administered when the initial dose has worn off, the frequency of muscle pain increases when compared with a single dose.

The exact cause of muscle pain is unknown, although it is thought that fasciculations produced by depolarisation of the motor nerve endplate are involved in the pathogenesis. However, it has been shown that the visible extent of the fasciculations does not correlate with the severity of muscle pain. The fact that muscle injury does occur is shown by the occurrence of myoglobinuria in severe cases.

Following minor surgery the patient may be more disturbed by the muscle pains that the discomfort associated with the procedure. It is possible, however, to reduce the incidence and severity of muscle pain following the use of suxamethonium. The most frequently described method is to pretreat the patient with a small dose of nondepolarising muscle relaxant, e.g. 3–5 mg d-tubocurarine, 1 min before induction.

Three other methods which have been described are:

1. Pretreatment with a small dose of suxamethonium (0.1 mg/kg).

2. Administration of diazepam, 0.15 mg/kg i.v. prior to induction.

3. The administration of dantrolene, approximately 2 h preoperatively.

FURTHER READING

Bastron, Deutsch 1976 Anaesthesia and the kidney. Grune and Stratton, New York

Churchill-Davidson H C 1978 A practice of anaesthesia, 4th edn. Lloyd-Luke, London

Gray T, Nunn J F, Utting J E (eds) 1980 General anaesthesia, 4th edn. Butterworths, London

Strunin L 1977 The liver and anaesthesia. W B Saunders, London

Sykes M K, McNicol M W, Campbell E J M 1976 Respiratory failure, 2nd edn. Blackwell Scientific Publications, Oxford

22

Postoperative pain

Postoperative pain is unique because it is a self-limiting condition with progressive improvement over a relatively short time-course. Previous experience influences the patient's response to treatment as do individual variations in demand, response, pain threshold and motivation.

MEASUREMENT OF PAIN

Because there is a subjective element in the estimation of pain, whether by patient or observer, measurement presents particular problems. The linear analogue score is the most widely used system. A 10 cm horizontal line is drawn on paper, the two ends of which are said to represent no pain, and the most excruciating pain imaginable. The patient marks on the line the degree of pain experienced at that moment. The distance of the mark from the end of the line is used as a score of pain severity. More recently, a device has been described for monitoring postoperative sequelae electronically using a visual display of lights with which patients record sedation, nausea and pain on a linear analogue system.

None of these methods is perfect. More objective assessment may be obtained from use of respiratory function tests, in particular FEV_1 and PEFR, both of which are reduced by the presence of pain, but these measurements are affected only by thoracic or abdominal surgery.

Many patients demonstrate a placebo effect, and experience analgesia in the absence of active treatment. Psychological factors are important in the experience of pain.

It cannot be stressed too highly that there is enormous variation in pharmacological responses and therefore in demand, patients varying from extreme stoicism to the opposite extreme (see Table 22.1).

Table 22.1 Factors influencing analgesic requirement

1. Site — see Table 22.2
2. Sex — female patients require opioids earlier, but total demand is equal
3. Age — elderly patients' opioid requirements are low
4. Personality — analgesic requirements increased in patients with a neurotic personality
5. Previous experience — reduces demand, especially if the same operation is undertaken
6. Response of patient — huge variation in response to a given dose of drug — especially marked with opioids
7. Motivation — analgesia achieved more easily after surgery for benign conditions than after palliative cancer surgery

REQUIREMENT FOR ANALGESIA

Table 22.2 describes the average severity of pain associated with various operative procedures, and provides an indication of the duration of the postoperative period during which opioid analgesics are usually required.

Table 22.2 Duration and severity of postoperative pain

Site of operation		Duration of opioid use	Severity of pain (0–4)
Abdominal —	upper	48–72 h	3
	lower	up to 48 h	2
	inguinal	up to 24 h	1
Thoracotomy		72–96 h	4
Limbs		24–36 h	2
Faciomaxillary		up to 48 h	2
Body wall		up to 24 h	1
Perineal		24–48 h	2
Hip surgery		up to 48 h	2

METHODS OF PROVIDING PAIN RELIEF

Systemic administration

Many drugs used systemically to provide analgesia are listed in Table 22.3.

Table 22.3 Analgesic drugs — classification

Opioids		Antipyretic and anti-inflammatory analgesics	
Opium derivatives	Morphine	Salicylates	Acetylsalicylic acid
Morphine derivatives	Diamorphine		Mefenamic acid, etc.
	Dihydrocodeine	Anilines	Acetanilide, Paracetamol
	Codeine		
Benzomorphinan family	Pentazocine	Indoles	Indomethacin
	Phenazocine		
Synthetic opioids	Fentanyl	Pyrazolines	Phenylbutazone
	Pethidine		Oxyphenbutazone
	Phenoperidine		
	Meptazinol		
Methadone derivatives	Dipipanone	New synthetic compounds	Diflunisal, etc.
	Dextromoramide		
	Dextropropoxyphene		

Adequate analgesia is obtained only if the notional pain threshold for a particular patient has been exceeded, and subsequently the level of drug in the biophase necessary to achieve this should not be allowed to diminish below threshold (see Fig. 22.1). As a result of recent improvements in the accuracy and sensitivity of measuring plasma concentrations of drugs, it has been possible to establish 'minimum effective analgesic concentrations' for some opioids including pethidine and morphine. These effective plasma concentrations are relatively constant for an individual patient but vary widely between patients. In addition, there is enormous pharmacokinetic variability in response to i.m. injections and therefore, as shown in Figure 22.1, there may be pain breakthrough between periods of analgesia with the conventional method of pain relief, viz. intermittent intramuscular injection.

It is customary to prescribe antiemetics simultaneously on demand as most opioids cause nausea to a greater or lesser degree.

Intramuscular opioids

Intramuscular administration of opioids on a 'PRN' (as required) basis is the method used most commonly for prescribing postoperative analgesia. However, this often fails to provide adequate pain relief. Intramuscular injection may result in variable absorption, particularly in the patient with poor

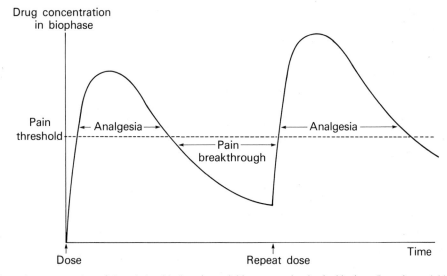

Fig. 22.1 Schematic representation of the relationship between opioid concentration in the biophase (bound to opioid receptors) and time after i.m. injection. Analgesia results only if the biophase concentration exceeds the 'pain threshold' concentration, which varies in different patients.

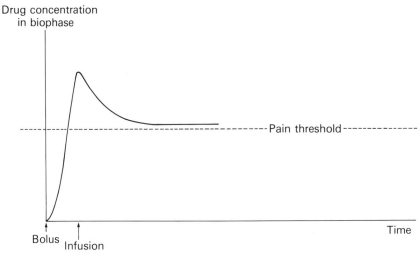

Fig. 22.2 Schematic representation of opioid concentration in the biophase after an i.v. bolus injection followed by a continuous i.v. infusion which maintains the biophase concentration above the 'pain threshold'.

peripheral perfusion. Patients may be unaware of the availability of analgesia; availability should be stressed by the anaesthetist during the preoperative visit. There may be a considerable delay between the request for analgesia and administration while controlled drugs are checked and drawn into a syringe. Because absorption from muscle is relatively slow, a further delay occurs between administration and onset of effective analgesia. Thus, there may be prolonged periods of 'breakthrough' pain if analgesics are prescribed on a 'PRN' basis (Fig. 22.1).

Regular administration of i.m. opioids provides improved analgesia, although care must be taken to avoid overdosage in debilitated patients and those at the extremes of age.

Continuous intravenous opioids

Continuous i.v. administration of opioids, although less convenient than the i.m. route, may provide considerable benefits and is attracting increasing interest. In general terms, a loading dose (or fast infusion) is used initially to generate a therapeutically effective concentration of drug which is maintained by a slow infusion using accurate equipment such as a motor driven syringe pump (Fig. 22.2). For an average 70 kg man a loading dose of 10–15 mg of papaveretum and an infusion of 4–20 mg/h may be required It must be stressed that there is enormous variation in individual response (2 to 10-fold). Results from this technique are generally good, and titration

of analgesia is possible with patient co-operation. However, this technique demands close monitoring, particularly of the cardiovascular and respiratory systems, and the patient must be nursed in a high dependency unit.

Patient-controlled methods. Bolus administration of i.v. opioids on a patient demand basis has been used successfully with devices such as the 'Cardiff Palliator' (Fig. 22.3). This system comprises an accurate source of infusion, coupled to an i.v. cannula and controlled by a patient–machine interface device (Fig. 22.4). Safety features are incorporated in the design which limit the preset dose and the number of doses which can be administered, and provide a mandatory time period between doses and a means of

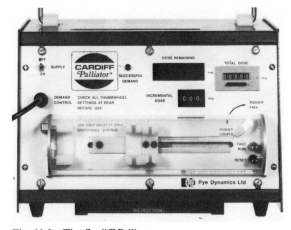

Fig. 22.3 The Cardiff Palliator

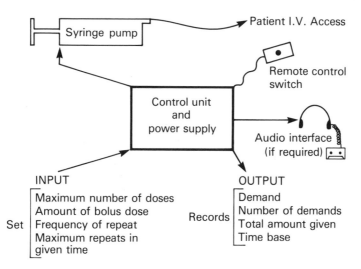

Fig. 22.4 Schematic diagram of a patient-controlled analgesia device.

avoiding accidental triggering. Detailed information is given to the patient prior to operation and on awakening he has the ability to administer a bolus of analgesic on demand — usually by a push-button or similar control. Time limits and dosage are preset according to the drug used. This system has been used principally with pethidine, delivering boluses of approx. 10–20 mg (for a 70 kg patient). Kinetically, this technique may allow pain breakthrough on an intermittent basis. When a patient falls asleep, administration of drug ceases, and analgesic levels decrease. On awakening, he may be in considerable pain, but the safety mechanisms prevent him from administering an adequate number of doses to produce analgesic plasma levels of drug. To eliminate this problem, other designs (Fig. 22.5) incorporate a

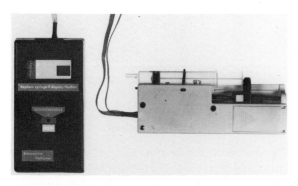

Fig. 22.5 A small, battery driven, patient-controlled device delivering a basal continuous infusion and patient-triggered bolus injection.

low background level of infusion which may be patient-supplemented on an intermittent basis. Other devices currently available incorporate respiratory monitoring and infusion cut-outs, and patient interaction devices with a cassette/headphone system.

Sublingual opioids

A technique increasing in popularity is the use of the sublingual route for opioid administration. Most experience has been gained using buprenorphine. Although sublingual administration requires alert co-operation, good analgesia can be provided without injections, making this route popular with patients and convenient for nursing staff.

Sublingual buprenorphine has a gradual onset and offset with a kinetic profile similar to oral administration, and as buprenorphine-receptor dissociation is slow, its duration of action exceeds twice that of morphine.

As buprenorphine is a partial agonist, it may cause dysphoria and withdrawal phenomena if mixed with an agonist such as morphine, if, for example, one has been used intraoperatively and the other is prescribed in the postoperative period. Hence, it is preferable when using buprenorphine to use it exclusively.

Oral opioids

Oral opioids may be used in patients capable of swallowing. Slow release morphine sulphate provides

Table 22.4 Drugs used systemically for postoperative pain relief and antiemesis

Drug		Dose i.m. (healthy 70 kg patient)
Opioids		
Morphine		10 mg 4 hrly
Papaveretum		20 mg 4 hrly
Pethidine		100 mg 3 hrly
Buprenorphine	(sublingual)	0.4 mg 6 hrly
Antiemetics		
Prochlorperazine		12.5 mg 6 hrly
Perphenazine		5 mg 6 hrly
Cyclizine Tartrate		50 mg 6 hrly
Metoclopramide		10 mg 6 hrly
Moderate analgesics		
Pentazocine		60 mg 4 hrly
Dihydrocodeine		50 mg 4 hrly

satisfactory analgesia lasting 6–8 h, although longer periods have been claimed.

Because drug is lost in first pass metabolism, drug concentrations are lower after oral than after i.v. administration of the same dose.

Doses of systemic drugs used commonly in alleviation of postoperative pain are summarised in Table 22.4.

Problems with opioids. Jaundice has been reported following the use of opioids. However, this is likely to result from poor aseptic techniques after parenteral administration and there is little evidence to suggest delayed toxicity from breakdown products or conjugated derivatives following clinical dosage of opioids.

The most common problems found with normal use of opioids are nausea and vomiting.

Respiratory depression has been well documented, although its presence is not always noticeable.

Psychotomimetic effects occur. These are usually dose-related and in general are seen more commonly with n-allyl derivatives (e.g. pentazocine).

Muscular rigidity may be encountered, particularly with fentanyl, although it may also occur with pethidine.

Constipation is well known following opioid use and is a particular problem with oral administration of codeine.

In the field of postoperative pain relief, the time course of opioid use is short enough to minimise the problem of drug dependence.

Morphine and papaveretum are known to cause release of histamine which make their use inadvisable in asthmatic patients. Morphine may cause spasm of the sphincter of Oddi and should be used with caution after biliary surgery.

All opioids may reduce arterial pressure to some extent and degrees of sedation vary between individual drugs. Meptazinol, a recently developed opioid, is claimed to have little sedative action and only slight respiratory depression, but otherwise is similar to pethidine.

Claims have been made for the improved efficacy of opioids when administered in combination with other drugs. Evidence exists that morphine is more effective as an analgesic when combined with diazepam, probably because of the simultaneous treatment of the affective component of pain. Other mixtures of drugs which have been used for analgesia include morphine combined with hydroxyzine and dexamphetamine.

Nefopam hydrochloride, a new analgesic compound unrelated chemically to the benzomorphinan class (which comprises morphine, pethidine and pentazocine) appears to be free from the problems of addiction and respiratory depression, while analgesic potency is reported to be good. This agent is still in the early stages of clinical evaluation.

Nonopioid drugs

Other systemic agents which may be useful, especially in the later postoperative period, include the anti-inflammatory drugs, e.g. phenylbutazone and aspirin, or their more recent derivatives, including the new antiprostaglandin agents, e.g. diclofenac, ketoprofen.

In addition, the anaesthetist should consider the continuing effect of opioids administered as part of the anaesthetic technique, which may provide analgesia continuing into the early postoperative period. Some volatile anaesthetic agents, e.g. trichloroethylene, may provide an analgesic effect for a short time postoperatively

Local and regional techniques

Direct injection of local anaesthetic agents close to peripheral nerves or major nerve trunks or nerve roots may produce analgesia by blocking the conduction of afferent impulses. Opioids injected into the subarachnoid or extradural spaces also produce profound analgesia by an action on opioid receptors in the substantia gelatinosa of the spinal cord.

Methods using local anaesthetic drugs

Spinal nerve block. Conduction block of nerve roots adjacent to the spinal cord can be achieved either by the subarachnoid or extradural route. Subarachnoid anaesthesia may provide analgesia in the immediate postoperative period, particularly if local anaesthetic agents of prolonged duration are used, e.g. bupivacaine. However, repeated lumbar punctures would be required to produce a continuing block.

Extradural anaesthesia is more useful in the postoperative patient because a catheter can be introduced safely into the extradural space (see p. 325) and repeated injections made as required.

Bupivacaine by the extradural route may produce analgesia lasting up to 4 h from a single dose. Bupivacaine plain 0.25% injected at L2–3 provides good analgesia following lower abdominal or perineal surgery, e.g. hysterectomy or transurethral resection of prostate. Upper abdominal procedures require a higher block. Approx. 15 ml of 0.5% bupivacaine produces analgesia up to T7.

Etidocaine is a newer agent which also has a long duration of action and has been used extradurally. Profound motor blockade accompanies its sensory effects.

Very careful patient monitoring is required following subarachnoid or extradural anaesthesia because of the risk of hypotension from sympathetic blockade, and respiratory arrest by excessive cephalad spread of local anaesthetic agent. Continuous infusions have been used into the extradural space but have gained little popularity.

Caudal block. Caudal administration of local anaesthetic drugs is extremely useful for child day-case surgery, e.g. circumcision, or in patients undergoing anal or perineal surgery. Suitable dosage of local anaesthetic solutions for use by the caudal route are described in Table 22.5.

Table 22.5 Doses of bupivacaine for caudal analgesia

	Adult	Child
Bupivacaine 0.25% plain	0.3–0.4 ml/kg	0.5–0.7 ml/kg (or 0.1 ml/yr/segment ±0.2 ml)

N.B. Dosage of bupivacaine should *never* exceed 2 mg/kg

Other regional blocks. Paravertebral blocks may be used to provide analgesia after thoracic or abdominal surgery. Local anaesthetic solution is injected into the region of the paravertebral space to block the dorsal sensory nerve roots as they emerge from the vertebral foramina. This technique may be performed using single or repeated injections, or with an indwelling catheter for repeat dosage.

Intercostal blockade can be achieved by injection (usually at the angle of the rib) of the intercostal nerves as they pass around the chest wall beneath the inferior border at the ribs. Pneumothorax is a particular risk and bilateral block is not recommended. Some spread of analgesia occurs across dermatomes, but in general multiple blocks are necessary. For example, a block used for pain relief after subcostal incision (e.g. cholecystectomy) requires blocks of T4–8 or 9 to provide satisfactory results.

It is vital to have access to an i.v. route with all techniques involving local anaesthetics, as inadvertent intravascular injection may precipitate cardiovascular and respiratory collapse.

Local nerve block. Other techniques involving local anaesthetics include the individual nerve blocks, e.g. sciatic, ulnar, etc. Bupivacaine or etidocaine have an action of sufficient duration to provide analgesia during the immediate postoperative period. This is useful particularly in orthopaedic procedures where a nerve block is often appropriate intraoperatively. Dorsal nerve block of the penis may be used for analgesia following circumcision.

Methods using opioids

The use of opioids by the subarachnoid or extradural routes has increased rapidly in recent years. There appears to be great variation in individual response, the dose required, and the occurrence of unwanted side-effects. Drugs used commonly by these routes include morphine, pethidine and fentanyl, although other opioids are under investigation. It is essential to use drug solutions free of preservative. (The commonly available opioid solutions for systemic use include a preserving agent which is neurotoxic.)

Opioids by extradural or subarachnoid routes tend to give generalised analgesia irrespective of the level of injection, unlike local anaesthetics where the level of injection and volume of solution determine the level of subsequent analgesia. There is variation in the delay before onset of analgesia with different opioid drugs, which may result from differences in lipid solubility or transport within the cerebrospinal fluid. The dura mater itself provides a barrier to transport. Thus, extradural opioids are administered in higher doses than those required by the subarachnoid route.

A cause of considerable concern is the occurrence of delayed respiratory depression which may take place up to 18 h after injection of spinal opioids. Thus close monitoring is mandatory. It is thought that the action of opioids in this respect is a function of their binding to opioid receptors in the spinal cord, and any delay in onset is likely to be a reflection of delays in transport to this site and subsequent receptor occupancy. The respiratory depression, but not the analgesia, is reversed by naloxone.

Doses of opioid drugs used by subarachnoid and extradural routes are indicated in Table 22.6. A

Table 22.6 Opioid drugs used by subarachnoid and extradural routes

Route	Drug	Dose	Duration
Subarachnoid	Morphine	0.5–1 mg	up to 18 h
Extradural	Morphine	2–5 mg	up to 24 h
	Pethidine	25–50 mg	1–2 h
	Fentanyl	0.1 mg	2–4 h
	Phenoperidine	1 mg	2–4 h
	Diamorphine	2.5 mg	up to 12 h

All values are quoted for a healthy 70 kg patient, injectate volume of 5–15 ml, for analgesia following abdominal surgery.

combination of local anaesthetic and opioid techniques may be employed. A mixture of local anaesthetic and opioid drugs may be injected intrathecally to provide a potent regional nerve block during operation, and analgesia for 24–48 h in the postoperative period. It may be preferable to insert an extradural catheter preoperatively, and to use extradural injection of a local anaesthetic agent for intraoperative regional anaesthesia, followed by opioid injections, repeated as necessary, to provide postoperative analgesia. The use of both techniques requires careful monitoring in a high-dependency unit.

Intraoperative techniques

Certain manoeuvres during operation may provide analgesia in the postoperative period. Surgical nerve section has been used at thoracotomy. Intercostal nerves are transected, resulting in analgesia in the region of the incision. Destruction of nerves using cryotechniques has been reported. The nerve is surrounded by an ice ball produced by intense subzero temperatures at the end of a probe. The neuronal disruption produced by this method is temporary, and sensation returns after some months although it may be accompanied by unpleasant paraesthesiae which may lead to persistent neuralgia.

Miscellaneous

Ice packs have been used in dentistry and may add to analgesia following wisdom tooth extraction.

Acupuncture should be mentioned, but for details readers are referred to monographs on the subject.

Transcutaneous electrical stimulation has been used with varying degrees of success. A small alternating current is passed between two surface electrodes at low voltage and at frequencies between 0.2 and 200 Hz. Evidence is accumulating that this technique acts by increasing c.s.f. levels of endorphins, particularly β-endorphin. Acupuncture appears to work in a similar way. However, it is likely that both methods also involve activation of the 'pain gate' (see p. 93) via counter irritation. Currently, pharmacological evaluation is taking place of parenteral administration of synthetic endorphin analogues. However, most of these appear to be metabolised quickly. At least four opioid receptors exist, some of which appear to offer the possibility of analgesia without untoward side-effects if suitable ligands can be found.

Problems

Sporadic pain resulting from contraction of smooth muscle, e.g. tubal spasm following laparoscopy, may be relieved by drugs such as hyoscine bromide. Dental pain may be particularly difficult to relieve and anti-inflammatory analgesics are often useful.

Special consideration should be given to painful procedures during the postoperative period (e.g. chest physiotherapy after laparotomy), and additional short-term analgesia may be needed to cover these, e.g. an opioid i.v. or Entonox inhalation.

Phantom limb pain following amputation may be very difficult to manage. Even cordotomy may not provide relief and systemic analgesics are of little value.

FURTHER READING

Beecher H 1959 Measurement of subjective responses. Oxford University Press

Bond M 1979 Physical and psychological methods of relieving pain. In: Pain — its nature, analysis and treatment, part 3. Churchill Livingstone, Edinburgh

Bullingham R 1982 Extradural and intrathecal narcotics. In: Atkinson R S, Langton Hewer C (eds) Recent advances in anaesthesia and analgesia, 14. Churchill Livingstone, Edinburgh

Covino B, Smith G 1984 Acute pain. Butterworths, London

Laurence D 1980 Clinical pharmacology, 5th edn. Churchill Livingstone 1980, Edinburgh

Mendelson G 1977 Acupuncture analgesia — a review of clinical studies. Australian and New Zealand Journal of Medicine 7: 642

Smith G 1984 Pain — general perspectives. In: Nimmo W S, Smith G (eds) Opioid agonists and agonists/antagonists. Excerpta Medica, Amsterdam

Smith G 1984 Postoperative pain. In: Lunn J (ed) The quality of care in anaesthetic practice, MacMillan, London

Vickers M, Schnieden H, Wood-Smith F 1984 Systemic analgesics. In: Drugs in anaesthetic practice, 6th edn. Butterworths, London

White D C 1982 Relief of postoperative pain. In: Atkinson R S, Langton Hewer C (eds) Recent advances in anaesthesia and analgesia, 14. Churchill Livingstone, Edinburgh

23

Local anaesthetic techniques

Local anaesthesia techniques used most commonly by trainee anaesthetists include subarachnoid block (SAB), (also termed spinal anaesthesia), extradural block (also termed epidural block), brachial plexus block and intravenous regional analgesia (also termed Bier's block) and these will be described briefly in this chapter. For a description of other local anaesthetic blocks, the reader should consult the standard textbooks, e.g. *Regional Block* by Moore, *Illustrated Handbook in Local Anaesthesia* by Eriksson.

Local anaesthesia may be used as an alternative or as an adjunct to general anaesthesia. The use of long-acting local anaesthetic drugs produces useful analgesia in the immediate postoperative period and this may be extended by the use of catheter techniques (especially with extradural block) into the whole of the postoperative period.

SPINAL ANAESTHESIA (SAB)

Spinal anaesthesia is produced by the injection of local anaesthetic solution into the subarachnoid space where it mixes with c.s.f.

The specific gravity (Sp. gr.) of c.s.f. is 1.004. The majority of local anaesthetic solutions used for performing SAB are of sp. gr. 1.024 or greater as a result of mixing with 5% or 6% dextrose, and are termed *hyperbaric* solutions. Although *hypobaric* solutions are described, these generally behave in the subarachnoid space as if they were *isobaric* with respect to c.s.f.

The movement of hyperbaric solutions within the subarachnoid space is determined by gravity, and the anaesthetist must take into account the position adopted by the patient and the curvature of the spinal cord (Fig. 23.1). As lumbar puncture is performed at

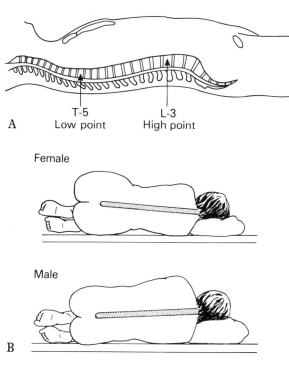

A T-5 Low point   L-3 High point

Female

Male

B

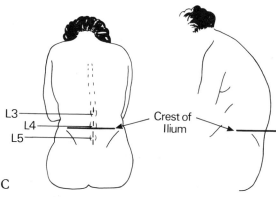

L3
L4
L5   Crest of Ilium

C

Fig. 23.1 Spinal curvature in (**a**) supine, (**b**) lateral, (**c**) sitting position.

either L3/4 or L4/5, hyperbaric solutions spread both in a caudad and cephalad direction if the patient is in the horizontal position.

Factors influencing the spread of solutions within the c.s.f. are listed in Table 23.1 and are described in greater detail below.

Table 23.1 Factors influencing spread of hyperbaric spinal solutions

Factor	Effect
Position of patient	Sitting position produces perineal block. In lateral position, block more pronounced on dependent side
Spinal curvature	Because of lumbar lordosis, solutions may spread up to T4 with patient horizontal and supine.
Speed of injection	Rapid injections cause dilution with c.s.f. thereby reducing the effect of gravity. Produces a higher level of block but may be less intense.
Barbotage	Dilutes the local anaesthetic, increases the height of block but may reduce the intensity. Vigorous barbotage may produce a solution too weak to produce any block.
Interspace chosen	Higher the interspace, higher the block
Volume of local anaesthetic	Larger volumes produce higher blocks
Dose of drug	The larger the dose and concentration, the more intense the block and the longer the duration.
Sp.gr. of drug	Hyperbaric solutions move under the influence of gravity.
Fixation	The concentration of local anaesthetic decreases below a blocking concentration after 15–20 min. Subsequent alteration in patient's position does not cause further spread of block.

Physiological effects

Differential nerve blockade

As spinal anaesthetic solutions spread away from the site of injection the concentration of the solution declines as mixing with c.s.f. occurs. Since small fibres are blocked by weaker concentrations of local anaesthetic solution, a differential blockade of fibres occurs. Sympathetic fibres are blocked to a level two segments higher than the upper segmental level of sensory blockade. Motor blockade tends to extend to within two segments caudal of the upper level of sensory block. Thus sensory levels of spinal anaesthesia to T3 are associated with total blockade of the T1–L2 sympathetic outflow.

Respiratory system

Low spinal blocks have no effect on the respiratory system and thus the technique is used frequently for patients with chest disease.

Blocks extending as high as the roots of the phrenic nerve (C 3.4.5) cause total apnoea.

Blocks reaching the thoracic level cause loss of intercostal muscle activity. Total loss of intercostal activity has little effect on tidal volume (because of diaphragmatic compensation) but there is a marked decrease in vital capacity resulting from a 48% decrease in expiratory reserve volume. However, a thoracic block leads to reduction in cardiac output and pulmonary artery pressure, and increased ventilation/perfusion imbalance results in a decrease in Pa_{O_2}. Thus awake patients with a high spinal block should always be given oxygen-enriched air to breathe.

Cardiovascular system

The cardiovascular effects are proportional to the height of the block and result from denervation of the sympathetic outflow tracts (T1 to L2). This produces dilatation of resistance and capacitance vessels resulting in hypotension. In awake patients, compensatory vasoconstriction above the height of the block may compensate almost completely for these changes, thereby maintaining arterial pressure, but loss of consciousness produced by the smallest dose of anaesthetic drug may abolish this compensation with consequent profound hypotension.

Hypotension is augmented by: (a) the use of head-up posture; (b) any degree of hypovolaemia — pre-existing or induced by surgery.

It is common practice to minimise hypotension during spinal or extradural anaesthesia by 'preloading' the patient with 500–1000 ml of Hartmann's solution i.v. before or during the institution of the block. This compensates for the 'relative' hypovolaemia induced by increased capacitance of the circulation.

Bradycardia may occur because of: (a) Neurogenic factors in awake patients, i.e. vasovagal syndrome; (b) block of the cardiac sympathetic fibres (T1–T4).

SAB has no direct effect on the liver or kidneys, but reductions in hepatic and renal blood flow occur in the presence of hypotension associated with high spinal blocks.

Gastro-intestinal system

The vagus nerve supplies parasympathetic fibres to the whole of the gut as far as the transverse colon. Thus a spinal or extradural anaesthetic causes sympathetic denervation (proportional to height of block) and unopposed parasympathetic action leading to a constricted gut with increased peristaltic activity. This is regarded by some as advantageous for surgery.

Nausea, retching or vomiting may occur in the awake patient and are produced by: (a) unopposed parasympathetic activity; (b) hypotension.

If nausea or retching occurs, the anaesthetist must measure arterial pressure and heart rate immediately and take appropriate measures.

Indications for SAB anaesthesia

Sympathetic, sensory and motor blockade may be produced more consistently with a lower dose of drug than extradural block. However, it is not customary in Europe to use catheters in the subarachnoid space (unlike the extradural) and therefore prolonged analgesia cannot be produced. SAB is most suited to surgery below the umbilicus and in this situation a patient may remain awake. Surgery above the umbilicus in the presence of a SAB generally necessitates a general anaesthetic in addition in order to abolish unpleasant sensations from visceral manipulation resulting from afferent impulses transmitted by the vagus nerves.

Uses

1. For prostatectomy where a 'bloodless' field is desired.

2. For open · prostatectomy and gynaecological surgery, in combination with the Trendelenburg position and usually a general anaesthetic.

3. For rapid onset of analgesia in obstetrics, e.g. forceps delivery, removal of retained placenta. Extradural analgesia is less predictable and has a slower onset of action.

4. For patients with medical problems, a low SAB may be the anaesthetic of choice, e.g.

   a. Metabolic disease — diabetes mellitus, thyrotoxicosis.

   b. Respiratory disease — a low SAB has no effect on respiration and obviates the use of anaesthetic drugs with respiratory depressant properties. Active cough reflexes during surgery may be important in maintaining a clear chest.

   c. Cardiovascular disease — a low SAB may be ideal for patients with ischaemic heart disease or congestive failure in whom a small reduction in preload and afterload may be beneficial. SAB is highly effective in preventing cardiovascular responses to surgery e.g. hypertension, tahycardia, which are undesirable, particulary in patients with ischaemic heart disease.

5. For vaginal or operative obstetric delivery (Table 23.2), where general anaesthesia has particular risks (see Chapter 31).

Contraindications to SAB and extradural anaesthesia

1. Anticoagulant therapy — an absolute contra-indication.

2. Hypovolaemia.

3. Increased likelihood of contamination with skin organisms:

   a. sepsis on skin of back:

   b. colostomy, ileostomy.

4. Emergency abdominal surgery, particularly patients with intestinal obstruction. These patients are often dehydrated and surgical incisions may extend above the umbilicus.

5. Pre-eclamptic toxaemia. Although extradural analgesia has been used in this condition, there may be a platelet count of less than 100×10^9/litre and this usually precludes extradural or subarachnoid analgesia.

6. Active bacterial or viral infections of the peripheral or central nervous system. However, SAB and extradural analgesia are not contraindicated by the presence of *Herpes zoster* infections or by the presence of genital herpes. In these conditions, viraemia is associated only with primary infection.

7. Chronic neurological disease, disseminated sclerosis, peripheral neuropathy, and poliomyelitis. Resurgence of neurological signs may be ascribed to the spinal anaesthetic.

Performance of spinal block (Fig. 23.2)

1. Preoperative visit. This allows:

   a. Selection of patients who would benefit from this technique.
   b. Careful explanation of the procedure to the patient.
   c. Assessment of the patient's cardiovascular, haematological, and respiratory status.

2. An intravenous infusion must be instituted through a large i.v. cannula before lumbar puncture is performed. Preloading with crystalloid solutions reduces hypotension but caution must be exercised in patients with congestive cardiac failure or if the bladder is to be filled with glycine solutions prior to cystoscopy.

3. Correct positioning of the patient. This aids rapid performance of lumbar puncture. If positioning is likely to be painful (e.g. fracture of femur) ketamine 0.5 mg/kg may be given i.v. prior to positioning. The positions in which patients may be placed are summarised in Table 23.3.

4. A full sterile technique (with gown, gloves and surgical drapes) is adopted. All drugs should be drawn into syringes directly from sterile ampoules which are double wrapped and autoclaved only once. Repeated autoclaving reduces the efficacy of heavy cinchocaine.

5. Selection of spinal needles 22 G and 25 G should be available. A diamond point or pencil point Whitacre needle (with side holes) may be used. Disposable introducer needles (18 G) are used, particularly with a 25G spinal needle, for bracing the spinal needle and reducing contamination of the spinal needle tip by skin.

6. Selection of drug: bupivacaine 0.5% plain may be used as an isobaric spinal solution. Two commercial hyperbaric solutions are available in the U.K.: cinchocaine 5 mg/ml in 5% dextrose and mepivacaine 4% in dextrose 9.5%. The duration of action is similar ($1\frac{1}{2}$–$2\frac{1}{2}$ h).

7. Selection of block. Classically, five types of block exist using hyperbaric solutions (see Table 23.3).

8. Spread of spinal analgesic solution (Table 23.1). The specific gravity, viscosity and temperature of the spinal solution and speed of injection modify the spread of solution in c.s.f. Barbotage (the repeated aspiration of c.s.f. into the syringe containing local analgesic drug, and reinjection) is not employed at the

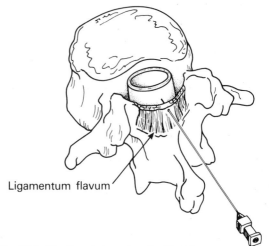

Fig. 23.2 Needle entering subarachnoid space.

Ligamentum flavum

present time. In the lateral decubitus position the presence of a markedly gynaecoid pelvis leads to tilting of the spine and cephalad spread of hyperbaric spinal solutions. With the patient supine, the thoracic curvature of the spine leads to pooling of the solution and limitation of the level of block to T4. If the level of puncture site chosen is on the sacral side of the lumbar curvature, confinement of the solution to the sacral roots is likely on placing the patient supine (Fig. 23.1). A lumbar lordosis may be eliminated by asking the patient to flex the hips once the supine position has been assumed.

9. Vasopressors should be available. Ephedrine is the best choice because it combines chronotropic and inotropic effects with vasoconstriction. The dose of ephedrine is 10–15 mg i.v. initially followed by 5 mg aliquots. Agents with pure α-stimulating effects, e.g. methoxamine, are not indicated initially but may be used if ephedrine fails to produce the desired response. Small doses of methoxamine (2 mg) should be used, as in this situation, patients tend to be sensitive to pure α-stimulants. Ephedrine, 30–50 mg i.m. has been employed prophylactically before instituting a block.

10. Monitoring: patients who are nervous or who become hypotensive during spinal analgesia are prone to bradycardia. Measurement of arterial pressure and heart rate and monitoring of e.c.g. is mandatory. Increased vigilance is required if the patient's posture is changed rapidly, e.g. during a change from lithotomy to supine position.

Table 23.2 Spinal anaesthetic techniques in obstetrics

Procedure	Comments	Type of block	Upper level of analgesia	Volume of hyperbaric cinchocaine (ml)
Vaginal delivery	Pain from uterine contractions not affected	Saddle block	S1	0.6–0.8
Vaginal delivery	Pain from uterine action abolished. Abdominal muscles relaxed.	Medium spinal block	T10	1
Caesarean section	Beware of hypotension. Large volumes of crystalloid solutions, e.g. Ringer lactate, may be required to prevent hypotension. Ephedrine if necessary.	High spinal block	T7–T6	1.2–1.5

Table 23.3 Techniques of spinal anaesthesia (SAB). The volumes of other hyperbaric spinal solutions are similar to those shown for cinchocaine

Type of block	Upper level of analgesia	Surgical indications	Position during lumbar puncture	Optimal puncture site	Volume of hyperbaric cinchocaine (ml)
Saddle block	S1	Cystoscopy External genitalia (not testes) Perineal/anal surgery	Sitting. Maintain for 5 min and do not tilt head down for 15-min (period of fixation)	L4–5 L5–S1	0.8–1
Low spinal anaesthesia	L1–T12	Above plus lower extremities and transurethral prostatectomy	Sitting or lateral decubitus	L3–L4	1–1.2
Medium spinal anaesthesia	T10–T8	Lower abdominal surgery Hernia not involving intra-abdominal manipulations. Open prostatectomy Appendicectomy Hip surgery	Sitting or lateral decubitus	L3–L4 L2–L3	1.2–1.5
High spinal anaesthesia	T4	All abdominal surgery	lateral decubitus	L2–L3	1.5–2
Unilateral	Intended to minimise sympathetic blockade. Probably impossible to achieve in practice. May be present at 5 min postinitiation of block but block usually develops to bilateral after a further 15 min.				

Spinal needles

Choice of needle gauge is influenced by two factors:

1. The relationship between needle gauge and postspinal headache. The incidence of postspinal headache is related to needle size. 18 G needles are associated with a 75% incidence in young patients whilst the use of a 25 G needle reduces the incidence to 1 to 2%. Parturient patients are particularly prone to develop spinal headache and a 25 G needle is mandatory.

2. Pathology or ageing of the vertebrae and ligaments. The elderly patient may have calcified supraspinous ligaments (necessitating a lateral

approach to the subarachnoid space) or may have collapsed vertebrae or a lordotic or scoliotic spine which mitigate against successful lumbar puncture. In general, greater success is achieved with the larger, stiffer 22 G needle than the 25 G. Fortunately, the elderly have a low incidence of headache following spinal analgesia.

Complications

Acute

1. Hypotension — significant hypotension should be anticipated with SAB. Although a saddle block should produce no change in arterial pressure, fixation of the block (see Table 23.1) takes 15–20 min and a head-down posture within this period may lead to sympathetic block.

2. Phantom limb pain may occur for the first time in amputees under SAB .

3. Severe itching in patients with disseminated sclerosis or diabetic neuropathy.

4. Patient confusion in respect of limb position.

Middle term

1. Headache — spinal headache normally occurs 2–7 days after lumbar puncture and may persist for up to 6 weeks. It should be treated initially by conservative means — bed rest, large fluid intake, analgesics; subsequently by the use of extradural infusion of sterile saline, and if these measures fail, the use of an extradural blood patch.

2. Urinary retention — frequently associated with the surgical procedure.

3. Labyrinthine disturbances.

4. Cranial nerve palsy. VI nerve palsy may occur and is usually temporary. More common with larger needles.

5. Meningitis and meningism.

6. Transverse myelitis and cauda equina syndrome resulting from adhesive arachnoiditis. Fortunately these conditions, giving rise to permanent neurological damage or paraplegia, are extremely rare.

EXTRADURAL (EPIDURAL) BLOCK

Extradural blockade may be performed in the sacral (caudal block), lumbar, thoracic, or cervical regions. The commonest route employed is the lumbar. The thoracic route is useful for abdominal or thoracic surgery particularly when a catheter is used to provide postoperative analgesia.

Although extradural block is similar in many respects to subarachnoid block, there are important differences and these are summarised in Table 23.4.

Table 23.4 Differences between subarachnoid and extradural block

	SAB	Extradural
Dose of drug employed	Small. The drug has no action other than within the spinal cord	Large. Systemic absorption occurs with possible c.n.s. effects (drowsiness or fits) and cardiovascular effects (myocardial depression and peripheral dilatation)
Rate of onset of action	Fast — 2–8 min	Slow: 20–40 min
Site of action	On spinal cord and spinal nerve roots	Various: 1. Diffusion across dura into c.s.f. 2. Diffusion into c.s.f. via spinal nerve root dural cuffs 3. Paravertebral nerve blocks
Success rate	100% if lumbar puncture successful	Missed segments, total failure not uncommon
Extent of block	May be extensive — dependent on positioning	Dependent on *dose* injected (rather than volume) Position of patient has small effect.
Intensity of block	May be complete	Rarely complete block of all nerve pathways
Segmental block	No	Yes
Addition of vasoconstrictor	Prolongs block in lumbar and sacral segments. With lignocaine and bupivacaine effects are variable in individual patients. With amethocaine block is prolonged reliably with phenylephrine but not with adrenaline	Prolongs block with lignocaine. No significant effect with bupivacaine

Anatomy

The anatomy of the extradural space is described in detail in Chapter 1.

Physiological effects

The physiological effects of extradural blockade are similar to those following SAB. However, there may be important differences resulting from the much larger volumes of anaesthetic solutions used, as there is appreciable systemic absorption leading to myocardial depression. These effects are complicated by the use of adrenaline-containing solutions.

In summary the cardiovascular effects comprise:

1. A reduction in cardiac output with plain solutions but an increase with adrenaline-containing solutions.
2. A reduction in heart rate with plain solutions but maintenance of heart rate or tachycardia with adrenaline-containing solutions.
3. A greater decrease in mean and diastolic arterial pressures with adrenaline than with plain solutions (although systolic arterial pressure may be greater with adrenaline-containing solutions).
4. Extremely severe myocardial depression with plain solutions in the presence of haemorrhagic hypovolaemia — this is much less marked with adrenaline-containing solutions.

Indications

1. Cervical: chronic pain relief.
2. Thoracic: pain relief. Postoperatively following thoracotomy or upper abdominal surgery. Local analgesic or opioid drugs may be used. Opioids are used frequently in the management of chest injury with fractured ribs.
3. Lumbar:
   a. Continuous extradural analgesia in obstetric pain relief.
   b. To reduce blood loss during pelvic surgery. Venodilatation is produced. Thus if the operative site is positioned above the level of the right atrium, veins empty and bleeding tends to be reduced.
   c. To produce constriction of the gut (by the same mechanism as SAB — vide supra). Extradural analgesia facilitates the execution of procedures including total cystectomy by providing better access to the bladder and reduced blood loss.
   d. The use of neostigmine following neuromuscular blocking agents leads to increased leakage from gut anastomoses whilst extradural analgesia provides muscular relaxation and obviates the need for anticholinesterases at termination of anaesthesia.

Intraoperative

1. As sole technique: suitable for transurethral procedures, hernia repair and anal surgery.
2. In combination with i.v. drugs: premedication with moderate doses of papaveretum i.v. When a satisfactory block has been established, sedation during operation should be provided by opioid analgesic drugs since an extradural technique may fail to block all segments.
3. In combination with general anaesthesia for major surgery. Only light anaesthesia is required as extradural block provides analgesia and muscular relaxation. In addition blood loss is reduced and the block may be continued to provide postoperative analgesia, providing adequate supervision is available.

If a steep head-down tilt is anticipated, extradural block should be accompanied by light general anaesthesia.

Vasovagal episodes may occur in awake supine patients undergoing surgery under local analgesic techniques. Neurogenic factors may cause bradycardia in awake patients even with adequate extradural blockade, whilst light general anaesthesia abolishes these effects.

Equipment

Extradural anaesthesia is performed usually using a Tuohy needle (Fig. 23.3). The needle (8 cm long) is marked at 1-cm intervals and has a Huber point which allows a catheter to be directed along the long axis of the epidural space. The Portex disposable catheter has a blind distal end with terminal side holes.

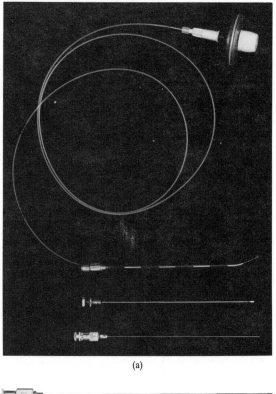

(a)

(b)

Fig. 23.3 (a) 16 G Tuohy extradural needle (above) and 25 G spinal needle (below). Through the extradural needle has been passed a Portex catheter protruding 1 cm beyond the tip of the needle which angulates the catheter upwards. The Tuohy needle is marked at 1 cm intervals. Between the two needles is the stilette for the extradural needle. A bacterial filter is attached to the proximal end of the catheter. (b) Close-up view of Tuohy extradural needle.

Technique of lumbar extradural blockade

Identification of the extradural space

Odom's indicator and Macintosh's balloon rely on the presence of a subatmospheric pressure in the extradural space. However, methods dependent on resistance to injection of air or saline have become the most popular means of identifying the space.

The pressure in the extradural space is not constant, but fluctuates and is least in the thoracic region as a result of communications by valveless veins between the extradural and intrathoracic spaces.

With the patient in the left lateral position, a skin weal is raised with local anaesthetic over the appropriate lumbar interspace and a small skin

incision (2 mm) is made in the centre of the chosen space. The thumb of the left hand is placed on the spine of the vertebra on the cephalad side of the chosen space. This provides a landmark and allows the index finger of the left hand to guide the needle, which is grasped between middle and index finger of the right hand. The right thumb is used to steady the needle. The needle is introduced into the supraspinous ligament, the stilette is removed and a syringe containing air or saline attached firmly. Saline is incompressible and produces a better feel than air when injected. However, the use of saline makes recognition of dural puncture more difficult. The ligamentum flavum is identified, usually by an increased resistance to injection and the extradural space by sudden loss of resistance to injection on subsequent advancement. If prolonged analgesia is required an extradural catheter is inserted; only a 2–3 cm length of catheter is placed in the space. Unilateral block or absence of analgesia may occur if excessive lengths of catheter are inserted through the needle, as the catheter may pass out through an intervertebral foramen.

Should the catheter be aspirated? Extradural veins are fragile and may collapse on application of a large degree of suction. A better method of detecting presence of the catheter in an extradural vein has been suggested. 2–5 ml of saline are injected via the catheter and the proximal end is left open to atmosphere at a level below the patient. The catheter is observed for the presence of blood at the point of entry at the skin. If the catheter is aspirated gently and blood is present, placement in an extradural vein is likely. The catheter should be removed 1 cm and flushed with 5 ml of 0.9% saline. If after 2 min, further aspiration does not produce blood, local analgesic solution is injected through a bacterial filter. If blood is present in the catheter, it is removed and placed in another space.

Aspiration of clear fluid at this stage indicates a dural tap unless saline or local analgesic has been injected into the extradural space prior to catheter placement. If so, the fluid aspirated should be tested for sugar. If dural tap occurs, the needle is removed and a catheter is placed in an adjacent space.

Failure to aspirate c.s.f. at this stage does not exclude the presence of the catheter in the subarachnoid space and a test dose is advocated by many for two purposes: (a) to detect accidental subarachnoid injection; (b) to detect the presence of the catheter in an extradural vein.

The following are suggested test doses: lignocaine 1.5% 4 ml, bupivacaine 0.5% 2 ml. There may be considerable delay in the production of muscular weakness following the use of local analgesics as test doses, even if injected into the subarachnoid space. A test dose designed to produce muscular weakness in, say, 5 min should be similar to the dose employed for SAB. The addition of adrenaline 1:200 000 to the test dose produces tachycardia and hypertension if the catheter is placed in a vein. This effect is rapid in onset, but transient.

Dosage

Pregnancy. Requirement for local analgesic is one-third that of nonpregnant patients.

For abdominal surgery in a 70 kg nonpregnant adult.

	Volume (ml)	Position of patient for block
Lignocaine 1.5%	10–30	Supine
Bupivacaine 0.5%	15–20	Supine
Bupivacaine 0.75%	10–18	Supine

Bupivacaine plain solution 0.75% is recommended for surgical procedures (but *not* in obstetrics) as it causes more profound muscular block than lower concentrations of the drug.

Complications of extradural block

Serious

1. Dural tap leading to:
   a. Total spinal anaesthesia }
   b. Postspinal headache } vide infra
2. Toxicity of local analgesic agents
3. Hypotension. Mechanisms:
   a. Systemic absorption
   b. High sympathetic block
   c. Bradycardia with a sympathetic block to T 1–4
4. Respiratory insufficiency
5. Inadvertent injection of chemical irritants
6. Haematoma formation
7. Extradural abscess
8. Trauma to spinal cord and nerve roots

Less serious

1. Nausea and vomiting
2. Prolonged analgesia or paraesthesia
3. Shivering
4. Horner's syndrome

Very rare

1. Introduction of a foreign body
2. Implantation dermoid

Total spinal anaesthesia. In contrast to SAB, relatively large volumes of solution are used in extradural blockade. Inadvertent injection into the subarachnoid space may:

1. Travel cephalad in the c.s.f. In the supine position, pooling of drug at T5 level (T4 dermatome) tends to occur due to the curvature of the thoracic spine.
2. Cause respiratory failure by phrenic nerve paralysis and by direct medullary depression.
3. Cause severe hypotension.
4. Cause epileptiform convulsions by systemic absorption of drug or by direct spread in c.s.f. to brain.

The possibility of such drastic changes should always be considered in response to either the initial injection or a subsequent 'top-up' injection. Provided skilled resuscitation is undertaken rapidly, a total spinal is always followed by complete recovery, and continuation of surgery is not contraindicated. However, prior to performing an extradural block, the following are *essential*:

1. Resuscitation equipment must be available.
2. An i.v. infusion *must* be established.
3. Vasopressors (ephedrine and methoxamine) should be available.
4. Thiopentone should be available. This is preferred to diazepam as an anticonvulsant.
5. Facility to provide IPPV safely for several hours.
6. Personnel skilled in dealing with the problems caused by total spinal blockade.

Postspinal headache. Postspinal headache occurs in 75% of patients when a 16 or 18 G needle has been used and a dural tap performed. The frequency of this complication can be reduced by employing the following measures:

1. In obstetric practice, c.s.f. leakage is increased by straining during the second stage of labour. This is

minimised if obstetric forceps are used to assist vaginal delivery.

2. When analgesia is no longer required the catheter is left in situ and 1.5 litre of Hartmann's solution is infused over 24 h, via a bacterial filter.

3. The patient is kept well hydrated with oral or i.v. fluids as appropriate.

Anticoagulants and SAB or extradural anaesthesia

The spinal canal acts as a rigid box and an expanding haematoma within the canal compresses the spinal cord, resulting in loss of neurological function unless the compression is relieved at a very early stage by surgery. Decompression within 6 h is completely effective in virtually all patients, but after 12 h is almost totally ineffective.

Bleeding deficiences. 1. Oral anticoagulants. The half life of coumarin-type drugs is 1–4 days and 2–3 weeks for diphenadione so anticoagulation should be stopped at an appropriate time prior to surgery if SAB or extradural anaesthesia is to be used.

2. Platelets. The platelet count should probably be in excess of 150×10^9/litre.

3. Heparin. The half life of heparin given i.v. is 58–160 min depending on dose. When given s.c. blood concentrations vary widely; in some patients plasma levels are in the anticoagulant range. At present it is regarded as imprudent to use SAB or extradural analgesia with 'minihep' regimens.

4. Intraoperative heparinisation. Extradural analgesia and SAB offer advantages for major vascular surgery but the routine use of heparin introduces the theoretical risk of haemorrhage if an extradural catheter is in place. The precise risk is unknown since prospective trials would require in excess of 10 000 cases. Some large series (3000 patients) have been conducted under extradural analgesia without haematoma formation.

BRACHIAL PLEXUS BLOCK

Anatomy

The brachial plexus is enveloped by an extension of the prevertebral fascia from the cervical vertebrae. This sheath extends to the distal axilla.

The anterior scalene muscle arises from the anterior tubercle of the transverse processess of C3, 4, 5 and 6.

This muscle inserts into the scalene tubercle of the first rib, and separates the subclavian vein from the subclavian artery. The artery lies posterior to this insertion. The middle scalene muscle arises from the posterior tubercles of the transverse process of the lower 6th cervical vertebra. Its insertion is separated from the anterior scalene muscle by the subclavian groove along which travels the subclavian artery. (Fig. 23.4).

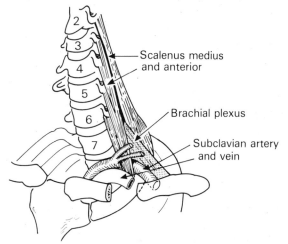

Fig. 23.4 Root of neck.

The roots of the brachial plexus pass out between the anterior and posterior tubercles of the transverse processes of the cervical vertebrae. They travel towards the first rib in the interscalene space formed by the scalene muscles. As the roots pass down through the space they merge to form the trunks of the plexus. Together with the subclavian artery these invaginate the scalene fascia to form the subclavian perivascular sheath which becomes the axillary sheath below the level of the clavicle. The presence of a fibrous envelope from the cervical vertebrae to several centimetres distal to the axilla allows brachial plexus block to be carried out at several levels. The choice of site depends on the distribution of analgesia required, the site of surgery, and the physical state of the patient.

The musculocutaneous nerve supplies an area over the lateral side of the forearm and it arises high in the axilla. The axillary nerve arises from the posterior cord and leaves the neurovascular bundle at the level of the pectoralis muscle. Both nerves may be missed with an axillary block.

The intercostobrachial nerve (T2) supplies the upper inner aspect of the arm and runs superficial to the sheath; it may be a cause of tourniquet pain.

Techniques of brachial plexus block

Axillary approach (Fig. 23.5)

The patient lies supine and places the palm of the hand of the arm to be blocked under the occiput. This allows the upper arm to be abducted 90° from the trunk and the forearm to be pronated. An i.v. cannula is inserted into the back of the opposite hand to provide venous access. The skin of the axilla is cleansed.

The aim of injection is to push the analgesic solution as high as possible into the proximal part of the axillary sheath. Thus injection is made as high in the axilla as possible.

The axillary artery is the landmark for injection. A single injection is made just above the vessel, with the needle inclined cephalad. A definite click may be felt as the sheath is penetrated. Eliciting paraesthesia is not necessary to confirm correct placement of the needle. If a nerve stimulator is used, muscle twitching in the arm indicates correct positioning, although muscle contraction may occur with the exploring needle outside the perivascular sheath if a large voltage is used. When properly positioned, pulsation of the needle is seen and after aspiration to obviate intravascular injection, the analgesic solution is deposited. The volume of solution injected varies with the patient's age, weight, and the level of anaesthesia required; 25–40 ml of solution may be required to produce anaesthesia which includes the musculocutaneous and axillary nerves. 2–3 ml of solution are retained in the syringe and injected subcutaneously as the needle is withdrawn to block the intercostobrachial nerve.

An i.v. infusion extension may be placed between the needle and syringe. This allows pulsation of the needle to be seen and avoids displacement of the needle if the syringe should be changed. The needle used may be a standard 21 or 23 G hypodermic needle, or if a nerve stimulator is employed, an insulated needle should be used which provides an electrical stimulus only at the tip.

The head of the humerus tends to kink the axillary perivascular sheath. This is most pronounced in the position in which the block is performed, i.e. with the arm abducted. Thus, as soon as injection is made, the arm is adducted to lie by the patient's side. Manual compression of the perivascular sheath against the humerus just below the site of injection prevents distal spread of solution and should be instituted at the time of injection and continued for some minutes after the arm is returned to the patient's side.

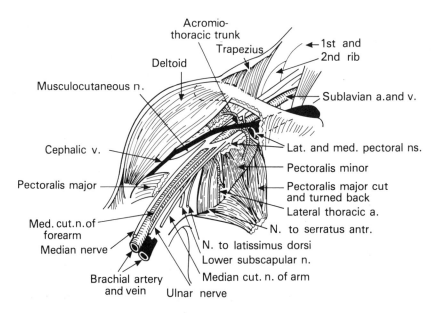

Fig. 23.5 Relations of the brachial plexus in the axilla.

Alternatively, a tourniquet may be placed high in the axilla. Some anaesthetists recommend that the arm should be raised by the patient once the injection has been made. Failure to obtain proximal spread of solution leads to failure to anaesthetise the musculocutaneous and axillary nerves.

Direct block of the musculocutaneous nerve can be made without separate skin puncture by inserting the needle superior to the entire neurovascular bundle and injecting 5 ml of solution into the substance of the coracobrachialis muscle.

Dose. 1. Large males in excess of 80 kg: 25–40 ml of lignocaine or prilocaine 1.5% with adrenaline 1:200 000.

2. Smaller males and females; 20–25 ml of lignocaine or prilocaine 1.5% with adrenaline 1:200 000.

3. Children 19–25 kg: 9–14 ml of prilocaine 1% with adrenaline.

These agents produce analgesia within 20 min and the duration of block is $1\frac{1}{2}$–2 h.

Bupivacaine with adrenaline provides long-lasting blocks which provide postoperative analgesia well into the postoperative period (duration 3–12 h).

Advantages. 1. Obviates phrenic, vagus, recurrent layngeal nerve, and stellate ganglion block which are complications of the supraclavicular routes.

2. Obviates SAB or extradural injection and pneumothorax which may occur with supraclavicular approaches.

3. There is no need to produce paraesthesia, so nerve damage and patient discomfort are avoided.

Disadvantages. 1. Cannot be used if the patient cannot abduct the arm.

2. Large volumes of solution are required (approaching maximum recommended limits).

3. Intravascular injection is possible. Careful aspiration is necessary prior to injection. Severe toxic reactions result if a major portion of the dose is injected into a vessel.

4. The technique may be difficult in obese patients.

5. The method is contraindicated if active infection or malignancy is present in the ipsilateral limb or axilla.

Supraclavicular brachial plexus block

Classical method. This block is performed at the site where the plexus crosses the first rib.

The patient lies with the head turned away from the site of injection. A point is located 1 cm above and immediately lateral to the midpoint of the clavicle. A fine needle, 5 cm in length is inserted at this point inclined at 80° to the skin and directed backwards, inwards and downwards ('b.i.d.'). Paraesthesia indicates contact with the plexus. Firm resistance indicates contact with the first rib. In the absence of paraesthesia the needle is 'walked' along the rib. It is possible to explore all three main divisions of the plexus, producing paraesthesia in the upper and lower arm and both sides of the hand. Eight to 10 ml of 1.5% lignocaine or prilocaine with adrenaline 1:200 000 is injected into each division. The limitations of this technique are as follows:

1. The point of injection often does not lie over the first rib.

2. The incidence of pneumothorax is 0.5–6%.

3. The subclavian perivascular space is deep and very narrow in its anteroposterior dimension. Thus the needle is directed across the space at its narrowest diameter, with reduced chance of successful block.

4. The trunks of the plexus tend to lie one on top of the other not one behind each other in a horizontal plane. Consequently large volumes of solution may be deposited outside the sheath causing block of phrenic, vagus, recurrent layngeal and sympathetic nerves — the last causing Horner's syndrome.

Winnie's perivascular technique. The patient lies with the head turned away from the site of injection. He reaches for his knee, lowers the clavicle and then relaxes the arm and shoulder. On raising the head slightly, the clavicular head of sternomastoid is brought into prominence. Beginning at the lateral border of this muscle the finger explores laterally across the anterior scalene muscle until the interscalene groove is found. This groove is followed towards the clavicle until the subclavian artery is palpated as it emerges from between the scalene muscles. The finger is kept on the artery and a $1\frac{1}{2}$-in 21 G needle is inserted above the finger and directed in a caudal direction only. Thus the needle follows the longest dimension of the interscalene space. A mild click may be felt as the sheath is entered. Paraesthesia, usually in the hand, confirms correct placement of the needle. Twenty ml of local anaesthetic solution provides equivalent motor and sensory loss compared with that produced by 30 ml in the axillary perivascular space. The advantages of this technique are:

1. The possibility of pneumothorax is minimised by use of a short needle, direction of insertion and single injection.

2. The first rib is located reliably.

3. Paraesthesia is often produced before contact with the rib.

4. Smaller doses of local analgesic are required.

5. Inadvertent i.v. injection is unlikely.

6. SAB or extradural block is obviated.

However, it has the following disadvantages:

1. Because of the remote risk of affecting the phrenic or recurrent laryngeal nerves, bilateral blocks should not be undertaken.

2. Paraesthesia should be elicited. This causes the patient discomfort, but if not elicited, reduces the success rate by 15%.

Winnie's interscalene brachial plexus block

The roots of the brachial and cervical plexuses travel between the scalene muscles in the interscalene space. The major part of this space is above the subclavian artery and ideally suited for plexus blockade.

Method. The patient lies with the head turned away from the side of injection. A line is taken from the level of the cricoid cartilage (C6 level) laterally to the interscalene groove which is identified just lateral to sternomastoid. At this point a $1\frac{1}{2}$-in 22 G needle is introduced at right angles to all planes of the skin. The direction of the needle is slightly caudal, posterior and medial. Advancement produces paraesthesia or the needle comes up against the transverse process of cervical vertebrae.

In the adult, 20 ml of solution injected at this level produces anaesthesia of the cervical and brachial plexuses. Ulnar nerve block may be delayed or absent with this volume, but not if the volume is increased to 40 ml. However, a small volume may be combined with ulnar nerve block at the elbow if a minimal dose of drug is required.

Advantages. 1. The block is easier to perform in the obese patient than other approaches to the brachial plexus.

2. Ideal for shoulder manipulations where high

block and good muscle relaxation with small doses are produced.

3. Pneumothorax is obviated.

Disadvantages. 1. Slow onset or absence of ulnar nerve block.

2. SAB and extradural injection may occur.

3. Vertebral artery injection may occur. In this case, the drug is taken straight to the brain. Fatalities have occurred with small volumes of local analgesic solution injected here.

4. Bilateral blockade must be avoided because of frequent phrenic nerve block.

INTRAVENOUS REGIONAL ANALGESIA

This technique depends upon exsanguination of the limb and injection of dilute anaesthetic solution into the vascular compartment where it diffuses to large nerve trunks but also exerts an action at terminal nerve fibres. The method is suitable for analgesia both of upper and of lower limbs. A tourniquet applied to the calf reduces the dose required for analgesia of the distal lower limb.

Technique

An i.v. needle or cannula is placed into a distal vein of the limb which is subsequently exsanguinated and a recently calibrated tourniquet applied. A double cuff may be used to prevent pain under the inflated cuff. The cuff is inflated to 100 mmHg above systolic arterial pressure. Local anaesthetic solution is injected *slowly* into the exsanguinated limb. Rapid injection or the use of a proximal vein result in high intravascular pressures which may exceed the tourniquet pressure and introduce local anaesthetic solution directly into the systemic circulation. Prilocaine is the least toxic and thus the drug of choice.

The duration of analgesia produced by i.v. regional analgesia depends not so much on the potency of the drug injected as on the duration of cuff inflation; thus the use of prilocaine (with a relatively low potency) is appropriate. Accidental bolus injection of prilocaine is associated with rapid clearance from the circulation. The dose of prilocaine is 3 mg/kg of 0.5%

Table 23.5 Volumes of prilocaine for i.v. regional analgesia

Weight of patient (kg)	Dose of prilocaine (mg)	Final injection volume 0.5% solution
70	210	42 ml
60	180	36 ml
50	150	30 ml
40	120	24 ml

plain solution (Table 23.5). Methaemoglobinaemia is not a problem and the drug is less likely to cause c.n.s. toxicity than lignocaine. On i.v. injection, prilocaine leaves the vascular compartment more rapidly than lignocaine or bupivacaine. In general, compounds poorly protein bound, e.g. prilocaine, and compounds that are highly lipid-soluble distribute rapidly between blood and tissues.

Cuff deflation. The cuff must not be deflated within 20 min of injection of local anaesthetic solution otherwise high peak plasma concentrations of drug occur within 30 s of deflation. To obviate this, cyclical inflation and deflation may be underaken.

If tourniquet pain is a problem, where a double cuff has been used, the lower may be inflated and the upper deflated after onset of the block.

Contraindications. 1. Severe neurological disease, or vascular disease of the limb where the use of a tourniquet is contraindicated.

2. Haemolytic disease or sickle cell disease.

3. Absence of skilled personnel who can recognise and treat complications.

4. Absence of full resuscitation equipment.

Precautions. The patient should be starved prior to use of this technique and i.v. access established in the contralateral limb. Treatment of systemic toxicity of local anaesthesic drugs is discussed in Chapter 14.

Several fatalities have occurred recently with this technique in the U.K., either because of lack of familiarity with the technique, faulty tourniquet equipment or inexperience in emergency resuscitation.

LOCAL ANAESTHESIA FOR HERNIA REPAIR (Fig. 23.6)

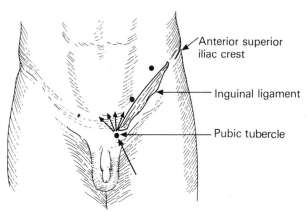

Fig. 23.6 Landmarks for inguinal hernia repair.

Local anaesthetic solution is injected at three points:

1. Through a weal 1.5 cm medial to the anterior superior iliac spine, a needle is inserted perpendicular to the coronal plane until a snap is felt as the needle penetrates the aponeurosis of external oblique. After aspiration, 30 ml of lignocaine 0.5% (or prilocaine 0.5%) with adrenaline 1:200 000 is injected to block ilio-inguinal and iliohypogastric nerves. The needle is withdrawn, continuing to inject 5–10 ml of solution.

2. At the spine of the pubis, a needle is passed intradermally and subcutaneously along the line of the incision and also up towards the midline to block nerve fibres overlapping from the contralateral side — 20 ml solution is used.

3. Through a weal 1.5 cm above the midpoint of the inguinal ligament, a needle is inserted perpendicular to the coronal plane to penetrate the aponeurosis of external oblique. At this point, 20 ml is injected to block the genital branch of the genitofemoral nerve.

The surgeon may be requested to infiltrate the peritoneum in the neck of the sac if the patient feels discomfort.

FURTHER READING

Bromage P R 1978 Epidural analgesia. W B Saunders, London
Cousins M J, Bridenbaugh P O 1980 Neural blockade in clinical anesthesia and management of pain. J B Lippincott Co, Philadelphia

Eriksson E 1979 Illustrated handbook in local anaesthesia, 2nd edn. Lloyd-Luke, London
Greene N M 1981 Physiology of spinal anesthesia, 3rd edn. Williams-Wilkins, Baltimore
Moore D C 1979 Regional block, 4th edn. Charles C Thomas, Springfield, Illinois

24

ENT anaesthesia

Two hundred and fifty thousand ear, nose and throat operations are performed in the United Kingdom each year, accounting for approx. 5% of the workload of an anaesthetic department. Patients are usually young and healthy and the average hospital stay is short (less than three days). Many operations are performed as day cases, thereby reducing the need for inpatient admission.

Children and young adults are frequently apprehensive and require reassurance. Some may have an atopic history which influences the choice of premedication and anaesthetic technique. Older patients may have hypertension or ischaemic heart disease and require careful preoperative assessment.

Smooth anaesthesia combined with a clear airway is essential since coughing and straining result in venous congestion which may persist into surgery and cause increased bleeding. Partial obstruction of the airway may lead to hypoxia, hypercapnia and unduly light anaesthesia.

THE SHARED AIRWAY

Special problems are caused when the airway is shared by both anaesthetist and surgeon. If bleeding is anticipated, the airway *must* be protected by the use of an endotracheal tube and the oropharynx packed to obviate contamination of the larynx with blood, pus and other debris. Techniques which rely on insufflation of anaesthetic vapours to an unintubated, unprotected trachea are no longer in common use and are not described.

Sometimes, a Boyle Davis gag may compress the endotracheal tube and cause partial airway obstruction. During IPPV this is detected by a decrease in compliance and increased inflation pressure and in the spontaneously breathing patient by decreased movement of the reservoir bag.

At the end of the procedure the pack must be removed and the pharynx cleared of blood and debris before the trachea is extubated with the patient in a head-down lateral position.

TONSILLECTOMY

Each year 100 000 adenotonsillectomies are performed in the U.K. with a rate of 8 per 1000 children under the age of 15. This frequency is 50% of that 15 years ago. In 1968 there were 6 deaths, a mortality rate of 1 in 28 000.

It is customary to prescribe a premedication prior to tonsillectomy. This is administered most conveniently to the younger child as a syrup (trimeprazine 3 mg/kg or diazepam 0.4 mg/kg are effective). Most anaesthetists combine this with atropine 0.1–0.3 mg orally (except in hot weather) to decrease salivation during operation. Induction of anaesthesia may be either by inhalation or intravenous route, whichever is appropriate for the individual child. Oral tracheal intubation is advisable, performed either under deep volatile anaesthesia or facilitated by suxamethonium; on occasions it may be difficult to maintain a patent airway because of respiratory obstruction produced by enlarged tonsils.

Relaxation provided by suxamethonium may assist the surgeon who guillotines (as opposed to dissects) tonsils before achieving haemostasis. The frequent use of diathermy to control bleeding excludes the use of ether.

Analgesia should be given at the end of surgery, if none has been given previously, so that the child awakens in a pain-free state. Tracheal extubation is performed with the patient slightly head down in a lateral position after suction has ensured that the pharynx is free from blood.

Blood loss during tonsillectomy is not usually measured but may be deceptively large. Particular care should be exercised in the 3–4 yr-old child, weighing 13–15 kg. In this age range, blood transfusion is required after the loss of only 100 ml of blood.

The postoperative bleeding tonsil

Diagnosis is made usually on the basis of clinical signs of hypovolaemia — tachycardia, pallor and sweating. Swallowing is not uncommon, followed by vomiting of a large quantity of blood. Anaesthesia for such a child is difficult and the assistance of an experienced anaesthetist must be sought.

An i.v. infusion is essential and blood transfusion is required. After resuscitation, the patient is placed head-down in a lateral position and suction apparatus is positioned within grasp. After preoxygenation, a small dose of thiopentone (2–3 mg/kg) is given followed by suxamethonium 1 mg/kg and cricoid pressure applied, although this may make laryngoscopy difficult. Alternatively, a gaseous induction with halothane in oxygen may be used and pharyngeal suction and tracheal intubation undertaken under deep halothane anaesthesia. When bleeding has been controlled surgically the stomach is emptied with a nasogastric tube. At the end of the procedure the trachea is extubated with the child in a lateral position.

It should be emphasised that induction of anaesthesia with thiopentone must *never* be attempted before adequate resuscitation has been undertaken and the intravascular volume restored.

ADENOIDECTOMY

Adenoidectomy is often combined either with tonsillectomy or examination of the ears under anaesthesia. Premedication is similar to that for tonsillectomy and anaesthesia is induced either by inhalation or by the i.v. route. Oral tracheal intubation is advisable either under deep anaesthesia or facilitated by suxamethonium, and a small throat pack is inserted by the surgeon. The adenoids are curetted and the postnasal space is packed to achieve

haemostasis. After 3 min, this pack is removed, and after removal of the throat pack, the patient is turned into the lateral position and the trachea extubated.

MICROLARYNGOSCOPY

The operating microscope has revolutionised the treatment of laryngeal disorders. The Kleinsasser laryngoscope is supported on the chest by rests and the operating microscope allows detailed examination and assessment of the larynx.

Premedication with pethidine and promethazine has been suggested if there is no evidence of airway obstruction. The most popular technique uses a Coplan's tube (5 mm i.d., 31 cm long, constructed from soft plastic, with a 10 ml cuff volume). Anaesthesia is induced with thiopentone followed by a nondepolarising muscle relaxant; the vocal cords are sprayed with 3 ml lignocaine 4% to assist smooth anaesthesia and to minimise the possibility of postextubation laryngospasm. The Coplan's tube is passed nasally. The lungs are ventilated artificially with 66% N_2O in O_2 supplemented either with a volatile agent or analgesic drug. The small diameter tube does not impede the surgeon's view and allows good access to the larynx. The cuff prevents contamination of the trachea with blood or debris.

At the end of the procedure, the pharynx is cleared with suction under direct vision, muscle relaxants are antagonised and tracheal extubation performed in a lateral position. Oxygen is administered to minimise hypoxia from laryngeal stridor.

Other techniques used for microlaryngoscopy include the use of:

1. Topical analgesia to the larynx with insufflation of N_2O/O_2 and halothane via a fine catheter.

2. Neuroleptanalgesia combined with topical analgesia.

3. Venturi ventilation with O_2 using a catheter and a Sanders injector. Hypnosis is maintained with increments of a rapidly metabolised induction agent.

4. A conventional or Pollard's endotracheal tube and controlled ventilation.

The lumen of the Pollard's tube differs in size at the proximal and distal ends. It is constructed of latex reinforced with a nylon spiral. The proximal internal diameter is 10 mm, narrowing to 5, 6 or 7 mm for the distal laryngeal portion.

In children, microlaryngoscopy is performed using spontaneous ventilation via an oral endotracheal tube one size smaller than would normally be used. The larynx should be sprayed with a measured quantity of lignocaine to prevent postoperative laryngospasm. Occasionally the surgeon requests that he observe the larynx without an endotracheal tube in situ; in these circumstances the tube is removed during deep anaesthesia, allowing examination to take place during emergence.

LARYNGECTOMY

The incidence of carcinoma of the larynx is 3–4 per 100 000 population. Many tumours may be treated with radiotherapy and therefore surgery is relatively uncommon for this condition. Airway obstruction by tumour is the major anaesthetic problem; alcohol and smoking are aetiological factors which may influence anaesthesia.

Respiratory function should be assessed preoperatively although this is difficult to measure accurately if there is airways obstruction. Chest physiotherapy should always be prescribed since it aids clearance of secretions pre- and postoperatively.

When respiratory obstruction is present, opioid or sedative premedication should always be avoided. If awake intubation is contemplated, successful topical anaesthesia of the mouth and pharynx requires an anticholinergic agent in addition. There is a risk of mechanical obstruction on induction of anaesthesia so if an i.v. agent is used, it should be given slowly in minimal dose until consciousness is lost. If subsequently the patient's lungs can be inflated using a face mask, suxamethonium may be given to facilitate tracheal intubation; if not, anaesthesia is deepened slowly with nitrous oxide and halothane in oxygen until laryngoscopy is possible. If there is any doubt regarding the patient's ability to maintain a patent airway following loss of consciousness, the anaesthetist must *not* use an i.v. induction even with the smallest dose of thiopentone; instead an inhalational technique should be used and if there is a progression to severe respiratory tract obstruction, awake intubation should be employed. A selection of noncuffed endotracheal tubes should be available as

the lumen of the trachea may be narrowed at the level of the cords or subglottically. Tracheal intubation may be more difficult if preoperative radiotherapy has reduced the mobility of the floor of the mouth.

Monitoring of e.c.g. and arterial pressure should be instituted in the anaesthetic room before induction of anaesthesia, which is maintained using controlled ventilation with nitrous oxide in oxygen supplemented by a volatile agent or opioid analgesic. Induced hypotension is often used to facilitate dissection of the neck (see Chapter 35). When the larynx has been dissected free, it is important to check that a sterile e.t. tube and compatible connections are available before the trachea is divided. The patient's lungs are ventilated with 100% oxygen for 2 min, the tracheal tube is withdrawn into the larynx, the trachea is divided and a second endotracheal tube is placed rapidly in the trachea and secured firmly. This tube should be placed correctly within the shortened trachea to prevent inadvertent one-lung anaesthesia.

At the end of surgery, residual neuromuscular blockade is antagonised and the endotracheal tube changed for a laryngectomy or tracheostomy tube. Adequate humidification is essential postoperatively. Enteral nutrition is provided via a nasogastric tube.

PHARYNGOLARYNGECTOMY

Pharyngolaryngectomy is performed for tumours of the postcricoid region. The pharynx and larynx are removed and the stomach mobilised and anastomosed in the neck behind the tracheostomy. There are two surgical approaches: in one, after initial laparotomy, the stomach is passed through a mediastinal tract which is formed by blunt dissection; in the other more common procedure the stomach is mobilised via a thoraco-abdominal incision to be anastomosed in the neck. Thus several problems may arise:

1. Difficulty in intubation.
2. Temperature loss resulting from a large surgical incision, a prolonged operative procedure and extensive blood loss.
3. Pneumothorax if the pleura is damaged during dissection.
4. Rupture of the trachea causing difficulty in ventilation and mediastinal emphysema.

LASER SURGERY

The laser is used to strip polyps or tumours from the vocal cords accurately and with immediate control of bleeding. There are two anaesthetic problems:

1. *Damage to the endotracheal tube.* It has been found that in the presence of oxygen PVC microlaryngoscopy tubes may be ignited by the intensity of the laser beam. This may be prevented by wrapping the tube in protective silver foil. Aluminised silicone is being developed to overcome this problem.

2. *Retinal damage.* The DHSS recommend that all personnel should wear protective spectacles to prevent retinal damage.

NASAL OPERATIONS

Preparation of the nose with local anaesthetic

In 1942 Moffatt described a method of topical anaesthesia of the nose using cocaine as an alternative to spraying or packing the nose. There were three advantages to his method: minimal patient discomfort during preparation, a low risk of cocaine toxicity and a bloodless surgical field. In 1952 Curtiss simplified Moffatt's method as follows:

The patient lies supine with his head extended fully over the end of a trolley and supported by an assistant. A round-ended angulated needle is inserted with its tip directed along the floor of the nose. When the angle of the needle is reached, the tip is directed towards the roof of the nose and 2 ml of solution deposited when the tip has made contact. The procedure is repeated in the second nostril. The patient remains in this position for 10 min and is advised not to swallow any solution which may have trickled into the pharynx. Then he sits upright and spits out any residual solution.

Analgesia is produced by accumulation of cocaine in the region of the sphenopalatine ganglion, thereby blocking most of the sensory supply to the nose, including the anterior ethmoidal nerve. The columella is not affected, and requires a separate injection. Arterial blood supply to the nose accompanies the nerve supply, and is therefore constricted by the cocaine, producing good haemostasis.

Preparation of the nose in this manner enables any operation to be performed and dispenses with the need to use hypotensive techniques to control surgical bleeding.

Anaesthetic technique for nasal operations

Adequate premedication is essential and may be given either orally or i.m. A smooth induction is desirable to avoid coughing and straining. Suxamethonium or a nondepolarising muscle relaxant may be used for tracheal intubation. The larynx is not sprayed with local anaesthetic before intubation in order that full laryngeal reflexes return as soon as possible after surgery.

Anaesthesia may be maintained using either spontaneous or controlled ventilation, depending on the duration of surgery. It is important to use a nonkinking tracheal tube and to pack the pharynx with 2-inch ribbon gauze so that blood, pus or debris does not contaminate the larynx. The presence of the pack should be marked in writing on the strapping which secures the tube to remind the anaesthetist to remove it at the end of the operation.

The patient is positioned 10° head up and all connections are checked before surgery begins. An e.c.g. should be used to detect the presence of arrhythmias which may occur frequently during operations on the face. When surgery has been completed, the pack is removed, the pharynx cleared and the patient is turned into a lateral position for tracheal extubation.

Preparation of the nose is omitted frequently for nasal polypectomy and diathermy of the turbinates because the nasal mucosa can be shrunk to such a degree that surgery becomes difficult.

For submucosal resection of the nasal septum, or rhinoplasty (altering the external shape of the nose), the use of a Magill oral connector allows a flush fitting connection which does not intrude into the operative field; a good nasal preparation minimises bleeding and improves operating conditions.

Epistaxis

Surgical intervention may be necessary to control bleeding from the nose and may involve packing the nose or postnasal space, or ligation of the maxillary artery.

The patient is often elderly, may be hypertensive and may have been sedated heavily with either barbiturates or benzodiazepines which render further premedication unnecessary. Before induction of anaesthesia, it is essential that the blood volume is restored. The problems inherent in bleeding from the upper airway and a stomach containing swallowed blood are similar to those of the bleeding tonsil, and the anaesthetic technique used is similar.

The sinuses

Bacterial infection of the paranasal sinuses occurs when the self-cleansing mechanism becomes impaired and mucus accumulates and stagnates. Antral washouts and intranasal antrostomies are performed to aid restoration of normal mucosal activity. In a Caldwell Luc operation a radical antrostomy is performed via a buccal incision above the canine tooth.

In all these procedures, the airway is protected by means of an oral endotracheal tube and pharyngeal pack. Ethmoidectomy may require hypotensive anaesthesia.

Maxillectomy

Excision of the maxilla for tumour is a major procedure and hypotensive anaesthesia is used to reduce bleeding; e.c.g. monitoring using a CM_5 lead is advisable. Accurate measurement of arterial pressure requires radial artery cannulation (p. 261). A pack or obturator is inserted into the maxillectomy cavity at the end of surgery; first a mould is fashioned from a rapidly setting plastic compound in situ and additional debris may be deposited in the pharynx as a result. The patient is usually anaesthetised on a second occasion one week later to insert the permanent prosthesis.

EARS

Myringotomy

Examination of the ears together with myringotomy and insertion of grommets is frequently carried out in children who have secretory otitis media. This operation may be performed as an outpatient.

Premedication with trimeprazine or diazepam often settles the fretful child who cannot understand why he has been starved. Either inhalational or i.v. induction may be used and anaesthesia is maintained with spontaneous respiration via a face mask for myringotomy alone; if adenoidectomy is performed, oral endotracheal intubation is essential. The use of nitrous oxide increases middle ear pressure significantly, especially when combined with IPPV, and this may alter the appearance of the tympanic membrane.

Middle ear surgery

Smooth anaesthesia is essential for operations on the middle ear. Coughing, straining or bucking increase venous pressure and produce oozing which may persist for some time. Premedication may be given orally or i.m., omitting atropine for hypotensive anaesthesia. After induction of anaesthesia with thiopentone, suxamethonium is used to facilitate intubation with a nonkinking oral endotracheal tube; the trachea and larynx are sprayed with lignocaine to aid tolerance of the tube. Often, sufficient reduction in arterial pressure is obtained using nitrous oxide in oxygen with halothane or enflurane in combination with d-tubocurarine and IPPV. Small doses of a β-blocker to reduce heart rate are often effective adjuvants. A 10° head-up tilt aids venous drainage. When induced hypotension is used, CM_5 e.c.g. and accurate arterial pressure monitoring are essential using either a Dinamap or direct intra-arterial measurement.

The middle ear is a closed cavity and nitrous oxide diffuses rapidly into the middle ear causing an increase in pressure. The maximum pressure is reached approx. 40 min after induction. There is concern that this may cause grafts to become dislodged. Such complications have led some authors to suggest that O_2/N_2 should be used in place of O_2/N_2O gas mixtures.

Bandaging the ear at the end of surgery involves movement of the head. This should be anticipated and supervised by the anaesthetist to prevent undue movement which may lead to gagging on the tracheal tube. If labyrinthine function has been disturbed, an antiemetic may be necessary to control postoperative vertigo and vomiting.

FURTHER READING

Atkinson R S 1976 Anaesthesia for endoscopy. In: Atkinson R S, Langton Hewer C (eds) Recent advances in anaesthesia and analgesia, 12. Churchill Livingstone, Edinburgh

Brown T C K, Fisk G C 1979 Anaesthesia for ear nose and throat operations. In: Anaesthesia for children. Blackwell Scientific Publications, Oxford

Davis I, Moore J R M 1979 Nitrous oxide and the middle ear. Anaesthesia 34: 147

Flood L M, Astley B 1982 Anaesthetic management of acute laryngeal trauma. British Journal of Anaesthesia 54: 1339

Hospital Inpatient Inquiry Series, MB4, 13. DHSS Office of Population Censuses & Surveys, Welsh Office, E.N.T., Table 251.629/4658004

Pearman K J 1979 Cocaine: a review. Journal of Laryngology & Otology 93: 1191

Morrow W F, Morrison J D 1975 Anaesthesia for eye, ear, nose and throat surgery. Churchill Livingstone, Edinburgh

Smith B L, Manford M L M 1974 Postoperative vomiting after paediatric adenotonsillectomy. British Journal of Anaesthesia 46: 373

25

Ophthalmic anaesthesia

The anaesthetist plays a crucial role in the production of suitable operating conditions for ophthalmic surgery. Careful attention to details of technique is therefore essential, particularly for intraocular procedures; e.g. cataract extraction, intraocular lens implantation, corneal grafting.

Many patients requiring surgery of the eye are at the extremes of age, and this presents associated problems for the anaesthetist. Ophthalmic surgical procedures may be categorised into: (a) intraocular; (b) extraocular.

INTRAOCULAR SURGERY

Surgical requirements

When the globe is opened, intraocular pressure (IOP) becomes equal to atmospheric pressure. In the presence of a raised IOP, the sudden reduction in pressure on incision of the globe may lead to expression of ocular contents, including iris and vitreous, through the wound. The sudden release of pressure may also cause disastrous expulsive haemorrhage from the short ciliary blood vessels in the posterior aspect of the eye.

Thus, control of IOP is essential, and moderate reduction is usually desirable for most procedures involving opening of the globe. Retinal detachment surgery is also facilitated by some reduction in IOP to allow the positioning of plombs, straps, etc. However, in corneal graft surgery, excessive reduction in IOP may cause difficulty in suturing. Complete immobility of the eye is essential for the microsurgical techniques which are now undertaken commonly for the majority of intraocular procedures.

Meticulous attention to the control of intra-operative IOP is essential for certain patients who are at particular risk of ocular complications, including: those who have high myopia or diabetes; those who are aphakic; those with only one functioning eye, and adults of less than about 60 yr of age. Particular care is necessary also in lens implant surgery as bulging of the vitreous, or loss of vitreous, may render the implant procedure impossible.

The factors controlling IOP are similar to those controlling intra-cranial pressure, as both involve manipulation of the volume of contents contained in a semirigid container. When the eye is opened, IOP is equal to atmospheric and the *volume* of contents (particularly intra-vascular volume) assumes prime importance.

Control of intraocular pressure

The main factors involved in the regulation of IOP include: external pressure, volume of arterial and venous vasculature (choroidal volume), and volumes of aqueous and vitreous.

External pressure

Accidental pressure on the eye should be avoided; for example from anaesthetic masks or retractors. Relaxation of the extraocular muscles with non-depolarising muscle relaxants may help to reduce IOP, but the evidence for this effect is contradictory. However, suxamethonium causes a transient increase in IOP (see below).

Vascular (or choroidal) volume

Variation in volume may result from vaso-constriction, or dilatation of the choroid, or changes in central venous pressure transmitted to the eye via its valveless venous drainage.

Venous pressure. Changes in venous pressure are transmitted to the ocular vasculature and are accompanied by immediate changes in ocular pressure and vascular volume. Raised venous pressure also impedes aqueous drainage by increased back pressure on the veins which drain the canal of Schlemm (Fig. 25.1), causing a further secondary gradual increase in IOP. During anaesthesia, venous pressure is influenced mainly by posture and transmitted intrathoracic pressure. A 15° head-up (antiTrendelenburg) tilt causes a significant decrease in IOP.

Situations mimicking a Valsalva manoeuvre (e.g. airway obstruction, coughing or retching) cause an immediate increase in venous and arterial pressures reflected by immediate elevation in ocular pressure and vascular volume. These conditions must therefore be avoided.

Intermittent positive pressure ventilation (IPPV) produces a small increase in venous pressure secondary to the elevation in mean intrathoracic pressure, but this may be overcompensated by ability to regulate arterial P_{CO_2}.

Arterial blood gases. Arterial P_{CO_2} is a major influence in the control of choroidal vascular volume and IOP. A reduction in Pa_{CO_2} constricts the choroidal vessels and prevents forward displacement of the vitreous. If the eye is intact, this results in a reduction in IOP, and if open, reduces the likelihood of prolapse of vitreous or other contents. Elevation of Pa_{CO_2} results in a proportional and linear increase in IOP. Recent work suggests that increased Pa_{CO_2} may result also in raised central venous pressure.

Hypoxia produces intraocular vasodilatation and an increase in IOP.

Arterial pressure. Stable values of arterial pressure within the physiological range have little effect on IOP. However, when systolic arterial pressure

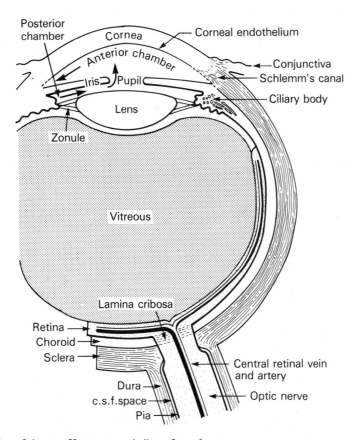

Fig. 25.1 Cross-section of the eye. Heavy arrows indicate flow of aqueous.

decreases below 85–90 mmHg, IOP diminishes progressively and profoundly towards atmospheric pressure, which is reached at a systolic arterial pressure of 50–60 mmHg. Sudden increases or decreases in arterial pressure produce rapid parallel but transient fluctuations in IOP and are therefore undesirable. The arterial pressure oscillations are buffered by expression of venous blood from the eye and, more slowly, by changes in aqueous volume. It should be noted that the effects of changes in venous pressure on IOP cannot be buffered by compression of the arterial vasculature of the eye.

Aqueous and vitreous volume

Control of aqueous volume is important in the treatment of glaucoma, but has less importance during surgery since the rate of change is relatively slow.

Reduction of vitreous volume by osmotic dehydrating agents (mannitol or sucrose) may be useful for controlling IOP during surgery. Mannitol (20–60 g) should be started 45 min before surgery. The diuresis produced necessitates catheterisation of the bladder. The usual precautions should be taken in administration of mannitol to patients with cardiovascular disease. Sucrose 50% (1 g/kg) i.v. produces a fairly rapid decrease in IOP (within 5 min) without a diuresis.

Reduction in IOP using acetazolamide, which reduces aqueous production and facilitates drainage, is of questionable benefit during surgery since it leads to increased intrachoroidal vascular volume. Thus, when the eye is open, a tendency to prolapse of contents may still exist.

Effects of anaesthetic drugs on IOP

Premedication. Drugs used for premedication have little effect on IOP, with the exception of those which may alter Pa_{CO_2}. The use of the opioid analgesics is unnecessary and their inherent properties of producing vomiting, retching, and respiratory depression are undesirable. Anticholinergic agents (in the doses used in premedication) have no effect on the glaucomatous eye provided that existing topical treatment is maintained. The commonly used anxiolytic and antiemetic drugs have little effect on IOP.

Induction agents. Thiopentone causes a moderate but transient decrease in IOP. Etomidate produces an immediate and prolonged decrease in IOP of approx. 40% from baseline values with little effect on cardiovascular stability, and the decrease in IOP persists for at least 20 min. The IOP does not seem to be affected by the myoclonic movements which may occur with this agent.

Ketamine may produce an increase in IOP and is therefore contraindicated if intraocular surgery is undertaken.

Muscle relaxants. Suxamethonium produces an increase in IOP which is maximal 2 min after injection, but the pressure returns to baseline by 5 min. This effect is thought to be caused by increased tone of the extraocular muscles and intraocular vasodilatation. Pretreatment with a small dose of nondepolarising muscle relaxant to prevent muscle fasciculation does not obtund this elevation of IOP reliably. Suxamethonium may be used safely if the eye is intact as IOP will return to normal before the incision is made. The problems involved in using suxamethonium in the presence of a penetrating eye injury are discussed below.

Nondepolarising muscle relaxants have no direct effects on IOP, but may produce alterations secondary to cardiovascular changes. Thus, tubocurarine causes a marked decrease in IOP but no change occurs with pancuronium, alcuronium or fazadinium.

Volatile agents. Both halothane and enflurane cause a decrease in IOP, this effect being more marked with enflurane. The effect of trichloroethylene is disputed, but it probably causes a small reduction in ocular pressure. Ether and isoflurane also decrease IOP. The mechanism of these changes is unknown. Nitrous oxide has no effect in the absence of air in the globe.

Opioids. Opioids cause a moderate reduction in IOP in the absence of significant respiratory depression.

Suggested techniques for elective intraocular surgery

Table 25.1 summarises a suitable technique for adults. Premedication by the oral route (e.g.

Table 25.1 Suggested technique for anaesthesia in elective
intra-ocular surgery in adults

Premedication (oral)	Diazepam 0.1–0.2 mg/kg +/– hyoscine 0.6 mg (omit in elderly)
Induction	Fentanyl 1–2 μg/kg Etomidate 0.3 mg/kg Suxamethonium 100 mg
Spray larynx and trachea	Lignocaine 4% (3–4 ml)
IPPV (moderate hyperventilation)	N_2O/O_2 + halothane 0.5% or enflurane 1% Alcuronium 10–15 mg
Antiemetic	Perphenazine 2–3 mg i.m. (20 min before completion of surgery)
Reversal	Atropine 1.2 mg Neostigmine 2.5 mg

diazepam) is satisfactory. In young children, trimeprazine syrup (3–4 mg/kg) is an appropriate sedative and antiemetic. Usually sedative premedication is not given to babies or patients undergoing 'day-case' surgery. Anticholinergic agents are not essential in adults but are desirable in young children. Hyoscine 0.6 mg orally may be used in adults under 65 years of age, and is both sedative and antiemetic.

Induction of anaesthesia may be preceded by fentanyl (1–2 μg/kg). This reduces the doses required of induction and maintenance agents but has little effect on the cardiovascular system. It may also reduce the likelihood of coughing after extubation of the trachea.

The benefits of etomidate induction (reduction of IOP, cardiovascular stability and rapid recovery) are offset by the high frequency of pain on injection. The addition of 1–2 ml (20–40 mg) of lignocaine 2% to a 20 mg ampoule of etomidate helps to reduce this problem. The use of a large vein is also helpful. The advantages of etomidate are particularly noticeable in the elderly, unfit patient. It is unwise to use etomidate in children because of pain on injection, and thiopentone is a satisfactory alternative in both adults and children.

Suxamethonium provides ideal conditions for endotracheal intubation with minimal risk of coughing or straining, and usually the transient increase in IOP has passed when the surgical procedure commences.

Topical anaesthesia of the larynx and trachea

should be undertaken with a lignocaine spray before the trachea is intubated as this may help to reduce postoperative coughing. Patients should not eat or drink for 3 h subsequently because of the danger of aspiration. Topical local anaesthetic is unnecessary in children and indeed may cause increased coughing after tracheal extubation.

Ventilation — spontaneous or controlled?

The choice of spontaneous or controlled ventilation is controversial. There is no doubt that for the 'high risk' eye, the combination of moderate hyperventilation and a 15° head-up tilt provides excellent conditions. IPPV with muscle relaxation virtually guarantees that no coughing or straining occurs whilst the eye is open, and reduction in Pa_{CO_2} can be achieved. In addition, smaller doses of anaesthetic agents are required with consequently improved cardiovascular stability and more rapid recovery from anaesthesia.

Spontaneous ventilation requires deeper levels of anaesthesia to ensure that coughing or straining on the endotracheal tube do not take place when the eye is open. Carbon dioxide retention, hypotension and slow recovery from anaesthesia are often associated with this technique. If a head-up tilt and a nonrebreathing circuit are utilised, operating conditions may be adequate for many procedures, but the technique is unpredictable and may be unsatisfactory for the 'high risk' eye.

Thus, IPPV is the method of choice to ensure good operating conditions for every patient. It has few disadvantages except for occasional delay in resumption of spontaneous ventilation following hyperventilation. Administration of the non-depolarising relaxant before the action of suxamethonium has ceased ensures that no coughing or straining takes place. No technique is completely reliable in preventing coughing following antagonism of residual neuromuscular blockade and tracheal extubation. Continuation of the volatile agent until reversal is helpful. It is the surgeon's responsibility to ensure watertight closure of the wound.

An antiemetic should be administered i.m. approx. 20 min before the end of the procedure and further doses should be given during the postoperative period.

Perphenazine is an excellent antiemetic for adults and also produces a useful degree of sedation. Conservative dosage (2–3 mg) avoids extrapyramidal side-effects. Caution is advised in patients with cardiovascular disease or dehydration, as hypotension may be produced on occasions. Perphenazine should not be given i.v. and is not suitable for children; a small dose of cyclizine may be substituted.

Opioid analgesia is not usually required, but, if necessary, a small dose of papaveretum (with an antiemetic) is satisfactory.

Penetrating eye injury

The anaesthetic management of the patient with a penetrating injury causes potentially great problems to the anaesthetist, and experienced help should always be sought. If an increase in IOP is produced during induction of anaesthesia, loss of ocular contents may occur. As repair is carried out as an emergency procedure, the patient may have a full stomach. However, suxamethonium is contraindicated, as it produces an increase in IOP. Thus, the choice of muscle relaxant for tracheal intubation must balance the risks to the eye(s) against those of pulmonary aspiration. If it is anticipated that endotracheal intubation will be uneventful, a large dose of nondepolarising agent can be substituted for suxamethonium in the usual 'crash induction' technique. Care should be taken not to exert pressure on the injured eye with the mask during preoxygenation. Vecuronium, atracurium or pancuronium are suitable choices of nondepolarising relaxant. However, if difficulties with endotracheal intubation are anticipated, suxamethonium should be used despite the risk to the eye. If intubation is difficult and ventilation with a face mask is not efficient, the resulting hypoxia and hypercarbia produce far more risk to the eye than a single dose of suxamethonium.

Spraying of the larynx with local anaesthetic is undesirable in the emergency patient as airway protective reflexes are obtunded. Management is otherwise as for an intraocular procedure, but extubation of the trachea should be performed with the patient on his side and almost awake.

EXTRAOCULAR SURGERY

The most common procedures are squint surgery, examination under anaesthesia (EUA) and dacrocystorhinostomy (DCR).

Squint surgery

Any technique of anaesthesia with endotracheal intubation is satisfactory. Traction on the extraocular muscles or pressure on the globe may provoke bradycardia via the oculocardiac reflex, which is mediated by the vagus. Prevention of the reflex by premedication with atropine is only partially effective, and careful intraoperative monitoring of heart rate is essential. Treatment of the bradycardia consists of cessation of traction and/or i.v. atropine, although the atropine may itself cause arrhythmias. Patients with squint may have an increased risk of developing malignant hyperpyrexia (see p. 287).

EUA

EUA is undertaken mainly in children as day cases, and repeated anaesthetics at fairly short intervals may be required. Inhalational anaesthesia by mask is often satisfactory, but may limit surgical access. Endotracheal intubation provides ideal access. The view expressed in the past that this might induce laryngeal oedema and postextubation stridor is now disputed. Ketamine is a very appropriate agent for small children as intervention to maintain the airway is seldom required, but premedication with atropine is mandatory to reduce the risk of secretions provoking laryngeal spasm. IOP under ketamine anaesthesia is normal or slightly raised, and this is useful if repeated pressure measurements are required (as in buphthalmos) as falsely low pressure readings are avoided.

DCR

The main complication during DCR is haemorrhage which obscures the surgical field. Preparation of the nose with cocaine paste or other vasoconstrictor is helpful, and a throat pack is mandatory, as blood trickles into the nasopharynx. Hypotensive anaesthesia has been used to improve operating conditions in this procedure, but seems unjustified. The surgeon may infiltrate the operation site with adrenaline and the precautions indicated below should be noted.

DRUG INTERACTIONS

Patients with eye disease, especially glaucoma, are often receiving medication which may pose potential problems to the anaesthetist.

1. Acetazolamide, a carbonic-anhydrase inhibitor, is used both acutely and chronically in the treatment of glaucoma. It is a diuretic and may produce dehydration and, less commonly, electrolyte imbalance.

2. Adrenaline is used topically in the long-term treatment of glaucoma, or intraoperatively by the surgeon to reduce bleeding. Systemic absorption may be significant and caution is necessary in the use of volatile agents, particularly halothane. Hypercapnia should be avoided.

3. Ecothiopate iodine (phospholine iodide) is a potent anticholinesterase used in the treatment of glaucoma. It depletes pseudocholinesterase and thus prolongs the action of suxamethonium.

4. Timolol maleate (Timoptol), a topical β-blocker, is used in some patients with raised IOP. Systemic absorption may be significant and precautions should be taken as for patients on oral β-blockers.

FURTHER READING

Adams A K, Jones R M 1980 Anaesthesia for eye surgery: general considerations. British Journal of Anaesthesia 52: 663
Arthur D S, Dewar K M S 1980 Anaesthesia for eye surgery in children. British Journal of Anaesthesia 52: 681
Barry Smith G 1983 Ophthalmic Anaesthesia. Edward Arnold, London
Foulds W S 1980 The changing pattern of eye surgery. British Journal of Anaesthesia 52: 643
Holloway K B 1980 Control of the eye during general anaesthesia for intraocular surgery. British Journal of Anaesthesia 42: 671
Jay J L 1980 Functional organization of the human eye. British Journal of Anaesthesia 52: 649

26

Day case anaesthesia

Day-stay surgery comprises the admission of a patient, surgical treatment, recovery and discharge occurring within the same day. This concept has become popular since 1960 for the reasons noted in Table 26.1.

Table 26.1 Advantages of day stay surgery

Party	Advantage
Patient	Shorter waiting time for operation than as inpatient. Recovery in own home
Surgeon	Shortens inpatient operation waiting lists. Lower infection rate
Health economist	No 'hotel' costs and lower nursing costs, therefore economical
Nurses	No night or weekend duty
Child	Avoids psychological trauma of prolonged separation from parents and home
Relatives	No repeated hospital visiting

Although there are few disadvantages with this system, it is essential that any complications are reported by the patient, and some relatives feel insecure if left alone at home with a patient. The fear of increased medicolegal risk has not proved to be justified.

In addition to surgical indications, anaesthesia for day-stay patients may be required for haematological, radiological and other investigations.

TYPES OF UNIT

There are three common types:

1. A unit within a hospital complex, but with separate wards and operating theatre. This is functionally the most flexible type as it may be adapted to the varying requirements of day patients.
2. A unit with a separate ward, but utilising the hospital's main operating theatre complex.
3. The third type, which is common outside the United Kingdom, comprises a separate centre with its own operating theatres and wards remote from a conventional hospital.

In many hospitals lacking special units, day-stay patients are admitted to the ordinary wards.

Whatever the system employed, the staff and facilities for surgery, anaesthesia and recovery should be of the same standard as for inpatients and complete facilities for resuscitation must be provided.

Standing arrangements should exist for admitting a day-patient immediately to a standard hospital bed if he is not fit to be discharged at the end of the day.

PATIENT SELECTION

Selection of patients for day surgery is dependent on both the surgical procedure and also the physical state of the patient. Practically any surgical procedure expected to last less than 1 h may be undertaken provided that undue haemorrhage and severe postoperative pain are not anticipated. Patients should be of a fitness rating of ASA grade I or II, although very short examinations under anaesthesia may be performed on grade III patients (see Table 15.1). It is essential that the home background is adequate and that relations or friends are available to provide postoperative monitoring and care.

Initial selection is made by the surgeon who advises operation. In some centres, the patient may then be assessed immediately at an outpatient anaesthetic clinic. Where selection is delegated to the surgeon, he must instigate appropriate investigations. However, cancellation of surgery after a patient's admission to a day care unit rarely results from incorrect selection, but more often is occasioned by recent ingestion of food, an upper respiratory tract infection or the disappearance of the lesion requiring surgery.

The letter calling the patient for surgery should contain an outline of what he (or she) should expect (see Table 26.2). It should also stress that the patient must:

1. Refrain from eating and drinking for 6 h before operation (modified for infants, where 3–4 h abstention is preferable to avoid hypoglycaemia).

2. Bring current medication to hospital so that it may be identified.

3. Be accompanied home.

4. Have company in the house on the night of operation.

5. Abstain from alcohol for 24 h after operation.

6. Not drive a car or work machinery for 24 h after operation.

Although minor behavioural changes have been noted for up to 48 h after anaesthesia, most anaesthetists consider a 24-h abstention from driving as reasonable.

Abstention from food is very important and although early studies suggested that patients may ignore this instruction, this has not been confirmed recently.

Fear of the risks involved has prompted some anaesthetists to insist that the patient signs a special consent form indicating agreement to these limitations.

In some centres, patients are asked to complete a questionnaire providing details of medical history and medication. This is brought with the patient on admission and speeds clerking (Table 26.3). Such a form is particularly valuable for children if the person accompanying the child is not a parent.

ADMISSION

Patients should be admitted to the day ward in adequate time for history-taking and examination. The results of any investigation requested as an outpatient should be noted. The patient should receive an identity wristlet and their name should be entered in the nursing record. The operation site should be marked.

Premedication

There is some controversy regarding premedication, both sedative and antisialagogue. Sedative pre-

Table 26.2 An example of an explanatory letter sent to the parents of day surgical children at Leicester Royal Infirmary

---

DAY CASE SURGERY FOR CHILDREN

Dear Parent,

Your child requires a minor operation which can probably be done in a single day in hospital, thus reducing the unpleasantness of a long hospital stay.

In order to make the visit to hospital as happy as possible, your help would be appreciated in making things run as smoothly as they can. The following notes are provided to give you some idea of what to do in preparation for the visit.

Please do explain to your child, if old enough, that he is going into hospital, but do not enter into elaborate details which will only confuse and frighten him, and may well be wrong. Try to present the hospital admission as an interesting experience. Try to control your own natural anxiety. If you are obviously worried, then your child will think that something awful is about to happen.

On the day of the operation you will be asked to arrive in good time to enable the necessary preparations to be made.

Most of the operations will be done under general anaesthesia. It is essential that your child should have nothing at all to eat or drink for some hours before the operation. The exact arrangements depend on the child's age. Please follow the instructions below.

On arrival in the ward, there will be some essential paperwork to complete.

Your child will then be seen by a member of the surgical team and an anaesthetist. Normally there will be NO injections or medicines to take on the ward before the operation.

Children are taken to the operating theatre in their beds or cots. You may, if you wish, accompany them as far as the theatre entrance. However, the design of our theatres is such that parents cannot come into the anaesthetic rooms.

Anaesthesia and surgery will take a variable time, depending on the operation, but all children are kept in the recovery area of the theatre suite, under careful supervision until they are safely awake again.

If the operation is likely to cause any pain afterwards a pain-killer will be given while the child is still asleep. This may result in your child being quite sleepy after the operation.

Before discharge from hospital children are again visited by an anaesthetist and surgeon, at which time instruction for postoperative care will be given.

EATING AND DRINKING BEFORE OPERATION — MORNING CASES

1. *Children over 4 years of age*
   Nothing to eat or drink after midnight on the day before operation.
2. *Children between 2 and 4 years of age*
   Wake when you go to bed and give a milk drink and biscuits. After this — nothing to eat or drink.
3. *Children less than 2 years of age*
   Wake very early on the morning of operation and give a milk drink (up to $\frac{1}{2}$ pint of milk). This must be completed by 6.00 a.m.

REMEMBER

1. The aim is to make the admission as pleasant as possible.
2. If you do not understand anything, please ask for more details.
3. If you have any helpful suggestions for improving the service, please let us know.

HOSPITAL FOR SICK CHILDREN
Ambulatory Services
Outpatient surgery
Instructions:
— Check one answer to each question
— Please complete this side only
— Please bring this form with you on the day of surgery

	Yes	No	Don't Know
1. Has your child ever been in hospital?	☐	☐	☐
2. Has he been in this hospital before?	☐	☐	☐
3. Has your child ever had an anaesthetic?	☐	☐	☐
4. Did your child have any problems with the anaesthetic?	☐	☐	☐
5. Does your child have any allergies?	☐	☐	☐
6. Was the allergy due to:			
a) A drug or medicine?	☐	☐	
b) Any type of food?	☐	☐	
c) Other things?	☐	☐	
7. If he had an allergy, did he have:			
a) A skin rash or hives?	☐	☐	☐
b) Wheezing or trouble breathing?	☐	☐	☐
c) Hay fever or a runny nose?	☐	☐	☐
d) A high fever?	☐	☐	☐
8. Has this child had a head cold or cough within the past week?	☐	☐	☐
9. Does your child wear a dental plate or bridge?	☐	☐	☐
10. Has your child had a cortisone type drug within the past two years?	☐	☐	☐
11. Is your child receiving any medicine just now?	☐	☐	☐
12. Is there anyone in the family with a bleeding problem?	☐	☐	☐
13. Has the patient had any minor injuries, operations, or tooth extraction followed by an unusual amount of bleeding?	☐	☐	☐
14. Does the child bruise easily on body areas other than the legs?	☐	☐	☐
15. Has your child been exposed to any infectious disease within the past month?	☐	☐	☐
16. Has your child ever had:			
Diabetes	☐	☐	☐
Asthma	☐	☐	☐
Cystic fibrosis	☐	☐	☐
Tuberculosis	☐	☐	☐
Rheumatic fever	☐	☐	☐
Rheumatism	☐	☐	☐
Heart disease	☐	☐	☐
Liver disease	☐	☐	☐
Anemia	☐	☐	☐
Convulsions or fits	☐	☐	☐
Glaucoma	☐	☐	☐
Jaundice	☐	☐	☐
17. Is there any problem about your child not mentioned so far?	☐	☐	☐
18. Has anyone in your family ever had a problem with an anaesthetic?	☐	☐	☐

IF ANY QUESTIONS ABOVE RECEIVED A 'YES' ANSWER GIVE DETAILS BELOW:

_____
_____
_____
_____
_____

DATE COMPLETED:_____
SIGNATURE OF PARENT:_____

Proposed Procedure:_____
_____
History of Present Illness:_____
_____
_____
_____
_____
_____
_____
_____

Physical Examination:
Under 6 years —   Over 6 years —
  length_____cm   height_____cm
Weight:_____   Blood Pressure:_____
Temperature:_____   Hemoglobin:_____gm%
Pulse:_____   Sickle Cell Test:_____
Respirations:_____   Urinalysis:_____
Nose and Throat:_____
_____

Heart:_____

Lungs:_____

Other Physical Findings:_____
_____
_____
_____

Diagnosis: Date: Physician Signature

_____   _____

medicant drugs produce a 'hangover' effect which delays recovery and thereby departure from a day ward and often prevents discharge from a half-day ward. Preoperative explanation and psychotherapy usually render the use of sedatives unnecessary, but they may be required for the very anxious or retarded patient. Children over 5 yr are usually co-operative and do not require sedation. In children under 5 yr, the greatest cause of distress is usually separation from the mother and if the theatre design allows it, the mother's presence in the anaesthetic room obviates this problem. If this is not possible, an oral premedication may be given 1–2 h before surgery. Some authors have prescribed diazepam 0.5 mg/kg for young children, given by the mother at home. Children under 1 yr seldom require sedation.

Premedication with anticholinegic drugs is usually avoided in adults. In paediatric practice, their use is controversial and the same considerations discussed in Chapter 32 apply to outpatient as to inpatient paediatric practice.

Table 26.3 Example of form for completion by the parents, used by the Toronto Hospital for Sick Children. (Reproduced by permission)

Induction of anaesthesia

Induction of anaesthesia with i.v. agents in unpremedicated patients requires slightly larger doses than normal. The incidence of excitatory phenomena (coughing, movement, or breath-holding) is much greater than in premedicated patients and care must be exercised to avoid moving any part of the patient, attempting to insert an oral airway too early, or increasing the dose of volatile agents too rapidly. Unpremedicated patients are more likely to experience cutaneous pain on i.v. injection with methohexitone, and particularly etomidate.

All the common i.v. induction agents have been used in day case patients. The factors affecting their suitability are shown in Table 26.4.

The agents currently available are not ideal induction agents, but nonetheless sleep doses of methohexitone (1.5 mg/kg) and thiopentone (5 mg/kg) are popular. The use of ketamine for outpatients is controversial. As premedication is usually avoided, emergence phenomena are particularly likely to occur, so it is rarely used in adults. It is said that emergence effects are rare in children, although many paediatric nurses would disagree. The i.m. route (8–10 mg/kg) is convenient in the unco-operative small child without visible veins.

Children may be allowed to choose the method of induction, but where veins are prominent, the i.v. route is preferable. If the child has chosen a gas induction, 66% N_2O in O_2 with the gradual introduction of 1–2.5% halothane is acceptable. The fastest rate of gaseous induction is produced by the use of 50% cyclopropane in oxygen, although the popularity of this technique has declined as a result of the general avoidance of explosive agents.

Rectal methohexitone (10% methohexitone in water = 100 mg/ml) in a dose of 25 mg/kg administered through a lubricated 14 G cannula, has been recommended for the preschool child. Close monitoring of the patient is required during the slow induction, which may take up to 11 min and occasionally longer. The anaesthetist must be available immediately with ventilatory support if required. After 30 min, the rate of recovery is the same as that for children given i.v. methohexitone.

Endotracheal intubation

It has been shown that provided an unduly large tube is not used, endotracheal intubation does not produce subsequent airway problems at home, even in children. However, as patients are young, healthy and mobilise quickly, suxamethonium is particularly prone to produce 'scoline pains'. Prior administration of a small dose of a nondepolarising neuromuscular blocking agent (e.g. gallamine 20 mg) reduces the incidence, but a larger dose of suxamethonium (up to 2 mg/kg) is required for equivalent relaxation. When artificial ventilation is intended, a medium length competitive agent (e.g. alcuronium or atracurium) may be used from the outset, *provided* that the anaesthetist is *experienced* and that difficulty in intubation is not anticipated.

Maintenance of anaesthesia

The technique used for maintenance is less important than the choice of anaesthetic agents. Maintenance by inhalation with spontaneous respiration, a total i.v. technique, and a nitrous oxide/oxygen/muscle relaxant technique supplemented by short-acting opioids or volatile agents have all been used successfully. The principle employed is that every sedative agent used should be either excreted rapidly or metabolised rapidly to inactive metabolites. When analgesia is required, short-acting analgesics, e.g. fentanyl (or alfentanil) should be used.

Table 26.4 Side-effects of the induction agents

Agent	Awakening	Hangover effect	Pain on injection	Smoothness of induction	Severe Reactions common
Thiopentone	Rapid	+ +		+ +	
Methohexitone	Rapid	+	+		
Althesin	Rapid	+		+	+
Propanidid	Very rapid			+	+ +
Etomidate	Rapid		+ +		
Disoprofol	Rapid		+	+ +	?

Of the volatile agents, enflurane is theoretically preferable to halothane as it has a lower blood/gas solubility and recovery of consciousness is slightly quicker. However, there is no difference between these two agents in respect of recovery to 'street fitness'. Isoflurane appears promising.

Local analgesia

Local analgesic techniques are particularly valuable in day surgery. These include local infiltration, Bier's block (i.v. regional analgesia for the forearm and hand), blocks of nerve trunks (e.g. axillary brachial plexus block) or spinal nerve blockade, e.g. caudal block. Subarachnoid anaesthesia has been performed, although this is rare in the United Kingdom.

Local anaesthesia may be employed in many patients without the use of sedatives. However, the use of a local anaesthetic technique in combination with general anaesthesia enables a lighter depth of unconsciousness to be maintained and provides prolonged analgesia postoperatively, reducing the requirement for systemic analgesics. A common and successful example is the use of caudal anaesthesia with light inhalational analgesia for circumcision. A penile dorsal nerve block is an alternative local technique.

Monitoring during anaesthesia

There is no reason to accept a lower standard of monitoring than that employed for inpatient surgery. Observation of the patient's colour, respiration and general state, and of the functioning of the anaesthetic machine, is practised and arterial pressure should be monitored regularly using sphygmomanometry.

The e.c.g. should be monitored routinely.

Reusable, so-called 'disposable', 3 or 4 contact e.c.g. back pads (e.g. the Deseret EKG pad) permit economical and rapid connection to the e.c.g. amplifier. In the absence of an e.c.g., a pulsometer is valuable.

Recovery

Recovery of unconscious patients should be undertaken by trained nursing staff. There should be one nurse to each unconscious patient. Standard resuscitation equipment (oxygen masks, suction equipment, defibrillator) and standard resuscitation drugs must be available. The patient must recline on a bed or trolley capable of tilting to a Trendelenburg position. The anaesthetist must be available to deal with complications.

Patients should not leave the recovery area until they are awake with restoration of all protective reflexes. Babies should be awake before leaving the operating theatre.

Analgesia

Providing recovery of consciousness is rapid, the patient is soon able to take simple oral analgesics (aspirin or paracetamol). These drugs usually provide adequate analgesia, and the patient is advised to continue with them at home. When a nerve block has been used, simple analgesics should be ingested before the block is expected to wear off (e.g. 4 h for caudal bupivacaine).

There remains a small number of patients for whom systemic analgesia (e.g. pethidine 1 mg/kg) is required, with the disadvantage that the consequent sedation may delay discharge. Occasionally it is necessary for community nurses to administer strong analgesics to the patient at home under the supervision of the general practitioner.

Complications

Although modern, well-organised day stay surgery is well tolerated by patients (only 9% of patients in one study wished to stay longer, and only 1.4% in another study would refuse further surgery as a day case), there is a relatively high incidence of minor complications (Table 26.5).

Table 26.5 Complications of day case surgery. Percentage of patients reporting symptoms in three studies

Symptom %	Ogg (1972)	Study Routh (1979)	Dawson (1980)
Headache	27	38	
Drowsiness	26	39	
Muscle stiffness	15	24	
Nausea	22	17	30
Vomiting	8	6	20
Dizziness	11	15	
Sore throat	6	15	
Injection site pain	17	3	

Nausea is a common minor complication of anaesthesia particularly when opioids have been employed. It is especially common in patients susceptible to travel sickness. Some anaesthetists employ antiemetic drugs routinely.

Migraine sufferers are particularly likely to develop headache. Deep anaesthesia and the use of volatile agents may be predisposing factors.

Nonetheless, the commonest complaint is of pain at the operation site.

Discharge

Every patient should be seen by the anaesthetist before discharge. Although day stay patients are generally healthy, surgery is relatively minor and is of short duration (less than 1 h), nonetheless a decision is required for every patient regarding discharge.

Elaborate tests have been devised to compare the hangover effects of different agents. These are research tools and are not necessarily relevant to the fitness of a patient for discharge. The patient who is ready to go home is obviously conscious, communicating well, and steady on his feet. Enquiry should be made for pain, headache or nausea and treatment prescribed if necessary.

After circumcision, with or without a caudal block, micturition is often delayed. As the child is more likely to pass urine in familiar surroundings, he is allowed to go home, with instructions to the parents to contact their general practitioner should the child become distressed (which rarely occurs).

To reinforce previous written instructions, patients must be warned against driving, operating machinery and ingesting alcohol for 24 h. They must be accompanied home and if a child is being taken home by car, a second adult is required to prevent distraction of the driver.

FURTHER READING

Burn J M 1979 A blue print for day surgery. Anaesthesia 34: 790
Dawson B, Reed W A 1980 Anaesthesia for adult surgery outpatients. Anaesthesia for day-care surgery; a symposium in 4 parts. Canadian Anaesthetists' Society Journal 27: 409
Edelist G, Urbach G 1980 Organisation of the outpatient surgical facility. Anaesthesia for day-care surgery; a symposium in 4 parts. Canadian Anaesthetists' Society Journal 27: 406
Korttila K 1981 Recovery and driving after brief anaesthesia. Der Anaesthesist 30: 377

Ogg T W 1972 An assessment of postoperative outpatient cases. British Medical Journal 4: 573
Routh G S 1979 Day care surgery under general anaesthesia in a purpose-built unit. Anaesthesia 34: 809
Shah C P 1980 Day care surgery in Canada. Anaesthesia for day-care surgery; a symposium in 4 parts. Canadian Anaesthetists' Society Journal 27: 399
Steward D J 1980 Anaesthesia for paediatric outpatients. Anaesthesia for day-care surgery; a symposium in 4 parts. Canadian Anaesthetists' Society Journal 27: 412

27

Neurosurgical anaesthesia

Anaesthesia for intracranial operations requires conditions which maintain perfusion of the brain with blood. This is dependent upon cerebral perfusion pressure (CPP = mean arterial pressure minus intracranial pressure).

Anaesthesia must also facilitate surgical access by reducing brain volume and minimising surgical haemorrhage.

PHYSIOLOGY OF INTRACRANIAL PRESSURE AND CEREBRAL BLOOD FLOW

The intracranial contents comprise the brain (weighing approx. 1400 g), the c.s.f. (approx. 75 ml) and blood (approx. 130 ml). Although these compartments of the brain volumes are essentially fluid and therefore incompressible, both blood and c.s.f. communicate with extracranial compartments allowing a certain degree of adaptability of intracranial pressure to changes in intracranial volume.

Volume-pressure relationship

In the presence of an expanding intracranial lesion, the intracranial pressure (ICP) changes from its normal value when the adaptive mechanisms of venous blood displacement and c.s.f. displacement have been utilised fully.

Figure 27.1 shows that between points 1 and 2 intracranial pressure is normal, although the volume change that can be tolerated is reduced progressively. Beyond point 2, compliance is lost and an increase in volume of any intracranial content results in a very steep increase in intracranial pressure, seen at points 3 and 4.

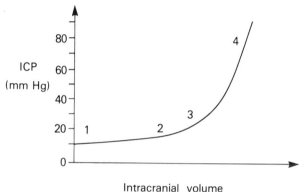

Fig. 27.1 The intracranial pressure/volume relationship.

When the growth of a lesion is slow and its siting allows maximum accommodation, large volumes of tumour may be found in the presence of relatively normal ICP. Lesions which grow quickly soon exhaust the displacement mechanisms and lead to severe elevations of ICP.

Intracranial volumes

The volume occupied by the brain may be increased by tumour, abscess or haematoma, and augmented by oedema or hyperaemia. C.s.f. is formed at approx. 0.4 ml/min irrespective of ICP up to pressures of 200 mmH$_2$O. It is reabsorbed in the arachnoid villi by a purely mechanical process dependent on the pressure gradient between c.s.f. and venous blood in the sinuses.

Intracranial blood volume is increased by cerebral vasodilatation and by obstruction of venous return. The effect on ICP of neck flexion, neck rotation and compression of the jugular veins is shown in Figure 27.2. The normal ICP is 100–150 mmH$_2$O (or 7–10

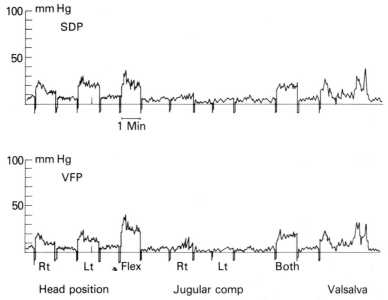

Fig. 27.2   Effect of head movement (right, left lateral movement and flexion), right, left and combined jugular compression and Valsalva manoeuvres on ICP.(SDP — Subdural pressure, VFP — Ventricular fluid pressure).

mmHg) throughout the c.s.f. in the horizontal position. Jugular bulb pressure is approximately equal to atmospheric pressure. In the erect posture there is an initial decrease in ICP (and increase in lumbar c.s.f. pressure), but ICP is restored rapidly as a result of the decreased rate of absorption of c.s.f. by the arachnoid villi.

C.s.f. pressure is related directly to airway pressure. Large increases in ICP are produced by coughing, straining and the use of positive end-expiratory pressure (PEEP). The effect of positive pressure ventilation seen in Figure 27.3 is caused probably by transmission of intrathoracic pressure throughout jugular and vertebral veins.

ICP recordings show fluctuations related to the arterial pulse and respiration. These oscillations reflect changes in the size of the arterioles and to a lesser extent of the choroid plexus. Their amplitude is increased when ICP is elevated and when there is cerebral vasodilatation.

From the relationship beween ICP and intracranial volume illustrated in Figure 27.1, it is evident that as the decompensated stage is approached, the brain becomes more vulnerable to the effects of any cerebral vasodilator, e.g. ketamine, halothane or carbon dioxide, or any other cause of increased intracranial volume, e.g. poor posture. A feature of this phase of the volume-pressure relationship is the appearance of

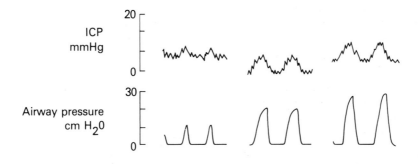

Fig. 27.3   Effects of change in airway pressure on ICP.

Lundberg A waves on the ICP recording. These are plateaus of large increases in c.s.f. pressure (up to 80 mmHg) often superimposed on a relatively normal baseline pressure. These waves have a duration of 5–20 min. A transient increase in Pa_{CO_2} often precedes the development of A waves, although other factors may be responsible. B waves, with a frequency of approximately 1/min, and C waves of 6/min are also seen in these patients (Fig. 27.4).

Cerebral blood flow

Two-thirds of the CBF is transmitted through the carotid arteries and one-third through the vertebral arteries.

Autoregulation

Normally, CBF is approx. 50 ml/100 g of brain tissue per min, and is maintained at this constant rate over a wide range of CPP. The cerebral arteries constrict as the systemic arterial pressure increases and dilate as it diminishes. This phenomenon is termed auto-regulation, and in man is effective between mean arterial pressures of 60–130 mmHg; below and above these limits, CBF varies passively with perfusion pressure. Although autoregulation appears to be an intrinsic response of cerebral arteriolar smooth muscle, the sympathetic nervous system influences the range of pressures over which autoregulation is effective.

Autoregulation occurs when CPP is decreased by either hypotension or raised ICP. In states of raised ICP, CBF is preserved until ICP exceeds 30–40 mmHg; then the Cushing response of hypertension maintains perfusion at the cost of further increases in ICP.

The lower limit of autoregulation during hypotension depends on the cause of hypotension. Hypotension resulting from haemorrhage leads to a loss of autoregulation at higher pressures than during drug-induced hypotension. Halothane hypotension allows autoregulation to lower pressures than trimetaphan and much lower than sodium nitroprusside.

Hypertensive patients have a high range of autoregulation limits (e.g. 90–160 mmHg) and cervical sympathetic stimulation produces a similar elevation. This is illustrated in Figure 27.5.

When the upper limit of autoregulation is exceeded, breakthrough focal haemorrhages and oedema are produced.

Autoregulation is impaired or abolished by hypoxia and this impairment persists for some time in the posthypoxic brain. Hypercapnia, acute intracranial disease and trauma, and drug induced hypotension to very low levels all lead to a persisting loss of autoregulation. Hyperventilation has been shown to restore autoregulation in some patients in whom the disease process had produced a loss of autoregulation at normocapnia.

Metabolic regulation of cerebral blood flow

Increases in specific regional cerebral blood flows are encountered during increased mental activity or voluntary muscle effort. Both global cerebral blood flow and cerebral metabolism are greatly increased by the intense activity of a grand mal convulsion.

The regulation of regional CBF to match the metabolic demand of the brain is thought to be mediated by local changes in concentrations of vasodilator metabolites, lactic acid and carbon dioxide, which may act via pH and K^+ in the region of the terminal arterioles. Pain and anxiety also increase CBF and cerebral metabolism; these effects are probably related to the enhanced neuronal function and catecholamine release in the brain associated with arousal.

Metabolic depression leads to a reduction in

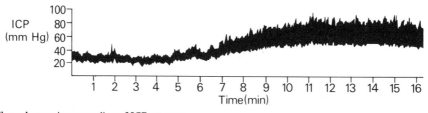

Fig. 27.4 Lundberg A wave in a recording of ICP pressure.

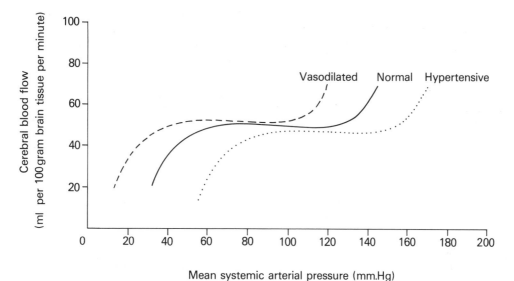

Fig. 27.5 Autoregulation curves in normal, hypertensive and drug induced hypotensive states.

cerebral blood flow and may be induced by hypothermia, barbiturates, Althesin and etomidate.

Carbon dioxide and blood gas changes

The effect of changes in Pa_{CO_2} on cerebral blood flow are shown in Figure 27.6. The greatest response in CBF is at normal Pa_{CO_2}, where a change of 1 kPa results in a 30% change in blood flow. Hyperventilation below 4kPa has less effect and below 2.6 kPa it is minimal. Little further vasodilatation takes place with hypercapnia in excess of 10 kPa.

Hyperventilation below 2.6 kPa is associated with increased desaturation of jugular bulb venous blood,

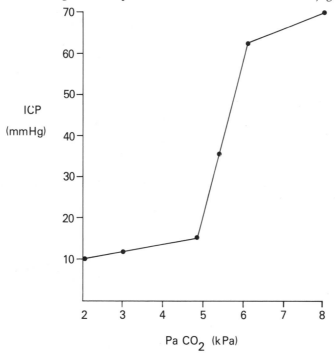

Fig. 27.6 Effect on ICP of change in Pa_{CO_2}.

slow waves on the e.e.g., increasing drowsiness, and evidence of anaerobic glycolysis.

The response of the cerebral circulation to hyperventilation is modified by the arterial pressure. High perfusion pressures are associated with increased responsiveness to hyperventilation whereas hypotension to 50 mmHg abolishes the effect of increased or decreased Pa_{CO_2}.

Oxygen

Hypoxia below Pa_{O_2} of 7 kPa is necessary before cerebral vasodilatation occurs. Further hypoxia produces marked vasodilatation. The vasoconstrictor effect of hypocapnia is preserved in the presence of arterial hypoxaemia.

CEREBRAL METABOLISM AND CMRO$_2$

Although regional metabolic requirements of the brain vary with the level of cerebral activity, the overall energy consumption of the brain is relatively constant in sleep or active intellectual work. This activity is high; the brain consumes 20% of the oxygen used by a resting subject. To support this metabolism, the brain relies on glucose supplies; there is no store of substrate. There is also active metabolism of aminoacids including glutamate, aspartate and γ-aminobutyric acid in addition to the release and inactivation of neurotransmitters.

The energy production of the brain may be equated with its rate of oxygen consumption. The cerebral metabolic rate for oxygen (CMRO$_2$) is the product of the cerebral blood flow and the arteriovenous oxygen content difference.

When there is a failure in oxygen or glucose supply, ATP production falls short of ATP utilisation and CMRO$_2$ does not reveal the nature or extent of this deficit.

Knowledge of regional blood flow and CMRO$_2$ is an inadequate guide to cellular oxygenation because of the considerable tissue heterogeneity in pathological conditions. Tissue Po_2 measurements are undergoing rapid development and in the future it may be possible to monitor Po_2 at selected cortical sites. Alternative approaches have been developed using fluorimetric techniques to measure NADH$^+$, dual-beam spectrophotometry of cytochrome oxidase redox changes, and optodes (fluorescent oxygen sensitive compounds). Potassium, hydrogen ion, and glucose can also be monitored by tissue electrodes.

EFFECTS OF DRUGS AND TECHNIQUES

The following are under the anaesthetist's control and have profound effects on the neurosurgical patient.

Arterial carbon dioxide tension

Carbon dioxide is the most potent cerebral vasodilator and CBF changes associated with it are linearly related to cerebral blood volume. The decrease in ICP produced by hypocapnia leads to gradual redistribution of the intracranial contents, resulting in an increase in c.s.f. volume which tends to restore ICP; nevertheless, hypocapnia provides good operating conditions at craniotomy. There is no advantage in reducing Pa_{CO_2} below 4 kPa.

Hypercapnia increases ICP as a result of increased CBF and vascular engorgement. Autoregulation is abolished.

Arterial pressure changes

Hypertension

Many neurosurgical patients have focal or global loss of autoregulation and therefore cannot withstand hypertension. Even patients with preserved autoregulation should be protected from hypertensive episodes.

It is recognised that hypertensive incidents occur in response to endotracheal intubation, skin incision and other nociceptive stimuli, and also at the end of anaesthesia. Only gradual restoration of normal arterial pressure should be permitted after deliberate hypotension, and control of arterial pressure with maintenance of hypocapnia is desirable in patients with disturbances of autoregulation.

Hypertensive episodes produce the added risk of haemorrhage, especially during aneurysm surgery.

Hypotension

Although reduction in arterial pressure reduces brain bulk at pressures below the limit of autoregulation, it is generally wise to avoid hypotension until satisfactory decompression of the brain has been achieved.

Effect of anaesthetic agents

Inhalational agents including nitrous oxide, are cerebral vasodilators and tend to increase CBF and ICP. Hyperventilation almost always prevents the increase in ICP caused by the volatile agents and nitrous oxide.

Despite increasing CBF, all the inhalational anaesthetics with the possible exception of nitrous oxide, are mild metabolic depressants.

Thiopentone, Althesin and etomidate produce a reduction in $CMRO_2$ and CBF, and consequently in ICP. Ketamine increases $CMRO_2$, CBF and ICP, although these effects can be prevented by concurrent use of diazepam.

The commonly used opioids have little direct effect on intracranial haemodynamics, although their effect can be devastating if ventilatory depression is permitted to occur.

The muscle relaxants in common use do not affect cerebral metabolism or cerebral blood flow directly; however their effects on arterial pressure, cardiac output and venous pressure cause indirect effects.

Diazepam has been found to cause a moderate reduction in cerebral metabolism and cerebral blood flow.

Effect of anaesthetic technique

Increase in central venous pressure is transmitted directly to the intracranial veins and also increases c.s.f. pressure; consequently a slight head-up posture is often indicated. Insufficient expiratory time, high expiratory resistance, coughing, or straining on the endotracheal tube increase ICP.

Cerebral venous pressure may be reduced only slightly by a subatmospheric expiratory phase and generally if the patient is well relaxed, has a free expiratory pathway and an adequate expiratory time there is little to be gained from a negative phase. PEEP increases ICP, although the effects are usually less than might be expected.

ANAESTHESIA FOR NEUROLOGICAL INVESTIGATIONS

Precise anatomical localisation of intracranial pathology almost always requires sophisticated radiological investigations. The development of computerised axial tomography in 1973 revolutionised neuroradiology and made pneumo-encephalography a rarely used technique.

The majority of neuroradiological investigations require the use of contrast medium which carries some intrinsic risks. Nevertheless, as these investigations are essential before surgery, they are justifiable even when performed on very ill patients.

Contrast material occasionally produces anaphylactic or other hypersensitivity reactions and resuscitation facilities should always be available in the X-ray department. Metrizamide is used for intrathecal injection. It is said to be less likely than Myodil to cause anaphylactic reactions but may cause epileptiform convulsions. Known epileptics and patients receiving butyrophenone or phenothiazine derivatives are said to be particularly susceptible to this complication.

Local anaesthetic techniques may be used, with or without sedation, in co-operative adult patients. Small children and nervous, confused or disorientated adult patients usually require general anaesthesia.

Respiratory depressants must be avoided in patients with space-occupying lesions. Many neurosurgical patients require several anaesthetics and therefore agents which are known to produce occasional sensitivity reactions on repeated use should be avoided.

Any patient having a general anaesthetic for neuroradiology requires the same degree of care and the same precautions as when definitive neurosurgery is to be performed.

Computerised axial tomography (CAT)

CAT involves scanning the head with a beam of X-rays and a large number of detectors. The X-rays and detectors rotate through 180° around the patient's head and the data is processed by computer to yield tomographic anatomical slices of the head. In many instances contrast medium is injected to highlight tumour areas.

CAT scanning is not uncomfortable but requires

complete immobility of the patient for 1–6 min (depending on the generation of scanner).

Because of the apparent simplicity of the procedure, it is easy to allow stuporose patients to develop airway obstruction, and patients with multiple trauma to deteriorate during the investigation. It is essential to have the fullest supervision of ill patients undergoing CAT scan.

The choice of general anaesthesia depends on the neurological state of the patient. Endotracheal intubation and controlled ventilation are recommended for seriously ill or head-injured patients, whereas inhalational anaesthesia with spontaneous ventilation or continuous i.v. sedation is satisfactory for many patients.

Arteriography

Arteriography of the cranial vessels is performed either by direct puncture or by retrograde femoral catheterisation. The investigation may be limited to the carotid or vertebral systems or may include all vessels.

In many units, routine carotid arteriography is performed using local analgesia and sedation, but vertebral and panarteriography is performed under general anaesthesia. A technique using endotracheal intubation, muscle relaxation and hyperventilation has been shown to improve the quality of the radiographs; ventilation to a Pa_{CO_2} of 4 to 4.6 kPa is adequate. Occasional hypotension and hypertension have been reported during carotid arteriography, but more frequent circulatory changes are seen during vertebral arteriography.

Air encephalography and ventriculography

These investigations involve the injection of air, oxygen or nitrous oxide into the lumbar subarachnoid space or directly into the cerebral ventricle. The passage of the gas is governed by the position of the patient. It is usual to take radiographs using several different patient positions.

The use of air contrast has been condemned by some anaesthetists when nitrous oxide anaesthesia is being administered, because dissolved nitrous oxide diffuses into the air in the ventricular system and thereby increases its volume and pressure. To overcome this problem, the use of nitrous oxide as a contrast medium has been advocated. However the time available for radiography is limited by the greater solubility of nitrous oxide.

Hypotension and bradycardia are seen frequently during encephalography and may be associated with changes in breathing pattern.

In co-operative patients, local analgesia and sedation are recommended. General anaesthesia must avoid hypotension and hypercapnia. Controlled ventilation using pancuronium is often preferred in order to maintain normotension.

Myelography and other investigations

These studies are usually performed under local analgesia, but occasionally general anaesthesia is necessary. Caution is required where there is a lesion in the region of the foramen magnum or upper cervical spine, since there may be abnormal sympathetic tone.

ANAESTHESIA FOR NEUROSURGERY

The conduct of anaesthesia should aim to provide good operating conditions with an easily retractable brain and minimal blood loss.

Preoperative assessment

The care of the patient begins some days before major surgery. It is essential to recognise those patients who have an increased ICP, as the adverse effects of anaesthesia are greatly magnified. The presence of papilloedema, depression of consciousness and the degree of neurological deficit must be assessed. If there has been vomiting, there may be dehydration and electrolyte abnormalities, but no attempt should be made to hydrate fully patients with intracranial hypertension before surgery. The general medical condition of the patients and their fitness for anaesthesia must also be assessed.

Many patients are receiving steroid, anticonvulsant or antihypertensive drug therapy. Patients with grossly increased ICP should have ventricular drainage or mannitol therapy before operation. If gliomas or other causes of cerebral oedema are present, steroid thrapy (e.g. betamethasone 8 mg every 6 h) should be instituted.

Blood should be cross-matched as there is often more than 1 litre of haemorrhage at surgery and replacement with large volumes of crystalloid solutions is contraindicated.

The preoperative visit also allows assessment of the suitability of either the radial or dorsalis pedis artery for cannulation.

Alert patients are naturally apprehensive before a craniotomy and, as opioid and sedative premedication are usually contraindicated, it is important that reassurance and explanation are kind and thoughtful. Atropine 0.6 mg reduces oral secretions, and is frequently prescribed, while diazepam calms the patient and is used widely for premedication of neurosurgical patients. Diazepam has little effect on ICP, is a useful anticonvulsant, and in modest dosage produces little respiratory depression.

Induction of anaesthesia

With suitable preoperative care, few patients arrive in the anaesthetic room with grossly increased ICP. The induction technique should prevent hypoxia and hypercapnia and employ agents which reduce ICP, e.g. thiopentone or Althesin. The depth of anaesthesia achieved at induction should limit the responses of arterial pressure and ICP to laryngoscopy and intubation. A β-adrenergic receptor blocker administered at this stage may also be used to attenuate further the pressor responses. Preoxygenation, hyperventilation and full muscular relaxation should be achieved before attempting intubation in order to avoid coughing and straining.

Rapid gentle intubation of the trachea should be performed after spraying the larynx and upper trachea with local anaesthetic solution (e.g. lignocaine 4%). A nonkinkable endotracheal tube is recommended and should be fixed to the face with meticulous care, after checking that it is positioned correctly. A nasogastric tube is a useful precaution in long operations which may be associated with gastric dilatation. A pharyngeal pack is necessary in patients in whom a leak of blood or c.s.f. into the nasopharynx is anticipated.

Monitoring

1. Arterial pressure and heart rate. Direct cannulation of the radial artery at the wrist or the dorsalis pedis artery is usually indicated. This permits arterial pressure and heart rate to be displayed and provides access for arterial blood gas analysis. Newer noninvasive techniques are improving in reliability and may lessen the need for invasive monitoring in some patients.

2. Electrocardiogram.

3. Temperature — oesophageal or rectal.

4. Central venous pressure. A central venous line is indicated in operations where severe bleeding is expected. Where the sitting position is used it is considered essential in certain centres that the catheter is placed in the right atrium or ventricle.

5. A precordial or oesophageal stethoscope is useful and is indicated especially in operations performed in the sitting position, and in craniotomies in infants.

6. Expired carbon dioxide concentration.

7. Other monitoring may include ICP, e.e.g. or a processed derivative, blood gas measurements and measurements of CBF.

Transfusion and heat loss

An i.v. infusion should be commenced using compound sodium lactate and should incorporate a blood warming device. It is useful to prepare a second separate infusion for use with mannitol or hypotensive agents.

Heat loss is reduced by the use of a 'space rescue' blanket — a polyester sheet surrounded by laminates of aluminium foil. The impermeable material prevents heat loss from convection and evaporation and the aluminium prevents radiant heat loss. Alternatively, the patient may be placed on, and covered by, water circulation blankets.

Neurosurgical patients are at great risk of developing postoperative deep vein thrombosis. As there is some anxiety regarding the use of prophylactic heparin or dextran 70, because of the risks of bleeding, mechanical methods should be used for minimising stagnation of blood in the legs.

Iatrogenic injury

Care must be taken to protect the eyes by covering the closed lids with waterproof nonirritant adhesive plaster. There must be no stretching of peripheral nerves, and vulnerable skin pressure areas including the forehead, ears and nose must be protected.

Position for surgery

The surgical position is chosen to provide operative access and should allow good venous drainage from the site of operation by elevation of the head above the heart. Care should be taken to avoid excessive flexion or rotation of the neck, which might obstruct the neck veins.

Most craniotomies are performed in the supine brow-up position; temporal and posterior fossa craniotomies are satisfactory in the lateral or lateral/prone position with some rotation of the neck depending on the site of the lesion. The full prone position gives adequate exposure for many posterior fossa and cervical spine operations, but meticulous care must be taken to support the body on the iliac crests and the chest in order to leave a free, uncompressed abdomen and vena cava.

In many centres, the sitting position is still preferred to provide optimal access for posterior fossa surgery, despite a 5% reported incidence of marked postural hypotension, necessitating vasopressor therapy in 40% of patients. Air embolism occurs in 2 to 40% of patients (depending on the sensitivity of the method of detection). The author believes that the use of the sitting position for posterior fossa surgery should be discouraged strongly and that it should not be used for cervical spine surgery.

It is kinder to shave the head under anaesthesia with the patient in the surgical position rather than before operation. Finally the patient should be inspected to check the position of the endotracheal tube, its fixation and that of the anaesthetic tubing and other equipment.

Maintenance of anaesthesia

The basic technique for most craniotomies is hyperventilation with 70% nitrous oxide in oxygen to an arterial P_{CO_2} of 3.3 to 4 kPa. Muscle relaxation is maintained with incremental doses of a nondepolarising neuromuscular blocking agent given regularly to prevent any possibility of coughing or straining. An adequate depth of anaesthesia may be maintained if nitrous oxide is supplemented with fentanyl or phenoperidine. It is arguably safer to supplement anaesthesia with halothane or an alternative volatile agent during hypocapnia than to allow an excessively light patient to suffer hypertensive episodes during surgical stimulation.

Currently there is great interest in the replacement of inhalational 'anaesthetic agents by a total i.v. technique. Barbiturates, Althesin and etomidate lower intracranial pressure and in expert hands, problems of hypotension and delayed recovery do not seem to be unacceptable.

Active reduction in intracranial pressure

When the ICP is high or when the dura is tight and the brain swollen, the ICP must be lowered by pharmacological and occasionally mechanical means.

Mannitol in a 20% solution may be given in a dosage of 0.25–0.5 g/kg body weight. In this dosage, serum osmolality increases of over 10 mmol/kg may be expected and the acute effects on ICP are comparable to those achieved by higher doses. Effective reduction of ICP occurs within 5 min of commencing the infusion, and the improvement in the volume-pressure relationship lasts for up to 2 h. Mannitol is also helpful in making the brain softer and more easily retractable.

A disadvantage of mannitol is the associated transient hypervolaemia which may increase surgical bleeding.

Loop diuretics (e.g. frusemide in a dose of 1 mg/kg) produce a brisk diuresis and a reduction in brain bulk. In less urgent situations 30% glycerol may be given by mouth. Unfortunately high concentrations of glycerol produce haemolysis and haemoglobinuria when administered i.v.

When osmotic therapy is anticipated, a catheter should be placed in the bladder.

ICP reduction may also be achieved by ventriculostomy. In patients in whom only a small increase of ICP is present and there is communicating hydrocephalus, e.g. aneurysm surgery, drainage may be achieved via an indwelling lumbar spinal needle. However drainage should be limited in volume and to a rate of less than 5 ml/min, otherwise arterial hypertension and cardiac arrhythmias are common and a rebound increase in ICP may occur.

Recovery from anaesthesia

Patients who are expected to have a high risk of developing convulsions should be given phenytoin 250 mg by slow i.v. injection during anaesthesia. When cerebral oedema is anticipated following surgery, betamethasone or dexamethasone therapy should be commenced.

At the end of the operation, problems may arise as a result of depression of consciousness, damage to cranial nerves which limit the patient's ability to maintain a safe airway, and central respiratory depression.

After major procedures in which oedema is expected, or where autoregulation is likely to be grossly impaired, it is wise to continue hyperventilation into the postoperative period.

In patients in whom spontaneous ventilation is to be preferred, residual neuromuscular blockade should be antagonised with neostigmine and atropine. The increased sensitivity of neurosurgical patients to opioids makes it advisable to administer naloxone routinely to reverse residual effects.

The ability of the patient to breathe and maintain an airway spontaneously must be assessed and no carbon dioxide retention, hypoxia or asphyxia permitted otherwise serious brain swelling will occur.

SPECIFIC OPERATIONS

Intracranial vascular surgery

Before operation, hypertension should be treated and after subarachnoid haemorrhage epsilon aminocaproic acid (Epsikapron) therapy instituted to reduce the risk of further haemorrhage.

Induction of anaesthesia as described above should prevent surges of arterial pressure. After dural exposure, c.s.f. may be withdrawn via a needle in the lumbar subarachnoid space.

The author's policy regarding ventilation is to maintain normocapnia, as extremely low grey matter blood flows are encountered when hypocapnia is superimposed on the vasoconstriction associated with intracranial aneurysms.

The use of the operating microscope and hypotensive anaesthesia provide excellent operating conditions for surgical dissection of the aneurysmal sac and have led to the gradual abandonment of

hypothermia in most neurosurgical units in the United Kingdom.

Halothane may be used as the primary hypotensive agent, or used in addition to infusion of nitroprusside or trimetaphan.

Hypophysectomy

Removal of the pituitary gland is performed for tumours of the gland and for treatment of metastatic hormone-sensitive tumours. Hormone replacement with cortisone should be commenced before operation; other hormone problems, e.g. diabetes insipidus or mellitus may require therapy postoperatively.

Tracheal intubation in patients with acromegaly can be difficult and endotracheal tube introducers and an extra long laryngoscope blade should be available. Patients with carcinomatosis are often anaemic and cachectic and may have multiple bone metastases, pleural effusions and ascites. They should quickly be rendered as healthy as possible and the anaesthetic risk accepted, as there is often a gratifying response to surgery.

After hypophysectomy, a few patients develop severe hypothalamic disturbances of temperature and circulatory regulation.

AIR EMBOLISM

Air embolism occurs in 2 to 40% of patients in the sitting position, the reported incidence being related to the sensitivity of the method of detection. The severity of the embolism is determined by the rate and volume of air entrained and the ability of the circulation to withstand the insult. Air bubbles expand in the presence of nitrous oxide whilst 100% oxygen reduces the hazard.

Detection

Monitoring with a stethoscope reveals a drum-like resonance to the heart sounds and this becomes 'millwheel' with larger volumes of air. The Doppler ultrasonic flowmeter is the most sensitive detection device but many instruments are still unshielded from diathermy interference.

Expired carbon dioxide concentration decreases and arterial pressure and e.c.g. changes are common.

Pulmonary artery pressure increases during embolism before circulatory collapse. This haemodynamic variable is measured commonly in the U.S.A.

Treatment of air embolism comprises surgical sealing of the open veins, accompanied by jugular vein compression and an increase in intrathoracic pressure. A G-suit may be used to increase venous pressure, and aspiration of the right heart via a catheter enables air to be removed directly. Oxygen, vasopressors and external or internal cardiac massage may also be required.

HEAD INJURIES

Anaesthetists are involved in the care of head injuries because they are asked to provide anaesthesia for extracranial surgery in patients who have suffered minor head injuries, anaesthesia for intracranial surgery in more severe head injuries, and also to assist or supervise the resuscitation and medical care of comatose patients.

Anaesthesia for head injuries

All patients with head injury have some oedema of the brain with damage to its blood vessels and some degree of loss of autoregulation. An anaesthetic with a volatile agent using spontaneous ventilation is likely to produce a severe increase in ICP and neurological deterioration in the patient. Patients having minor procedures performed require the same anaesthetic standards as those undergoing neurosurgery.

First aid

Unconscious patients should be nursed in the semiprone position; the airway should be cleared of blood, vomit, false teeth, etc. It is essential to take great care when moving the head or neck as cervical spine injuries are commonly associated with head injuries. If cough and swallowing reflexes are impaired, endotracheal intubation is mandatory. It is wise to pass a large nasogastric tube, and, as far as possible, empty the stomach. Hypotension is rare in closed head injuries and suggests associated injuries.

Clinical assessment using the Glasgow coma scale (Table 27.1) should include an initial baseline

Table 27.1 The Glasgow coma scale is based upon eye opening, verbal and motor response. Each response on the scale is given a number (high for normal and low for impaired responses). The responsiveness of the patient is expressed by summation of the numbers. The lowest score is 3; the highest is 15.

Eyes	Open	Spontaneously	4
		To verbal command	3
		To pain	2
	No response		1
Best motor response	To verbal command	Obeys	6
		Localises pain	5
	To painful stimulus*	Flexion-withdrawal	4
		Flexion-abnormal (decorticate rigidity)	3
		Extension (decerebrate rigidity)	2
		No response	1
Best verbal response**		Orientated and converses	5
		Disorientated and converses	4
		Inappropriate words	3
		Incomprehensible sounds	2
		No response	1
TOTAL			3–15

*Apply knuckle to sternum, observe arms
**Arouse patient with painful stimulus if necessary

assessment, and additional investigations may be required including X-ray, scans, and arterial blood gas analysis.

Mannitol should not be used routinely but may help to prevent deterioration during patient transfer or postpone 'coning' when a patient appears to be deteriorating rapidly.

Immediate surgery is required in those patients in whom there is a rapid decline in conscious level or the sudden development of unilateral neurological signs. Most operations are performed for suspected or proven haematoma, depressed fractures and c.s.f. rhinorrhoea not associated with simple malar fractures.

Intensive care

Special care is necessary in all patients with head injury where airway care is required, if a laparotomy has been performed and in those with combinations of head and chest, spinal or jaw injury.

Control of raised ICP

Many patients with severe head injury develop an elevation of ICP. This may result from the development of a subdural or extradural haematoma, but occurs also in patients with no mass lesion, or in patients whose haematoma has been drained. In the first 24 h following head injury, the cerebral vasculature in damaged areas of brain dilates (vasoparesis), resulting in an increased cerebral blood volume. Later, both extracellular and intracellular oedema develop, increasing the volume of fluid inside the skull. Measures to control raised ICP are designed either to reduce cerebral blood volume, or to decrease the volume of intracerebral water.

Position. In order to encourage venous drainage, the patient should be nursed with the head and shoulder elevated at about 15° to the horizontal. The head should be straight, as kinking of neck veins occurs if cervical rotation is permitted.

Oxygenation. An arterial oxygen tension of at least 13 kPa should be maintained. Secondary cerebral damage may occur if areas of damaged brain with impaired capillary blood flow are subjected to hypoxaemia, and further cerebral vasodilatation occurs if Pa_{O_2} decreases below 7 kPa.

Controlled ventilation. Elective controlled hyperventilation is used widely in patients whose head injury results in persistent intracranial hypertension. It is also indicated in hyper- or hypoventilating or hypoxic patients, e.g. where $Pa_{CO_2} < 3$ kPa, or $Pa_{O_2} < 10$ kPa with an $F_{I_{O_2}}$ of 0.4. Neurological indications include status epilepticus or decerebrate spasms which have not responded to conventional therapy, and combined head and chest injuries.

When controlled ventilation is instituted, it is essential to prevent coughing and straining, and achieve good oxygenation and moderate hypocapnia (Pa_{CO_2} 3.5–4 kPa). Arterial oxygenation and carbon dioxide clearance must be maintained with the minimal airway pressure and the least value of PEEP, whenever the latter is necessary in the presence of severe lung dysfunction.

When elective ventilation is required, continuous ICP monitoring must be instituted.

Sedation. In the patient receiving IPPV, sedation is usually necessary, despite the resulting difficulty in clinical assessment of the nervous system. A continuous infusion of an opioid agent (e.g. papaveretum 10–20 mg/h) is often sufficient to prevent arterial hypertension, coughing and straining. Neuromuscular blocking agents may be useful if moderate doses of opioids are inadequate to prevent transient elevation of ICP, and are most effective if administered as a continuous infusion. Bolus doses of i.v. anaesthetic agents may be required in addition immediately before turning or physiotherapy.

Steroids. The use of steroids in patients with head injury is controversial. At present, it is thought that they do not influence control of ICP, or the eventual outcome of the patient.

Diuretics. Mannitol 0.25–0.5 g/kg, administered over 15–30 min, may be used to reduce the volume of intracranial water if the general trend of ICP is rising. Mannitol extracts water from normal brain, and does not reduce cerebral oedema per se. Serum osmolality must be monitored if frequent doses of mannitol are administered, and if the value exceeds 320 mmol/kg, further mannitol should be withheld. Frusemide or bumetanide may be used, and these agents reduce c.s.f. formation in addition to reducing intracerebral water. Serum electrolyte concentrations should be monitored closely.

Fluid balance. Normal fluid requirements and appropriate electrolytes should be administered. Dehydration does not assist in control of ICP.

The development of diabetes insipidus should be suspected if urine output increases in the absence of diuretic administration. Confirmation may be obtained by biochemical analysis of urine, and measurements of serum electrolytes and osmolality. Vasopressin should be administered as necessary.

Metabolic depression. When the management described fails to control ICP, but there are grounds for hope that the patient's condition may be reversible, metabolic depression may be undertaken using an infusion of an i.v. anaesthetic agent.

It is necessary to monitor directly arterial and central venous pressure to ensure that volume replacement is adequate. Access to a large vein is essential as dopamine may be required occasionally to counteract drug-induced circulatory depression.

Pentobarbitone, Althesin, thiopentone, gamma hydroxybutyric acid and etomidate have all been used. In all instances the cerebral perfusion pressure should be maintained at 60–70 mmHg using circulatory support if necessary.

Phenytoin has protective effects on the brain as a result of its anticonvulsant properties and perhaps its ability to reduce c.s.f. K^+ accumulation during hypoxia.

Although the use of these agents is often valuable in helping to control ICP, there is little evidence at present that this form of therapy has produced any great improvement in the outcome of these very ill patients.

Anticonvulsants

Anticonvulsants are required prophylactically in patients with depressed skull fractures with dural penetration, in those with early convulsions, and following acute subdural haematoma. Usually, phenytoin suffices, but if fits persist diazepam, phenobarbitone or other agents may be required. The metabolism of the brain is increased greatly during convulsions and therefore all fits must be treated vigorously. Monitoring the e.e.g. is helpful.

FURTHER READING

Campkin T V, Turner J M 1980 Neurosurgical anaesthesia and intensive care. Butterworths, London

Greenbaum R 1976 General anaesthesia for neurosurgery. British Journal of Anaesthesia 48: 773

Horton J M 1975 The immediate care of head injuries. Anaesthesia 30: 212

Jennett B, Teasdale G 1981 Management of head injuries. F A Davis, Philadelphia

Jones P W 1981 Hyperventilation in the management of cerebral oedema. Intensive Care Medicine 7: 205

Levy W J, Shapiro H M, Maruchak G, Meathe E 1980 Automated e.e.g. processing for intraoperative monitoring: a comparison of techniques. Anesthesiology 53: 223

McDowall D G 1975 The influence of anaesthetic drugs and techniques on intracranial pressure. In: Gordon E (ed) A basis and practice of neuroanaesthesia. Excerpta Medica, Amsterdam

Marshall L F, Smith R W, Shapiro H M 1979 The outcome with aggressive treatment in severe head injuries. Journal of Neurosurgery 50: 20

Silver I A 1979 The significance of clinical assessment of brain tissue oxygenation in different pathological conditions: an overview. Federation Proceedings 38: 2495

28

Anaesthesia for thoracic surgery

In the early 20th century, thoracic surgery was confined predominantly to the treatment of tuberculosis and empyema. Advances in anaesthetic practice permitted thoracoplasty, and subsequently lung resection and pneumonectomy, to be performed with increasing safety. With the introduction of antibiotics and antituberculous agents, surgical intervention has become progressively less common for pulmonary tuberculosis and bronchiectasis. The most common conditions presenting currently for thoracic surgery are carcinoma of bronchus, carcinoma of oesophagus, metastatic disease, and a variety of benign processes.

PREOPERATIVE ASSESSMENT

General assessment of the preoperative patient is considered in Chapter 15. In this section, only assessment of factors specific to thoracic surgery are discussed.

History

Dyspnoea

This common symptom may indicate disease of lungs or airways, cardiac disease or anaemia. Attempts should be made to relate dyspnoea to a specified degree of activity, e.g. climbing a flight of stairs, walking on the level, etc. The degree of dyspnoea in an individual may vary considerably, particularly if it is associated with disease of small airways, e.g. asthma or chronic bronchitis, when it may be accompanied by wheezing. Dyspnoea may result also from mucosal oedema, secretions, premature small airway closure, or alveolar fibrosis and infiltration.

Cough

A dry cough usually indicates irritation of the large airways, but if persistent, may be caused by serious pathology, e.g. compression of the trachea or main bronchi by glands. A productive cough is of greater importance, as material in the bronchial tree may spread infection, or cause obstruction and collapse of areas of lung. Sputum should be obtained for bacteriological examination

Haemoptysis

Large haemoptyses are uncommon, but have important anaesthetic implications, as the area responsible may require isolation using an endobronchial intubation technique in order to prevent contamination of the entire respiratory tree. Bronchiectasis and cavitating tuberculosis may cause severe haemoptysis, as may certain tumours, particularly after biopsy. Minor degrees of haemoptysis are common in inflammatory and neoplastic disease of the lung.

Dysphagia

Severe dysphagia has two important sequelae; the patient rapidly becomes malnourished and cachectic, and the oesophagus above the lesion dilates and may contain large volumes of previously ingested food which may be regurgitated when the patient becomes unconscious.

Examination

Physical examination of the patient is discussed in Chapter 15. Careful examination of the respiratory system is essential in patients presenting for thoracic surgery.

Cyanosis may be present, either centrally because of severe pulmonary disease, or peripherally in the distribution of superior vena caval drainage if that vessel is obstructed. Asymmetry of chest wall movement should be noted, together with any deviation of the trachea. If an intercostal drain is in place, the presence of an air leak should be noted, and its magnitude assessed. Stridor may be present if there is major obstruction of the trachea.

Percussion may demonstrate the presence of a pleural effusion or a major area of lung collapse.

Auscultation may reveal mild tracheal stridor, or partial obstruction of a main or lobar bronchus. More generalised airways obstruction is indicated by widespread rhonchi, often heard only during expiration. Fine crepitations suggest disease of peripheral airways or alveoli, while coarse crepitations are associated more usually with secretions in large airways, and may disappear after coughing.

The mouth and neck should be examined carefully. Features which suggest difficult endotracheal intubation are likely to result in severe hindrance to the introduction of an endobronchial or double lumen tube. Loose, prominent or capped teeth may interfere with, or be damaged during, rigid bronchoscopy or oesophagoscopy.

Preoperative investigations

Routine

Full blood count, serum urea and electrolytes, and blood glucose estimations are requested normally. A coagulation screen and liver function tests may be indicated. An e.c.g. is essential.

Radiological

Good quality posteroanterior and lateral X-rays of chest are helpful in demonstrating localised disease of the lungs, and distortion of the tracheobronchial tree. Tomography provides more detailed information on a lesion or malformation of the bronchial anatomy. Computerised axial tomography (body scan), nuclear magnetic resonance imaging and radionuclide scanning are used increasingly. Bronchography, using radio-opaque contrast medium to display the tracheobronchial tree, is employed particularly in patients with bronchiectasis. A barium swallow is required to define lesions of the oesophagus.

Pulmonary function tests

Objective assessment of pulmonary function is essential to assess the extent of impairment of lung function and as an aid in predicting the ability of a patient to survive pneumonectomy.

Reduction in forced vital capacity (FVC) indicates a restrictive defect. A low forced expiratory volume in one second (FEV_1), reduced FEV_1/FVC ratio, and decreased peak expiratory flow rate (PEFR) suggest the presence of obstructive disease of the airways. Additional information may be obtained by displaying flow-volume loops (see Chapter 2, Fig. 2.9). Reversibility of airways obstruction should be ascertained by repeating these tests after administration of a bronchodilator e.g. salbutamol. Measurement of gas transfer using carbon monoxide, and in particular, calculation of the gas transfer coefficient (gas transfer per unit of ventilated lung volume) provides information on gas exchange which may be useful in predicting the extent of postoperative hypoxaemia. Arterial blood gas analysis is necessary in all patients with moderate or severe lung disease in order to select an appropriate inspired oxygen concentration during and after surgery, and to detect patients with hypercapnia, in whom excessive inspired oxygen concentrations may reduce respiratory drive.

Regional lung function is assessed using radioisotope techniques, and aids decisions concerning pulmonary resection; overall lung function is unlikely to be impaired significantly if the resectable area has poor function.

Interpretation of lung function tests is not always easy, particularly with regard to prediction of postoperative problems. It is important to consider measurements in comparison with those predicted for a patient on the basis of height and weight (see Appendix, XIb, pp. 563–4). In general, if the FVC, FEV_1/FVC, and gas transfer are less than 50% of predicted values, prognosis after pneumonectomy is poor. If PEFR is less than 70% of predicted, or FEV_1/FEV less than 60%, complications following any form of pulmonary surgery may be anticipated. However, many factors not amenable to measurement are likely to influence the outcome, including motivation of the patient, coexisting nonpulmonary disease, and the occurrence of surgical complications.

PREPARATION FOR SURGERY

If possible, patients should stop cigarette smoking in order to reduce bronchial secretions. Antibiotics may be required if infected sputum is present. Bronchodilator drugs, preferably inhaled, may reduce airway obstruction considerably. Occasionally, corticosteroids may be required to reduce bronchospasm.

Preoperative physiotherapy is used to help clear bronchial secretions, and to encourage all patients to practice breathing exercises which are required in the postoperative period.

Rehydration, electrolyte correction and i.v. nutrition are often necessary in patients with oesophageal obstruction. Oesophageal lavage may be advisable in patients with a grossly dilated oesophagus.

Perioperative digitalisation is used in a number of centres for older patients undergoing thoracotomy. Low-dose heparin therapy has become popular to reduce the incidence of deep venous thrombosis and its sequelae.

An explanation should be given to the patient of the procedure which is to be undertaken, and of the postoperative environment. In particular, it is wise to warn the patient of the presence of chest drains and postoperative pain.

Premedication

The choice of premedication, if any, is one of personal preference, although an anticholinergic agent is advisable prior to endobronchial instrumentation.

DIAGNOSTIC PROCEDURES

Fibreoptic bronchoscopy

The fibreoptic bronchoscope (Fig. 28.1) may be introduced through the nose, injecting local anaesthetic solution through the injection port under direct vision as the instrument is advanced. In the anaesthetised patient, the bronchoscope may be introduced through an endotracheal tube by insertion through a diaphragm (Fig. 28.2) which minimises leakage of air during ventilation. Artificial ventilation should be maintained throughout bronchoscopy. Ventilation is impaired significantly unless the internal diameter of the endotracheal tube is more than 2 mm larger than the diameter of the bronchoscope. Techniques of ventilation using jet devices may be dangerous if expiration through the endotracheal tube is impeded by the presence of the bronchoscope, resulting in very high pressures in the lower trachea and bronchi.

Rigid bronchoscopy

Although fibreoptic bronchoscopy has become popular recently, the rigid bronchoscope remains the

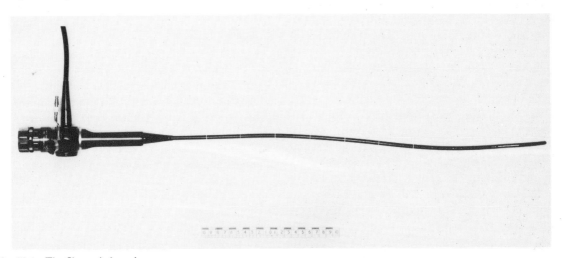

Fig. 28.1 The fibreoptic bronchoscope.

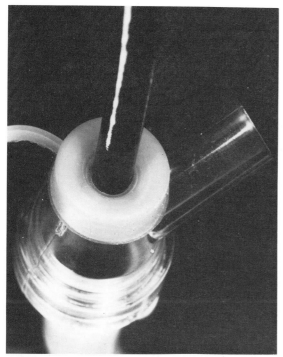

Fig. 28.2 Diaphragm used to ensure an airtight seal during fibreoptic bronchoscopy in patients receiving IPPV.

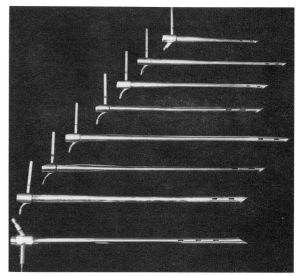

Fig. 28.3 Negus bronchoscopes.

preferred instrument of thoracic surgeons for location of bronchial tumours and for removal of foreign bodies or dilatation of strictures. Although this instrument may be used by the skilled practitioner under local anaesthesia, rigid bronchoscopy is carried out more commonly during general anaesthesia.

The rigid bronchoscope is essentially a long, tapered, metal tube. The most commonly used is the Negus (Fig. 28.3). An appropriate sized bronchoscope is chosen, and the patient's head positioned on one pillow with the neck slightly flexed. The head is extended on the neck. A gauze swab is placed on the patient's upper teeth or gums, and the middle finger of the bronchoscopist's left hand positioned on the patient's upper left second incisor (or the corresponding position in the edentulous patient). The bronchoscope is held in the right hand and introduced into the mouth alongside the operator's left middle finger, ensuring that the instrument is in the midline at the alveolar margin. The index finger and thumb of the left hand support the bronchoscope as it is advanced, keeping it clear of the teeth. The bronchoscope is passed backwards in the mouth until the uvula is visualised. The tip of the bronchoscope

and the portion at the alveolar margin are now both in the midline. Maintaining this midline position, the proximal end of the bronchoscope is angled downwards, thus lifting the tip, until the epiglottis is seen. The tip is passed beneath the epiglottis, then forwards and upwards until the vocal cords are visible, and finally into the trachea.

The head of the table may now be lowered, or the pillow removed carefully, so that the whole trachea comes into view. On advancing the instrument, the carina is seen. To pass the bronchoscope into one of the main bronchi, the head is rotated to the opposite side in order to bring the bronchus into line with the mouth. The appearance of the carina and main bronchi as seen through a bronchoscope are shown in Figure 1.15.

Rigid bronchoscopy may induce bronchospasm or cardiac arrhythmias, and interfere with ventilation. Thus, the anaesthetic technique should provide adequate analgesia and muscle relaxation, to permit introduction of the instrument and abolish reflexes from stimulation of the respiratory tract. Adequate gas exchange must be maintained. Rapid recovery of consciousness is desirable to enable the patient to cough up secretions or blood.

Topical analgesia is used occasionally, the technique being similar to that described for endotracheal intubation in Chapter 19.

Inhalational anaesthesia using halothane or ether is used by some anaesthetists for rigid bronchoscopy in children. The child is anaesthetised deeply using the volatile agent, and bronchoscopy performed with the patient breathing air spontaneously through the instrument. The depth of anaesthesia lightens progressively, fairly rapidly with halothane but more slowly if ether is used, and the bronchoscope may have to be removed intermittently to allow the level of anaesthesia to be deepened.

More commonly, i.v. anaesthesia is used. Following preoxygenation, light narcosis is induced using an i.v. anaesthetic agent, e.g. methohexitone. Suxamethonium is used to provide muscle relaxation. The lungs are inflated with oxygen by face mask, and bronchoscopy undertaken. Incremental doses of i.v. anaesthetic agent and suxamethonium are given as indicated. Artificial ventilation is achieved usually using an injector, which produces a high pressure jet of gas down the bronchoscope. Either oxygen of Entonox may be used as the driving gas. The jet of gas entrains air and produces inflation of the lungs. Expiration occurs through and round the bronchoscope. An appropriate size of jet must be selected (Table 28.1). Recently, high frequency positive pressure ventilation (HFPPV), at rates of 100–300 breath/min, has been used during bronchoscopy. This technique eliminates air entrainment and allows ventilation with an undiluted anaesthetic gas mixture.

Table 28.1 Appropriate sizes, and typical maximum inflation pressures, with Venturi bronchoscope injectors

Patient	Size (s.w.g.)	Pressure (cmH$_2$O)
Adult (poor compliance)	14	50
Adult	16	25
Child (over 12 yr)	17	20
Child (under 12 yr)	19	15

Oesophagoscopy

Fibreoptic oesophagoscopy is undertaken normally in the sedated patient. The rigid oesophagoscope is inserted under general anaesthesia. Features of importance to the anaesthetist are the potential of regurgitation on induction of anaesthesia, and the risk of damage to teeth or the cervical spine as the instrument is introduced. A 'crash induction' should be used, and ventilation controlled after endotracheal intubation. The cuff of the endotracheal tube may require deflation temporarily to enable the oesophagoscope to pass through the cricopharyngeal sphincter.

The most serious complication of oesophagoscopy is perforation of the oesophagus, and a chest X-ray is required following the procedure before any fluids are allowed by mouth.

Mediastinoscopy

This procedure permits direct inspection and biopsy of mediastinal lesions, in particular lymph nodes. The mediastinoscope is introduced through a small suprasternal incision (Fig. 28.4). Complications include haemorrhage, pneumothorax, haemothorax, air embolism and recurrent laryngeal nerve damage. The most commonly used anaesthetic technique employs tracheal intubation and controlled ventilation.

Bronchography

This is performed usually using the oil-based radio-opaque contrast medium propyliodine (Dionosil) to outline the tracheobronchial tree. Bronchography may be undertaken in the conscious patient under local anaesthesia, either by injecting contrast medium through a catheter placed in the trachea, or by allowing it to trickle over the back of the tongue. General anaesthesia is required for children and uncooperative adults.

The commonest indication for bronchography is investigation of the extent of bronchiectasis. The patient may already have compromised respiratory function and copious infected sputum. A sedative premedication with atropine is usually prescribed, and anaesthesia induced either with an i.v., or in young children, an inhalational agent. The trachea is intubated, and anaesthesia maintained with a nitrous oxide/oxygen mixture. This may be supplemented with a volatile agent (halothane or enflurane) if spontaneous ventilation is employed. This technique is used because it permits contrast medium to be inhaled gently into the bronchi, whereas positive pressure ventilation tends to disperse the contrast medium distally to bronchioles and alveoli. When the patient is anaesthetised to a depth at which the cough reflex is depressed, contrast medium is injected via a catheter introduced through the tracheal tube. The patient is tilted to enable filling of the various segments of the lung. Twenty to 30 ml of contrast medium may be required for bronchograms of each lung.

Many anaesthetists prefer to control ventilation during bronchography. Following endotracheal intubation, either a nondepolarising muscle relaxant is administered, or suxamethonium is used intermittently as required. Contrast medium is introduced through a catheter, and the lungs ventilated gently by hand to move contrast into the bronchi. It is important not to ventilate vigorously at this stage.

Following bronchography, the contrast medium is aspirated through the endotracheal tube. The patient is allowed to waken with the cough reflex restored before the trachea is extubated.

CHEST WALL INTEGRITY

If chest wall integrity is lost, either as a result of trauma or surgical intervention, abnormal chest wall movement and gas distribution occur. In the patient with a damaged chest wall, e.g. crush injury, paradoxical movement of the chest wall is seen, with inward movement of the rib cage during inspiration and the reverse during expiration. During inspiration, the lung on the unaffected side expands, but fills with gas partly from the trachea, and partly from the lung on the abnormal side, which deflates.

During expiration, the normal lung deflates, but part of the expired gas passes into the lung on the affected side, which expands. This pattern of ventilation, termed 'pendulum breathing' or Pendelluft, results in progressive hypoxaemia and hypercapnia. A similar pattern occurs if the chest wall is opened surgically. Thus spontaneous ventilation is inappropriate if integrity of the chest wall is to be lost, and positive pressure ventilation should be employed.

ONE-LUNG ANAESTHESIA

Distribution of ventilation and perfusion

In the awake, spontaneously breathing subject in the lateral position, the dependent lung is better perfused than the upper lung because of gravity (Fig. 28.5). The dependent diaphragm is pushed higher than the upper during expiration by the weight of the abdominal contents. As a result, it contracts more efficiently, so that ventilation of the dependent lung is also better than that of the upper lung. Thus, ventilation and perfusion are reasonably well matched in both lungs. However, in the anaesthetised patient, functional residual capacity (FRC) is reduced and the upper lung receives greater ventilation, whereas perfusion remains better in the lower lung. Similarly,

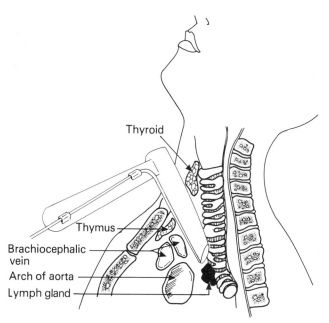

Fig. 28.4   Insertion of mediastinoscope through a suprasternal incision. Note the proximity of large blood vessels.

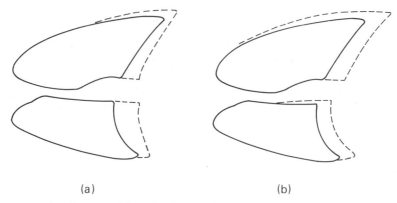

Fig. 28.5 Ventilatory excursion of upper and dependent lungs in the lateral position during (a) spontaneous breathing in the conscious patient and (b) IPPV. See text for details.

during controlled ventilation, the upper lung is ventilated preferentially as the compliance of the dependent lung is reduced by the weight of the abdominal contents and mediastinum.

In order to improve surgical access, the upper lung may be allowed to collapse, whereupon it acts as a source of true shunt, since it still receives a proportion of the right ventricular output, but no ventilation. The dependent lung receives the major portion of pulmonary blood flow, and the entire minute ventilation. Ventilation and perfusion are unlikely to be matched perfectly throughout the dependent lung, and the total calculated intra-pulmonary shunt therefore varies from 25 to 40% when the upper lung is collapsed. Paradoxically, higher values tend to be found in patients with normal lungs, since a diseased lung, even if it contains a focal lesion, tends to have a reduced blood supply. During pulmonary surgery, the more diseased lung is uppermost, and the dependent lung receives an increased proportion of total pulmonary blood flow. In contrast, a patient undergoing oesophageal surgery may have two healthy lungs, and intrapulmonary shunt during one-lung anaesthesia may be very high.

Increased intrapulmonary shunting causes a decrease in arterial oxygen tension. Although there is no degree of hypoxaemia which may be regarded as safe, it is generally felt that an arterial P_{O_2} of approximately 9 kPa is acceptable; this results in an oxygen saturation of approximately 90%. In order to achieve this or a higher Pa_{O_2} during one-lung ventilation, a number of techniques can be employed. It is generally recommended that an inspired oxygen concentration of 40% be provided initially on switching to one-lung anaesthesia. Higher con-

centrations may be necessary if there is clinical or blood gas evidence of hypoxaemia. However, concentrations of oxygen in excess of 60% are unlikely to produce a substantial increase in Pa_{O_2}, and may, unexpectedly, increase intrapulmonary shunt by decreasing the normal hypoxic vasoconstriction in poorly ventilated areas of the dependent lung. Although blood flow to the unventilated lung decreases because of an increase in vascular resistance, this does not occur to a significant extent in the first few hours after lung collapse, and a large intrapulmonary shunt persists throughout the course of one-lung anaesthesia.

Blood flow through the collapsed lung may be reduced by restricting intra-alveolar pressure, thereby encouraging blood flow through the dependent lung. Thus, positive end-expiratory pressure (PEEP), which might be expected to improve arterial oxygenation by increasing FRC in the dependent lung, has been found to increase shunt by diverting blood to the unventilated lung. In some patients, it may be necessary to supply oxygen under a small positive pressure (3–5 cmH$_2$O) to the unventilated lung. This permits diffusion oxygenation of the blood perfusing that lung, and reduces arterial hypoxaemia.

Because of the increased inspired oxygen concentration required to prevent arterial hypox-aemia, only 40–60% nitrous oxide should be administered. In order to ensure adequate anaesthesia, this should be supplemented with a volatile agent (halothane or enflurane), i.v. opioid drugs, or a combination of the two. A recent innovation has been the use of opioids administered through an extradural catheter to provide intra-operative analgesia, although a volatile agent should be used in conjunction with nitrous oxide in order to prevent awareness.

Although dead space:tidal volume ratio may diminish when one-lung ventilation is commenced, the increase in intrapulmonary shunt results in impaired carbon dioxide excretion. The net result is that carbon dioxide elimination remains essentially unchanged if minute ventilation is kept constant on changing to one-lung ventilation.

Apparatus for one-lung anaesthesia

Bronchial blockers

A bronchial blocker is simply a suction catheter with an inflatable balloon at its distal end. It is used to isolate, and to permit aspiration of secretions from, one lung or lobe. After introduction through a bronchoscope, the balloon is inflated, and an endotracheal tube inserted to permit ventilation of the unblocked areas of lung. Bronchial blockers are seldom used now, having been superseded by double-lumen tubes, but they have occasional indications, e.g. for control of haemorrhage.

Single lumen endobronchial tubes

Some single lumen endobronchial tubes may be introduced blindly into position, while others are designed to be inserted under direct vision over a bronchoscope. These latter types are useful if bronchial anatomy is distorted. A single lumen tube is passed into the main bronchus of the nonoperated lung. This lung can be isolated by inflation of the balloon at the distal end of the tube, or both lungs can be ventilated, although unequally, by deflation of this balloon, and inflation of the tracheal cuff.

In infants, endobronchial intubation may be required occasionally, and can be achieved by the use of an endotracheal tube cut 1 cm longer than normal, and of the same diameter or 1 mm smaller than would be used for endotracheal intubation.

Double lumen tubes

Double lumen tubes (Fig. 28.6) are the commonest type of endobronchial apparatus in current use. Their purpose is to provide separate channels for ventilation and suction of both lungs. The lumen on one side is shaped at its distal end to enter and occupy one or

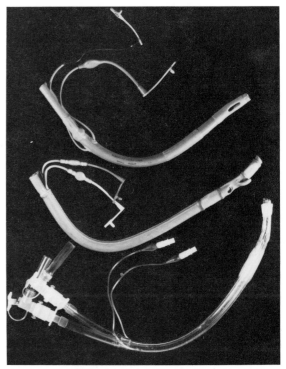

Fig. 28.6 Double lumen tubes. Top to bottom: right-sided Robertshaw, Carlen (left-sided, with carinal hook), left-sided Bronchocath (disposable, PVC).

other main bronchus, while the second lumen ends in the trachea. In order to permit clamping and transection of the main bronchus during pneumonectomy, a right-sided tube is used for operations on the left lung, although it may occlude the upper lobe bronchus despite the slit in the bronchial cuff (Fig. 28.7), because the location of the right upper lobe bronchus is variable. A left-sided tube is used when surgery of the right lung is planned, or when nonpulmonary surgery is undertaken. Double lumen tubes may be awkward to introduce through the larynx, and may not enter the desired bronchus if the anatomy is distorted. However, when correctly positioned, they permit access to both lungs, provide even ventilation, and are less likely to be dislodged than a single lumen tube.

THORACOTOMY

Anaesthetic technique

(Modifications to the technique described here are required in the presence of a bronchopleural fistula,

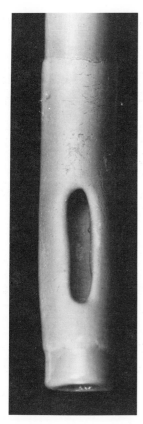

Fig. 28.7 Orifice in endobronchial lumen of right-sided Robertshaw double lumen tube to permit ventilation of right upper lobe.

empyema, lung cyst or pneumothorax. These modifications are detailed in the appropriate sections of this chapter.)

Induction of anaesthesia may be achieved using an appropriate i.v. agent. Although some anaesthetists prefer to use suxamethonium if a double-lumen tube is to be introduced, others use a large dose of nondepolarising relaxant (e.g. pancuronium 0.1 mg/kg, alcuronium 0.3 mg/kg), as comparable relaxation ensues in 2–3 min, and thoracotomy is seldom of shorter duration than that of the relaxant.

A large gauge i.v. cannula is essential for infusion of fluids and blood (which is usually required).

Maintenance of anaesthesia is achieved normally using a combination of nitrous oxide/oxygen, i.v. opioid and volatile anaesthetic. The choice may be influenced by the need for one-lung anaesthesia. The depth of anaesthesia required is comparable to that for abdominal surgery.

Monitoring

Monitoring of e.c.g., heart rate and arterial pressure is mandatory. Arterial pressure may be measured indirectly with a sphygmomanometer or oscillotonometer, although in the lateral position pressure recordings from the dependent arm may be unreliable because of compression by the thorax. Direct arterial pressure measurement using an intra-arterial cannula is indicated in the poor risk patient, or if severe haemorrhage or mediastinal retraction are anticipated. This technique also allows sampling for blood gas analysis, and is useful if severe hypoxaemia is expected. Central venous pressure monitoring may be necessary when major surgery, associated with heavy bleeding, is planned. Monitoring of temperature is important in children, or if prolonged surgery is anticipated in adults. In these situations, a warming blanket and blood warmer should be used, and inspired gases require warming and humidification.

Position

Pulmonary surgery is undertaken normally with the patient in the lateral position (Fig. 28.8), with the diseased side uppermost. Care must be taken to avoid nerve damage in the upper arm by avoiding excess traction, and a pillow should be placed between the legs to prevent pressure damage.

Some surgeons prefer the patient to be positioned prone, in the Parry Brown position (Fig. 28.9). The shoulders and pelvis are supported to prevent pressure on the abdomen, which increases intra-abdominal pressure, impairs expansion of the lung bases, and reduces venous return to the heart. The arm on the operated side hangs over the edge of the operating table so that the scapula is pulled away from the site of surgery. This position allows drainage of secretions from the diseased lung towards the trachea without soiling the other lung.

Oesophageal surgery is undertaken usually with the patient in the lateral or semilateral position.

At the end of thoracotomy, the pleural cavity is drained (not always after pneumonectomy) to ensure that air or fluid does not accumulate in the postoperative period. If the lung has been collapsed, it is reinflated before the thorax is closed so that re-expansion may be confirmed under direct vision.

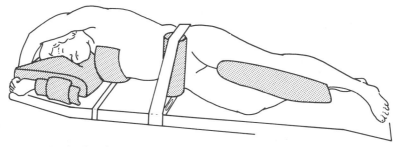

Fig. 28.8 Patient in lateral position for thoracic surgery.

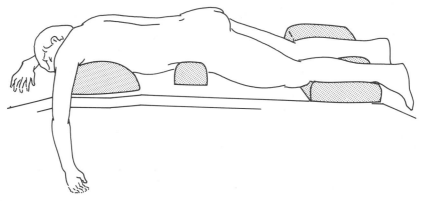

Fig. 28.9 Patient in Parry Brown position for thoracic surgery.

Following closure of the thorax, the drains are connected to an underwater seal, which permits drainage of air or fluid with minimal resistance, and allows measurement of drained fluid or blood. As IPPV is continued, air is expelled from the pleural space, and the lung expands to fill the cavity.

It is usual to allow patients to breathe spontaneously following thoracotomy, and residual effects of neuromuscular blocking drugs are therefore antagonised. Secretions are aspirated via a suction catheter passed through the tracheal tube. When adequate spontaneous ventilation has returned, and the patient has regained control of reflexes, pharyngeal secretions are aspirated and the tracheal (or double lumen) tube removed.

Postoperative care

Pulmonary function may be reduced considerably following thoracotomy. The lungs may be affected by chronic disease, a lobe or lung may have been excised, and the remaining lung tissue has been manipulated and retracted, resulting in patchy oedema and contusion, and an increase in pulmonary secretions. Blood or infected material from a resected area may contaminate the remaining lung. Pain from the incision and chest drain sites inhibits chest wall movement, and, together with any accumulation of fluid or air in the pleural cavity, may reduce expansion and encourage atelectasis and collapse.

Although mechanical ventilation in the post-operative period permits expansion of the lungs, aspiration of secretions and adequate analgesia and sedation (without fear of respiratory depression), there are disadvantages, particularly after pulmonary surgery. Air leaks from the surface of the lung or from the resected bronchial stump may be augmented by IPPV. Continued endotracheal intubation may result in increased risk of chest infection. However, elective mechanical ventilation is necessary occasionally in debilitated patients following oesophageal resection, and in patients with severely impaired lung function following pulmonary surgery.

In all patients, adequate oxygenation and ventilation should be ensured. An increased inspired oxygen concentration of 40% (unless the patient is chronically hypercapnic) is advisable to prevent arterial hypoxaemia, together with humidification of the inspired gases to prevent inspissation of secretions, and physiotherapy to aid lung expansion and coughing. Effective analgesia is essential. An opioid analgesic administered intermittently by the i.m. route is easy to prescribe, but provides sporadic analgesia, and may cause respiratory depression. Patient-controlled i.v. infusions of opioid analgesic drugs provide more continuity of analgesia. Blockade of the intercostal nerves during thoracotomy either with a local anaesthetic agent or using cryoanalgesia reduces the requirements for systemic analgesic drugs. Paravertebral or extradural nerve block with a local anaesthetic agent is extremely effective, while extradural or intrathecal opioids may provide profound analgesia with virtually no cardiovascular complications, although there is a high risk of late respiratory depression. Extradural catheter techniques permit administration of repeated doses of drug, but require careful monitoring, and should be contemplated only if the patient is nursed in a high dependency or intensive care area.

SURGERY RELATED TO THE LUNG

Removal of inhaled foreign body

Inhalation of foreign bodies is not uncommon in children. Obstruction of the larynx results in acute obstruction, but smaller objects wedge more distally and may result either in valvular obstruction with emphysema of the affected lobe or segment, or more commonly in total obstruction leading to distal consolidation and collapse. Eighty per cent of foreign bodies lodge in the right lung. There may be considerable reaction and oedema at the site of obstruction, particularly when an irritant object, e.g. a peanut, has been inhaled.

The patient may have a degree of respiratory obstruction, pulmonary infection and hypoxaemia. An inhalational induction is preferable in children, particularly if respiratory obstruction is present, and a selection of endotracheal tubes should be available. Removal of the foreign body is performed through a rigid bronchoscope, and may be extremely difficult, particularly if bronchial oedema is present. Laryngeal stridor is not uncommon during recovery, and the patient must be observed closely for at least 12 h.

Lobectomy

The usual indications for lobectomy are:

1. *Bronchial neoplasm.*
2. *Bronchiectasis.* Lobectomy is indicated if haemoptyses occur repeatedly or infection cannot be controlled.
3. *Infection.* Although it is now relatively rare, tuberculosis is the most common infective condition under this heading.

Lobectomy may be a straightforward procedure with few surgical problems, but it may be difficult and result in severe haemorrhage in the presence of invading tumour, chronic infection or pleural adhesions. In many centres, isolation of the affected lung is achieved using a single or double lumen endobronchial tube in the healthy lung. This permits aspiration of secretions, deflation of the affected lung when required, and reflation of the remaining lobes before closure of the chest. When the lobe has been removed, the bronchus is clamped and divided, and the remnant either sutured or stapled. The pleural cavity may be filled with saline, and inflation of the affected lung to a pressure of 30–40 cmH$_2$O is undertaken to ensure that no significant air leak exists. Depending on the experience and requirements of the surgeon, bronchial division and closure may not require cessation of ventilation of the affected lung for any significant period of time, and an endotracheal tube may be satisfactory unless there is a need to protect the healthy lung from secretions, or sleeve resection of the main bronchus is anticipated because of tumour close to the origin of the lobar bronchus.

Pneumonectomy

Bronchial carcinoma not confined to a single lobe is the normal indication for this operation. Pneumonectomy may be performed either in the prone or lateral position. Endobronchial intubation is usually selected if the lateral position is used. Mediastinal manipulation may result in arrhythmias, and haemorrhage may be considerable. The main bronchus is divided and sutured, and tested for air leaks as described above.

Following pneumonectomy, the pleural space fills with serosanguinous fluid, and this is allowed to accumulate. Thus, the pleural cavity is not always drained. If a drain is inserted at operation, it is connected to an underwater seal, and left open to drain air and fluid while the patient is returned to the supine position. After a chest X-ray has confirmed that the mediastinum is central, the drain is clamped, but the clamps are removed for a short period every hour during the 24 h following surgery to ensure that neither air nor excess fluid is accumulating. If the pleural space is not drained, on return to the supine position at the end of surgery, a needle is inserted through the chest wall, connected to a three-way stopcock and manometer, and air removed or injected until the intrapleural pressure is normal, indicating that the mediastinum is central. The risks of leaving the cavity undrained are that air may accumulate under pressure if the bronchial stump leaks, and that massive haemorrhage may go unrecognised. Drainage may, however, increase the risk of infection.

Normally, the empty pleural space fills gradually with serosanguinous fluid, and fibrosis subsequently occurs, pulling the diaphragm into the thorax and the mediastinum across to the operated side. If fluid accumulates too rapidly, mediastinal distortion and compression of the remaining lung result in a combination of hypotension, right ventricular failure and hypoxaemia. Central venous pressure is often high because of mediastinal distortion, although the patient is usually hypovolaemic because of fluid loss. Mediastinal displacement causing cardiorespiratory distress can occur also if the space fills too slowly with fluid as air is absorbed.

Sputum retention and respiratory failure are not uncommon after pneumonectomy — mortality is increased significantly if mechanical ventilation is required. Arrhythmias and pericarditis are also frequent complications, probably because of mediastinal manipulation. The incidence of supraventricular arrhythmias is reduced if the patient is digitalised during the perioperative period.

Other complications of major surgery, e.g. myocardial infarction, renal failure, may occur. The mortality following left pneumonectomy is 7–10%, and may be as high as 20% after excision of the larger right lung.

Bronchopleural fistula

A connection between the tracheobronchial tree and the pleural cavity may result from trauma, neoplasm, rupture of an intrapulmonary cavity (e.g. abscess), or from breakdown of a bronchial stump or anastomosis after surgery. Bronchopleural fistulae are almost always complicated by the collection of infected fluid in the pleural cavity. This results in a number of problems of importance to the anaesthetist. The patient may be cachectic and dehydrated, and pulmonary function may be impaired considerably. Careful preoperative assessment is essential, although surgical intervention may be urgent. In addition to factors related to the general condition of the patient, two specific dangers exist:

1. The remaining healthy lung is at risk of contamination by the infected contents of the pleural space.

2. Positive pressure applied to the affected bronchial tree may result either in passage of the inspired gas out through the chest drain resulting in little or no effective alveolar ventilation, or, if the drain is only partially patent, in an increase in intrapleural pressure with the danger that infected material may be squeezed into the tracheobronchial tree with consequent pulmonary contamination.

Only anticholinergic premedication is prescribed. The patient is placed in a semisitting, semilateral position with the affected side dependent. Endobronchial intubation is essential if possible. The optimum method of induction of anaesthesia is controversial. Some anaesthetists feel that an inhalational induction is the safest technique, as spontaneous ventilation can be maintained until the endobronchial or double-lumen tube is in position and the damaged lung isolated. However, deep anaesthesia is required, and this may have cardiovascular complications in the semirecumbent position. In addition, prolonged attempts at intubation may result in coughing, which increases intrapleural pressure and may spread infected material through the lungs. Consequently, many anaesthetists who are practised at endobronchial intubation prefer to preoxygenate the lungs, induce anaesthesia with an i.v. agent, and produce muscle paralysis with suxamethonium. Intubation is carried out when spontaneous respiration has ceased.

When the tube is in position, the healthy lung is ventilated, and infected material from the affected bronchial tree aspirated. A nondepolarising muscle relaxant is administered, and one-lung anaesthesia maintained as described above. Following surgery, attempts are made to restore spontaneous ventilation, although this may be precluded by the patient's condition.

Drainage of empyema

An empyema is a collection of purulent material in the pleural cavity. It is associated usually with an infective process in the lung, although it may occur also after oesophageal perforation or as a complication of thoracotomy. Initial treatment is with appropriate antibiotics and drainage through an intercostal drain. This is inserted under local anaesthesia. Drainage may be incomplete, however, and a chronic empyema may develop with fibrosis of the surrounding pleura. Resection of one or more ribs may be required in order to obtain satisfactory drainage. An empyema is often accompanied by a bronchopleural fistula, and this determines anaesthetic management (vide supra).

Lung cysts and bullae

These are thin-walled, air-filled cavities within the lung which may be congenital, the consequence of previous infection, or the result of emphysema. Their connection with the bronchial tree may be valvular. Large cysts may present problems during unrelated surgery. IPPV may result in rupture of a thin-walled cyst. Enlargement of the cyst may occur if a valvular connection is present. Nitrous oxide may also enlarge a cyst because nitrogen is less soluble in blood.

Rupture of a cyst results very rapidly in respiratory distress. Gross enlargement of a cyst may produce a similar effect. The two may be indistinguishable clinically, and a chest drain should be inserted if respiratory distress occurs. A persistent air leak is likely to develop if an enlarged cyst is drained, and may also follow rupture of a cyst.

During anaesthesia for resection of a lung cyst, attention must be given to prevention of rupture of the cyst, in addition to the problems associated with thoracotomy. Endobronchial blocking or intubation permit selective ventilation of the normal lung, although endotracheal intubation and gentle positive pressure ventilation is regarded by some anaesthetists as a satisfactory technique.

Lung abscess

The majority of lung abscesses are amenable to treatment with antibiotics, and usually rupture into a bronchus from which the contents are expectorated, or into the pleura resulting in an empyema and bronchopleural fistula. Surgery for an abscess may result in its rupture during anaesthesia. A double-lumen tube should be used to ensure that contamination of the unaffected lung does not take place, and so that infected material can be aspirated.

Pleurectomy and pleurodesis

Pleurectomy is performed through an anterolateral thoracotomy. Pleurodesis is achieved by the introduction of iodised talc through a thoracoscope, or by abrasion of the pleura with a gauze swab through a small thoracotomy incision. The usual indication for these procedures is repeated spontaneous pneumothorax.

The patient presenting for pleurectomy may have a pneumothorax, and may have underlying pulmonary disease. If the pleural cavity is not drained, the pneumothorax may be increased in size by nitrous oxide, or by IPPV if an air leak is present or a lung cyst ruptured. However, the time period between induction of anaesthesia and exposure of the pleural cavity is short. It is seldom necessary to avoid the use of nitrous oxide, and gentle IPPV may be used until the chest wall is open. A double lumen tube is not necessary unless a large air leak is present. Haemorrhage may be considerable, and postoperative pain is severe.

NONPULMONARY SURGERY

Diaphragmatic hernia

Anaesthesia for repair of a congenital diaphragmatic hernia in the neonate is discussed in Chapter 32. A congenital hernia may present in adults, but the condition is associated more commonly with trauma in adult life. It may be possible to repair the hernia from the abdomen, but thoracotomy is often necessary. The lung may be compressed by distended bowel, and pulmonary function impaired as a result.

Electrolyte abnormalities may be present because of intestinal obstruction. If the stomach has herniated into the thorax, the risk of reflux of gastric contents is increased.

Repair of hiatus hernia

A hiatus hernia may require repair using a thoracic approach through a left thoracotomy. The patient may be obese. It should be assumed that regurgitation of gastric contents may occur because of incompetence of the lower oesophageal sphincter. Antacids should be continued preoperatively, and H_2-antagonists may be given with premedication to increase pH of the gastric contents. Preoxygenation of the lungs should be carried out before induction of anaesthesia, and cricoid pressure applied until the airway is secure. An endotracheal tube is usually adequate, and is easier and faster to position than a double lumen tube. However, in some centres, a left-sided double lumen tube is used and the left lung deflated to permit better surgical access. One-lung anaesthesia in the patient with normal lungs may result in severe hypoxaemia (vide supra).

Oesophageal myotomy

Oesophageal myotomy (Heller's operation) is indicated in the presence of achalasia. This disorder of oesophageal motility results in gross dilatation of the oesophagus and the collection in it of large volumes of undigested food. The patient may have pulmonary disease as a result of repeated aspiration of oesophageal contents. The principal risk during anaesthesia is that of aspiration, and the anaesthetic management is similar to that described for repair of hiatus hernia.

Surgery for carcinoma of oesophagus

Inoperable carcinoma of oesophagus causes progressive obstruction, resulting eventually in complete dysphagia. Insertion of an oesophageal tube (e.g. Celestine) may provide some palliation. Bypass of the tumour can be accomplished by mobilisation of the stomach through a laparotomy and, after passing the stomach behind the sternum, anastomosis to the upper oesophagus in the neck.

Tumours of the middle and lower thirds of the oesophagus may be resectable. This is a major procedure, undertaken in a patient who may be cachectic, hypoproteinaemic and anaemic. In addition, pulmonary function may be impaired by repeated aspiration of oesophageal contents. Preoperative nutrition, either enteral or parenteral, may be advisable in the cachectic patient. Premedication should be appropriate for the nutritional state of the patient.

Carcinoma of the lower third of the oesophagus is resected through a left thoracoabdominal incision. If the lesion is in the middle third, the operation may be performed in two stages; initially, abdominal organs are mobilised through a laparotomy, and the patient is then turned into the left lateral position in order that the resection can be completed, and the anastomosis performed, through a right thoracotomy. Irrespective of the surgical approach, a left-sided double-lumen tube is used and the lung on the side of the thoracotomy collapsed intermittently to allow surgical access to the oesophagus. Haemorrhage can be considerable, and cardiovascular problems may result from retraction of the vena cava or heart. An indwelling arterial cannula and central venous catheter are required. The procedure is often of prolonged duration, and precautions should be taken to prevent hypothermia.

FURTHER READING

Churchill-Davidson H C 1978 Thoracic anaesthesia. In: Churchill-Davidson H C (ed) A practice of anaesthesia. Lloyd-Luke, London
Fordham R 1978 Pulmonary ventilation. In: Churchill-Davidson H C (ed) A practice of anaesthesia. Lloyd-Luke, London

Gothard J W W, Branthwaite M A 1982 Anaesthesia for thoracic surgery. Blackwell Scientific Publications, Oxford
Kaplan J A (ed) 1983 Thoracic anesthesia. Churchill Livingstone, New York

29

Anaesthesia for cardiac surgery

The cardiac surgical theatre, with its profusion of personnel, monitors and support equipment, is often intimidating to the trainee anaesthetist. However, the principles of anaesthetic care are similar to those pertaining elsewhere, the only essential differences lying in the specific operations undertaken and the fact that essential organ perfusion is achieved artificially when the heart itself is the object of surgery. Operations are termed 'open heart' when the function of the heart and the lungs are assumed by an extracorporeal pump and gas exchange unit (cardiopulmonary bypass, or CPB). During 'closed' operations, cardiac and pulmonary functions remain intact, and anaesthetic management is similar to that for thoracic surgery (Chapter 28).

Excluding the insertion of pacemakers, approx. 15 000 cardiac operations are undertaken each year in the U.K. in N.H.S. hospitals. These include: 3000 for congenital abnormalities, 4500 for acquired valvular disease, 6000 for ischaemic heart disease plus a miscellany of aortic and pericardial surgery.

Congenital cardiac abnormalities

These occur at a rate of 6–8 per 1000 live births. Correction of almost a third of these lesions, including patent ductus arteriosus or coarctation, may be undertaken by 'closed' operation but the remainder, including atrial and ventricular septal defects, valve abnormalities and cyanotic lesions such as Fallot's tetralogy require CPB.

Acquired valvular disease

This type of cardiac lesion has become less common as a result of the reduced incidence of rheumatic fever. Stenosis or incompetence still occur and most commonly involve the mitral and aortic valves. Although closed valvotomy is possible, surgery usually comprises replacement with an artificial valve. This may be a mechanical prosthesis with a ball or tilting disc, or a tissue valve (usually a pig valve) specially mounted and prepared (heterograft). Less commonly, a human valve (homograft) is used. Prosthetic valves are reliable but necessitate the patient receiving anticoagulants for life. This is not usually necessary when porcine heterografts are used and although there are some doubts about their durability, these valves are becoming more popular.

Ischaemic heart disease

The concept of revascularising ischaemic myocardium was introduced about 15 yr ago with the insertion of a portion of saphenous vein from aorta to coronary artery distal to a stenosis (Fig. 29.1). Since then, coronary artery bypass grafting has become the most commonly performed cardiac operation. However, there is some controversy regarding the indications for this operation. Although angina is relieved in 80–90% of patients, life expectancy is not increased in all groups when compared with medical treatment. Only in left main and triple vessel disease has life expectancy been shown clearly to have been prolonged as a result of surgery.

ASSESSMENT OF RISK

The mortality rate associated with cardiac surgery is diminishing but is still significant. Several units have

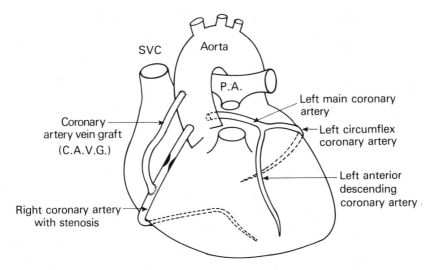

Fig. 29.1 Diagrammatic representation of coronary arteries and CAVG. 'Triple' vessel disease includes right, left circumflex and left anterior descending arteries.

achieved a mortality rate of 1–2% with uncomplicated coronary vein grafts but valve surgery is usually associated with a mortality of 5–6%. When more extensive surgery is undertaken, e.g. multiple valve replacement or coronary artery vein graft (CAVG) plus valve replacement, mortality rate increases to 12–15%.

Patients with an increased risk of perioperative complications may be identified during preoperative assessment. Patients who are classified as the New York Heart Association's functional class III or IV, in which symptoms occur with minimal activity or at rest, may be expected to experience problems. Increased risk is associated with the following factors:

1. Age > 65 yr.
2. Unstable angina or infarction within 6 months prior to surgery.
3. Emergency surgery or reoperation.
4. Poor left ventricular function as shown by:

   (a) LVEDP > 18mmHg
   (b) ejection fraction < 40%
   (c) cardiac index < 2 litre/min/m^2
   (d) dyskinetic wall motion.

5. Raised pulmonary artery pressures (mean PAP > 25 mmHg especially after exercise).
6. Evidence of right ventricular failure.
7. Other system disease, e.g. diabetes.

EXTRACORPOREAL CIRCULATION (ECC)

The essential components of ECC comprise:

1. Pumps
2. An oxygenator
3. Connecting tubes and filters
4. Fluid prime of these components

These are normally arranged as shown in Figure 29.2. Blood from the venous side of the circulation, usually from the vena cavae, is drained by gravity to a venous reservoir and thence to a gas exchange unit (oxygenator), where oxygen is delivered to, and carbon dioxide removed from, the blood. This 'arterialised' blood is pumped into the arterial side of the circulation, usually into the ascending aorta. The heart and lungs are thus 'bypassed' or isolated and their function maintained temporarily by mechanical equipment remote from the body. Most systems include a heat exchanger in the oxygenator to vary the temperature of blood rapidly, and suction to drain redundant or spilled blood in or around the bypassed heart and return it to the venous reservoir for oxygenation and thence to the circulation.

Pumps (Fig. 29.3)

The majority of pumps are of the roller variety, which displace blood around the circuit by intermittent compression of the circuit tubing during each sweep.

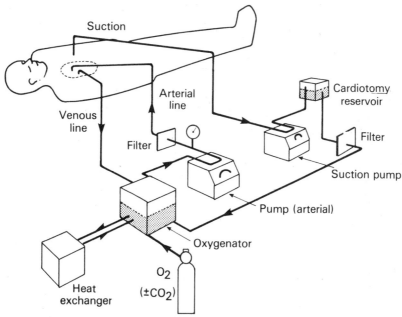

Fig. 29.2 Components of extracorporeal circuit.

Traditionally, these pumps have produced a 'continuous' or steady arterial wave form, but by intermittent acceleration of the roller head, a 'pulsatile' wave form may be achieved which mimics normal physiological blood flow and is claimed to reduce postoperative organ dysfunction.

Oxygenator

There are two types of oxygenator:

1. Direct contact oxygenators

Disc oxygenators consist of rotating discs which dip into blood; the film of blood on the disc is rotated through a flow of oxygen. These have been superseded by the 'bubble' oxygenator in which oxygen is bubbled through venous blood (Fig. 29.3). Bubble oxygenators are the most commonly used devices at present. They are produced relatively cheaply, are disposable and are of small internal volume. They usually include a venous reservoir and an integral heat exchanger. However, 'bubbling' results in damage to red cells and platelets, and consumption of coagulation factors. Their use is limited to a few hours as the extent of damage is time-dependent.

2. Membrane oxygenators

These comprise a semipermeable membrane which separates gas and blood phases, and through which

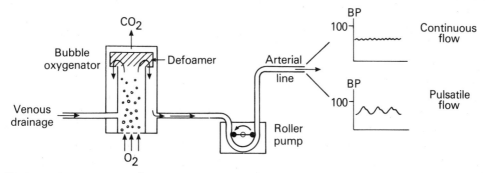

Fig. 29.3 Diagrammatic representation of oxygenator and arterial pump.

gas exchange occurs. In comparison with bubble oxygenators, damage to blood components is reduced. Membrane oxygenators have been used in certain circumstances to support the circulation for several days. Because of expense and the requirement for an additional pump to drive venous blood through the oxygenator, membrane oxygenators have not been adopted widely.

Connecting tubes, filters, manometer, suction

These must be sterile and nontoxic, and should damage blood as little as possible during passage through the circuit.

A defoaming unit is included in bubble oxygenators but, in addition, a unit should be incorporated in the arterial line to remove gas emboli which would pass directly to the aorta. Suction pumps are supplied to vent blood collecting in the pulmonary circulation or left ventricle during bypass, and also to remove spilled blood from the pericardial sac. The blood is collected in the 'cardiotomy' reservoir, filtered and returned to the main circuit. This suction also causes damage to blood components.

Fluid prime

Originally it was anticipated that connection of the circulation to an external circuit would necessitate the extracorporeal circuit being filled with anticoagulated whole blood. However, this is expensive and may lead to incompatibility reactions. In addition, it became clear that the use of whole blood to fill the external circuit was unnecessary, as the body tolerates a relatively low haematocrit. As the volume of the ECC may be no more than 2 litre when CPB is commenced and the patient's blood mixes with an ECC comprising clear fluid (fluid prime), the haematocrit decreases to approx. 20–25%. Although oxygen content is reduced, availability may be increased by improved organ blood flow resulting from reduced blood viscosity. In certain patients (low body weight, children, or those with a low preoperative haemoglobin in whom dilution would reduce the haematocrit to below 20%), blood may be added to the prime. In the normal adult, 'clear' primes are used almost exclusively and comprise crystalloid solutions, e.g. dextrose or Ringer lactate. Most cardiac surgical units have individual recipes for addition to the prime, e.g. plasma, dextran, mannitol, sodium bicarbonate and potassium, to achieve an isosmolar solution of physiological pH.

PREOPERATIVE ASSESSMENT

The majority of patients presenting for cardiac surgery have undergone comprehensive cardiological investigation and are usually receiving medications. In addition to the routine investigations undertaken prior to any operation, certain specialised techniques are employed to assess the cardiac lesion and degree of resultant dysfunction. The results of these investigations permit the anaesthetist to identify patients at particular risk in whom extra care and monitoring are required.

Exercise electrocardiography

Various stress protocols are employed whereby a standard exercise test is used to provoke ischaemic changes and symptoms. Changes in rhythm, rate, arterial pressure and conduction are recorded. The anaesthetist identifies the most useful e.c.g. leads to monitor during surgery and notes the rate pressure product (heart rate × systolic arterial pressure) at which evidence of ischaemia occurs.

Cardiac catheterisation

Considerable information may be obtained from catheterisation:

1. Evidence of failing function or of gradients across stenosed valves may be identified by pressure monitoring.

2. Oximetry of blood at different sites indicates if shunts are present (Fig. 29.4).

3. Cardiac output may be measured.

4. The injection of radiopaque dye into aorta or ventricles assesses incompetence of valves and the efficiency of ventricular contraction (ejection fraction) and wall motion.

The ejection fraction (EF) =

$$\frac{\text{end-diastolic volume} - \text{end-systolic volume}}{\text{end-diastolic volume}}$$

5. Injection of dye into coronary arteries defines the anatomy of the coronary circulation and the degree of patency or sites of stenosis.

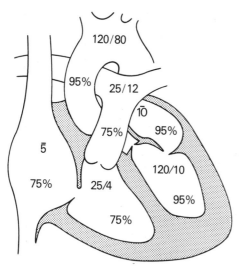

Fig. 29.4 Diagram of catheterisation values in normal adult: pressures (mmHg) and oxygen saturations.

Echocardiograph

Ultrasound is used to identify myocardial motion and valvular function. Although ventricular function may be assessed and EF estimated, this technique is most useful in identifying the degree of valvular abnormality.

Radionuclide imaging

By imaging the activity of an appropriate radioisotope as it passes through the heart or into the myocardium, ventricular function and myocardial perfusion may be assessed. Technetium images blood volume and may be used to demonstrate abnormal wall motion and EF. Thallium, which is taken up by the myocardium, may be used to assess regional blood flow. These techniques may be employed before and after exercise and/or therapy.

Preoperative drug therapy

Digitalis. Most centres discontinue digoxin 24–48 h before surgery to diminish digoxin associated arrhythmias after surgery.

β-Blocking agents. Continued administration of these drugs up to the time of surgery is desirable unless evidence of overdosage is present. Discontinuation may increase the risk of preoperative infarction.

Calcium antagonists (e.g. nifedipine). These drugs have a negative inotropic effect but as with the β-blockers, it is probably preferable to continue therapy throughout the preoperative period.

Nitrates should be continued, and may be included in the premedication if indicated.

Diuretics should be continued until the day before surgery.

Anticoagulants are usually stopped several days before surgery to permit coagulation to return towards normal. If a high risk of embolism is present, anticoagulants should be continued and coagulation defects treated postoperatively.

Other investigations prior to surgery

Haemoglobin. Should be adequate (> 11 g/dl) to prevent excessive haemodilution on bypass.

Coagulation. Prothrombin time should be measured prior to surgery. Specific defects require correction before surgery or alternatively the appropriate blood products should be made available.

Electrolytes. Serum K^+ in particular should be within normal limits.

Urea and creatinine. Raised levels indicate an increased risk of renal failure postoperatively. Adequate urine output should be ensured after operation.

Liver function tests. Abnormal values may indicate evidence of congestive cardiac failure.

Pulmonary function tests. In patients complaining of dyspnoea, spirometry should be undertaken to measure vital capacity and forced expiratory volume. If FEV_1/FVC is less than 60%, more extensive tests are indicated including assessment of the effect of bronchodilators and arterial blood gas analysis.

MONITORING

Extensive and accurate monitoring is essential throughout the perioperative period for the safe practice of cardiac surgery.

E.c.g.

E.c.g. should be monitored throughout the perioperative period. The ideal system is one which allows simultaneous multiple lead monitoring or at least switching between lead II and V_5 for accurate identification of ischaemia. Rate and rhythm should also be observed.

Systemic arterial pressure

Arterial cannulation is mandatory, and not only permits direct measurement but also facilitates sampling of arterial blood for biochemical analysis. The preferred site is a radial artery.

Central venous and left atrial pressures

Right-sided filling pressure should be monitored by a cannula placed into the superior vena cava.

Controversy exists regarding the necessity to monitor left heart filling pressure in all patients. If time permits, a direct left atrial line can be inserted at surgery as an aid to terminating bypass and improving postoperative care but it is often desirable to insert a flow-directed pulmonary artery catheter at or before induction to measure pulmonary capillary wedge pressure (PCWP). In the U.S.A. there is enthusiasm for commencing full invasive monitoring prior to anaesthesia but most anaesthetists in the U.K. undertake this only in poor risk patients.

Cardiac output (CO)

CO may be measured by thermal or dye dilution, most conveniently in association with measurement of PCWP and PAP using a pulmonary artery catheter. There is no doubt that calculation of cardiac output and cardiac index together with the derivatives of stroke work, pulmonary and systemic vascular resistances and tissue oxygen flux, permits the most accurate assessment of cardiological therapy.

E.e.g.

A simple guide to cerebral activity and perfusion may be obtained from the cerebral function monitor although interpretation is difficult in the hypothermic patient.

Temperature

Core temperature should be monitored from the nasopharynx. It is helpful also to monitor the peripheral temperature from the first toe to assess core-peripheral temperature gradients and peripheral perfusion.

Biochemical analysis

Facilities should be available for immediate analysis of blood gases, acid–base balance and serum potassium.

Haematological analysis

Rapid measurement of packed cell volume and coagulation status should be available. Activated clotting time (ACT) can be measured quickly in the operating theatre using the Haemochron apparatus (normal = 100–120 s) but access to the haematology laboratory should be rapid for assessment of a full clotting screen. It is also salutory to measure free haemoglobin on occasion as an indicator of erythrocyte damage during extracorporeal circulation.

Display

E.c.g., pressure waveforms, and a digital output of heart rate and pressures should be displayed clearly on a screen visible to both surgeon and anaesthetist. The facility to produce a hard copy of e.c.g. and pressures is necessary for records and accurate diagnosis.

PATHOPHYSIOLOGICAL CONSIDERATIONS

The anaesthetist should have a clear understanding of the fundamental principles of cardiac physiology. Accurate monitoring reveals alterations in cardiac function and permits the anaesthetist to manipulate those factors which ensure adequate pump output (Fig. 29.5) and myocardial blood supply.

Preload and contractility determine the amount of work that the heart can perform. In the failing heart the afterload determines how much work is expended in overcoming pressure compared with that used to provide forward flow. Thus, cardiac output may be increased either by increasing preload or contractility, or by reducing afterload. However, oxygen consumption is raised by increasing heart rate, contractility, preload and afterload.

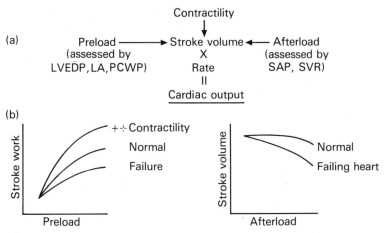

Fig. 29.5 Important aspects of mechanical function.

Augmentation of cardiac output by increasing preload or contractility may thus have a detrimental effect on oxygen balance. Reduction of afterload, however, may increase cardiac output while simultaneously reducing oxygen demand.

Adequate coronary perfusion demands maintenance of diastolic aortic pressure at adequate levels. Oxygen supply to the myocardium occurs predominantly in diastole and is dependent on the gradient between diastolic aortic pressure and intraventricular pressure, and on the diastolic time. The portion of myocardium most at risk of developing ischaemia is the left ventricular endocardium and a useful index of oxygen balance is the endocardial viability ratio (EVR) (Fig. 29.6). Normally the EVR exceeds 1, but if the ratio decreases below 0.7, ischaemia is likely to develop.

A useful clinical measurement of oxygen demand is the rate pressure product (RPP) (heart rate × systolic arterial pressure). This simple index may predict the point at which ischaemia occurs in the conscious exercising patient. During anaesthesia, RPP is kept below the conscious ischaemic value.

Care of the patient suffering from ischaemic heart disease therefore necessitates attempts to reduce oxygen demand and maintain oxygen supply. In general, patients with valvular stenosis require adequate preload and do not tolerate rapid reduction in peripheral resistance. Aortic stenosis presents a high afterload to the left ventricle and also renders coronary perfusion particularly sensitive to systemic hypotension. Incompetent valves tend to perform better if afterload is maintained at a low level.

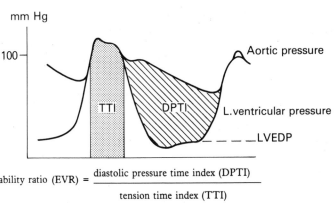

Fig. 29.6 Endocardial viability ratio (EVR) = $\dfrac{\text{diastolic pressure time index (DPTI)}}{\text{tension time index (TTI)}}$

$= \dfrac{O_2 \text{ supply}}{O_2 \text{ demand}} =$

Abnormal heart rates are not tolerated well by a heart with any valvular lesion.

ANAESTHETIC TECHNIQUE

There is no single preferred anaesthetic technique for cardiac surgery. The choice of particular agents is less important than the care with which the drug is administered and its effects monitored.

Premedication

As far as the patient is concerned, the most important preoperative preparation is a full explanation of what is about to occur and the development of rapport with and confidence in the nursing and medical staff.

Most patients (particularly those with poor cardiovascular reserve) may be sedated preoperatively with an oral benzodiazepine (lorazepam 2–4 mg, temazepam 20–30 mg). Opioid premedication may diminish cardiovascular and respiratory reserve.

In the particularly anxious patient, heavy sedation may be required to prevent increases in heart rate and arterial pressure prior to operation. Tranquillisers, e.g. diazepam, may be commenced on a regular basis several days before operation and premedication undertaken with papaveretum (10–20 mg) and hyoscine (0.2–0.4 mg) i.m. 1–2 h prior to transfer to theatre.

Atropine is best avoided in cardiac patients because of its potent chronotropic effects. Patients receiving glyceryl trinitrate (GTN) may benefit from its administration as a skin paste at the time of premedication. GTN increases alveolar dead space, and oxygen therapy should be given by mask during transfer from the ward.

Induction

All drugs and equipment should be prepared and ready and the theatre and bypass circuit available for immediate use prior to the arrival of the patient in the anaesthetic room. Two anaesthetists should be present at induction.

Before induction, e.c.g. electrodes should be applied and the e.c.g. displayed, arterial pressure recorded and large gauge venous cannulae inserted under local anaesthesia. Preoxygenation should be commenced.

Induction may be undertaken with the standard agents in small doses (e.g. thiopentone 1–3 mg/kg), or the use of large doses of opioids (e.g. morphine 1–4 mg/kg, fentanyl 10–50 μg/kg) in combination with benzodiazepines to obtain unconsciousness. Exponents of the latter technique claim greater cardiovascular stability especially if the use of nitrous oxide is avoided, and this may be valuable in the poor risk patient. A combination of these techniques may be used: consciousness is obtunded by an opioid in moderate dose and hypnosis then produced by a small dose of an induction agent.

As consciousness is lost, a muscle relaxant is administered and ventilation supported when necessary. Pancuronium (0.1–0.15 mg/kg) is used commonly, although it may cause tachycardia. The objective is to undertake endotracheal intubation without cardiovascular stimulation and thus adequate analgesia/anaesthesia is required. It is customary to spray the cords and trachea with local anaesthetic solution. A low pressure high volume cuffed endotracheal tube should be used. Positive pressure ventilation is continued usually with 50% nitrous oxide in oxygen.

Percutaneous cannulation of the radial artery and internal jugular veins is performed. Two central lines are advisable, one for monitoring, the second for infusions. Nasopharyngeal and peripheral temperature probes are applied and a urinary catheter inserted. Mechanical ventilation is continued with a circuit containing a humidifier.

Previously identified 'poor risk' patients may require more extensive monitoring of pressures and cardiac output prior to induction, and these are established under local anaesthesia. Induction should be undertaken in theatre with the full team ready for immediate surgery. Adequate sedation must be provided during insertion of invasive monitoring lines.

Maintenance—prebypass

During this period, surgical procedure involves preparation of the patient, skin incision, sternotomy, and insertion of arterial and venous bypass cannulae. Anaesthetic management is designed to maintain stability of heart rate and arterial pressure, particularly at moments of profound stimulation, notably skin incision and sternotomy. Additional i.v. analgesic drug or inhalational anaesthetic should be given prior to stimulation. Large doses of morphine or fentanyl are required to obtund the effects of surgical stimulation. The use of inhalational agents, e.g. halothane or enflurane, is most effective, although their negative inotropic actions may be undesirable and arrhythmias precipitated, particularly in those with poor ventricular function.

The alternative to deepening anaesthesia/analgesia is to counteract hypertension with vasodilators (phentolamine 1–2 mg, or infusion of sodium nitroprusside 1–5 μg/kg/min or glyceryl trinitrate 0.5–5 μg/kg/min) and to treat tachycardia with β-blockers (practolol 2–5 mg or oxprenolol 0.25–1 mg).

Whatever method is employed the rate pressure product should not be allowed to exceed approx. 12 000 or the critical ischaemic level determined previously during preoperative assessment.

Arterial blood gases, serum K^+, and haematocrit should be measured when surgery is under way and conditions are stable. If possible, the activated clotting time (ACT) should be estimated. Before cannulation for bypass lines, heparin (3 mg/kg) should be injected into a secure central line of proven patency. In some units, the surgeon injects heparin directly into the left atrium prior to cannulation. ACT measurement should be repeated 5 min after injection of heparin; the value should exceed 3 times normal. Cardioplegia should be prepared, and stored at 4°C.

When preparations are complete, the bypass pump commences and circulation is assumed by the extracorporeal circuit.

Maintenance — on bypass

Two factors complicate the provision of anaesthesia during cardiopulmonary bypass. Firstly, the dilutional effect of the crystalloid prime reduces the concentration of drugs administered previously, and secondly, by short circuiting the lungs, bypass prevents the continuation of inhalational anaesthesia. Therefore, anaesthesia is maintained usually by the administration of bolus doses of opioids (e.g. morphine 5–10 mg) and muscle relaxant drugs to the circulation at the start of bypass. Additional adjuvants include benzodiazepines (e.g. lorazepam 2–4 mg or

midazolam 5–10 mg), a continuous i.v. infusion of a short acting anaesthetic agent (e.g. etomidate) or more rarely the administration of a volatile agent into the gas flow of the oxygenator. When full pump oxygenator flow is reached and ventricular ejection ceases, ventilation is suspended and the lungs maintained in inflation with a slight positive pressure (5 cmH$_2$O). If possible, air should be employed for this manoeuvre as the nitrogen present helps to reduce atelectasis.

Surgery is usually preceded by cross-clamping the aorta to isolate the heart and prevent backflow. In the case of valvular surgery, the appropriate valve is exposed, excised and a new valve sutured in place. During coronary artery vein grafting, the distal anastomoses are usually completed first and, following release of the cross-clamp to permit restoration of myocardial perfusion, the proximal anastomoses are constructed using a portion of the aorta isolated by a side-clamp (Fig. 29.7).

Myocardial preservation

Most surgical techniques on the heart require an immobile heart with empty chambers. On bypass, the aorta is cross-clamped between the aortic cannula and the aortic valve, thus isolating the heart from the flow of oxygenated blood. During aortic cross-clamping, the myocardium is at risk of ischaemic damage unless measures are taken to reduce myocardial oxygen consumption. Currently, techniques of myocardial preservation include hypothermia to reduce basal metabolic rate and cardiac arrest to reduce oxygen requirements to a minimum. Arrest is achieved by injecting 500–1000 ml of cardioplegic solution around the coronary arteries and arresting the heart in diastole. Many cardioplegic solutions are available, but the majority contain potassium and a membrane stabilising agent, e.g. procaine. Cooling is achieved by the use of ice-cold cardioplegia and by pouring cold fluid (4°C) into the pericardial sac and into the heart chambers if they have been opened.

If the heart is cooled to 15°C it withstands total ischaemia for approx. 1 h. The technique used most commonly at present involves moderate hypothermia of the body to 28–30°C and local cooling of the myocardium itself to a temperature of 15–18°C. This technique is very successful but depends on meticulous attention to detail. If prolonged cross-

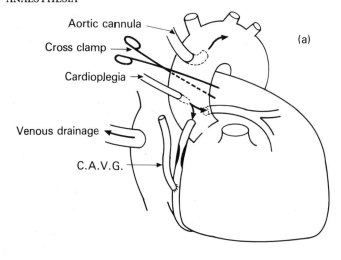

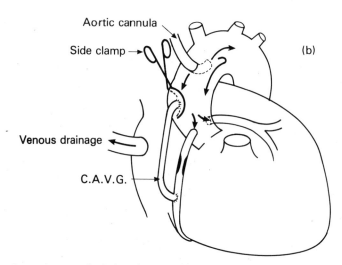

Fig. 29.7 Arrangement of cross-clamp, cardioplegia and anastomoses.

clamp times are required, cardioplegic cooling must be repeated if evidence of spontaneous cardiac contraction is seen or the temperature of the heart increases above 18°C.

Perfusion on bypass

At normothermia, a pump flow of 2.4 litre/min/m² of body surface area is required to prevent inadequate perfusion of the body. The pressure achieved within the vascular system is dependent on pump output and systemic vascular resistance. Controversy exists regarding optimum perfusion pressure. It has been suggested that essential organs, in particular brain, are damaged if perfusion is maintained below 50 mmHg mean arterial pressure. In many centres, however, anaesthetists ignore low pressures, and claim to produce no increased neurological problems.

Following the institution of bypass, there are usually marked decreases in peripheral resistance and arterial pressure, which in most instances resolve spontaneously in 5–10 min. If this does not occur, arterial pressure may be increased by raising systemic resistance with a sympathomimetic agent, e.g. methoxamine 1–5 mg. Frequently, the systemic resistance increases during and after bypass as a result of increasing plasma levels of catecholamines, renin-angiotensin and thromboxane. If the mean arterial pressure exceeds 100 mmHg, the use of vasodilators may be required.

Perfusion is difficult to assess clinically, especially in the hypothermic patient and often the most useful monitor of adequate organ perfusion is the urine output. The cerebral function monitor may also be useful in assessing when pressure and perfusion are inadequate.

Coagulation control. Adequate anticoagulation must be maintained during CPB. If the Haemochron is available, ACT should be measured every 30 min and extra heparin administered if ACT decreases below 400 s. If this facility is not available, half the initial dose of heparin should be given every hour.

Oxygen delivery. Arterial blood samples should be obtained regularly, and blood gases and haematocrit measured. Temperature corrections should be applied to blood gas data.

Oxygen carriage is dependent on haemoglobin concentration in addition to adequate oxygen tension. Haematocrit may be permitted to decrease to 20% but further reduction should be prevented by the addition of packed cells or blood to the bypass circuit.

Acid-base balance. The development of metabolic acidosis suggests that perfusion is inadequate and if necessary (base deficit > 6–8 mmol/litre), sodium bicarbonate should be administered.

Serum potassium. Serum K^+ should be maintained at approx. 4.5 mmol/litre by the administration of KCl (10–20 mmol).

Restoration of spontaneous heart beat

When the cross-clamp has been removed, oxygenated blood again flows into the coronary arteries washing out cardioplegia and repaying the oxygen debt. In most instances, the heart regains activity spontaneously; in a minority of patients it commences beating spontaneously in sinus rhythm, but usually reverts to ventricular fibrillation. Internal defibrillation is required to convert fibrillation to sinus rhythm and is successful only if pH, oxygenation and temperature are approaching normal values. The heat exchanger in the oxygenator is used to raise the temperature of blood but peripheral temperature is often depressed for some time. If a spontaneous heart beat cannot be maintained, pacing wires should be attached to the epicardium to initiate activity artificially.

At this stage full bypass flow is maintained and although the heart is beating there is little ejection from the ventricles. It is wise at this time to pause, ensure that all air has been vented from the heart chambers, wait until core temperature exceeds 36°C and rest the heart before it is required to pump again.

Termination of bypass

When body temperature exceeds 36°C, metabolic indices are normal and a regular heart beat present, the establishment of spontaneous cardiac output is attempted. This is undertaken by diverting an increasing volume of venous return into the right atrium past the extracorporeal cannulae by constricting the venous return line to the pump. Blood is now passing again through the pulmonary circulation and mechanical ventilation should be recommenced. One hundred per cent oxygen should be employed, as the gas exchanging efficiency of the lung is unknown at this stage and in addition any air bubbles which have not been vented enlarge in volume if nitrous oxide is introduced.

If pump flow has been pulsatile, it is advisable to revert to a continuous output at this time and any output or ejection from the left ventricle is seen as a 'blip' on the arterial pressure trace after a QRS complex is noted. If the myocardium is contracting satisfactorily, pump flow is reduced cautiously and the heart, now receiving all the venous return, achieves normal output. At this time 5 mmol $CaCl_2$ (repeated if necessary) may provide a useful if temporary inotropic stimulus.

Although arterial pressure is the most easily measured index of successful termination of bypass, it should be remembered that this is a derivative of cardiac output and peripheral resistance. The former is measured fairly easily and where there is doubt regarding pump efficiency, cardiac output (and thus cardiac index) should be assessed.

Peripheral resistance may be derived when cardiac output is measured but is assessed clinically by observing peripheral perfusion, core-peripheral temperature gradient and urine output. Peripheral resistance is increased consistently during bypass and much of the care of patients henceforth is directed towards producing increased peripheral dilatation and perfusion.

If ECC is discontinued successfully, preload should be optimised (left atrial pressure 12–15 mmHg) by infusion of as much as possible of the residual fluid contained in the pump circuit. This is facilitated by the administration of vasodilators, e.g. SNP or GTN. If cardiac output is inadequate, the circulation is reassumed by the extracorporeal pump and the heart allowed more time to recover.

Low output

If the heart is unable to generate sufficient output to maintain body perfusion after the preload has been optimised, further action is required. An increase in contractility is produced by inotropes. The simplest is a bolus of $CaCl_2$ but the most commonly employed is dopamine (2–20 μg/kg/min) by infusion. Adrenaline (0.05–0.2 μg/kg/min) and, if heart rate is slow, isoprenaline (0.02–0.2 μg/kg/min), may be indicated in some patients.

Although all these drugs augment cardiac output they tend to precipitate tachyarrhythmias. Adrenaline and dopamine also cause vasoconstriction in high doses. In addition, all these agents increase myocardial oxygen demand. They may precipitate infarction in patients with ischaemic heart disease.

An alternative approach is to assist output by reducing the afterload with vasodilators. As described previously, reduced afterload not only reduces oxygen demand, but, in the failing ventricle, augments forward flow into the aorta. Diastolic pressure must not be reduced excessively (< 65 mmHg) since oxygen supply to the ventricle is jeopardised. Infusion of fluid may be required during dilatation to maintain preload at adequate levels. In acute low output syndromes, vasodilators are usually prescribed in addition to inotropes and the drugs may have a cumulative effect in raising cardiac index, permitting a reduction in the dosage of inotropes. Sodium nitroprusside is currently the most commonly used vasodilator (reduces both preload and afterload) but recent evidence suggests that it may cause a 'steal' from areas of ischaemic myocardium. Glyceryl trinitrate, which predominantly reduces preload, does not appear to have this effect and is becoming the dilator of choice in patients with myocardial ischaemia.

The success of these manoeuvres should not be measured by the level of arterial pressure attained but by evidence of increased flow to tissues, i.e. increased cardiac output and peripheral temperatures, and increasing urine output. It should be remembered, however, that both drugs may affect ventilation/perfusion ratios adversely and may aggravate hypoxaemia.

If these pharmacological methods fail to produce an adequate cardiac output, the intra-aortic balloon pump (IABP) may be used.

Intra-aortic balloon pump. The principle of the IABP is illustrated in Figure 29.8. If the balloon in the aorta is inflated immediately after systole,

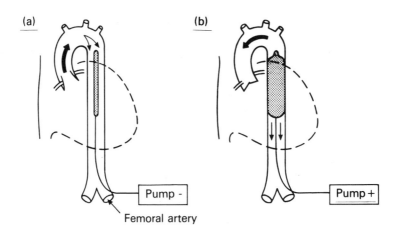

Fig. 29.8 Intra-aortic balloon pump (IABP).

diastolic filling pressure is augmented and myocardial oxygen balance improved. Inflation also displaces blood from the aorta and increases peripheral flow. The balloon is deflated immediately before systole and this creates a low pressure in the aorta as ventricular output commences, reducing afterload (and thus oxygen consumption) and at the same time augmenting output. The use of the IABP has decreased recently as surgery, anaesthesia, and in particular myocardial preservation techniques have improved. However, it may be remarkably successful in some patients with a persistent low output syndrome.

Coagulation control

When the bypass cannulae have been removed, residual effects of heparin are antagonised with protamine. Traditionally 1.5 mg protamine has been administered per 1 mg heparin given, but this does not take into account the short half life of heparin (1.5–2 h) and recent work suggests that much smaller doses of protamine may be adequate to regain normal coagulability after a bypass lasting 1–2 h. The dosage may be titrated using the ACT. The drug should be given slowly (5–20 min) especially if there is residual hypovolaemia or raised pulmonary vascular resistance. Protamine may produce systemic hypotension rapidly, as a result of peripheral vasodilatation, and it may increase pulmonary vasoconstriction to levels which embarrass right ventricular output. In excessive dosage, it also has anticoagulant effects.

Heparin is not the only factor causing bleeding during and after bypass. Contact of blood with bubbles in the oxygenator and with foreign surfaces in the bypass circuit and suction tubing causes consumption of clotting factors and of platelets. Thus if heparin appears to have been reversed satisfactorily and unexplained bleeding persists, a full clotting screen should be performed, including estimation of platelet numbers. Clotting factors may be replaced by the infusion of fresh frozen plasma and/or cryoprecipitate, and platelet concentrate should be infused if the platelet count is less than 60×10^9/litre.

From the surgical standpoint, the period following termination of bypass is concerned with prevention of haemorrhage and closure of the chest with drains in situ. The anaesthetist's aim, in addition to the maintenance of patient comfort, is to ensure the efficiency of myocardial pumping, oxygen balance and peripheral perfusion together with correction of metabolic, biochemical, haematological or temperature abnormalities.

CONTROL OF THE CIRCULATION AFTER BYPASS

Despite the use of measures to protect the myocardium during bypass, the heart suffers some deterioration in function and has reduced contractility for several hours. Thus it operates on a lower Frank Starling curve (Fig. 29.5) and requires a higher preload to produce the same output. Usually, a left atrial pressure of approx. 15 mmHg is optimal. The contractility of the myocardium improves in the first 3–4 h after bypass and this increased efficiency permits reduction in preload.

In addition, the peripheral circulation remains vasoconstricted for several hours postoperatively. In patients with reasonable ventricular function, hypertension often occurs after bypass, especially in operations involving the aortic valve or revascularisation. The increased afterload results in additional myocardial oxygen consumption and tends to reduce cardiac output.

Reduction of peripheral resistance and systemic arterial pressure by a vasodilator (e.g. SNP or GTN) protects suture lines from damage, decreases oxygen demand, increases cardiac output if preload is not reduced excessively, improves peripheral perfusion and accelerates warming. The use of vasodilators in the early postoperative period is increasing and is now regarded as beneficial in more than 50% of patients.

Other aspects of maintenance post-bypass

In addition to maintaining cardiac function and oxygen supply to the tissues during this period, the anaesthetist should ensure that normality is regained as soon as possible, and maintained, in respect of the following:

1. Temperature

Core temperature is raised easily on bypass via the oxygenator. However, the efficiency of rewarming the peripheral tissues depends on the patient's weight, total flow rate and peripheral perfusion. After bypass there is often a decrease in core temperature (afterdrop). More efficient rewarming and reduction in afterdrop may be achieved by the use of a water circulating mattress.

2. Biochemical monitoring

Essential monitoring includes blood gases, acid-base balance, serum K^+ and haematocrit.

3. Cardiac rhythm

Heart block. Epicardial pacing lines should be inserted if AV dissociation occurs. Infusion of isoprenaline may improve ventricular rate and output as a temporary measure.

Supraventricular arrhythmias. Direct current cardioversion is the most convenient treatment when the chest is open. After chest closure, digoxin is the most commonly used drug but verapamil has recently been shown to be of value.

Ventricular arrhythmias. The threshold for arrhythmias is reduced by hypokalaemia, and serum K^+ should be maintained at approx. 4.5 mmol/litre. If ventricular arrhythmias persist, lignocaine is the drug of choice although β-blockers may be useful, but should be administered cautiously.

Transfer to postoperative ITU

It is normal to prolong the same level of support and monitoring undertaken during surgery into the postoperative period. The duration of this care depends on the individual patient's response to surgery and speed of recovery.

Transfer of the patient from theatre to the intensive care unit may involve journeys along corridors and into lifts. It is essential that controlled ventilation is continued and e.c.g. and arterial pressure monitored during transfer. Hypertension often occurs as a result of stimulation during movement, as anaesthesia for the latter part of surgery is maintained at a light level. In addition, infusion of vasodilators may be interrupted during transfer. A bolus dose of opioid (e.g. morphine 5–10 mg) is often advisable prior to moving.

POSTOPERATIVE INTENSIVE THERAPY

The surgical team should have a well practiced routine for the care of patients after surgery. Ventilation of the lungs with a volume-preset ventilator and full cardiovascular monitoring should be recommenced immediately.

The principles of care in this phase are similar to those described for the period of anaesthesia after termination of bypass.

Haemodynamic care

On return to ITU, most patients are cold, vasoconstricted and exhibit a tendency to hypertension. Attention is directed towards achieving vasodilatation, reduction of afterload and maintenance of preload. Blood is required if the haematocrit is less than 35%. Urine output should be maintained with diuretics if necessary but usually a spontaneous diuresis occurs in response to the crystalloid load received in theatre. Potassium concentrations should be monitored carefully, and abnormalities corrected.

The majority of patients stabilise and regain adequate peripheral perfusion over the succeeding 3–4 h, permitting the level of cardiovascular support to be reduced.

In a minority of patients, low cardiac output requires the continued use of inotropes, vasodilators and, if necessary, IABP for some time.

Blood loss

This should be measured accurately. If excessive (300–400 ml/h), it may be necessary to re-operate on the patient. Attention to the coagulation system is required and further protamine or coagulation factors prescribed as necessary. The most sinister complication of excessive bleeding is cardiac tamponade which requires rapid thoracotomy and evacuation of blood from the chest. If deterioration is rapid, this must be undertaken in the ITU.

Ventilation

Respiratory dysfunction is manifest as an increase in venous admixture. This is common after cardiac surgery and persists for several days. Usually ventilation is assisted for 12–18 h after operation in order to obviate the work of breathing and maximise oxygenation. Adequate analgesia is prescribed more safely, and return to theatre, if required, is more convenient and rapid. However, recent experience suggests that the time of mechanical ventilation may be reduced safely and continued only for the period of postoperative haemodynamic instability which in most patients lasts 4–6 h. Thus when the patient's arterial pressure and peripheral perfusion are satisfactory, the temperature exceeds 36°C core and 30°C peripheral, urine output is more than 30 ml/h, blood loss less than 100 ml/h, the patient is conscious and can maintain satisfactory blood gases with an inspired oxygen concentration of less than 40%, a trial of spontaneous ventilation is indicated. If respiratory volumes are adequate and the patient is not distressed, the trachea may be extubated.

There are some patients in whom these criteria are not achieved, and ventilation is continued. High inspired oxygen levels should be avoided if possible by the use of PEEP to maintain an arterial oxygen tension of approx. 10 kPa (75 mmHg) if cardiovascular function permits.

Analgesia

The anaesthetic technique employed determines the timing of administration of postoperative analgesia. Even after high dose opioid techniques, patients usually show some sign of response in the first 2–3 h after surgery. It is useful to assess cerebral function at this stage in case damage has occurred, but it is inadvisable to distress the patient, as reflex hypertension may occur. The most commonly used method of pain relief is the use of i.v. opioids either by bolus or continuous infusion. Often the addition of a tranquilliser (diazepam 5 mg or midazolam 2–5 mg) is advantageous in maintaining the patient comfortable but rousable. Regional analgesic techniques are not popular since coagulation defects are common but the use of pre-bypass intrathecal opioids and postoperative extradural analgesia has been reported.

Patients who have suffered cerebral damage or who require long-term cardiovascular support may be managed more easily by augmenting analgesia with an infusion of etomidate.

As important as pharmacological support is the human rapport which should be achieved between attending staff and patient.

FURTHER READING

Branthwaite M A 1982 Anaesthesia for cardiac surgery. Blackwell Scientific Publications, Oxford
Conahan T J 1982 Cardiac anesthesia. Addison-Wesley, California
Ionescu M I 1981 Techniques in extracorporeal circulation. Butterworths, London
Kaplan J A 1979 Cardiac anesthesia. Grune and Stratton, New York

Longmore D B (ed) 1981 Towards safer cardiac surgery. M T P Press, Lancaster
Tarhan S 1982 Cardiovascular anesthesia and postoperative care. Year Book Medical Publishers, Chicago
Ream A K, Fogdall R P 1982 Acute cardiovascular management: anesthesia and intensive care. J B Lippincott, Philadelphia

30

Emergency anaesthesia

Patients scheduled for elective surgery are usually in optimal physical and mental condition, with a definitive surgical diagnosis and with concomitant medical illness well-controlled. In contrast, the patient with a surgical emergency may have an uncertain diagnosis and uncontrolled concomitant medical illness, with consequent cardiovascular and metabolic derangements.

Thus a major principle governing the practice of emergency anaesthesia is that of careful preparation for all potential complications, including vomiting and regurgitation, hypovolaemia and haemorrhage and abnormal reaction to drugs in the presence of electrolyte disturbances and renal impairment.

PREOPERATIVE ASSESSMENT

The objective of emergency anaesthesia is to permit correction of the surgical pathology with the minimum of risk to the patient. This requires adequate and accurate preoperative evaluation of the patient's general condition, with particular attention to specific problems which may influence anaesthetic management.

It is essential to ascertain the likely surgical diagnosis, the magnitude of the proposed surgery, and how urgently surgery is indicated, as these dictate both the extent of preoperative preparation and the method of anaesthesia indicated.

A pertinent past medical and drug history is elicited. In particular, enquiry is made into the presence and severity of specific symptoms relevant to cardiopulmonary reserve: angina, productive cough, dyspnoea of effort, orthopnoea or nocturnal coughing bouts. The presence of such symptoms should provoke detailed enquiry into the cardiovascular and respiratory systems (see chapter 15 on preoperative assessment).

According to the urgency of surgery, physical examination may be selective to identify significant cardiopulmonary dysfunction or any abnormalities which might lead to technical difficulties during anaesthesia. Basal crepitations, triple rhythm and raised jugular venous pulse signify impaired ventricular function and limited cardiac reserve, which increase significantly the risk of anaesthesia. It is also important to exclude arrhythmias and heart sounds indicative of valvular disease, as these influence the patient's response to physiological change and thus the anaesthetic management. Assessment of respiratory function is particularly difficult as the patient in pain (with or without peritoneal irritation) may be unable to be co-operative in pulmonary function testing.

It is important to cultivate the habit of airway evaluation if a 'crash induction' is contemplated, since contingency plans are required for management of the patient in the event of failure to intubate the trachea.

Finally, a review of any laboratory investigations is made and urgent requests are made for further tests which may influence patient management.

Assessment of volaemic status

Assessment of the extent of the intravascular volume is essential since underestimated or unrecognised hypovolaemia may lead to circulatory collapse during induction of anaesthesia, which causes reduction in the sympathetically mediated increase in arteriolar and venous constriction. In any patient in whom fluid is sequestered or lost (e.g. peritonitis, bowel obstruction), or in whom haemorrhage has occurred (any trauma case), efforts shoud be made to quantitate the blood volume or extracellular fluid volume and correct any deficit.

Intravascular volume deficit. Assessment of blood loss may be made from the history and any measured losses, but more commonly, the anaesthetist has to rely on clinical evaluation. Useful indices include heart rate, arterial pressure (especially pulse pressure), the state of the peripheral circulation, central venous pressure and urine output. Table 30.1 describes approximate correlations between these clinical indices and the extent of haemorrhage, but it should be stressed that these refer to the 'ideal' patient. In young, healthy adults, heart rate and arterial pressure may be unreliable guides to volume status, and in elderly patients with widespread arterial disease, limited cardiac reserve and a rigid vascular tree (fixed total peripheral resistance), signs of severe hypovolaemia may become evident when blood volume has been reduced by as little as 15–20%.

In general, hypovolaemia does not become apparent clinically until blood volume has been reduced by at least 1000 ml (20% of blood volume). A reduction by more than 30% of blood volume occurs before the classical 'shock syndrome' is produced, with hypotension, tachycardia, oliguria and cold, clammy extremities. Haemorrhage in excess of 40% of blood volume may be associated with loss of compensatory mechanisms maintaining cerebral and coronary blood flow and the patient becomes restless and agitated, and eventually comatose.

In patients with major trauma, it is valuable to compare the clinical assessment of the extent of haemorrhage with the measured or assumed loss. A marked disparity between these two estimates leads not infrequently to a diagnosis of a further concealed source of haemorrhage.

Extracellular volume deficit. Assessment of extracellular fluid volume deficit is difficult, as considerable losses must occur before clinical signs are apparent, making clinical acumen and a high index of suspicion necessary to detect the subtle signs of lesser deficits.

Guidance is obtained from the nature of the surgical condition, the duration of impaired fluid intake, and the presence and severity of symptoms associated with abnormal losses (e.g. vomiting). At the time of the earliest radiological evidence of intestinal obstruction, there may be 1500 ml of fluid sequestered in the lumen of the bowel. If the obstruction is well established and vomiting has occurred, the deficit may exceed 3000 ml. At this stage, clinical signs are minimal but evident to the skilled observer.

For convenience, extracellular fluid volume loss may be graded into four degrees of severity; in each

Table 30.1 Clinical indices of extent of blood loss

Grade of hypovolaemia	1 minimal	2 mild	3 moderate	4 severe
Percentage blood volume lost	10	20	30	over 40
Volume lost (ml)	500	1 000	1 500	over 2 000
Heart rate (beat/min)	normal	100–120	120–140	over 140
Arterial pressure (mmHg)	normal	orthostatic hypotension	systolic below 100	systolic below 80
Urinary output (ml/h)	normal (1 ml/kg/h)	20–30	10–20	nil
Sensorium	normal	normal	restless	impaired consciousness
State of peripheral circulation	normal	cool and pale	cold & pale slow capillary refill	cold & clammy peripheral cyanosis
CVP (cmH$_2$O)	normal	−3	−5	−8

instance, loss is expressed as the percentage of the body weight lost as fluid. It may be seen from Table 30.2 that in minor degrees of extracellular fluid volume loss, diagnosis is dependent on two highly subjective signs; diminished skin elasticity, and reduced intraocular pressure. Loss of skin turgor is demonstrated best by pinching a fold of skin over a clavicle or tibia, areas where, under normal circumstances, there is little subcutaneous fat or redundant skin. Soft eyeballs resulting from lower intraocular pressure are assessed by asking the patient to close his eyes and look downwards; the examiner presses lightly on the eyeballs (above the tarsal plate), with the index finger of each hand.

Table 30.2   Indices of extent of loss of extracellular fluid

Percentage body weight lost as water	ml of fluid lost per 70 kg	Signs and Symptoms
Over 4% (mild)	Over 2 500	Thirst, reduced skin elasticity, decreased intraocular pressure, dry tongue, reduced sweating
Over 6% (mild)	Over 4 200	As above, plus orthostatic hypotension, reduced filling of peripheral veins, oliguria, nausea, dry axillae and groin, low CVP, apathy, haemoconcentration
Over 8% (moderate)	Over 5 500	As above, plus hypotension, thready pulse with cool peripheries
10–15% (severe)	7 000–10 500	Coma, shock followed by death

It should be noted that the presence of orthostatic hypotension indicates considerable deficit which, if not corrected, may lead to severe hypotension on induction of anaesthesia. Orthostatic hypotension should be elicited with caution.

Laboratory investigations may help to confirm the extent of extracellular fluid volume deficit. Haemoconcentration results in an increased haemoglobin level and an increased packed cell volume. As dehydration becomes more marked, renal blood flow diminishes, reducing renal clearance of urea, and consequently increasing the concentration of blood urea. Under maximal stimulation from ADH and aldosterone, conservation of sodium and water by the kidneys results in excretion of urine of low sodium content (0–15 mmol/litre) and high osmolality (800–1400 mosmol/kg).

After estimation of the extent of blood volume or extracellular fluid volume deficit, correction is accomplished with the appropriate fluid. Hartmann's solution (compound sodium lactate) and 0.9% saline are isotonic, remaining predominantly in the extracellular space, and are suitable for replacement of extracellular fluid losses. Haemorrhage is treated preferably by blood transfusion, but alternative fluids may be used.

The optimal time for surgical intervention is when all fluid deficits have been corrected, but if there are urgent indications for surgery (e.g. presence of gangrenous bowel), compromise is necessary. As a general rule, the demonstration of orthostatic hypotension indicates that further fluid replacement is required.

THE FULL STOMACH

Of all the hazards of emergency anaesthesia, vomiting or regurgitation of gastric contents, followed by aspiration into the tracheobronchial tree whilst protective laryngeal reflexes are obtunded, is one of the commonest and most devastating.

Vomiting is an active process occurring in the lighter planes of anaesthesia, and is thus a problem during induction of, or emergence from, anaesthesia, but should not occur during maintenance if anaesthesia is sufficiently deep. In light planes of anaesthesia, the presence of vomited material above the vocal cords stimulates spasm of the cords which prevents material from entering the larynx. Apnoea may persist until severe hypoxia occurs, at which point the vocal cords open and ventilation resumes. Thus the presence of laryngeal reflexes provides a margin of safety provided that the anaesthetist clears the oropharynx of all debris before ventilation resumes.

In contrast, regurgitation is a passive process occurring at any time, is often 'silent' (i.e. not apparent to the anaesthetist), and if aspiration occurs, may be followed by minor pulmonary sequelae or fulminating aspiration pneumonitis. Because regurgitation occurs usually in the presence of deep anaesthesia or at the onset of action of muscle relaxant drugs, vocal reflexes are absent and the chances of aspiration are high.

In elective surgery, patients are usually starved of food and drink overnight, or for at least 4–6 h. However, in emergency surgery, it may be necessary to induce anaesthesia urgently before an adequate period of starvation occurs. In addition, the patient's surgical condition is often accompanied by delayed gastric emptying.

The most important factors determining the extent of gastric regurgitation are the function of the lower oesophageal sphincter and the rate of gastric emptying.

The lower oesophageal sphincter

The lower oesophageal sphincter (LOS) is an area (some 2–5 cm in length) of higher resting intraluminal pressure situated in the region of the cardia. The sphincter relaxes during oesophageal peristalsis to allow food into the stomach, but otherwise remains contracted. The structure cannot be defined anatomically but may be detected using intraluminal pressure manometry.

The LOS is the main barrier preventing reflux of gastric contents into the oesophagus, and its resting tone is affected by many drugs used in anaesthetic practice. Reflux is related not to the LOS tone *per se*, but to the difference between gastric and LOS pressure — this is termed the barrier pressure. Drugs which increase barrier pressure decrease the risk of reflux. Prochlorperazine, cyclizine, anticholinesterases, α-adrenergic agonists and suxamethonium increase barrier pressure. For many years it was thought that the increase in intragastric pressure during suxamethonium-induced fasciculations predisposed to reflux. However, recently it has been shown that there is a correspondingly greater increase in LOS pressure with a consequent increase in barrier pressure.

Anticholinergic drugs, ethanol, ganglion blocking drugs, tricyclic antidepressants, opioids and sodium thiopentone reduce LOS pressure and it is reasonable to assume that these drugs increase the tendency to gastro-oesophageal reflux.

Gastric emptying

Under normal circumstances, peristaltic waves sweep from cardia to pylorus at a rate of approx. 3 per min, although temporary inhibition of gastric motility follows recent ingestion of a meal. The rate of gastric emptying is proportional to the volume of the stomach contents, with approx. 1–3% of total gastric content reaching the duodenum per minute. Thus, emptying occurs at an exponential rate. The presence of fat, acid or hypertonic solutions in the duodenum significantly delays the rate of emptying (the inhibitory enterogastric reflex), but both the nervous and humoral elements of this regulating mechanism are still poorly understood. There are many pathological conditions associated with a reduced rate of gastric emptying (Table 30.3). In the absence of any of these factors, it is reasonably safe to assume that the stomach is empty provided that solids have not been ingested within the preceding 6 h, or fluids consumed in the preceding 4 h, and provided normal peristalsis is occurring.

Table 30.3 Situations in which vomiting or regurgitation may occur

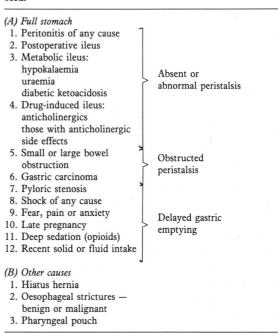

(A) Full stomach
1. Peritonitis of any cause
2. Postoperative ileus
3. Metabolic ileus:
   hypokalaemia
   uraemia
   diabetic ketoacidosis   } Absent or abnormal peristalsis
4. Drug-induced ileus:
   anticholinergics
   those with anticholinergic
   side effects
5. Small or large bowel
   obstruction   } Obstructed peristalsis
6. Gastric carcinoma
7. Pyloric stenosis
8. Shock of any cause
9. Fear, pain or anxiety
10. Late pregnancy   } Delayed gastric emptying
11. Deep sedation (opioids)
12. Recent solid or fluid intake

(B) Other causes
1. Hiatus hernia
2. Oesophageal strictures —
   benign or malignant
3. Pharyngeal pouch

Vomiting and regurgitation are encountered most frequently during induction of anaesthesia in patients with an acute abdomen or trauma. All patients with minor trauma (fractures and dislocations) must be assumed to have a full stomach as gastric emptying virtually ceases at the time of significant trauma as a result of the combined effects of fear, pain, shock and treatment with opioid analgesics. In all trauma patients, the time interval between ingestion of food and the accident is a more reliable index of the degree of gastric emptying than the period of fasting. It is not uncommon to encounter vomiting occurring up to 24 h after ingestion of food when trauma has occurred very shortly after the meal. Thus the 4–6 h rule is quite unreliable.

TECHNIQUES OF ANAESTHESIA

It is important to recognise any patient who may have significant gastric residue and is in danger of aspiration. The anaesthetic management of such a patient may be described in five phases; preparation, induction, maintenance, emergence and postoperative management.

Phase I — preparation

Whilst postponement of surgery in the emergency patient may be indicated in order to obtain investigations and institute resuscitation with i.v. fluids, there is usually no benefit to be gained in terms of reducing gastric contents. However, two manoeuvres are available:

1. Insertion of a nasogastric tube and aspiration of the stomach contents. This is useful when gastric contents are liquid, as in bowel obstruction, but is less effective when contents are solid.

2. Neutralisation of the pH of gastric contents (e.g. with sodium citrate) to reduce the chance of acid aspiration syndrome occurring in the event of inhalation. Although this is standard practice in obstetric anaesthesia, few anaesthetists employ this measure for emergency general surgery. The regimens which may be used are described in Chapter 31 (p. 416).

Phase II — induction

Crash induction

This is the most frequently employed technique for the patient with a full stomach, although it contravenes one of the fundamental rules of anaesthesia, notably that muscle relaxants are not given until control of the airway is assured. The decision to employ the crash induction technique balances the risk of losing control of the airway against the risk of aspiration. It is therefore imperative to assess carefully whether or not

difficulty is likely to be encountered in performing endotracheal intubation. The anaesthetist must have prepared a contingency plan for management of the patient should intubation fail. If preoperative evaluation indicates a particularly difficult airway, the anaesthetist should consider alternative methods of proceeding, e.g. local anaesthetic techniques or 'awake intubation' under local anaesthesia.

For crash induction to be consistently safe and successful it should be performed with meticulous attention to detail. The patient *must* be on a tipping trolley or table, preferably with an adjustable head piece so that the degree of neck extension/flexion may be altered quickly. Ideally, the patient's head should be in the classical 'sniffing position' with the neck flexed on the shoulders and the head extended on the neck. Failure to appreciate this point increases the frequency of difficult intubations.

The anaesthetist *must* be aided by at least one skilled assistant to perform cricoid pressure, assist in turning the patient, obtain smaller endotracheal tubes, supply stilettes for tubes, etc. Suction apparatus *must* be working and the suction catheter within reach of the anaesthetist's hand.

As with any anaesthetic, the machine should have been checked before commencing, ventilator adjusted to appropriate settings and all drugs drawn up into labelled syringes prior to induction. The patient should breathe 100% O_2 for 3–5 min while appropriate monitoring devices are attached and an i.v. infusion commenced (if not already in place). The optimal inclination of the operating table is debatable as some authorities recommend the reverse Trendelenburg (head-up) position (to prevent regurgitation), and some the classical Trendelenburg position (to prevent aspiration of any regurgitated or vomited material). It is the author's view that the optimum position is that in which the junior anaesthetist has gained greatest experience in performing intubation.

Preinduction measurement of heart rate, arterial pressure (and when appropriate central venous pressure), and inspection of the e.c.g. are made and a skilled assistant is positioned on the patient's right side to perform Sellick's manoeuvre (cricoid pressure). It is important that the assistant can identify the cricoid cartilage, as compression of the thyroid cartilage distorts laryngeal anatomy and may render endotracheal intubation very difficult. To perform Sellick's manoeuvre correctly, the thumb and forefinger of the right hand press the cricoid cartilage firmly in a posterior direction, thus compressing the oesophagus between the cricoid cartilage and the vertebral column. Because the cricoid cartilage forms a complete ring, the tracheal lumen is not distorted (Fig. 30.1).

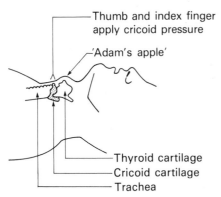

Thumb and index finger apply cricoid pressure

'Adam's apple'

Thyroid cartilage
Cricoid cartilage
Trachea

Fig. 30.1 Sellick's manoeuvre. The cricoid cartilage is palpated immediately below the thyroid cartilage.

Opinions differ on when cricoid pressure should be applied; some prefer to inform the patient and apply it just before administration of the i.v. induction agent; others apply it as soon as consciousness is lost.

With the assistant in position, a predetermined sleep dose of i.v. induction agent is given (usually thiopentone, 2–4 mg/kg or less in the presence of hypovolaemia). Without waiting to assess the effect of the induction agent, this is followed immediately by a paralysing dose of suxamethonium (1.5 mg/kg). As soon as the jaw begins to relax, laryngoscopy is performed and the trachea intubated with the aid of a stilette. Cricoid pressure *is maintained* until the endotracheal tube cuff is inflated and correct placement ascertained by auscultation of both lungs. The lungs are *gently* ventilated manually since excessive increases in intrathoracic pressure may have harmful effects on circulatory dynamics. One of the main disadvantages of the crash induction technique is the haemodynamic instability which may result if the dose of induction agent is excessive (hypotension, circulatory collapse) or inadequate (hypertension, tachycardia, arrhythmia). Unfortunately, selection of the correct dose is difficult and is dependent largely upon the experience of the anaesthetist. For sodium thiopentone, a dose of 4 mg/kg may suffice for

healthy, young patients, 2 mg/kg for the elderly, and less for the very frail. Alternatives are etomidate 0.1–0.3 mg/kg (which is less cardiodepressant than thiopentone) and methohexitone 1–1.5 mg/kg.

Inhalational induction

(With patient in left lateral head-down position.) In situations where there is reasonable doubt about the ability to perform intubation or to maintain a patent airway in a patient with a full stomach (for example the patient with faciomaxillary trauma or the child with epiglottitis), an inhalational induction may be used with oxygen and halothane, followed by an attempt at endotracheal intubation during spontaneous ventilation. If circumstances do not allow the lateral position then the supine posture with cricoid pressure may have to be accepted.

Awake intubation

Blind nasal intubation is a valuable skill which should be cultivated by all anaesthetists. It is most useful in patients likely to develop unrelievable airway obstruction when loss of consciousness occurs (e.g. trismus from dental abscess or angioneurotic oedema) although it may also be performed on unconscious patients. Before embarking on blind nasal intubation in the awake subject it is necessary to render the upper airway insensitive so that introduction of an endotracheal tube may be tolerated. This is accomplished in 3 stages:

1. The nasal mucosa is anaesthetised with cocaine solution 4% (maximum 2.5 ml/70 kg) which is sprayed into the more patent nasal passage. In addition to providing surface anaesthesia this also shrinks the nasal mucosa and greatly reduces the chance of bleeding.

2. The superior laryngeal branch of the vagus nerve is blocked as it sweeps around the hyoid bone. A 23 G needle is 'walked' off the inferior border of the greater cornu of the hyoid near its tip and approx. 3 ml of 1% lignocaine is deposited deep to the thyrohyoid membrane. A slight loss of resistance is felt as this membrane is penetrated by the needle. Successful bilateral block of the superior laryngeal nerve produces anaesthesia of the inferior surface of the epiglottis and the laryngeal inlet as far down as the vocal cords.

3. Anaesthesia of the tracheal mucosa below the vocal cords is best accomplished with a transtracheal injection of local anaesthetic. A 21 G needle is introduced in the midline through the cricothyroid membrane. Entry into the trachea is confirmed by aspiration of air and a bolus of 3–5 ml of lignocaine 1% is injected rapidly. Invariably this results in a bout of coughing which aids spread of the local anaesthetic over the inferior surface of the vocal cords. Anaesthesia of the upper airway should now be complete but it is emphasised that the patient will now be at risk from pulmonary aspiration should vomiting or regurgitation occur. It follows that this technique should be employed in the emergency situation only after full consideration of potential benefits have been carefully balanced against the risk of aspiration.

If a standard curved endotracheal tube is advanced through the nose it enters the trachea in approx. 50% of patients without special manipulation. In the other 50% of patients, certain manoeuvres increase the chances of success.

With the patient's head in the 'sniffing the morning air' position, a well lubricated tube is inserted gently into the anaesthetised nostril and advanced towards the nasopharynx. The tube should be rotated slowly between thumb and forefinger (pill rolling movement) and a distinct 'give' is felt on entry into the nasopharynx. As maximal vocal cord abduction occurs during inspiration, the tube is now advanced slowly in small steps coordinated with inspiration. Even with good upper airway anaesthesia, entry into the larynx often results in a violent cough but even if this occurs the position of the tube must be confirmed before general anaesthesia is induced.

If the endotracheal tube does not enter the trachea it must be situated in either the oesophagus, or one or other pyriform fossa or caught on the anterior commissure of the larynx. If it is in the oesophagus there will be an absence of breath sounds emanating from the end of the tube following complete insertion. The tube should be withdrawn into the pharynx and readvanced whilst the patient's head is extended slightly.

If the tip of the tube is lying in the pyriform fossa a slight bulge will be apparent in the neck just above the larynx, to the left or right of the midline. In this situation successful intubation is achieved by withdrawal of the tube a few cm, rotation towards the midline and reinsertion.

If the tube cannot be inserted completely and sustained pressure does not produce a bulge on either side of the larynx, it is almost certainly caught on the anterior commissure. It should be withdrawn a few cm and reinserted after slight flexion of the patient's head.

Regional anaesthesia

Anaesthetic expertise in the use of regional anaesthesia is lacking in many United Kingdom hospitals. This is unfortunate since local blocks are eminently suitable for emergency procedures on the extremities (e.g. to reduce fractures and dislocations).

Brachial plexus block by the axillary, supra-clavicular or interscalene approach is satisfactory for orthopaedic manipulations or surgical procedures involving the upper extremity. It satisfies surgical requirements for analgesia, muscle relaxation and immobility. There is minimal effect on the cardiovascular system and there is a prolonged period of analgesia postoperatively. Similarly, i.v. regional anaesthesia (Bier's block, p. 332) is useful for orthopaedic reductions; prilocaine plain (0.5%) is the drug of choice.

For regional anaesthesia of the lower extremity, techniques available include spinal and extradural anaesthesia. These techniques are contraindicated if there is doubt regarding adequacy of e.c.f. or vascular volume, as large decreases in arterial pressure may result from the associated pharmacological sympathectomy.

It is a common surgical misconception that spinal or extradural anaesthetic techniques are safer than general anaesthesia for patients in poor physical condition. It must be emphasised that for the *inexperienced* anaesthetist, these techniques are *invariably more dangerous* than general anaesthesia for the patient with moderate/major trauma or any intra-abdominal emergency condition.

Phase III — maintenance of anaesthesia

In emergency anaesthesia, there are strong arguments in favour of a balanced technique of anaesthesia combining:

1. Anaesthesia: loss of awareness.

2. Analgesia to attenuate autonomic reflexes in response to the painful stimulus.

3. Muscle relaxation.

If a crash induction has been performed, the patient's lungs are gently ventilated manually whilst heart rate and arterial pressure measurements are repeated to assess the cardiovascular effects of the drugs used and of the insult of endotracheal intubation. Nitrous oxide 50–66% (dependent upon the patient's condition) in oxygen contributes to loss of patient awareness but does not ensure it, and some anaesthetists advocate the use of either 0.5% halothane or 0.5–1% enflurane in addition.

When there is evidence of return of neuromuscular transmission (by clinical signs or use of a nerve stimulator) as suxamethonium is degraded, a nondepolarising myoneural blocking agent is administered. The choice is dependent upon the patient's condition and the effect of the induction of anaesthesia on the patient's cardiovascular status. Alcuronium is an appropriate drug for routine use in a dose of 0.25–0.3 mg/kg. A slight decrease in arterial pressure is often seen after administration, but this is usually transient and corrected easily with i.v. fluids. Pancuronium (dose 0.04–0.05 mg/kg) is useful in patients with hypovolaemia, as it tends to increase arterial pressure and heart rate. (The tachycardia it produces is undesirable in patients with ischaemic heart disease or valvular disease). Tubocurarine (0.3–0.4 mg/kg) is an alternative drug, but it often produces significant hypotension which is not usually desirable in emergency anaesthesia. The newer agents vecuronium and atracurium have virtually no cardiovascular effects in clinical doses and are ideal, particularly atracurium when renal impairment is present.

When the muscle relaxant has been administered, the endotracheal tube is connected to a mechanical ventilator and minute volume adjusted to produce normo- or slight hypocapnia. There are few accurate means of estimating ventilatory requirement, but a minute volume of 100 ml/kg/min at a tidal volume of 8–12 ml/kg should be employed initially. The inspiratory flow rate should be adjusted to minimise peak airway pressure.

Before the initial surgical incision is made, analgesia may be supplemented by small incremental doses of morphine 1–5 mg, papaveretum 2–10 mg, or fentanyl 25–100 μg.

The use of supplemental doses of analgesic and muscle relaxant drugs are described in Chapters 10 and 11. The trainee should be aware that during emergency anaesthesia, particularly for intra-abdominal or trauma surgery, much smaller doses of drugs are usually required. As a general rule, it is safe practice to administer half the dose which might be considered appropriate for an elective patient, and to determine further doses by assessment of the subsequent response. Particularly where there are poor or inadequate recovery room facilities, it is also a good general rule to err on the side of caution in the use of i.v. drugs and consider supplementing anaesthesia with a volatile agent.

Fluid management

During emergency intra-abdominal surgery there may be large blood and fluid losses which exceed the patient's maintenance fluid requirements. These include evaporative losses from exposed gut and mesentery, blood loss on to swabs and into suction bottles, and the poorly defined 'third space losses' caused by sequestration of fluid in inflamed and traumatised tissue. Intraoperatively, maintenance requirements are supplied with Hartmann's solution (compound sodium lactate) at 2 ml/kg/h. An appropriate volume of replacement for third space loss and evaporative gut loss is given in addition. This volume depends on the degree of surgical trauma but is normally in the range 2–7 ml/kg/h.

Haemorrhage in excess of 15% blood volume in adults or 10% in children is usually an indication for blood transfusion.

Phase IV — reversal and emergence

Any volatile agent is discontinued 15–20 min before surgery finishes. On insertion of the last skin suture, direct pharyngoscopy is performed and secretions/debris removed from the pharynx; if a nasogastric tube is in situ, it is aspirated and left unspigoted. Atropine and neostigmine are given in one bolus of 20 μg/kg and 50 μg/kg respectively, and ventilation is undertaken manually (with an F_{O_2} of 1.0) so that spontaneous respiratory activity may be detected. Because the risk of aspiration of gastric contents is as great on recovery as at induction, extubation of the trachea should not be performed until protective airway reflexes are intact. To demonstrate adequacy of reflexes, both level of consciousness and neuromuscular transmission should be assessed.

Level of consciousness. The patient should be awake and respond appropriately to verbal commands, e.g. eye opening.

Neuromuscular function. The adequacy of reversal of paralysis may be determined by observing the patient's ability to sustain a head lift for 5 s and ability to sustain a firm grip without fade (see Table 11.3). Preferably, a nerve stimulator is used to define reversal of neuromuscular transmission (see Chapter 11).

Immediately before tracheal extubation, the patient is turned to the lateral position (if possible) and asked to take a deep inspiration while gentle positive pressure is applied to the airway. At the peak of inspiration, the cuff is deflated and the endotracheal tube removed as the patient exhales, thus assisting removal of any secretions which may have accumulated above the cuff. Oxygen 100% is administered until a regular respiratory rhythm is re-established and the patient has demonstrated an ability to cough and maintain a patent airway. Breathing 40% O_2 he is transported in the lateral position to the recovery room and remains there until all vital signs are stable, postoperative shivering has ceased, core temperature is normal, and there is good perfusion as judged by warm extremities and good urine output.

If there is any doubt regarding the adequacy of ventilation after reversal of neuromuscular blockade, the patient is taken to the recovery room with the endotracheal tube in situ and this is removed from the trachea only when ventilation and gas exchange are adequate.

Phase V — postoperative management

Postoperatively the patient requires analgesics, e.g. morphine 0.2 mg/kg i.m. 4-hrly, or papaveretum 0.3 mg/kg 4-hrly. If there is continued concern regarding the metabolic or volaemic state of the patient, these dosages should be reduced considerably.

Fluid balance should take into account maintenance needs plus compensation for abnormal fluid loss (e.g. gastric aspirate, loss from intestinal fistulae, or from surgical drains). Normal maintenance fluid requirements in nonsurgical patients may be met by the infusion of 30–40 ml/kg/day of water, 1 mmol/kg/day of sodium and 1 mmol/kg/day of potassium. This may be achieved in the average adult by infusion of 2.5 litre of 0.18% saline/4% dextrose with 2 g KCl per litre, which provides 2500 ml of water, 75 mmol of sodium and 67 mmol of potassium, and 400 kcal (1.65 MJ). However, surgery is accompanied by release of ADH and aldosterone and fluid and electrolytes are sequestered in 'third spaces'. Failure to recognise this in the past has led to inadequate intraoperative fluid and electrolyte loading, with consequent postoperative hyponatraemia and oliguria. Thus, when there is doubt regarding the adequacy of intraoperative fluid or electrolyte administration, it may be necessary to give an additional 1 mmol/kg of sodium on the first postoperative day. Adequate replacement is confirmed by measurement of serum electrolyte concentrations.

Nasogastric aspirate and measurable enteric losses are replaced with equal volumes of 0.9% saline.

The need for further blood replacement is assessed by regular observation of vital signs and drainage measurements, and postoperative Hb or haematocrit measurements.

Prophylactic postoperative IPPV

Continuation of IPPV should be considered electively in a number of ill-defined circumstances, some of which are listed in Table 30.4.

Table 30.4 Indications for continuation of ventilatory assistance postoperatively

1.	Prolonged shock/hypoperfusion state of any cause
2.	Massive sepsis (faecal peritonitis, cholangitis, septicaemia)
3.	Severe ischaemic heart disease
4.	Extreme obesity
5.	Overt gastric acid aspiration
6.	Previously severe pulmonary disease

THE ANAESTHETIST AND MAJOR TRAUMA

The management of the patient with major trauma requires a multidisciplinary team effort. Successful treatment is often dependent on the efficacy of the initial resuscitation and rapid formulation of the correct priorities.

Immediate care

As soon as the patient arrives in the Accident and Emergency Department, resuscitation, diagnosis and specific treatment are required simultaneously.

The first priority for the anaesthetist is to establish the patency of the patient's airway. If upper airway obstruction is present, the pharynx is cleared of any debris, the jaw displaced forward (jaw thrust), and the neck extended gently. This manoeuvre must be performed very carefully in any patient with a potential cervical spine injury.

Once the airway is clear, attention is directed to the adequacy of ventilation and the need for tracheal intubation. If the patient is apnoeic, ventilation by mask with 100% oxygen is commenced immediately, as good oxygenation and correction of hypercapnia should be ensured before tracheal intubation is undertaken.

Patients with severe faciomaxillary trauma who are co-operative and awake despite their injuries may not require immediate tracheal intubation, but do need frequent and regular upper airway evaluation, to assess the rate of progress of pharyngeal or laryngeal oedema which may proceed to complete airway obstruction with alarming rapidity.

Once the airway is under control, ventilation is deemed adequate, and any obvious external bleeding has been arrested, the next priority is evaluation of the cardiovascular system: this may be divided into assessment of blood volume status and pump function.

Volume status

This has been described earlier in this chapter. Patients with major trauma often require urgent restoration of circulating blood volume. At least two large bore (14G) i.v. cannulae are inserted percutaneously into veins in one or two limbs, and at least one is attached to a blood warming coil. As soon as possible, a reliable CVP line is inserted. The right internal jugular vein is the preferred site for this purpose. Fluid is infused through the peripheral i.v. cannulae to produce a CVP of approx. 0–3 cm H_2O (manubrium being the zero reference).

Whilst whole blood is the ideal fluid for restoration of blood volume in haemorrhagic shock, substitute fluid should be given immediately while cross-matching is undertaken. If total exsanguination is imminent, type specific blood may be given, as the chance of a reaction is less than 1% in males, but over 2% in parous females. If the patient has 20–30% blood volume depletion, 2 litre of Hartmann's solution may be infused rapidly whilst cross-matching is in progress. If this does not increase perfusion and arterial pressure significantly, and blood is still not available, either plasma or a plasma substitute should be considered. Human plasma protein fraction is very expensive and probably has little advantage over Haemaccel. This is a 3.3% isotonic solution of degraded gelatin with a molecular weight of 35 000. Its half-life in the circulation is approx. 4 h in the normal patient, but is shorter in the presence of shock. Since 85% is excreted by the kidneys, Haemaccel promotes an osmotic diuresis and may therefore preserve urine output and renal function. Up to 1500 ml of Haemaccel may be given initially; in most circumstances this is adequate to restore circulating blood volume until cross-matched blood is available. Warmed, stored blood is administered subsequently to maintain urine output, arterial pressure and CVP.

Pump function

The commonest cause of pump failure in major trauma is the presence of a tension pneumothorax, but other possibilities include severe myocardial contusion and traumatic pericardial tamponade.

Tension pneumothorax causes compression of the mediastinum (heart and great vessels) and presents with extreme respiratory distress and shock, unilateral air entry, a shift of the trachea towards the normal side and distension of the veins in the neck, although the last sign may not be seen in hypovolaemic shock. It may be relieved immediately by insertion of a 14 G cannula through the 2nd intercostal space in the midclavicular line but this should be followed by standard chest drainage. If there is any suspicion of tension pneumothorax,

IPPV should not be commenced until decompression has been achieved, otherwise mediastinal compression is increased. Patients with blunt chest trauma and fractured ribs may develop a tension pneumothorax rapidly when positive pressure ventilation is instituted and consideration should be given to the prophylactic insertion of chest drains in such patients.

Definitive care

Whenever possible, hypovolaemia should be corrected before anaesthesia is induced, but when the rate of haemorrhage is likely to exceed the rate of transfusion, and continued transfusion results only in further bleeding (e.g. ruptured aorta), it may be necessary to induce anaesthesia in a hypovolaemic patient.

On arrival in theatre, the patient is placed on the operating table which is covered by a warming blanket at 37°C. One hundred per cent oxygen is given whilst at least two large-gauge cannulae are inserted (one connected to a blood warming coil), if this has not already been accomplished. In patients with major trauma, anaesthesia should be induced in theatre so that surgery can commence as soon as possible. Figure 30.2 illustrates standard monitoring which is necessary for the management of major trauma.

In the unconscious patient, the trachea may be intubated following a paralysing dose of suxamethonium. If the patient is conscious, despite being severely hypovolaemic, a controlled crash induction employing ketamine as the i.v. induction agent is preferred (although experienced anaesthetists may use extremely small doses of methohexitone). The dose of ketamine is critical and often very small doses suffice (0.3–0.7 mg/kg). If the dose is misjudged, cardiovascular decompensation may occur similar to that seen with other i.v. induction agents. The depressant effects of i.v. induction agents are exaggerated because the *proportion* of the cardiac output going to the heart and brain is increased. In addition, the rate of redistribution and/or metabolism is decreased as a result of reduced blood flow to muscle, liver and kidneys, and thus blood concentrations remain elevated for longer periods in comparison with healthy patients. Ketamine should not be used in patients with significant head injury.

Etomidate (0.1–0.3 mg/kg) is an alternative for normovolaemic or marginally hypovolaemic patients with head injury, but is more likely to attenuate compensatory mechanisms. Some experienced anaesthetists still regard cyclopropane 50% in oxygen as the best induction for severely hypovolaemic patients with or without head injury. Consciousness is lost rapidly following which endotracheal intubation may be undertaken with the aid of suxamethonium.

Following tracheal intubation, the lungs are ventilated at the lowest peak airway pressure consistent with an acceptable tidal volume. Pancuronium is given in small incremental doses of 1 mg to maintain relaxation. When the haemodynamic situation has stabilised and systolic arterial pressure exceeds 90 mmHg, consideration may be given to deepening anaesthesia. This should be undertaken cautiously and, in principle, agents which are rapidly reversible or rapidly excreted should be employed.

In the shock state, there is very rapid uptake of inhalational agents. As a result of chemoreceptor stimulation, the patient hyperventilates thus accelerating the rate of increase of alveolar concentration of anaesthetic gas. Similarly, reduced cardiac output and pulmonary blood flow decrease the rate of removal of anaesthetic agent from the alveoli, producing a rapid increase in alveolar concentration. Thus the MAC value is approached more rapidly than in normovolaemic patients.

Monitoring should be comprehensive in these patients (Fig. 30.2). When feasible, monitoring should be instituted before the induction of anaesthesia, although the urgency of the situation may preclude this. Blood may be sampled from the arterial line to monitor changes in blood gases, acid–base state, haemoglobin concentration, PCV and electrolyte values. Requirements for futher colloid replacement may be assessed from CVP measurement and urine output.

When surgical bleeding has been controlled, the patient's cardiovascular status should improve, but if hypotension persists despite apparently adequate fluid administration, other causes of haemorrhage should be sought (Table 30.5). It is important that the anaesthetist assesses the patient regularly during prolonged anaesthesia to exclude these latent complications of major trauma.

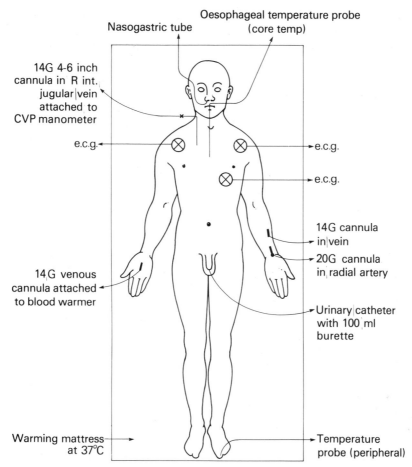

Fig. 30.2 Commonly used monitoring and resuscitation attachments in management of a patient with multiple injuries.

Massive transfusion

One definition states that an amount greater than 50% of the patient's blood volume be replaced rapidly before the transfusion is deemed massive, e.g. 5 unit blood in 1 h in a 70 kg adult.

Stored blood is an unphysiological solution with a pH of 7.2–6.6, serum potassium level of 5–25 mmol/litre and a temperature of 4–6°C. It contains citrate as an anticoagulant, and when stored for more than five days, has insignificant amounts of 2,3 DPG, thereby shifting the haemoglobin curve to the left. Blood stored for longer than 24 h has no functional platelets, with levels of factors V and VIII approx. 10% of normal and factor IX 20% of normal. Effete cells and platelets clump together forming debris which are potentially harmful when infused in sufficient quantity.

Table 30.5 Causes of persistent hypotension

1.	Continued overt bleeding
2.	Continued concealed bleeding — chest, abdomen retroperitoneal space, pelvis, soft tissues of each thigh } Surgical or medical (check platelets and clotting screen)
3.	Pump failure — haemothorax, pneumothorax, tamponade, myocardial contusion
4.	Metabolic problem — acidaemia (only correct pH less than 7.1) hypothermia (largely preventable) hypocalcaemia

406 TEXTBOOK OF ANAESTHESIA

Many of these disadvantages of stored blood are not a problem clinically; for example, citrate is removed by metabolic conversion in the liver (forming mostly bicarbonate), the transfused cells act as a 'potassium sink' and quickly mop up excess potassium and the post-transfusion alkalosis (resulting from citrate metabolism) may contribute to hypokalaemia in the post-transfusion period.

Indeed, when the transfused blood is warmed near to body temperature before infusion and a 20 μm filter is used to remove unwanted cellular debris, the commonest problem is that of haemostatic failure.

Transfusion of bank blood in quantities approaching the patient's blood volume causes a dilutional thrombocytopenia and some measure of clotting factor deficiency, both of which affect haemostasis adversely. These abnormalities may be detected by a platelet count, prothrombin time and partial thromboplastin time, reflecting disorders of extrinsic and intrinsic systems as a result of dilutional loss of factor V and VIII. Treatment should be directed at correcting the dilutional coagulation change and consists of fresh frozen plasma (1 unit for every 4 unit blood) and, occasionally, platelet concentrate for severe thrombocytopenia (platelet count below 30×10^9/litre). Requests for these expensive blood components should be made early as there is often delay in obtaining them, and it is better, if possible, to prevent the development of coagulation failure.

FURTHER READING

Campbell D 1979 The anaesthetist and trauma. In: Atkinson R S, Langton-Hewer C (eds) Recent advances in anaesthesia and analgesia, 13. Churchill Livingstone, Edinburgh

Campbell D 1977 Immediate hospital care of the injured. British Journal of Anaesthesia 49(7): 673

Clarke R S J, Carson I W 1980 Anaesthesia for trauma and major accidents. In: Gray T C, Nunn J F, Utting J E (eds) General anaesthesia, vol 2, 4th edn. Butterworths, London

Cotton B R, Smith G 1982 The lower oesophageal sphincter. In: Kaufman L (ed) Anaesthetic review 1. Churchill Livingstone, London

Giesecke A H 1981 Perioperative fluid therapy — crystalloids. In: Miller R D (ed) Anaesthesia, vol 2. Churchill Livingstone, London

Giesecke A H 1981 Anaesthesia for trauma surgery. In: Miller R D (ed) Anaesthesia, Vol 2. Churchill Livingstone, London, p 1247

Horsey P J 1982 Blood transfusion. In: Atkinson R S, Langton Hewer C (eds) Recent advances in anaesthesia and analgesia, 14. Churchill Livingstone, Edinburgh

Magill I W 1975 Lest we forget — blind nasal intubation. Anaesthesia 30(4): 476

Sellick B A 1961 Cricothyroid pressure to control regurgitation of stomach contents during induction of anaesthesia. Lancet 2: 404

Thornton J A 1980 Blood loss, colloid infusion and blood transfusion. In: Gray T C, Nunn J F, Utting J E (eds) General anaesthesia, 4th edn. Butterworths, London

Tunstall M E 1980 Inhalation of gastric contents. In: Gray T C, Nunn J F, Utting J E (eds) General anaesthesia, 4th edn. Butterworths, London

Walters F J M, Nott M R 1977 The hazards of anaesthesia in the injured patient. British Journal of Anaesthesia 49(7): 707

Wandless J G 1978 Emergency anaesthesia. British Journal of Hospital Medicine, May: 437

Wallace W A, Milne D D 1978 Intravenous regional anaesthesia. Hospital Update 3, 4: 137

31

Obstetric anaesthesia

Obstetric anaesthesia gained acceptance following the administration of chloroform to Queen Victoria to assist in the delivery of Prince Leopold in 1853. The anaesthetist was John Snow and the technique became known as chloroform 'à la Reine'. Prior to this, there had been a widespread belief that the pain of childbirth was good for the mother. This was based on a text from the Book of Genesis: 'In sorrow thou shalt bring forth children'. However the generally held belief nowadays is that childbirth should be a pleasant experience for the mother.

Most large hospitals in the U.K. and other Western countries have the services of an experienced anaesthetist in the maternity unit for 24 h each day. Smaller units may rely on the services of an 'on-call' anaesthetist who has other duties.

These anaesthetists administer anaesthetics for surgical procedures, provide analgesia for painful labour and assist in the management of diseases caused by or complicated by pregnancy.

MATERNAL MORTALITY

Triennial reports on Confidential Enquiries into Maternal Deaths provide information on deaths attributable to anaesthesia. It may be seen from Table 31.1 that although the actual number of deaths associated directly with anaesthesia has fallen from 50 to 30 per triennium in the years 1964–1978 there has been an increase in the percentage of true maternal deaths (resulting from anaesthesia) from 8.7 to 13.2%. This latter figure has remained the same over the period covered by the last two reports. However, it should be pointed out that the number of anaesthetics (general and regional) given for obstetric purposes over the period is unknown, and therefore this does not imply that the anaesthetic mortality rate in anaesthesia has either increased or remained unchanged.

The most common cause of death in 1976–1978 was inhalation of stomach contents (11 of the 30 reported deaths). The second most common cause of death was placement of the endotracheal tube in the oesophagus. The assessors commented that 'death was usually due to a combination of inexperience, low general standards of care in labour and in the operating theatre and poor administrative practices, in the form of unskilled assistance or isolation from fully equipped hospitals'. Four deaths were associated with extradural analgesia and it was concluded, 'that extradural analgesia should only be used by those properly trained to manage it and who are fully aware of the effects and hazards of regional blocks'.

PAIN RELIEF IN LABOUR

Labour is painful for most women and in the first stage this results from both uterine contractions and

Table 31.1 Deaths associated with anaesthesia in England and Wales from 1964 to 1978

	1964–66	1967–69	1970–72	1973–75	1976–78
Number of deaths directly associated with anaesthesia	50	50	37	31	30
Percentage of true maternal deaths from anaesthesia	8.7	10.9	10.4	13.2	13.2

dilatation of the cervix. In the second stage of labour, pain is caused by stretching, distension and tearing of fascia, skin and subcutaneous tissues and pressure on the skeletal muscles of the perineum.

With the use of bilateral paravertebral blocks it has been shown that the pain of the early part of the first stage of labour may be abolished by blocking T11 and T12 but abolition of pain caused by the strong contractions at the end of the first stage and during the second stage requires blockade of T10 and L1 in addition. Once the cervix is fully dilated, pain is appreciated by the impact of the presenting part on pain-sensitive structures in the pelvis, producing mild referred pain depending on the structure affected, e.g.

1. Pressure on bladder, urethra and rectum is referred to sacral segments.

2. Traction on uterine adnexae is referred to T10–L1.

3. Stretch and pressure on muscles and ligaments of pelvis is referred to lower lumbar and sacral segments.

The pain of stretching and tearing of the perineum can be abolished completely by bilateral pudendal nerve block.

The abolition of pain during labour is highly beneficial to both mother and fetus. Severe pain produces inhibition of gastro-intestinal function thus increasing gastric volume. In addition, urinary retention and inhibition of uterine activity may impair contractions. Pain-induced hyperventilation may be so severe as to cause marked respiratory alkalosis with consequent decrease in uterine blood flow. Maternal oxygen consumption is increased and both maternal and fetal metabolic acidosis may occur.

Various techniques have been used to alleviate labour pains for mothers who request it or for whom it is considered medically appropriate.

Systemic analgesia

In the absence of an obstetric extradural service, the commonest form of analgesia used during labour is intramuscular pethidine. This opioid is prescribed for approx. 70% of mothers in labour, and its use by midwives has been authorised by the Central Midwives Board in the U.K. since 1950. The timing of administration is usually at the discretion of the midwife; an initial dose of 100–150 mg is usually given followed by additional doses of 100 mg (to a maximum of 3) at approx. 3 hrly intervals to maintain adequate levels of analgesia.

The major disadvantage of this technique is that it is ineffective for 40–75% of mothers, possibly because it is given too late during labour, or in too small a dose.

Pethidine may occasionally cause maternal hypotension, but nausea and/or vomiting occurs in approx. 50% of mothers. Hypoxia (defined as a decrease in oxygen tension greater than 10% from control) has been demonstrated in some mothers who receive pethidine. This drug may also cause drowsiness and dissociation. It is claimed that these problems are reduced by patient-operated on-demand systems (see p. 314). Small bolus doses of pethidine are delivered to the patient when demanded at intervals of not less than 10 min. With this system it is claimed that 73% of mothers report adequate pain relief.

Pethidine crosses the placenta to a large extent following both i.m. and i.v. administration causing neontal respiratory depression which is maximum 3 h postinjection. Pa_{CO_2} in the neonate is increased for at least 24 h and metabolites of pethidine may be found in the urine of the neonate for up to 3 days. There is also depression of feeding and other neurobehavioural responses in babies of mothers given pethidine. Naloxone 40 μg administered to the baby reverses these effects but repeated doses are required to produce an adequate prolonged effect.

Other opioid analgesic drugs which have been used during labour include:

1. Pentazocine (which is approved by the Central Midwives Board for use by midwives), but the quality of analgesia is inferior to that produced by pethidine and its hallucinogenic properties are greater.

2. Diamorphine and morphine — these have been used more for their sedative properties but may result in an unacceptably high incidence of depressed neonates.

Inhalational analgesia

Inhalational analgesia is practised widely in the U.K. under the supervision of midwives. When used effectively, approx. 70% of mothers report considerable or complete pain relief.

Entonox

This is premixed 50% N$_2$O in oxygen and is contained in cylinders available in 500 litre size for domiciliary use or 2000 litre or 5000 litre sizes for hospital use.

It is important that the technique of administration of Entonox is taught during antenatal classes. The first 30 s of a contraction is not usually painful although the mother is aware of the onset of a contraction. This is important since the attainment of maximal analgesic effect from Entonox takes 45 s. The face mask should be applied as closely-fitting to the face as possible to avoid air leaks and consequent dilution of the gas mixture. Inhalation should begin as soon as the start of a contraction is felt and continue during the painful phase of the contraction; breathing should be deep and relatively slow. Rapid shallow breathing may result in hyperventilation producing a decrease in placental blood flow and possibly maternal tetany. When the contraction has terminated, inhalation may be discontinued resulting in rapid loss of analgesia. There is no restriction on the duration of administration during labour since cumulation does not occur.

However the quality of analgesia is not impressive. It has been shown that 30% of mothers given Entonox derive no benefit and only 50% obtain satisfactory analgesia. Furthermore the prior administration of pethidine does not increase the effectiveness of Entonox analgesia.

An alternative method of administration of Entonox is by continuous delivery from a nasal catheter supplemented by face-mask inhalation during contractions. This results in improved analgesia.

Trichloroethylene

This has been used in obstetric practice since 1952. It is delivered in a concentration of either 0.5% or 0.35% in air from accurate vaporisers, e.g. the Tecota Mark 6.

Analgesia does not occur until trichloroethylene has been inhaled for 4 min. Since the uptake and distribution of this agent is much slower than that of nitrous oxide, adequate blood concentrations are maintained between contractions. The technique of inhalation is essentially similar to that of Entonox. The higher concentration may be inhaled for the first few contractions, and subsequently the lower concentration to maintain analgesia. Trichloroethylene is cumulative over a period of time and its use in labour is not permitted for periods exceeding 6 h. It should not be used with soda-lime. The Central Midwives Board has withdrawn approval of the use of trichloroethylene during labour.

The quality of analgesia produced is similar to that produced by Entonox.

Methoxyflurane

This agent has been approved by the Central Midwives Board since 1970. It is administered intermittently during labour by means of a Cardiff Inhaler which delivers a concentration of 0.35% methoxyflurane in air. Analgesic blood concentrations develop within a few minutes but the levels decrease slowly between contractions. There is no risk of renal damage following the use of methoxyflurane when the drug is used in this manner. It has been shown that 90% of mothers are satisfied with the analgesia produced, but 30% dislike the odour of the drug.

The use of trichloroethylene and methoxyflurane has declined over the past few years, being superseded by Entonox or extradural analgesia.

Extradural analgesia by catheter technique

This is the most effective method of producing pain relief for the first stage of labour; 80% of mothers report total freedom from pain, and of the remainder, 15% report considerable relief. By using different volumes and concentrations of local anaesthetic it is possible to block sensory but not motor fibres from the uterus during the first stage and then to extend the block as labour progresses to cover all segments between T10 and S5. However, some anaesthetists prefer to produce the latter type of block from the outset.

The aim in providing an extradural block is to achieve a high rate of success in pain relief without unduly altering the course of labour. Extradural analgesia has been shown not to prolong the length of labour although uterine contractions may be inhibited temporarily if a hypotensive episode occurs (vide infra) or on injection of the first dose of local anaesthetic (or even saline) or if given early in spontaneous labour. However, if inco-ordinate uterine contractions are present, institution of an extradural block results frequently in a more normal pattern of uterine contractions. In addition, extradural analgesia results in a more normal biochemical environment for both mother and fetus.

Although top-up doses of local anaesthetic may be given by midwives in some institutions, the anaesthetist must give the first dose of drug, following a test dose. The agent most commonly used is bupivacaine, which may be used in one of three concentrations for obstetric analgesia. A concentration of 0.5% provides good pain relief in volumes of 6–10 ml. However, with this strength there is appreciable motor block, which may make nursing more difficult and which relaxes the pelvic floor muscles of the mother, interfering with normal descent of the fetal head. Bupivacaine 0.375% in an initial volume of 10 ml with top-up injections of 8–10 ml is a suitable alternative. Pain relief may be inadequate from the first dose in a small number of patients. A degree of motor block develops following subsequent top-up injections. A concentration of 0.25% in the range of 8–10 ml for top-up injections provides good sensory loss without motor weakness but requires increments at approx. 60 min intervals compared with 90–120 min for the other concentrations of bupivacaine. A common practice is to use 0.5% initially to abolish pain completely if labour is in progress, or 0.375% before contractions are perceived as painful, and then to provide continuous analgesia with top-up injections of 0.25%.

The indications for extradural analgesia are shown in Table 31.2 and a list of absolute and relative contraindications in Table 31.3.

There are certain refinements of technique which are of particular importance in obstetrics.

Table 31.2   Indications for extradural analgesia

Pain and maternal request	Multiple pregnancy
Inco-ordinate uterine action	Breech presentation
Pre-eclampsia	Forceps delivery
Premature labour	Caesarian section
Cardiovascular disease	
Diabetes	

Table 31.3   Contraindications to extradural analgesia

Absolute	Relative
Local sepsis	Previous LSCS
Anatomical deformity	Abruptio placentae
Ongoing neurological disease	
Bleeding tendency	
Anticoagulant therapy	
Hypovolaemia	

Maternal hypotension

This should be avoided at all costs. Hypotension may be expected during institution of the block if the mother is allowed to lie supine.

An i.v. infusion is mandatory before a block is produced. Preloading with 1 litre of Hartmann's solution while the block is being performed decreases the incidence of hypotension from 15% to 1%. Once the block has been established, the mother should be nursed either in the lateral position or if supine, in a lateral tilted position. Aortocaval occlusion in the supine position is the rule rather than the exception during the last few weeks of pregnancy. Venous return is maintained usually via alternative collateral routes and maternal hypotension is rare (2–3%) as any reduction in cardiac output is offset by increased peripheral vasoconstriction. However, impaired reflex vasoconstriction, e.g. following an extradural block, may result in hypotension. Tilting the mother to one side with a 15° wedge alleviates aortocaval occlusion. It is found that some mothers can only lie on one side during labour in order to prevent hypotension.

If hypotension does not respond either to i.v. fluids or to posture, a vasopressor should be used. The drug of choice in obstetrics is ephedrine in intermittent 5 mg doses i.v. Vasopressors with no inotropic effect, e.g. methoxamine, decrease uterine blood flow.

Dural puncture

The incidence of this complication varies from 0.2% with very experienced anaesthetists to approx 2–3% in average practice, although rates up to 10% have been reported in units with a large teaching commitment. It is caused by puncture of the dura with the peridural Tuohy needle or by the extradural catheter. If the dura is punctured, the anaesthetist should institute a continuous extradural block in an adjacent lumbar interspace and ensure a good block. The mother should be well hydrated and not allowed to strain during labour or delivery. Elective forceps delivery is advisable. After delivery, attempts should be made to obviate the occurrence of a spinal headache. The following routine is suggested:

1. The extradural catheter is left in situ and 1.5 litre of Hartmann's solution infused into the extradural space over 36 h.

2. The mother is kept well hydrated.

3. The patient is kept in bed and encouraged to adopt the prone position, although sitting up is allowed.

4. When the catheter is removed, light normal activity is allowed. If headache develops, conservative measures in the form of bed rest and analgesics are prescribed.

If the symptoms persist for 6 days an autologous blood patch may be utilised. For this technique two clinicians are needed, one to identify the extradural space and the other to draw from the patient 20 ml of sterile venous blood which is injected into the extradural space. The success rate for this technique is 90–100%.

Bloody tap

Puncture of a dural vein may be produced by the extradural needle, but is caused more commonly by passage of an extradural catheter. The incidence varies from 2.8% in general anaesthetic practice to 8% in obstetric practice, this higher incidence being related to the larger extradural veins present at term. These veins engorge further during uterine contractions and so passage of a catheter should be attemped only during a contraction-free interval. The incidence of a bloody tap is reduced further if 10 ml of saline is injected into the extradural space before introduction of the catheter.

If blood issues from the needle before the catheter is inserted, an alternative lumbar interspace should be approached. If a catheter is introduced and blood flows down the catheter it should be withdrawn partially until flow stops. If, after careful aspiration, no further blood appears the procedure may continue. However, it is customary to proceed to an adjacent lumbar interspace.

Inadequacy of analgesia

This may occur in up to 20% of patients and is manifest usually as either an unblocked segment or as a unilateral block. An unblocked segment usually presents as pain in the groin, worse during contractions. This may be relieved by injecting 3 to 4 ml of local anaesthetic through the catheter with the patient lying on the painful side. It may be advisable to use a stronger concentration of local anaesthetic for this top-up injection. If this fails to relieve the pain then subcutaneous infiltration in the painful area should be attempted.

If a unilateral block develops (incidence: 8–20% of blocks), the length of catheter in the extradural space should be shortened to no more than 1–2 cm. If a top-up injection with the patient lying on the painful side fails to relieve pain, a further attempt to provide good analgesia can be made by resiting the extradural catheter in an adjacent lumbar interspace.

Another cause of inadequate analgesia is passage of the catheter into the paravertebral space usually because an excessive length of catheter is used within the extradural space. Persistent backache results from occipitoposterior position of the fetus and may usually be relieved by a top-up injection with a stronger concentration of local anaesthetic. Suprapubic pain usually results from a full bladder and catheterisation may be necessary.

There are three simple rules for achieving a high success rate in using extradural catheters:

1. Make sure the patient adopts the best position possible before attempting a block.

2. 'Open' up the extradural space with an injection of saline before passing a catheter.

3. Never pass more than 2 cm of catheter into the extradural space.

The postpartum incidence of headache, backache or disturbances of micturition are no different after extradural analgesia than that experienced by mothers receiving other methods of pain relief. Nonobstetric complications of extradural blocks are discussed elsewhere but it is important to remember that neurological sequelae, e.g. foot-drop, can occur because of faulty positioning of the mother in the lithotomy position.

Other methods of pain relief

1. Extradural injection of opioids, including morphine, pethidine and fentanyl has been used for pain relief during and after delivery. There is no

evidence that there is any benefit from their use, which is therefore not recommended at the present time.

2. Intrathecal opioids have been tried in a limited number of patients but the same reservation concerning the nursing and monitoring of these patients applies as with the use of extradural opioids. The incidence of postspinal headache in obstetric patients is high (approx. 20%) despite the use of 25 G needles.

3. Transcutaneous nerve stimulation does not produce adequate analgesia and has not gained widespread acceptance.

ANALGESIA FOR VAGINAL DELIVERY

There are three techniques which abolish pain both from uterine contractions and also from the lower birth canal, i.e. total analgesia, notably lumbar extradural, caudal and subarachnoid spinal nerve block (SAB). Analgesia of the lower birth canal may be achieved by pudendal nerve block and the pain of uterine contractions by paracervical nerve block.

Extradural and SAB

If a lumbar extradural block is used during labour, analgesia extends usually to include all the sacral segments and some procedures (e.g. forceps delivery)

may be accomplished painlessly. If a forceps delivery is indicated when an extradural catheter is not in situ, then a 'one-shot' extradural technique or an SAB may be used. To perform a 'one-shot' extradural, the space is entered and a predetermined dose of local anaesthetic injected (after a test dose and careful aspiration). The agent most commonly used is 0.5% bupivacaine plain 10–15 ml. The major drawback is the length of time to onset of analgesia and the unpredictability of analgesia.

In contrast, spinal anaesthesia does not have these drawbacks. A dose of 1.0–1.2 ml of hyperbaric cinchocaine 0.5% provides good analgesia for vaginal delivery and also abolishes the pain of uterine contractions.

Emergency general anaesthesia for vaginal delivery should not be necessary.

Caudal analgesia

Although analgesia by the caudal route preceded that by the lumbar extradural route, the technique has not enjoyed consistent popularity because of several disadvantages. The greatest problem is a 10% failure rate in routine obstetric practice.

The ideal anatomy of the sacrum is shown in Figure 31.1. Unfortunately, many variations occur (Fig. 31.2) which are largely responsible for this high failure rate.

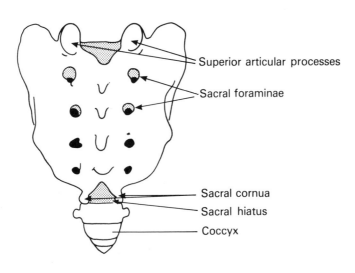

Fig. 31.1 Ideal anatomy of the sacrum.

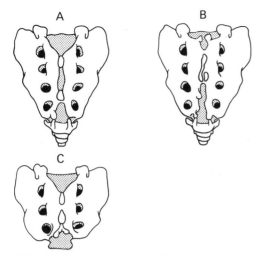

Fig. 31.2 Common variations in sacral anatomy.

Technique

The patient may be placed in one of two positions: (a) prone — suitably supported at the pelvis by pillows to flex the hips; or (b) lateral — as for lumbar block.

A wide area of skin is cleaned over the sacrum, coccyx and buttocks, protecting the sensitive perianal skin with a swab. The sacral cornua are palpated as two bony prominences which lie on each side of the sacral hiatus. A small intradermal weal of local anaesthetic is raised over the sacral hiatus and a 21 G needle is inserted through skin at an angle of approx. 70–80°, with the bevel facing anteriorly. A small click is felt as the needle passes through the sacrococcygeal membrane covering the sacral hiatus. At this point, the needle is depressed towards the natal cleft, making an angle of 10–20° to skin (Fig. 31.3) and gently advanced up the caudal canal a distance of not more than 2 cm. Aspiration for blood or cerebrospinal fluid is made and, if negative, a test dose of local anaesthetic injected. Injection should be easy and meet no resistance. After 5 min a dose of approx. 20 ml of 0.25% bupivacaine plain is injected to provide pain relief for the first stage of labour. A continuous caudal block may be produced using a Tuohy needle through which a catheter is inserted into the caudal canal (as for lumbar extradural techniques). The use of a stiff catheter or one containing a wire stilette may enable the catheter to pass as far as L5 but this increases the risk of either venous or dural puncture and is best avoided. A filter is attached to the end of the catheter and injections made as outlined previously. Top-up doses of 15–17 ml are required.

Indications and contraindications

These are similar to those for lumbar extradural block.

Complications. 1. Maternal hypotension — the incidence is the same as for the lumbar approach to the extradural space.

2. Dural puncture — the incidence is also similar to that following a lumbar approach. It should be remembered that the dural sac usually ends opposite the middle of S2 at the level of the posterior inferior iliac spines, but it may end as high as S1 or even as low as S3. In addition the upper level of the sacral hiatus is variable so care must be exercised. On no

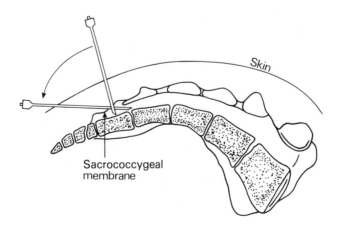

Fig. 31.3 Institution of a caudal block.

account must a needle be advanced more than 2 cm into the caudal canal.

3. Venous puncture — inadvertent puncture of a vein in the sacral venous extradural plexus occurs in 0.6% of patients, a much smaller incidence than that following lumbar approach.

4. Intraosseous injection — incidence 0.6%. A small amount of marrow may be aspirated. There is no resistance to injection and local anaesthetic is rapidly absorbed, leading to toxic reactions.

5. Toxic reactions — these may occur in both the mother and fetus as a result of the large volumes of local anaesthetic required to provide adequate pain relief, especially when a continuous technique is used.

Disadvantages. Failure of block — this is the most important disadvantage and may result from:

1. Anatomical variation of the sacrum. Various anomalies are shown in Figure 31.2. These range from a sacral hiatus that may be almost closed, asymmetrical or widely open, to a complete sacral spina bifida, which occurs in 0.3% of women. The volume of the sacral canal varies enormously, from 12–65 ml, depending on the A–P depth and lateral width of the canal. Patency and size of the sacral foraminae vary widely, and determine the volume of local anaesthetic required to produce a good block since the solution leaks out of these orifices.

2. Misplacement of needle. The commonest error is to place the needle superficial to the sacral hiatus, i.e. subcutaneously. The needle tip may be palpated in this position and a subcutaneous weal is obvious when a test dose is injected. The needle may be placed under the periosteum of the sacrum in which case needle placement is painful for the patient and there is resistance to injection. Lastly, the needle may be forced anteriorly between the sacrum and coccyx either into the rectum or into the presenting part of the fetus. Injection of local anaesthetic into the head of the fetus caused death in two of the four cases reported in the literature.

3. Infection. Although not documented, the use of the caudal route for a continuous block theoretically carries a high risk of infection because of proximity to skin which may be soiled by urine or faeces.

In summary, it is probably preferable to restrict the caudal technique to a single injection for analgesia during the second stage of labour. It should be used only in those patients in whom technical difficulties

are not anticipated. It is best avoided if the presenting part of the fetus has descended into the vagina. The indications for its use in such conditions are therefore few and analgesia may be produced preferably by SAB which provides more rapid and predictable analgesia. However, caudal analgesia may be considered in patients with a localised septic lesion in the lumbar region or in a patient who has a deformity of the lumbar spine.

Pudendal nerve block

Bilateral pudendal nerve block is used widely by obstetricians in the second stage of labour to provide perineal analgesia for low outlet forceps delivery. The pudendal nerve arises from the ventral roots of S 2,3 and 4, leaving the pelvis through the lower part of the greater sciatic foramen. It passes behind the spine of the ischium, lying posterior to the sacrospinous ligament, to re-enter the pelvis through the lesser sciatic foramen. It supplies the principal sensory nerves to the perineum, vulva and the lower two-thirds of the vagina.

Technique

The pudendal nerve may be blocked by either a transvaginal or transperineal approach.

Transvaginal (Fig. 31.4). This is the commonest approach unless the presenting part of the fetus is too low to permit its use.

The patient is placed in the lithotomy position, and after suitable antiseptic precautions, the operator's second and third fingers are introduced into the vagina to palpate the ischial spine. A 12.5 cm needle (usually of the guarded type) is passed along the line of the palpating fingers through the vaginal wall behind the ischial spine. The needle should be felt to pass into the tough sacrospinous ligament and as it passes through, loss of resistance is appreciated. The needle is steadied at this point, approx. 1.2–1.5 cm from the vaginal mucosa, and aspirated carefully for blood. The pudendal vessels are in close proximity to the nerve at this point, and puncture is common. If aspiration is negative, 10 ml of local anaesthetic solution are injected. The procedure is repeated on the other side. It is common practice to infiltrate in the line of an episiotomy.

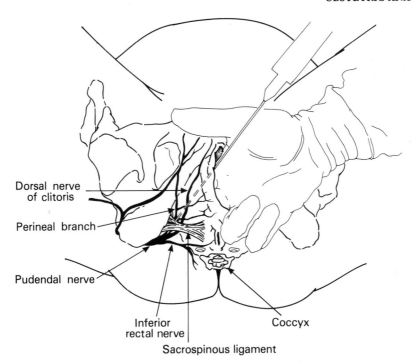

Dorsal nerve of clitoris

Perineal branch

Pudendal nerve

Inferior rectal nerve

Coccyx

Sacrospinous ligament

Fig. 31.4 Transvaginal pudendal nerve block.

Transperineal. This is used if the transvaginal route is contraindicated. With the patient in the lithotomy position, a skin weal is raised at a point midway between the anus and the ischial tuberosity. An unguarded needle is then advanced to the ischial spine which is palpated by a finger in the vagina. The needle is advanced until its point lies just behind the spine and after careful aspiration for blood, 10 ml of local anaesthetic solution are injected. The procedure is repeated on the other side.

It should be remembered that the sensory nerve supply to the vulva is derived from the ilio-inguinal nerve anteriorly and from the perineal branch of the posterior cutaneous nerve of the thigh posteriorly and these nerves may not be blocked with these techniques. Pudendal nerve block does not abolish the pain of uterine contractions and so delivery using this technique should be accompanied by the use of Entonox. One study has demonstrated a 50% failure rate of bilateral pudendal nerve block, and so it may be preferable to perform local infiltration for low outlet forceps delivery and use SAB or extradural anaesthesia for the more difficult forceps deliveries. However, the only contraindication to the technique

is patient sensitivity to local anaesthetics and the main complication, apart from failure, is toxicity resulting from i.v. injection and overdosage of local anaesthetic solution.

Paracervical nerve block

This block is effective in provision of analgesia during the first stage of labour, but its use has largely been abandoned because of the associated complications. The most important is a reduction in uteroplacental blood flow leading to fetal bradycardia, acidosis and occasional intrauterine death. These result from a direct vasoconstrictive effect of local anaesthetics on uterine arteries.

However, the block is practised frequently for termination of pregnancy on a day-care basis.

ANAESTHESIA FOR CAESARIAN SECTION

Anaesthesia for Caesarian section is either an elective, or more commonly an emergency procedure. Anaesthesia is identical in both instances. Until recently, general anaesthesia was the rule for Caesarian section but in many centres, regional block is displacing general anaesthesia as the preferred technique.

The aim of anaesthesia for Caesarian section is that it should be safe for both mother and fetus. The problems facing the anaesthetist include prevention of acid aspiration (the commonest cause of maternal death associated with anaesthesia) prevention of maternal hypotension and maintenance of placental blood flow.

More than 50% of pregnant patients at term have gastric contents with a volume exceeding 40 ml and in 50% of these patients the pH is less than 2.5. The development of acid aspiration syndrome in humans is said to require aspiration of only 25 ml of fluid of pH less than 2.5.

In order to neutralise gastric content, antacids are normally prescribed. The commonest regimen is mist. magnesium trisilicate given to all mothers in labour at 2-hrly intervals with an additional dose being given prior to surgery. However, doubt has been cast on the efficacy of this regimen as it has not been shown to decrease maternal mortality from aspiration of gastric contents.

It has been postulated recently that layering of gastric contents may occur in pregnant women at term, and that unless the patient is turned through 360° to mix stomach contents adequately, gastric acid material may still be aspirated on regurgitation. It has also been shown that aspiration of particulate antacids may also cause a syndrome identical to that of acid aspiration syndrome (or Mendelson's syndrome).

A nonparticulate antacid regimen in the form of 30 ml of 0.3 M sodium citrate is effective when given not more than 50 min before induction of anaesthesia in raising the pH of gastric contents above 2.5. In addition aspiration of sodium citrate into the lungs of dogs produces only minimal tissue changes.

The major disadvantage to the use of antacids is the associated increase in volume of gastric contents. The H_2-receptor blockers, which inhibit basal and nocturnal acid secretion by the stomach, may have a role in obstetric practice in the future. Preliminary studies have shown that cimetidine given regularly during labour has an effective action in 96% of patients in raising gastric pH above 2.5. Ranitidine, a newer, longer acting H_2 receptor-blocker with less side effects than cimetidine, has been evaluated prior to Caesarian section and shown to be equally effective. It must be remembered however that these drugs do not produce their effect immediately. Consequently, if anaesthesia is required within 2 h of administration of cimetidine, it is still necessary to administer antacids. At present the safety of H_2-receptor blockers in labour has not been established fully.

Gastric emptying is delayed in pregnancy and during labour, and no woman in labour should receive solid food. The tone of the lower oesophageal sphincter is also reduced during pregnancy, probably as a result of hormonal changes, rendering regurgitation more likely (as evidenced by heartburn).

To avoid maternal hypotension, every mother requiring anaesthesia should be transported in the lateral position to the operating theatre. During surgery, a 15° tilt is essential to prevent aortocaval occlusion and this may be achieved either by tilting the table or by placing a wedge under the patient's buttocks and pelvis. Whether the tilt is to the right or to the left probably makes no difference in an uncomplicated elective section, but if there is evidence of fetal distress there are good theoretical reasons for tilting to the left.

Adequate oxygenation of the fetus must be assured and it has been shown that ventilating the mother's lungs with an inspired O_2 concentration of 60% produces optimal fetal oxygenation. Hyperventilation should be avoided as a pregnant mother at term has an arterial $P\text{CO}_2$ of 4.0 kPa and further reduction in Pa_{CO_2} results in a metabolic and respiratory acidosis in the fetus. This results from direct vasoconstriction of uterine blood vessels. In addition, vigorous hyperventilation may cause a reduction in maternal cardiac output.

Awareness during anaesthesia for Caesarian section is a significant risk when high inspired oxygen concentrations are used. However, awareness may be prevented by the use of inhalational supplements, the most common being 0.5% halothane. This has been shown not to cause any increase in blood loss during Caesarian section despite the uterine relaxant properties of this agent.

Placental transfer of anaesthetic drugs is also an important consideration in anaesthesia for Caesarian section. The placenta is rarely an absolute barrier to the passage of drugs. Most i.v., gaseous and inhalational anaesthetics are lipid soluble and cross the placental barrier readily by simple diffusion. Barbiturates are found in fetal blood a few seconds after administration to the mother, but unless given in very high doses, produce no demonstrable depressant effect on the neonate as judged by Apgar scores. Most induction agents have been studied and found suitable with the exception of Althesin which produces significantly depressed infants. Non-depolarising muscle relaxants are highly ionised in maternal blood and so one would not expect passage across the placenta. However using sensitive assays it has been shown that placental transfer does occur, albeit in small nonparalysing amounts. Small amounts of suxamethonium also cross the placenta, but unless the fetus has atypical pseudocholin-esterase, when prolonged apnoea may ensue, it does not produce clinical symptoms.

Technique of general anaesthesia

The presence of a skilled assistant for the anaesthetist is *mandatory*.

On arrival in the anaesthetic room, the patient is turned from the lateral position to supine with a 15° lateral tilt. Arterial pressure and heart rate are measured and the availability of cross-matched blood is confirmed. An i.v. infusion is established and preoxygenation with 100% oxygen is undertaken using a face mask. A range of cuffed endotracheal tubes is available, with introducers. A crash induction routine is then followed. A sleep dose of thiopentone is injected followed by a paralysing dose of suxamethonium. At the point of loss of consciousness cricoid pressure (see Chapter 30 and Fig. 30.1) is applied and endotracheal intubation performed following the onset of muscle paralysis.

After securing the tube, the lungs are ventilated artificially with 40% nitrous oxide and 0.5% halo-thane in oxygen. Paralysis is maintained with a nondepolarising relaxant when the effects of suxamethonium have terminated. On delivery of the baby, a bolus dose of 5–10 i.u. of syntocinon is injected i.v. and after clamping of the cord an opioid analgesic drug is given i.v. to the mother. Ventilation continues with 70% nitrous oxide in oxygen. At the end of the operation, residual neuromuscular block is antagonised with atropine and neostigmine.

Syntocinon is preferred to ergometrine for contraction of the uterus as it produces a small and transient decrease in arterial pressure followed by an increase. The central venous pressure remains elevated slightly for less than 30 min and there is no increase in the incidence of postoperative nausea and vomiting. The use of ergometrine, however, is associated with unacceptably high increases in arterial pressure, persistent elevation of the CVP for up to 60 min and an increased incidence of nausea and vomiting. There is no increased blood loss associated with the use of Syntocinon. If the bolus dose fails to produce adequate contraction, an infusion of Syntocinon may be given over 4 h.

Much has been written on the subject of the ideal induction to delivery (I–D) time. Provided aortocaval occlusion is avoided, maternal $F_{I_{O_2}}$ is of the order of 0.6 and there are no untoward complications, the I–D interval may be as long as 30 min without deterioration in neonatal outcome.

Local anaesthetic techniques

An alternative technique to general anaesthesia is to use a regional block, normally either a lumbar extradural block or SAB. These techniques may be used for elective Caesarian section, or, in the case of lumbar extradural, for emergency surgery if the block is already established. To ensure good conditions for surgery, the block must be high enough to obtund peritoneal sensation (i.e. to the level of T6) and low enough to block sensation from uterine contraction (i.e. at least S1). In addition the surgeon must be aware that he is operating on an awake patient and utilise rapid, gentle, and skilful surgery.

Following insertion of an extradural catheter, 10–12 ml of 0.5% bupivacaine plain are injected, with the patient in a sitting position (to block the sacral segments). After several minutes the patient is placed supine (with a wedge), and 15 min later the height of the block is assessed. Additional bupivacaine 0.5% is injected through the extradural catheter in a dose of 1.5 ml for each unblocked segment (up to a level of approx. T6). During these additional injections, the patient should be in a lateral position, the dependent side possessing the greater number of unblocked segments.

When an adequate level of sensory analgesia is obtained, surgery may commence. The patient should breathe oxygen-enriched air (e.g. using an MC mask). Nausea and vomiting may occur, normally related to hypotension (which should not be allowed to persist), handling of viscera (which can be minimised by the surgeon), or the use of ergometrine.

If an extradural has been used for analgesia during labour, the level of block may be extended by using 1.5 ml of 0.5% bupivacaine for each additional segment which requires blockade.

Spinal anaesthesia (SAB) is becoming more popular in obstetric practice. Its main advantage over extradural anaesthesia is speed of onset. There is also reduced exposure of the fetus to local anaesthetic since the total dose used is much smaller. The technique is simple to perform and is more reliable in producing a good block. However, these advantages have to be weighed against the incidence of spinal headache (up to 20% despite use of a 25 G needle) and the greater incidence of maternal hypotension.

A regional technique for Caesarian section minimises the hazards of regurgitation and aspiration in the mother. It also decreases operative blood loss and produces an infant with no respiratory depression. It allows the participation of the mother and, in more progressive units, of the father in the birth of their child.

Failed endotracheal intubation

Intubation of the oesophagus instead of the trachea plays a large part in maternal mortality associated with anaesthesia. Tracheal intubation in a pregnant patient may be difficult and every obstetric theatre should have a 'failed intubation' routine.

The following is suggested:

1. Maintain cricoid pressure.
2. Place the patient head down in the left lateral position.
3. Maintain oxygenation with 100% oxygen, by IPPV if the action of suxamethonium has not terminated.

4. Allow the patient to awaken, and summon help.

With further assistance, the alternatives will include:

5. Reattempt general anaesthesia with additional equipment, e.g. longer-bladed laryngoscope, bougies, etc.
6. Spinal anaesthesia.
7. Extradural anaesthesia if a catheter is in situ.
8. Inhalational anaesthesia.

This routine is not suitable when it is essential to proceed to surgery as rapidly as possible (e.g. fetal distress or maternal haemorrhage). In these circumstances, anaesthesia is probably best maintained as follows:

1. Maintain cricoid pressure.
2. Place the patient head down.
3. Maintain oxygenation using 40% oxygen in nitrous oxide and add a volatile anaesthetic agent.
4. Maintain anaesthesia with 60% N_2O in oxygen and a volatile agent which may be halothane, enflurane, ether or cyclopropane. The inexperienced anaesthetist is recommended to use the agent with which he/she is most familiar.

ANAESTHESIA IN SPECIAL CIRCUMSTANCES

The commonest condition requiring the services of an anaesthetist immediately postpartum is that of a retained placenta. Blood loss is usually minimised with the routine use of oxytocic drugs at delivery. An i.v. infusion should be in progress. Blood loss should be estimated and if minimal, either a 'one-shot' extradural block or spinal anaesthesia may be used. If blood loss is severe, the patient should be resuscitated adequately and general anaesthesia considered, the conduct of the anaesthesia being the same as for Caesarian section.

FURTHER READING

Bromage P R 1978 Epidural analgesia. W. B. Saunders, Philadelphia
Crawford J S 1978 Principles and practice of obstetric anaesthesia, 4th edn. Blackwell Scientific Publications, Oxford
Moir D D 1980 Obstetric anaesthesia and analgesia, 2nd edn. Bailliere Tindall, London

32

Paediatric anaesthesia and intensive care

Major differences in anatomy and physiology in the small infant have important consequences on many aspects of anaesthesia. These differences also cause different patterns of disease in small infants and children seen in the intensive care unit, in comparison with adult patients.

The physical disparity between the adult and child diminishes at 10–12 yr of age although major psychological differences continue through adolescence.

PHYSIOLOGY IN THE NEONATE

Respiration

At birth the alveoli are thick-walled and number only approx. 10% of the adult total. Lung growth continues by alveolar multiplication until the age of 6–8 yr. The airways remain relatively narrow up to this age, resulting in high airway resistance and low compliance, and leading to a high incidence of airway disease in the young.

Ventilation is almost entirely diaphragmatic with soft horizontal ribs contributing little to gas movement in comparison with the bucket handle movement in the adult.

The high airway resistance and low compliance result in a short time constant. As a result, the respiratory rate is rapid (approx. 32 breath/min). The metabolic cost of respiration is higher in the infant and may reach 15% of total oxygen consumption (Table 31.1).

The metabolic rate in infants is almost twice that of the adult and consequently alveolar minute ventilation is also greater, whilst FRC is a similar fraction of lung volume as that in the adult. Consequently, inhalational induction of anaesthesia

Table 32.1 Lung mechanics of the neonate compared with the adult

	Neonate	Adult
Compliance (ml/cmH$_2$O)	5	100
Resistance (cmH$_2$O/litre/s)	30	2
Time constant (s)	0.5	1.3
Respiratory rate (breath/min)	32	15

and awakening at the termination of anaesthesia are more rapid than in the adult. Similarly hypoxia occurs much more rapidly in a child.

The poor elastic qualities of the infant lung cause the closing volume (CV) to be greater than FRC until the age of 6–8 yr: thus airway closure occurs during tidal ventilation, leading to an increase in the alveolar-arterial oxygen pressure difference (A-aPO$_2$) and a normal Pa$_{O_2}$ in the newborn of approx. 9–9.5 kPa (70 mmHg).

Physiological dead space is approx 30% of tidal volume (V_D/V_T = 0.3) as in the adult but the absolute volume is small so that any increase caused by apparatus dead space has a disproportionately greater effect on a small child (Table 32.2). During anaesthesia, dead space should be kept to a minimum and the resistance of breathing apparatus should be kept low. Secretions resulting either from cholinergic activity or upper respiratory infection may cause respiratory difficulty.

Table 32.2 Respiratory variables in the neonate

Tidal volume (V_T)	7 ml/kg
Dead space (V_D)	V_T × 0.3 ml
Respiratory rate	Neonate 32 breath/min Age 1–13 (24 — age/2) breath/min

Cardiovascular system

Following the dramatic change from fetal to adult circulation at birth, the child establishes a high cardiac output (commensurate with the high metabolic value) of approx. 200 ml/kg/min, which is 2–3 times the adult value. The small ventricles result in poor ventricular compliance; thus increased cardiac output is produced by an increase in heart rate. Babies tolerate heart rates of up to 200 beat/min without evidence of cardiac failure (Table 32.3).

Table 32.3 Variation of heart rate with age

Age	Mean value	Normal range
Neonate	140	100–180
1 yr	120	80–150
2 yr	110	80–130
6 yr	100	70–120
12 yr	80	60–100

Bradycardia may occur readily in the presence of vagal stimulation or hypoxia and treatment with atropine or oxygen is required rapidly. Arrhythmias are uncommon in the absence of cardiac disease, and cardiac arrest usually occurs in asystole rather than ventricular fibrillation.

Systemic arterial pressure is low at birth (approx. 80/50 mmHg) because of the low systemic vascular resistance resulting from the large proportion of vessel-rich tissues in the child. The pressure increases within the first month to approx. 90/60 mmHg and reaches adult levels of 120/70 mmHg at approx. 16 yr of age.

Monitoring of the cardiovascular system

The cardiovascular system must always be monitored carefully in babies. Arterial pressure may be measured with a sphygmomanometer cuff or alternatively by an ultrasonic detector or an automatic oscillotonometer. Intra-arterial monitoring of arterial pressure is feasible in the neonate by percutaneous arterial catheterisation with a 22 G cannula. This invasive technique should only be utilised when regular blood gas estimations are required since the complication rate of arterial cannulation is significantly higher in children than in adults. Intermittent flushing has been shown to cause retrograde flow from the radial artery to the carotid artery with the risk of cerebral embolisation.

Continuous flushing should therefore be used and the volume of fluid administered measured carefully. Central venous pressure (CVP) monitoring is of value in the treatment of fluid imbalance and haemorrhage; the internal jugular or subclavian veins are suitable for the introduction of CVP catheters.

Blood volume

Variations of up to ± 20% of blood volume occur at birth depending on the stage at which the cord is clamped. The average blood volume at birth is 90 ml/kg. This decreases in the infant and young child to 80 ml/kg and attains the adult level of 75 ml/kg at the age of 6–8 yr. Blood losses of greater than 10% of blood volume should be replaced with blood.

Haemoglobin

At birth, 75–80% of haemoglobin is fetal haemoglobin (HbF). A decrease in blood volume and HbF occurs before adult haemoglobin (HbA) haemopoiesis is fully established at 6 months. HbF has a greater affinity for oxygen than HbA because of a lower content of 2,3-diphosphoglycerate (2,3-DPG) and the dissociation curve is shifted to the left (Fig. 32.1). The greater affinity of HbF for oxygen is overcome in the tissues of the fetus because of low tissue Po_2 and a metabolic acidosis; the acidosis, which persists into infancy (and the high CO_2 output as a result of the high metabolic rate) aid oxygen delivery to the tissues. Respiratory alkalosis caused by hyperventilation reduces oxygen availability and should be avoided both in the operating theatre and intensive care unit.

Blood for transfusion should be warmed and filtered. If required in small volumes, it may be given by syringe through a tap in the i.v. line. This system also allows rapid transfusion. In other cases, a burette type of infusion set should be used to minimise the risk of accidental overtransfusion and to permit careful monitoring of the volumes of blood administered.

Monitoring

As a result of the small blood volume of the neonate, haemorrhage should be monitored carefully. Swabs should be weighed, and all suction losses collected in

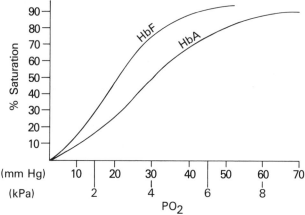

Fig. 32.1 Effects of HbF on oxygen dissociation curve.

a graduated container. Blood loss may also be measured by washing swabs and drapes in a fixed volume of fluid and measuring the haemoglobin content of the fluid.

Renal function and fluid balance

Body fluids constitute a greater proportion of body weight in the infant, particularly the premature infant, than the adult (Table 32.4).

Table 32.4 Distribution of water as percentage of body weight

Compartment	Premature	Neonate	Infant	Adult
E.c.f.	50	35	30	20
I.c.f.	30	40	40	40
Plasma	5	5	5	5
Total	85	80	75	65

The proportion of total body water present as extracellular fluid (e.c.f.) exceeds that of intracellular fluid (i.c.f.). This ratio gradually reverses with increasing age. Plasma volume remains constant, at approx. 5% body weight, throughout life.

The turnover of fluid is much greater in infants (15% total body water per day) than in adults. Thus, interruption in fluid intake in the infant results rapidly in dehydration.

The kidneys are immature at birth, both glomerular filtration and tubular reabsorption being reduced until the age of 6–8 months; as a result, there is inability to handle excessive water loads, and over-transfusion may lead to oedema and cardiac failure. There is also diminished ability to handle sodium

loads, which may occur with administration of excess sodium (e.g. sodium bicarbonate solutions.)

Immature renal function may lead to cumulation and toxicity of drugs excreted by the kidneys (e.g. digoxin and penicillin). Reduced doses or increased dosage intervals may be required in the neonate.

Fluid therapy

Normal maintenance requirements of fluid increase over the first few days of life (Table 32.5 and 32.6) and thereafter reduce more slowly.

Table 32.5 Fluid requirements in the first week of life

Day	Rate
1	0
2, 3	50 ml/kg/day
4, 5	75 ml/kg/day
6	100 ml/kg/day
7	120 ml/kg/day

Table 32.6 Maintenance fluid requirements

Weight	Rate
Up to 10 kg	100 ml/kg/day
10 to 20 kg	1000 ml + 50 × [wt (kg) − 10] ml/kg/day
20 to 30 kg	1500 ml + 25 × [wt (kg) − 20] ml/kg/day

Suitable solutions are $\frac{1}{4}$ strength saline for the neonate and infant up to 1 yr, thereafter $\frac{1}{2}$ strength saline or $\frac{1}{2}$ strength Ringer lactate. Because of the high metabolic rate, all fluids should contain at least 5% dextrose to avoid hypoglycaemia.

Clinical examination of skin turgor, tension of

fontanelles, arterial pressure and venous filling may aid the estimation of hydration, but electrolyte and haemoglobin concentrations and haematocrit, urine volumes and plasma and urine osmolalities should be monitored where problems of fluid balance exist (Table 32.7).

During surgery, fluid administration should be increased by 10–20%; intake should also be increased by 10% in babies nursed under radiant heaters because of increased insensible loss, and in babies with pyrexia. Plasma proteins may require replacement (either as plasma or plasma protein fraction) in severe dehydration.

Calculation of replacement fluids, as opposed to maintenance fluids, should also allow for additional losses of water, protein, and electrolytes which may occur with vomiting or diarrhoea. An i.v. infusion should be established for all but the briefest of procedures, to permit correction of preoperative dehydration and hypoglycaemia, to cover fluid requirements in the immediate postoperative period, and for administration of drugs.

Small doses of drugs should be given using either a 1 or 2 ml syringe or by dilution; overdilution should be avoided since excessive fluid administration may result. The drug and dilution should be labelled clearly on all syringes.

Intravenous fluids should be administered using a burette type of infusion set which (in the small infant) should deliver 60 drops per ml (Fig. 32.2), thus allowing the rate to be controlled down to very small volumes. Drip controllers of either mechanical or electrical type assist in the administration of small volumes (Fig. 32.3).

Temperature regulation and maintenance

The neonate has a surface area to volume ratio 2.5 times greater than the adult, and thus a greater area

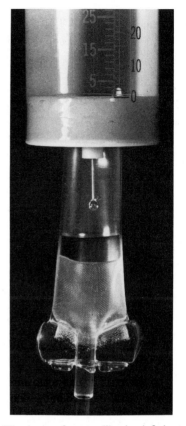

Fig. 32.2 Microburette for controlling i.v. infusion.

for heat loss. Heat is lost by conduction, by convection, and by evaporation from the skin and the respiratory tract. However, 70% of heat loss occurs by radiation to nearby surfaces e.g. the walls of an incubator.

In a thermoneutral environment, heat loss and energy expenditure are minimal. The temperature of such an environment is 34°C for the premature, 32°C for the neonate and 28°C for the adult. It is important therefore to raise the environmental

Table 32.7 Effects of dehydration in the young infant

	Mild	Moderate	Severe
Percentage loss of body weight	5%	10%	15%
Clinical signs	Dry skin & mucous membranes	Mottled cold periphery Loss of skin elasticity Depressed eyeballs & fontanelles Oliguria + +	Shocked Moribund Unresponsive to pain
Replacement	50 ml/kg	100 ml/kg	150 ml/kg

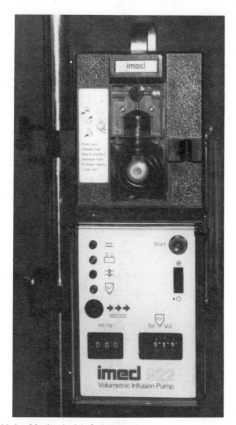

Fig. 32.3 Mechanical infusion pump.

temperature to reduce heat loss in the very young. Infants of less than three months old do not shiver to generate heat if exposed to cold, but depend on nonshivering thermogenesis. This is achieved by increasing metabolism of brown fat which is present in the neck and upper thoracic area, and surrounds the great vessels. This metabolism is controlled by the sympathetic nervous system. As with the muscular activity of shivering, the increase in metabolism causes an increase in oxygen consumption which may stress the immature respiratory system and may even induce respiratory failure. The control of brown fat metabolism is compromised by general anaesthesia, and so it is important to maintain body temperature by other means. A decrease in temperature may lead to respiratory depression, reduced cardiac output, prolongation of the action of drugs (especially the muscle relaxants) and lead to an increased danger of hypoventilation, regurgitation and aspiration in the postoperative period.

At birth, subcutaneous fat is minimal (almost absent in the premature) and so natural insulation is poor. Heat loss may be reduced during surgery by wrapping the limbs in orthopaedic wool or padding, or by using a space blanket or silver swaddler. The child should be placed on a heating blanket; water or heated air is preferable to an electric blanket to avoid the danger of electric shock, hot spots and interference with monitoring equipment. Overhead radiant heaters may be used (as in modern intensive care incubators) prior to surgery, but are inconvenient for the surgeon during surgery. Humidification and warming of inspired gases reduce heat losses from evaporation.

Malignant hyperpyrexia is extremely rare under 3 yr of age, although it has been reported in a child of 5 months.

Monitoring

Temperature should be monitored, even during the shortest procedure. An axillary probe is normally adequate. For longer surgery and in the intensive care area, core temperature should be monitored using a rectal, nasopharyngeal or oesophageal probe. The external auditory meatus should not be used in children because of the danger of damage to the tympanic membrane. If heating apparatus is in use, the temperature of the skin adjacent to the heating apparatus should be monitored closely and gradients of more than 10°C must be avoided at all temperatures to prevent burning. The core-skin temperature gradient is a useful monitor of cardiac output in the intensive care area. Decreases in cardiac output increase the gradient above the normal 3–4°C.

PHARMACOLOGY IN THE NEONATE

Central nervous system

At birth, the neurones are complete, but myelination is incomplete. In spite of this, the majority of body fat is contained within the central nervous system. Thus lipid soluble drugs (e.g. anaesthetics) reach high levels in the central nervous system more rapidly than in the adult. The blood-brain barrier is more permeable in the newborn period, allowing the passage of drugs (including barbiturates and opioids) which should therefore be given with caution and in small doses. Antibiotics cross more readily, which is of advantage in the treatment of meningitis, but bilirubin also crosses the blood-brain barrier leading to brain damage (kernicterus). The immaturity of the central nervous system (associated with the high metabolic rate) may be responsible for the increase in the minimum alveolar concentration of the inhalational anaesthetic agents in young children (Table 32.8).

Table 32.8 Minimum alveolar concentration of anaesthetic agents

Age	Halothane	Enflurane
0–3 yr	1.08	2.0
3–10 yr	0.9	1.9
Adult	0.76	1.7

Liver

The liver is partly immature at birth but rapidly becomes the centre of protein production and drug detoxification. In the neonate, there is a quantitative and qualitative difference in the plasma proteins with a reduction in plasma albumin. There is therefore less protein binding in the neonate, allowing more drug to remain active. Some drugs (e.g. diazepam and vitamin K) may displace bilirubin from protein and increase the likelihood of kernicterus in the neonate.

The enzymes responsible for glucuronidation are immature; as a consequence the opioids (and chloramphenicol) are metabolised slowly, with consequent increase in toxicity.

The immaturity of the liver microsomal enzymes may be responsible for the almost total absence of halothane-related hepatic damage in patients under 10 yr of age. By the age of 1–2 yr, the liver is double in volume relative to body weight compared with adults. This may result in the local anaesthetics being safer in youth than in later years.

Specific drugs in relationship to paediatric anaesthesia

Inhalational agents

The greater alveolar ventilation in relation to FRC, and the preponderance of vessel rich tissues, lead to more rapid increases in alveolar and brain concentrations of inhalational anaesthetics than in the adult. Induction is therefore more rapid, as is excretion of the agent at the termination of anaesthesia. The rapid increase in levels of depressant agents (e.g. halothane or enflurane) may lead to dramatic decreases in arterial pressure and cardiac output, particularly during controlled ventilation.

The minimum alveolar concentrations of inhalational anaesthetics are increased in the young (Table 32.8). This results in a more restricted therapeutic range between surgical anaesthesia and cardiovascular and respiratory depression. Great care should therefore be exercised in their use and the patient must be monitored closely.

Halothane. Halothane is the most commonly used agent in paediatric anaesthesia. It produces a smooth rapid induction of anaesthesia. The cardiovascular depressant properties are not normally marked in clinical anaesthesia, but are severe in the presence of cardiac failure. There is marked tendency for laryngeal spasm to occur during tracheal intubation or extubation at light levels of anaesthesia. Tracheal intubation should be undertaken at the level of surgical anaesthesia and the patient should be awake prior to extubation. However, extubation under deep anaesthesia is preferable in such types of surgery as intraocular. Hepatic dysfunction following halothane anaesthesia, even multiple anaesthetics, is extremely rare in children.

Enflurane. This does not produce as smooth an induction as halothane and can induce breath-holding, coughing and laryngospasm. Respiratory and cardiovascular depression leading to hypotension occur with enflurane: central nervous system excitation as shown on e.e.g. recordings occurs, and enflurane should not be used in children with a history of epilepsy.

Methoxyflurane. Methoxyflurane is metabolised to produce free fluoride; the levels of fluoride in children are less than those found in adults, probably as a result of sequestration of fluoride in bone. Dose-related renal failure remains a problem if the dose exceeds $1\frac{1}{2}$ MAC-hours. The drug is of value during endoscopy, since the slow recovery gives greater time to the endoscopist, while maintaining spontaneous ventilation. Laryngeal spasm occurs infrequently following methoxyflurane anaesthesia.

Cyclopropane. This is still used occasionally for rapid induction of anaesthesia but it is explosive and may cause laryngospasm on induction and tracheal extubation.

Nitrous oxide. Nitrous oxide is used as a carrier gas and supplement for most inhalational anaesthetics.

Because of the low solubility of nitrogen, an increase in the volume of air-containing spaces occurs during induction with N_2O/O_2. In the neonate this is important in lesions of the lung, especially pneumothorax and congenital lobar emphysema. Expansion of the bowel in diaphragmatic hernia, exomphalos or gastroschisis may increase diaphragmatic splinting following surgical correction. In necrotising enterocolitis, the gas within the bowel wall may expand, worsening the condition.

Intravenous agents
Thiopentone 5 mg/kg is still the most frequently used i.v. induction agent for children. Very young infants are extremely sensitive to barbiturates.

Methohexitone 1 mg/kg may cause pain on injection; this can be abolished by adding lignocaine (1 mg/ml) to the solution before injection. Methohexitone may also cause central nervous system excitation seen as muscular twitching, and the drug should be avoided in patients with epilepsy.

Barbiturates may be given rectally in increased dosage, e.g. thiopentone 30 mg/kg, methohexitone 25 mg/kg, as 10% solutions. Onset of sleep is pleasant but slow, taking 5–10 min, during which time the child must be observed closely for signs of respiratory obstruction or depression.

Althesin was used for i.v. induction but unexpected cardiovascular collapse occurred usually associated with bronchospasm. This happened on first exposure to the drug, although it was more common on subsequent administrations.

Etomidate has a rapid action and causes little cardiovascular or respiratory depression but does cause pain on injection; involuntary movements and coughing are common. Because of its rapid metabolism, it has been advocated as an infusion agent for total i.v. anaesthesia. This technique is not used frequently in children because of rapid fluctuations in depth of anaesthesia and the volume of infusion required.

Ketamine may be used i.v. in a dose of 2 mg/kg, or i.m. 10 mg/kg. In the very young, increased doses are required as a consequence of poor cortical development. Following i.v. induction, respiratory depression may occur, and breath-holding is not uncommon. There is a risk of aspiration at this time.

The presence of secretions or an airway in the mouth may cause laryngospasm because of increased airway reflex activity.

The psychic phenomena associated with emergence from ketamine anaesthesia in adults are less common in children and may be reduced further by premedication with diazepam and provision of a quiet, undisturbed recovery period. The analgesia and catatonia provided by ketamine is useful for skin grafting of burns and allows exposed skin grafts to become adherent while the child remains immobile following surgery. Ketamine tends to maintain or slightly increase intraocular pressure and can be used for examination of the eye under anaesthesia where the intraocular pressure is to be measured. Intracranial pressure is increased by ketamine and its use should be avoided where there is any possibility of pre-existing elevation of intracranial pressure.

Relaxants (see Appendix IX(a), p. 560)
Although it has been stated that the neonate is particularly sensitive to nondepolarising neuromuscular blockers, this is probably related to the more marked effect of small doses of relaxant on respiration because of poor respiratory reserve and dependence on the diaphragm, rather than a myasthenic response of neonatal neuromuscular function. Recent work shows a greater variation between neonates in their response to nondepolarising relaxants than occurs in the older child and adult, but the conclusion is that for surgical relaxation a 'scaled-down' adult dose should be used initially. Subsequent 'top-up' doses should be restricted to one-tenth of the initial dose. Residual paralysis or difficulty in reversal at the end of surgery is likely to be associated either with acid–base abnormalities or hypothermia, correction of which restores muscle activity to normal.

Curare (0.5 mg/kg) causes much less hypotension in the child than the adult. Histamine release does occur; thus there is a relative contraindication to the use of curare in the asthmatic child.

Pancuronium (0.1 mg/kg) is similar in action to curare but has the advantage of causing less histamine release. The tachycardia caused by pancuronium is a disadvantage in children, who normally have a rapid heart rate.

The neonate is said to be resistant to the

depolarising relaxant suxamethonium. The dose required is normally approx. twice that used in adults on a body weight basis, i.e. 2 mg/kg. This is related to the distribution of the drug in the relatively larger extracellular fluid space. Bradycardia occurring after administration of suxamethonium may be avoided by prior administration of atropine.

ANAESTHETIC MANAGEMENT

Preoperative preparation

Every patient should be visited by the anaesthetist prior to surgery. The procedure involved in anaesthesia should be explained to the patient, in the presence of a parent if possible, and in suitable language if the child is old enough to understand. Older children may express a preference for the type of induction and this should be used if possible.

The patient should be assessed for fitness for anaesthesia. Upper respiratory infections are common, as are other viral infections, e.g. measles, mumps or chickenpox. These are a contraindication to anaesthesia for nonessential operations, but not for a more urgent procedure. The presence of a pyrexia may indicate infection and is a contraindication to nonurgent surgery. The patient's weight should be noted as this is the most reliable and simple guide to drug dosage (Table 32.9). Veins should be examined with regard to i.v. induction and the establishment of i.v. infusions.

Table 32.9 Estimates of children's weights

Age	Body weight (approximate average values)
Neonate	3 (kg)
4 months	6 (kg)
1–8 yr	2 × age + 9 (kg)
8–13 yr	3 × age (kg)

Premedication

Premedication should be prescribed according to the needs of the patient. Many children do not require sedation or analgesia preoperatively, particularly the very young and outpatients. Secretions may contribute to respiratory obstruction in small airways and premedication with an antisialagogue may be required. Hyoscine (15 µg/kg) is an effective drying

agent with sedative and antiemetic properties. Atropine (20 µg/kg) is a most effective drug for prevention of arrhythmias from cardiovagal stimulation resulting from the oculocardiac reflex or endotracheal intubation, but is more useful for this purpose when given i.v. at the induction of anaesthesia. Atropine should not be given i.m. to patients with pyrexia, but may be used i.v. at induction.

If sedation with analgesia is required preoperatively, an opioid premedication (morphine 0.2 mg/kg, or papaveretum 0.3 mg/kg) may be prescribed. The resultant respiratory depression may impede inhalational induction of anaesthesia.

The majority of older children will require only sedation. The drugs used most frequently are trimeprazine 3 mg/kg, diazepam 0.2–0.4 mg/kg or droperidol 0.2–0.4 mg/kg administered orally.

Induction

Anaesthesia may be induced either by inhalation, i.v., i.m., or rectal administration of drugs. Inhalational induction may be accomplished rapidly with halothane or cyclopropane; these may be administered directly by mask or by placing the T-piece in the anaesthetist's hands. The latter technique reduces anxiety in the patient, but causes greater pollution of the atmosphere.

There is no place for the use of gas mixtures containing less than 30% O_2 to increase the rapidity of induction. If laryngeal spasm occurs, the already small reserves of oxygen are depleted further by such mixtures and very severe hypoxaemia may result.

The child should be monitored throughout an inhalational induction using a precordial stethoscope.

Intravenous induction may be virtually painless if 25 or 27 G needles are used. Intravenous injections in children may be difficult between the ages of 6 months and 2 yr because of increased subcutaneous fat. The veins are very mobile in children and the skin should be stretched tightly to stabilise the veins. An assistant is essential to hold and squeeze the arm and to distract and immobilise the patient.

Rectal induction is slow, taking up to 15 min, and requires supervision for a prolonged time while the patient is at risk of developing respiratory depression and obstruction.

Airway management

The physiological dead space of the young infant is small but the V_D/V_T ratio is the same throughout life (0.3). Any increase in dead space from anaesthetic apparatus is more significant in the infant, and therefore must be kept to a minimum.

The Rendell-Baker-Soucek mask is designed specifically to minimise dead space in infants. When holding the mask, it is important not to press (Fig. 32.4) upward on the tongue below the mandible as this may occlude the airway totally by pushing the tongue against the posterior pharyngeal wall. The chin should be supported by pressure on the mandible alone (Fig. 32.5).

The use of Ayres T-piece apparatus reduces dead space to a minimum and also has the advantage of a low resistance to expiration because of the absence of valves. The T-piece may be used for anaesthesia using spontaneous ventilation, but only for short periods in the very young as even the small increase in dead space causes an unacceptable level of rebreathing. The fresh gas flow should be calculated as 2.5 times the predicted minute volume.

Jackson Rees modified the T-piece by the addition of an open ended reservoir bag, and this allows the apparatus to be used for controlled ventilation. Alternatively, a ventilator may be attached to the expiratory limb for controlled ventilation. In this mode a fresh gas flow rate of 1000 ml + 100 ml/kg body weight per min results in an arterial PCO$_2$ of 4.8–5.3 kPa (35–40 mmHg). A minimum gas flow of 3 litre/min is required to operate the system satisfactorily.

The size of the small baby causes difficulty in maintenance of the airway during surgery with a mask. Most infants require endotracheal intubation. The reduction in cross-sectional area of the airway caused by a 3.5 or 4.0 mm tube in a small infant causes an increase in resistance of approximately 16 times, compared with a threefold increase in an adult with a 9.5 mm endotracheal tube. Thus controlled ventilation should always be undertaken in an infant subjected to tracheal intubation.

The very young are obligate nose-breathers and secretions caused by upper respiratory infection may lead to respiratory difficulty, particularly in the postoperative period. Enlarged tonsils and adenoids may cause difficulty with airway maintenance, particularly in the older child. This may be overcome by the use of an oropharyngeal airway.

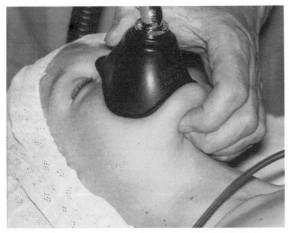

Fig. 32.4   Incorrect way of holding paediatric face mask.

Tracheal intubation

The anatomy of the infant may cause difficulties in endotracheal intubation. Infants have a relatively large head, short neck and large tongue. The mandible may be underdeveloped.

The larynx is higher in the neck (C3–4) than in the adult (C5–6) and is placed more anteriorly. The epiglottis is large, floppy and U-shaped and is not easily elevated using the conventional Macintosh laryngoscope in the valecula (Fig. 32.6). Intubation in the very young is easier if the epiglottis is elevated using a laryngoscope with a straight blade.

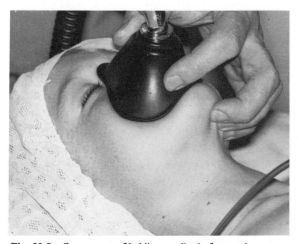

Fig. 32.5   Correct way of holding paediatric face mask.

INFANT LARYNX
U shaped epiglottis
Large arytenoids

ADULT LARYNX
Flat epiglottis

Fig. 32.6   The infant and adult larynx.

The internal diameter of an endotracheal tube for a child may be calculated from the formula:

$$\frac{\text{Age}}{4} + 4 \text{ mm}$$

The tube should be small enough to allow a leak during the application of positive pressure, otherwise pressure on the tissues of the glottis or cricoid may lead to oedema following extubation. This may cause stridor up to 8 h later and require reintubation. For this reason, intubation, although not entirely contraindicated, should be avoided in out-patients or day cases. Endotracheal tubes with shoulders (e.g. the Cole) may cause glottic oedema from pressure of the shoulder on the lax tissues of the glottis.

The endotracheal tube should be secured firmly to avoid accidental extubation or endobronchial intubation during anaesthesia. If adhesive tape is used the tube should be secured to the maxilla and not the mandible, which is extremely mobile in small children (except where this is not feasible, e.g. cleft lip and palate surgery).

The trachea of the infant is short (4 cm) at birth. Both lung fields must be auscultated to confirm correct positioning of an endotracheal tube. Although the angles between main bronchi and trachea are more nearly equal than in the adult, an endotracheal tube still tends to enter the right main bronchus. Preformed endotracheal tubes (e.g. the R.A.E. or Oxford) have the disadvantage of a fixed length, which may result in endobronchial intubation.

The narrowest part of the airway of the child is the cricoid ring. Because this is circular (unlike the diamond-shaped glottic opening which is the narrowest part of the adult airway) a cuff on the endotracheal tube is unnecessary if the correct size has been selected. Thus, in children up to 5–6 yr of age, the same sized tube may be used for either nasotracheal or orotracheal intubation.

Monitoring

Direct observation of the patient is the most important single method of monitoring. The anaesthetist may see changes in the patient's colour (cyanosis or pallor). Movement or lacrimation may be detected if anaesthesia is too light, or a change in respiratory pattern if respiratory obstruction occurs. A clear plastic drape permits observation of the patient during head and neck surgery when normal drapes totally obscure the small patient (Fig. 32.7).

The stethoscope, precordial or oesophageal, is the single most valuable monitoring device available to the anaesthetist and should always be attached prior

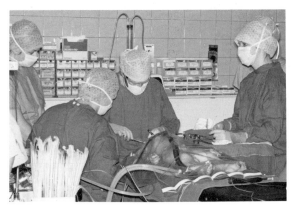

Fig. 32.7   Use of plastic surgical drapes to permit observation of child.

to induction. It allows continuous monitoring of heart sounds for rate, rhythm and intensity. In the infant, the intensity of sound varies with the stroke volume, and acts as a qualitative monitor of cardiac output. The stethoscope should always be used to check both lungs following intubation to confirm that endobronchial intubation has not taken place and it continues to give an indication of changes in ventilation during anaesthesia (Fig. 32.8).

The e.c.g. provides less information than the stethoscope but demonstrates any arrhythmias. An arterial pressure cuff and temperature probe should always be attached prior to induction.

It is important to have an i.v. infusion established, all monitoring apparatus attached and the patient

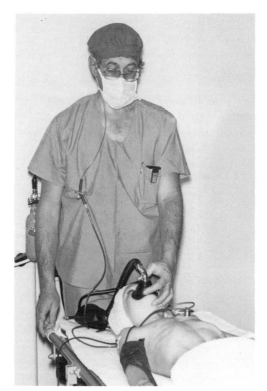

Fig. 32.8   Continuous use of precordial stethoscope.

positioned correctly prior to draping, since access to the patient may be extremely limited during surgery.

NEONATAL ANAESTHESIA

Additional problems are associated with anaesthetising the neonate because of size and immaturity. Temperature maintenance mechanisms are immature, and the patient must be kept warm during transport, induction and anaesthesia. The temperature should be monitored continuously, and the environmental temperature elevated throughout surgery. Venous access may be more difficult because of small mobile veins; scalp veins can be used in addition to limb veins. A flexible 24 or 22 G cannula should be used with a three-way tap for injection of drugs and blood. Any extension to the i.v. line should have a very small volume. Care must be taken to avoid overtransfusion. Burette infusion sets should be filled initially only to a volume of 10 ml/kg. Sedative premedication is not required for the neonate.

Atropine 0.015–0.02 mg/kg i.m. may be given to reduce secretions and prevent vagal stimulation during tracheal intubation and surgery. Vitamin K_1 1 mg should be given to reduce the neonatal bleeding tendency resulting from lack of vitamin K-dependent factors.

Ventilation by face mask should be carried out with extreme care to avoid inflation of the stomach.

The anatomy of the neonate may render tracheal intubation difficult. In the very small, weak or premature neonate, it is customary to perform intubation prior to induction of anaesthesia. This reduces the likelihood of aspiration of gastric contents and the need to ventilate by mask, with subsequent gastric distension. In addition, the baby is able to breathe should attempts to intubate fail.

The disadvantages of awake intubation are that it is often traumatic and it may be more difficult to see the larynx than in the anaesthetised child. A normal neonate requires a 3.5 mm tube, and a premature child a 3.0 mm or rarely a 2.5 mm tube.

Drugs should be prepared prior to anaesthesia and given from 1 ml or 2 ml syringes to avoid excessive administration of fluid. Cardiovascular monitoring must be continuous. Nondepolarising relaxants may be given in adult scaled doses initially (tubocurarine 0.5 mg/kg, pancuronium 0.1 mg/kg) but topping up doses should be only one tenth of the initial dose.

The neonate should not be allowed to breathe spontaneously under anaesthesia for any length of time; the inefficient respiratory system is easily depressed and the presence of a small tube greatly increases resistance. Controlled ventilation is carried out preferably by hand so that changes in compliance or resistance may be detected early.

Many neonatal surgical procedures affect pulmonary function. The major airways may be totally obstructed in repair of tracheo-oesophageal fistula, or compliance reduced greatly following the treatment of exomphalos or diaphragmatic hernia.

Bradycardia is usually a sign of hypoxia and should be treated by ventilation with 100% oxygen. Supplements of inhalational agents (halothane or enflurane) should be used in small doses to avoid hypotension, and should be discontinued well before the end of anaesthesia to avoid residual depression.

Relaxants should be antagonised by neostigmine and atropine. If there is any doubt regarding the quality of reversal, the temperature should be checked carefully and any abnormality in acid-base status treated appropriately. Any child whose respiration may be compromised following surgery should receive pulmonary ventilation electively. Opioid analgesics should be avoided postoperatively as they cause severe depression of respiration.

SPECIFIC OPERATIONS IN THE NEONATE

Pyloric stenosis

This occurs usually in babies of 3–8 weeks of age. In mild cases, the child may be well nourished and hydrated, but if severe, extreme dehydration and electrolyte imbalance are present, with hypokalaemia and severe alkalosis. Surgical treatment by pyloromyotomy is not an emergency and fluid and electrolyte imbalance should be corrected prior to anaesthesia. The child may have had a barium swallow and a nasogastric tube should always be passed and aspirated prior to induction; the patient should nevertheless be treated as though he has a full stomach. If an i.v. infusion is in progress, i.v. induction should be used, the trachea intubated after suxamethonium (1.5–2 mg/kg) and paralysis maintained with a long acting muscle relaxant or intermittent suxamethonium. Hyperventilation should be avoided to prevent worsening of the pre-existing alkalosis which may lead to slow onset of respiration at the termination of anaesthesia. The nasogastric tube should be aspirated prior to tracheal extubation.

Tracheo-oesophageal fistula and oesophageal atresia

The commonest form of this disorder is oesophageal atresia with a fistula between the trachea and the lower part of the oesophagus. The diagnosis may be made if the child aspirates secretions continually or chokes on his feed. The presence of a fistula may be detected by persistent pulmonary problems as a result of aspiration from the stomach. A large tube should be placed in the upper oesophageal pouch to aspirate secretions. Anaesthesia is similar to that for other neonates but particular problems are associated with intubation of the fistula and inflation of the stomach.

The position of the tube must be checked by auscultation.

During surgery large airways may be kinked or clamped accidentally, and surgical retraction may cause dramatic decreases in cardiac output by compression of the left and right atria or vagus nerve. Respiratory and cardiovascular systems should be monitored closely. The respiratory problems resulting from aspiration through the fistula do not resolve until after surgery but tracheobronchial toilet should be performed prior to and following surgery and postoperative elective ventilation may be required.

Diaphragmatic hernia

The usual presentation is that of severe acute respiratory distress and cyanosis, with a flat or scaphoid abdomen. Chest X-ray is usually diagnostic. Resuscitation should be initially by endotracheal intubation and controlled ventilation. Positive pressure ventilation must not be carried out using bag and mask, as expansion of the viscera in the hernia further compresses the contralateral lung and heart. Nitrous oxide should be avoided to prevent gas distension. Arterial or capillary blood gases should be monitored.

If the lungs expand well the trachea may be extubated postoperatively when blood gases are normal. Some infants have a hypoplastic lung on the side of the hernia, usually the left. If the hernia occurred early in fetal life there may, in addition, be some hypoplasia of the contralateral lung leaving inadequate pulmonary tissue to maintain life. Some children may survive following intensive care with controlled ventilation and a pulmonary arterial vasodilator, e.g. tolazoline. Bilateral chest drains should be inserted, as there is a danger of pneumothorax if high ventilatory pressures are required.

Exomphalos and gastroschisis

In these conditions there is herniation of the abdominal contents through the anterior abdominal wall. In exomphalos, the sac of the hernia is within the umbilical cord. In gastroschisis the hernia is lateral to the umbilicus and the bowel usually lacks any covering. If the defect is large there is a likelihood of dramatic loss of heat and fluid from exposed bowel. It may not be possible to return the bowel to the small abdominal cavity, and initially the bowel may be protected in a silastic pouch and gradually replaced into the abdomen over a few days.

Bowel obstruction

Obstruction may be the result of an atresia at any point from duodenum to anal canal. Malrotation, volvulus and reduplication of bowel may cause obstructive symptoms. Meconium ileus, a pre-monitory sign of cystic fibrosis, may cause neonatal obstruction, although the associated respiratory problems are not usually of significance in the neonate. The major anaesthetic problems are those of fluid and electrolyte imbalance and danger of regurgitation and aspiration.

Myelomeningocoele

This is a defect resulting from the failure of the neural tube to close in the fetus. If the defect is large, there may be severe problems of heat and fluid loss during surgery, and blood loss may be difficult to estimate because of mixture with c.s.f.

Hydrocephalus

Hydrocephalus may result from the closure of a myelomeningocoele or the associated Arnold-Chiari syndrome. A shunt procedure to drain excess c.s.f. into right atrium or into the peritoneal cavity may be required. Problems may be encountered in relation to raised intracranial pressure (ICP). In the very young with open fontanelles, tapping of the lateral ventricle may help reduce acute increases in pressure. Ketamine and volatile agents must be avoided. Hypertension resulting from raised ICP may disappear rapidly when ICP is reduced. Hypercapnia should be avoided at all stages. Blood loss is not usually a problem during shunt surgery.

Cleft lip and palate

This may cause airway problems which lead to difficult intubation, especially in association with Pierre Robin syndrome. Some surgeons treat these conditions during the neonatal period but it is more common to repair the cleft lip at 2–3 months and the palate at 18 months to 2 yr.

Atropine 20 μg/kg should be given, as secretions may be a problem. The airway should be monitored closely, as the endotracheal tube may be kinked or compressed by the gag used during cleft palate repair. A throat pack is inserted prior to surgery; its insertion and removal should be recorded. In some cases of Pierre Robin syndrome or mild micrognathia, closure of the soft palate may cause airway difficulty postoperatively, requiring endotracheal intubation for a day or two. Blood is usually not required during cleft palate surgery but should be available for cleft lip repair, as losses may exceed 10% of blood volume. Congenital heart disease is a commonly associated disorder in patients with cleft lip or palate.

POSTOPERATIVE CARE

When ventilation is adequate following recovery from anaesthesia, the child should be nursed in the lateral position and the airway, cardiovascular system and temperature monitored closely in an adequately equipped postoperative recovery area (see Chapter 20). The patient should be awake before return to the ward. Recovery from ketamine anaesthesia should take place in a quiet undisturbed manner. Diazepam 0.2 mg/kg may be required if there is evidence of psychological upset.

Laryngeal spasm

Laryngeal spasm is a relatively frequent complication of paediatric anaesthesia particularly following the use of volatile agents. Treatment comprises ventilation with 100% oxygen under positive pressure by bag and mask. If bradycardia occurs, the trachea should be reintubated rapidly and the lungs inflated with 100% oxygen. Laryngeal spasm may be avoided by extubating the trachea either when the patient is totally awake or when surgically anaesthetised. Extubation should not be carried out when the patient is only lightly anaesthetised or just beginning to cough. Under direct vision the pharynx should be cleared of all secretions as these may precipitate this particularly dangerous hazard.

Postoperative pain

Pain is frequent although not usually as protracted or severe a problem in children as in adult patients. Analgesics should be prescribed as a routine, with the exception of neonates and small infants. For severe pain, i.m. opioids are required while for less severe pain, milder drugs, e.g. paracetamol elixir orally, are preferable.

Local anaesthesia

Blocks which are suitable include extradurals (thoracic or lumbar) with or without a catheter, and caudal, intercostal, ilioinguinal and penile blocks. For the upper limb, axillary block, and for the lower limb femoral, lateral cutaneous nerve of thigh, or sciatic nerve block may be useful. A local block can be used as the sole technique of anaesthesia in the severely ill child, or in circumstances in which it may be desirable to avoid the metabolic upset associated with general anaesthesia, e.g. the severely dehydrated child with pyloric stenosis, or the neonate with a low imperforate anus where caudal anaesthesia has been shown to be useful. Local techniques should be performed on the young child only by experienced anaesthetists.

INTENSIVE CARE

The total reliance of the newborn on his diaphragm for adequate ventilation may result in a requirement for prolonged controlled ventilation if the diaphragm is paralysed or splinted by high intra-abdominal pressure. This may occur following surgery for gastroschisis or exomphalos, where abdominal growth is not adequate to contain the entire bowel. Severe splinting may also occur with distension of the bowel as a result of necrotising enterocolitis, bowel obstruction or gastro-enteritis.

Controlled ventilation may be required for babies with cardiac or respiratory failure. Institution of controlled ventilation may be necessary without the aid of biochemical blood gas information simply because of a clinical diagnosis of exhaustion.

The newborn tolerates relatively high ventilatory and intrathoracic pressures without a decrease in cardiac output because of his large right ventricle, which regresses slowly following the change from fetal to adult type of circulation. However, there is a danger of lung rupture leading to pneumothorax.

The immature respiratory system with small, easily obstructed airways, is the factor responsible for the majority of admissions to the intensive care unit. The child has little respiratory reserve and any increase in airway resistance or decrease in compliance may require respiratory support or assistance.

The method of choice for maintenance of the airway is nasotracheal intubation in preference to tracheostomy except when very prolonged airway control is required or a severe anatomical disorder of the upper airway or trachea is present. Narrow nasal tubes require meticulous care and attention to detail including fixation to prevent kinking or dislodgement of the tube and ulceration of the nares as a result of pressure. Humidification is of paramount importance if obstruction by secretions (requiring reintubation under emergency conditions) is to be avoided. If necessary the patient should be sedated to assist toleration of the endotracheal tube. Aspiration of secretions should be carried out regularly using soft atraumatic catheters no larger than half the diameter of the endotracheal tube. The duration of suction should be limited to a few seconds to prevent hypoxia. As with patients undergoing anaesthesia a child should not be allowed to breathe through a small endotracheal tube for prolonged periods without support either by positive pressure ventilation or continuous positive airway pressure (CPAP) Particular attention should be paid to adequate hydration of the patient in addition to humidification of inspired gas. The environmental temperature should be kept close to the neutral thermal environment to minimise oxygen requirements.

Respiratory distress syndrome (hyaline membrane disease)

This occurs particularly in the premature as a result of absence of pulmonary surfactant. This defect allows the alveoli to collapse, causing a decrease in compliance, and tachypnoea. Respiration is grunting in nature as the child breathes out against a closed glottis in an attempt to maintain alveolar patency. Mild cases may recover if the hypoxia is treated with humidified oxygen, and the acidosis is corrected. The arterial PO_2 should be maintained at a minimum of 9.5 kPa (70 mmHg). More severe cases require mechanical assistance to keep the alveoli patent either with spontaneous respiration using nasal catheters or endotracheal intubation to induce CPAP. The most severe cases require IPPV with PEEP.

Acute epiglottitis

This condition results from bacterial infection, usually by *Haemophilus influenzae*. The child usually presents between the ages of 2 and 7 yr. There is a rapid onset of severe respiratory obstruction and dysphagia resulting from glottic swelling. The patient cannot swallow saliva and has to sit to avoid choking. Toxaemia is usually present. Treatment is by endotracheal intubation under general anaesthesia, and antibiotic therapy. An i.v. infusion should be commenced and atropine 20 μg/kg given i.v. to avoid the effects of vagal stimulation when the inflamed epiglottis is stimulated during intubation. Anaesthesia is induced by inhalation of 100% oxygen with halothane with the child in the sitting position. This may be difficult and protracted in the presence of respiratory obstruction. Intubation may be extremely difficult because of the swollen epiglottis. In severe cases an ENT surgeon should be standing by to perform emergency tracheostomy if total respiratory obstruction occurs. Initially an oral tube should be used and this may be changed subsequently for a nasal tube when a clear airway has been established. Extubation is normally possible after antibiotic therapy for 24–48 h.

Laryngotracheobronchitis

This may be bacterial or, more commonly, viral in origin and is the most frequent cause of croup in children. It is a disorder of the larger airways. In mild conditions it may be treated with well humidified oxygen but if severe, the trachea should be intubated.

If hypoxia is present, IPPV may be necessary. Stridor and an increase in the work of breathing leading to physical exhaustion may necessitate intubation and ventilation on purely clinical grounds prior to the establishment of biochemical evidence of hypoxia. Profuse viscid secretions are a major problem. Humidification is of the utmost importance, and additional quantities of water should be instilled into the airways prior to the aspiration of secretions to maintain patency of the tube. If the cause is viral the course of the disease runs for 10 to 14 days during which time airway support may be required.

Bronchiolitis

This is a viral disorder of the smaller airways causing expiratory wheeze. Hypoxia tends to occur early and secretions are a problem. Tracheal intubation and ventilation are frequently required to treat hypoxia.

Cardiac arrest and resuscitation in children

The commonest causes of cardiac arrest in children are:

1. hypoxia
2. hypovolaemia
3. electrolyte imbalance
4. overdose of drugs.

Prevention of cardiac arrest and its sequelae may be achieved to a great extent by ensuring that all seriously ill children are well oxygenated, the circulating volume is maintained and electrolyte imbalances are monitored continuously and treated. Meticulous care should be taken with the doses of all drugs.

In children cardiac arrest is more commonly associated with asystole than ventricular fibrillation. Thus treatment with intracardiac adrenaline (1 in 10 000) should be used early, as acidosis reduces the effectiveness of catecholamines.

FURTHER READING

Arthur D S 1983 Local anaesthesia for paediatric surgery. In: Nimmo W, Henderson J J (eds) Practical local anaesthesia. Blackwell Scientific Publications, Edinburgh

Brown T C K, Fisk G C 1979 Anaesthesia for children. Blackwell Scientific Publications, Oxford

Hatch D, Sumner E 1981 Neonatal anaesthesia. Edward Arnold, London

Jackson Rees G, Gray T C 1981 Paediatric anaesthesia. Trends in current practice. Butterworths, London

Pang L M, Mellins R B 1975 Neonatal cardiorespiratory physiology. Anesthesiology 43: 171

Rackow H, Salanitre E 1969 Modern concepts in pediatric anesthesiology. Anesthesiology 30: 208

Rylance G 1981 Clinical pharmacology. Drugs in children. British Medical Journal 282: 50

Smith R M 1980 Anaesthesia for infants and children. C V Mosby, St Louis

Steward D J 1979 Manual of paediatric anaesthesia. Churchill Livingstone, Edinburgh

Steward D J (ed) 1981 Some aspects of paediatric anaesthesia. Biochemical Press, Amsterdam

Vivori E, Bush G H 1977 Modern aspects of the management of the newborn undergoing surgery. British Journal of Anaesthesia 49: 51

Winter R W 1973 The body fluids in pediatrics. Little, Brown, Boston

33

Dental anaesthesia

The term 'dental anaesthesia' usually encompasses the administration of a general anaesthetic, local anaesthetic or sedation technique to an outpatient in a dental hospital or dentist's surgery. Extensive dental surgery is carried out normally by oral surgeons upon hospital inpatients, and the anaesthetic considerations for this treatment are similar to those of general anaesthesia for ENT surgery. This chapter describes only the techniques appropriate to the former categories.

In 1976, 1.2 million dental anaesthetics were administered in England and Wales for extractions, and a further 129 000 for conservation work. This workload could not be accommodated in hospital practice and, for the foreseeable future, a substantial and major proportion of dental anaesthetics will be given to outpatients. Much of this work could be avoided if patients attended for regular dental treatment, but the attitude to conservation is complex and relates to the influence of education, custom and previous experiences of the patient.

Local anaesthetic blocks are safer than general anaesthetic techniques and patients should be encouraged to have dental work performed under local anaesthesia. It has been estimated that more than 60 million local anaesthetics are given annually in the UK. However, local techniques are contraindicated in some conditions, notably infection, but this is present only in a small proportion of patients presenting for surgery.

The estimated mortality rate of dental anaesthesia is 1/260 000 which compares favourably with the extrapolated mortality rate for general anaesthetics of 1/10 000. Much of this difference results from the fact that dental anaesthesia is of very short duration and the patients are usually young and healthy.

Most patients experience marked anxiety whilst undergoing dental treatment. In an attempt to reduce this, many combinations of drugs and techniques (including acupuncture and hypnotism) have been employed to produce mental relaxation without loss of consciousness. Currently, the two most popular techniques comprise sedation either with nitrous oxide/oxygen or with a drug administered i.v.

GENERAL ANAESTHETIC TECHNIQUES

Anaesthetic equipment

Historically, dental anaesthetists have used intermittent flow anaesthetic machines, but these are less accurate than continuous flow machines and are less familiar to most hospital anaesthetists. Continuous flow machines have the advantages of economy, simplicity, reliability, familiarity to junior anaesthetists, accuracy and flexibility.

The anaesthetic equipment and facilities which should be available in a dental outpatient surgery have been detailed in the Wylie report and include a basic anaesthetic machine (Fig. 33.1) with an oxygen failsafe device and inability to provide less than 20% oxygen, a vaporiser, a suitable range of masks, valves, laryngoscopes, endotracheal tubes and suction apparatus. All persons working in the anaesthetic area must be familiar with the emergency drug tray, the contents of which should be complete and unexpired. Lighting should be bright and enable the anaesthetist to see clearly the patient and the anaesthetic machine. The premises should be provided with easy access for emergency services.

It has been recommended that some provision be made for scavenging anaesthetic gases, particularly if volatile agents are used. Scavenging requires a

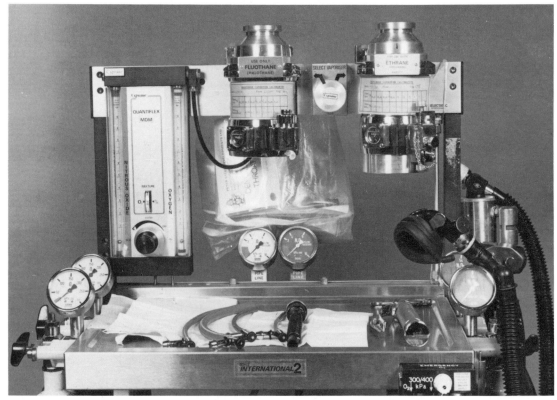

Fig. 33.1 Boyle international anaesthetic machine fitted with the Quantiflex rotameter head, with single dials to control both flow and mixture. This machine is ideal for both anaesthesia and relative analgesia. Note the reversed position of oxygen and nitrous oxide. This particular machine is also fitted with detachable vaporisers.

collecting device round the anaesthetic circuit valve (Fig. 33.2), and this may render the nasal mask rather cumbersome and awkward in use. The valve may be positioned at a different part of the circuit, but the efficiency of the circuit is impaired. For these reasons many anaesthetists rely solely upon good ventilation of the surgery.

Outpatient anaesthesia

Outpatient dental anaesthesia is undertaken for the same reason as other forms of outpatient surgery, i.e. speed, economy, convenience and because there are insufficient facilities to enable the surgery to be undertaken as inpatients. Only predominantly healthy patients should be considered for outpatient dental anaesthesia. Most hospitals have inpatient facilities for dental emergencies and patients with recognised risk factors should be admitted for treatment.

Selection of patients

The majority of patients requiring outpatient anaesthesia are children. There are two distinct groups:

1. Those too young to co-operate for local anaesthesia, or with oral infection which renders a local technique inadvisable.

2. Unco-operative children, many of whom are handicapped, who require conservation dentistry. These patients often require extensive work which should be undertaken with endotracheal anaesthesia.

Adults are less likely to require general anaesthesia for emergency dental work but when necessary the cause is usually infection.

Written consent should be obtained before undertaking treatment under general anaesthesia. This may be difficult to obtain with children, but a guardian's or parental consent is essential unless the condition is so serious that the child's life is in

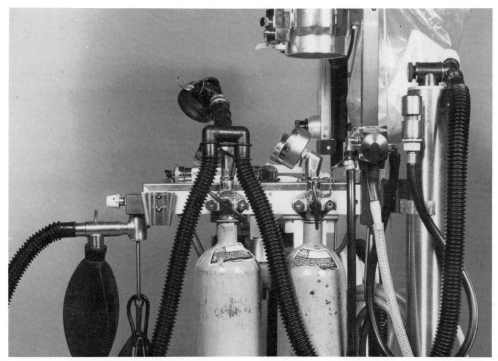

Fig. 33.2   View of anaesthetic machine showing the fitting of the active scavenging unit and the adapted breathing system.

danger, although this is virtually unknown in dental work. It should be remembered that most children presenting for either emergency or elective dental work have not been examined by a medical practitioner and the contact with the anaesthetist is the first meeting with a physician. It is common practice to ask the parent or guardian to complete a form with a series of questions about the health of the child, with particular emphasis on the respiratory and cardiovascular systems and the presence of known allergies (see Chapter 36). It is also essential to ensure that parents and adult patients are given both written and verbal instructions regarding the preparation and precautions which should be taken before and after surgery. It has been demonstrated that many outpatients presenting for surgery ignore instructions and one study noted that 9% of patients drove home, despite instructions to the contrary.

The anaesthetist should know the extent and likely duration of the proposed surgery. An attempt to assess the patency of the nasal airway should be made since if this is blocked, endotracheal intubation may be required. The dentist should have noted and brought to the attention of the anaesthetist the existence of loose teeth. However, it is sound practice to assume that some of the primary dentition of young children is likely to be loose, and great care should be taken in inserting gags and mouth props.

Induction of anaesthesia

The majority of anaesthetists use inhalational anaesthesia for induction in children, but some prefer to use i.v. agents, e.g. methohexitone. Some children find the insertion of an i.v. needle painful, and object strongly. Conversely, others dislike the anaesthetic mask and struggle to avoid inhalational anaesthesia. Usually, a combination of tact, persuasion and firmness suffices to induce acceptance of a mask.

Induction of anaesthesia with hypoxic mixtures of N_2O/O_2 (the so-called 'black gas') is now of historical interest only. The inspired concentration of oxygen should never be allowed to decrease below 30% at any time during anaesthesia. Halothane should be introduced early during induction in low concentrations and increased as rapidly as possible without provoking coughing. When the muscle tone of the lower jaw is diminished, the mouth prop or gag (Fig. 33.3) is inserted carefully.

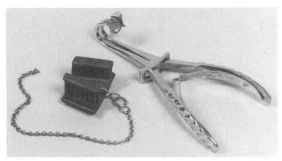

Fig. 33.3 The rubber mouth prop is usually placed in position before inducing intravenous anaesthesia. The Ferguson gag illustrated requires single handed ambidextrous manipulation to achieve maximum benefit. This requires practice.

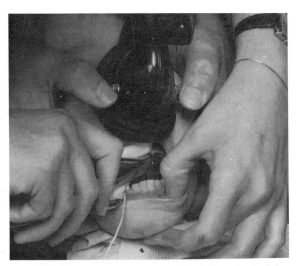

Fig. 33.5 The mouth can become crowded! The anaesthetist's hands support the head and lower jaw bringing it forward to maintain the airway. The mouth gag is concealed by the dentist's right hand. The dentist supports the lower jaw. Note the position of the throat pack, with the tail hanging from the mouth. In placing the throat pack, the tongue is not forced back, and the pack is positioned to prevent material from falling posteriorly and also to prevent oral breathing.

The introduction of a throat pack (Figs 33.4, 33.5) may be undertaken by either the anaesthetist or the dentist, although the latter is usually positioned in front of the patient and has a better view of the oral cavity. The anaesthetist must observe the reservoir bag and ensure that the airway is not compromised during placement of the pack. Correct placement is essential: the pack should not push the tongue back against the posterior pharyngeal wall and should prevent any debris passing into the lower pharynx or larynx. It should prevent oral breathing. A tail from the pack must always protrude out of the mouth to alert staff of its presence. At the end of the procedure,

the pack is removed, and the patient is transferred to the recovery room in the horizontal position on a trolley. Complete recovery must occur before the patient is discharged.

Problems

The most common difficulty is a problem with the airway, in the form of partial respiratory obstruction. Correct positioning of the jaw obviates much of the problem. It takes considerable practice to position the hands correctly. Initially the anaesthetist finds great difficulty in simultaneously holding the jaw, operating the gag, applying the mask and adjusting the flows of anaesthetic gases. The ideal position is to hold the jaw well forward with the middle and ring fingers of both hands, whilst both thumbs apply the mask. Once the patient is anaesthetised, the position may be maintained with one hand, thereby allowing the other to insert the gag and open it, while still maintaining an airway. If a clear airway is not possible despite altering the position of the jaw, endotracheal intubation should be undertaken.

Some children will have been crying and excessive salivation is not uncommon; this often results in some

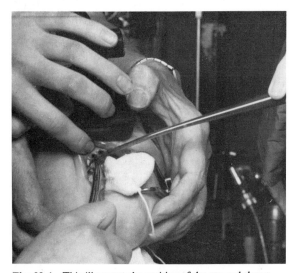

Fig. 33.4 This illustrates the position of the gag and throat pack. The suction is also in use. The nasal mask is positioned to avoid obstructing the external nares, but allowing access to the upper front teeth. Figures 33.4 and 33.5 demonstrate the advantages of the pack being placed by the dentist, who has a better view than the anaesthetist.

laryngospasm. Difficulty may then occur, as the spasm causes hypoventilation, diminished uptake of anaesthetic agents and reduction in depth of anaesthesia. Suction may be of some value, but care should be taken not to increase the extent of posterior pharyngeal stimulation.

Position — horizontal/sitting. There has been considerable controversy regarding the most appropriate position for patients during dental anaesthesia. There is a danger of fainting and resultant cerebral hypoxia in the patient sitting in an upright dental chair, although Tomlin, in a study of deaths following dental anaesthesia, maintained that there was little evidence to support this as a cause of mortality. In the horizontal or semisupine position (Fig. 33.6), material is more likely to fall posteriorly down the throat and it has been demonstrated that the

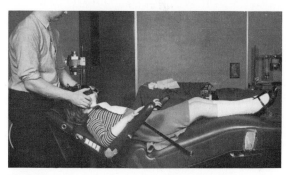

Fig. 33.6 The semisupine position. Note the position of the anaesthetist's fingers holding the jaw forward with both thumbs securing nasal mask. The anaesthetic machine, suction and dental equipment are to the left. This leaves the right side clear and gives the dentist sufficient room to gain access to all quadrants of the mouth.

nasal airway is less well maintained in this position, as the soft palate acts as a 'curtain' obstruction. This may result in hypoxia. On balance it would seem that the position should be the one with which the anaesthetist and dentist are most happy and familiar.

Arrhythmias. Arrhythmias have been reported in approx. 30% of patients undergoing general anaesthesia in the dental chair. Most of these abnormalities are benign, and are usually focal extrasystoles. Neither atropine premedication nor differing anaesthetic techniques have been shown to alter significantly the frequency of arrhythmia. It has been suggested that the patients most at risk are those with increased sympathetic activity, often manifest as tachycardia and a pale frightened appearance.

In the extremely rare event of cardiovascular collapse, with no evidence of peripheral perfusion cardiopulmonary resuscitation should be instituted immediately. Defibrillation should be undertaken as soon as possible, since ventricular fibrillation is more likely to be encountered than asystole.

Induction agents

The choice of i.v. induction agents is limited to those with a rapid rate of induction and short duration of recovery. Whilst many agents are available, the most commonly used drug is methohexitone. This is used as a 1% solution in an approximate dose of 1 mg/kg. Its disadvantages are pain on injection and occasional movements of the patient. For children this is probably the most popular drug as it produces a predictable response and few sensitivity reactions.

It is preferable to induce i.v. anaesthesia in the semi-reclining position.

Anaesthesia for adults

The majority of adults presenting for dental anaesthesia under general anaesthesia are suffering from oral infections which contraindicate the use of local anaesthesia. Thus the majority of patients present as emergencies, but there is a small number of adults who are unable or unwilling to submit to local techniques. In addition there are adult mentally handicapped patients who are unable to co-operate with the dentist. This last group present usually for a mixture of conservation and dental surgical work (often extensive) generally requiring endotracheal intubation.

Inhalational anaesthesia is not suitable for use in adult anaesthesia as it is not uncommon for some struggling to occur, and an i.v. induction is preferable. The most common reason for general anaesthesia is infection, often of one tooth, and this suggests that periodontal disease is present, which renders the tooth easily extractable. Thus a single tooth can usually be removed readily while the induction agent is effective. However, it is not always possible to extract the tooth readily and i.v. induction should always be followed by inhalation anaesthesia until surgery is complete. Before induction, it is usual to insert a mouth prop.

If infection is severe and trismus present, anaesthesia may not always relieve masseter spasm. It may be preferable in this case to assess adequacy of the airway by use of an inhalational induction. If access is too limited to allow extraction, antibiotics should be administered and the infection allowed to subside before surgery is undertaken.

Endotracheal anaesthesia

Formal endotracheal intubation is now undertaken much more commonly than in the past. Mental handicap, extended surgery, obstruction of nasal airways or difficulty in maintaining an airway are indications for endotracheal intubation. A formal decision to intubate may be made if surgery is scheduled to extend beyond 15 to 20 min.

Endotracheal intubation may be achieved during inhalational anaesthesia or by the use of an i.v. induction agent followed by a short-acting muscle relaxant. Conditions for intubation are arguably less ideal if inhalational methods are used, but suxamethonium pains are avoided. The tube may be passed either orally or nasally; the latter route allows access to both sides of the mouth without movement of the tube, and packing the throat is more secure. The pack may be placed more posteriorly than when no endotracheal tube is used; thus it is mandatory to ensure that some evidence of packing is obvious, e.g. by leaving a tail of the pack hanging from the corner of the mouth. Prior to extubation, the nasopharynx should be sucked out carefully under direct vision and the pack removed.

All children should be examined before discharge, particularly if a nasal tube has been used, as bleeding from disrupted adenoids may sometimes be troublesome. Advice regarding analgesia and postoperative care must also be given before discharge.

SEDATION TECHNIQUES

The anxiety experienced by the majority of patients undergoing dental treatment has encouraged a search for effective treatment. Nitrous oxide has become popular in the U.S.A. for this purpose. In the U.K. the Society for the Advancement of Anaesthesia in Dentistry was founded to establish satisfactory training facilities for dentists and dental anaesthetists using intermittent injections of i.v. methohexitone for sedation. With the introduction of the benzodiazepines, i.v. sedation has become more popular.

Relative analgesia

Relative analgesia is a misleading title. If painful operative dental surgery is undertaken, complete and not relative analgesia is necessary. However, the name was taken from the classical Guedel states of inhalation anaesthesia, relative analgesia being the name given to the first phase before the onset of anaesthesia. Relative analgesia is essentially a technique of inhalational sedation, using low concentrations of nitrous oxide (20–35%) in oxygen. The use of such low concentrations results in sedation without anaesthesia; there is no loss of consciousness, and reflex integrity is maintained. It should be understood that this is not an anaesthetic technique. Both the dental work and the relative analgesia should be undertaken by the dentist, as he knows when discomfort is to be expected and can maintain the necessary rapport with the patient.

Whilst almost any anaesthetic machine may be used for this technique, few are really suitable. Intermittent flow machines are probably too inaccurate for the low concentrations desired, and are wasteful of gases. Continuous flow machines do not have the safety features which specifically designed machines possess. Purpose-built machines may also be used as anaesthetic machines by the addition of a vaporiser.

Specific apparatus operates as a continous flow machine and does not function if the O_2 supply fails (or if the cylinder empties); the valve at the position of the anaesthetic reservoir bag is designed to admit room air if the machine switches off (as a result of failure of the O_2 supply). If the fresh gas flow is inadequate and the reservoir bag empties, air is admitted to the circuit as the valve will not allow rebreathing. From the foregoing it can be seen that the valve is not one which is familiar to anaesthetists.

The technique of relative analgesia consists initially of acclimatising the patient to the lightweight nasal mask, while inhaling oxygen. After a short period, nitrous oxide is introduced, initially in concentrations of less than 10% for a few breaths, then increased slowly whilst a steady stream of conversation is directed at the patient, indicating the sensations likely to be experienced (usually little until 10% N_2O is inhaled, although there are wide individual variations). The initial feelings comprise mild sedation, but part of this may result from suggestion by the dentist. The concentration is increased until the patient experiences a sense of floating, or paraesthesiae around the lips or fingers. At this point, the concentration of N_2O is decreased slightly, as this is probably just beyond the desirable point.

The advantages of this technique are that no preparation of the patient is required and the rapid uptake and elimination of N_2O ensures that no hangover effect is experienced. There are two disadvantages; equipment is expensive to install and to operate; it has also been suggested that in the absence of scavenging, the abortion rate is higher in female dental assistants in practices in which relative analgesia is used than those in which it is not used.

There are few contraindications to the use of relative analgesia, although expense prohibits universal use. The mask may be distressing to some patients, but this is usually overcome by gentle persuasion. The technique cannot be used in the presence of nasal obstruction. It has also been suggested that it should be avoided in patients with a serious psychiatric history or severe obstructive airways disease.

Intravenous sedation

With this technique, the patient is given a small dose of diazepam i.v. It is generally accepted that not more than 20 mg should be given to outpatients and sufficient time should be available to allow the drug to act before starting surgery. When teaching this technique to dentists, it is important to stress that a maximum dose should be selected which will not induce anaesthesia, as there is great patient variation in response to diazepam. The use of diazepam is associated with pain on injection ($>30\%$) and a substantial frequency of venous thrombosis. The introduction of an emulsion of diazepam ('Diazemuls') has reduced the frequency of both these complications. It is inadvisable to drive or to operate machinery within 24 h of administration, since the metabolites of diazepam are pharmacologically active.

Patients must receive written guidance regarding the duration of action of the benzodiazepines; nonetheless it has been shown that approx. 10% of outpatients ignore this advice.

The relative merits and disadvantages of i.v. sedation and relative analgesia are summarised in Table 33.1.

Table 33.1 A comparison of inhalational sedation and i.v. diazepam

	Relative analgesia	I.v. sedation
Advantages	No preparation	Simple equipment
	Rapid onset	Inexpensive
	Ease of control	Simplicity of use
	No escort required	
Disadvantages	Very expensive equipment	Venous access required
	Expensive to run	Injection may be painful
	Use of mask initially complicated	Slow onset
	Pollution	Prolonged action

CONCLUSION

It is appropriate to consider briefly the changes in dental anaesthetic practice which are likely to follow the relatively recent publication of reports on dental anaesthetic training. For some time it has been considered that it is not possible to train dental students to give safe anaesthesia without undertaking a considerably altered training programme as an undergraduate, and further training as a postgraduate.

In 1965 a Joint Subcommittee on Dental Anaesthesia was convened to consider the problem, and a report emerged in 1967. This led to the establishment with anaesthetists and dentists of a joint working party whose recommendations were published in 1969. No action was taken to implement the recommendations of these Committees.

In 1978, the Wylie report was published. The remit of this Committee was to consider the safety of patients under dental anaesthesia (all aspects including sedation techniques), to define the required training for a 'core anaesthetist', and to define the facilities required in any dental surgery where general anaesthesia is undertaken. It was the intention to institute the recommendations as a national policy, training programmes being subject to the joint approval of the Faculties of Dental Surgery and of Anaesthetists.

To implement the Wylie report, an interfaculty working party was formed under the chairmanship of Professor Seward, which reported in 1981. In Scotland similar steps were taken and published as the Spence report.

Unlike the earlier reports, there is firm resolve to implement their recommendations, though it is recognised that some time will be required, perhaps as long as 10 yr. The result is a profound change in the training of dental undergraduates and the provision of postgraduate training courses for dentists interested in dental anaesthesia. In general terms a substantial upgrading will be required of equipment and premises in which dental anaesthesia is undertaken. This will, in time, alter the demand for skilled dental anaesthetic services, although it is too early to predict the final result. It is interesting to note that the Wylie report acknowledges that no evidence exists to indicate that implementation of the proposals would result in improved safety.

FURTHER READING

Danziger A M 1980 Intubation and/or the supine position for dental outpatient. Anaesthesia 35: 70

Dinsdale R C W, Dixon R A 1978 Anaesthetic services to dental patients in England and Wales. British Dental Journal 144: 271

Editorial 1981 General anaesthesia for dentistry. British Dental Journal 151: 357

Langa H 1976 Relative analgesia in dental practice, inhalational analgesia sedation with nitrous oxide, 2nd edn. W B Saunders, Philadelphia

Muir V M J, Leonard M, Haddaway E 1976 Morbidity following dental extraction: a comparative survey of local and general anaesthesia. Anaesthesia 31: 171

Seward report 1981 Report of the Interfaculty Working Party formed to consider the implementation of the Wylie report. British Dental Journal 151: 389

Spence report 1981 Report of the Joint Working Party on Anaesthesia in General Dental Practice. British Dental Journal 151: 392

Sykes P (ed) 1979 Drummond-Jackson's dental sedation and anaesthesia, 6th edn. Society for Advancement of Anaesthesia in Dentistry, London

Tomlin P J 1974 Deaths in outpatient anaesthetic practice. Anaesthesia 29: 551

Wylie report 1978 Report of the Working Party on Training in Dental Anaesthesia. British Dental Journal 151: 385

34

Anaesthesia for miscellaneous procedures

MAJOR VASCULAR SURGERY

Anaesthesia for major vascular surgery is a complex subject; only the more important features are described here.

Elective repair of abdominal aortic aneurysm

During the preoperative visit, the anaesthetist should enquire particularly regarding symptoms of ischaemic heart disease, cerebrovascular disease, and pulmonary dysfunction. The clinical examination should seek evidence of systemic hypertension, lung pathology and renal dysfunction which may be present if there is involvement of the renal arteries in the aneurysm. Allen's test is performed to assess adequacy of radial and ulnar arteries in anticipation of cannulation of the radial artery for direct measurement of arterial pressure. It is normal practice to prescribe a sedative premedication; atropine should be avoided if there is evidence of ischaemic heart disease.

On arrival in the anaesthetic room, the patient should be placed on a warming blanket, and arterial pressure measured. In patients with myocardial disease, direct intra-arterial pressure and e.c.g. monitoring should be instituted prior to induction of anaesthesia. Following preoxygenation, induction is carried out by slow injection of an anaesthetic agent. After muscle relaxation, the trachea is intubated (see below) and IPPV continued using humidified gases.

The following procedures are performed before surgery commences:

1. E.c.g. monitoring.
2. Intravenous cannulation with at least one 14 G cannula for infusion of warmed fluids.
3. Cannulation of radial artery for direct measurement of arterial pressure.
4. Central venous catheterisation for measurement of right atrial pressure.
5. An oesophageal or tympanic membrane temperature probe is placed in position.
6. Bladder catheterisation for monitoring of urine output.

Stress points

There are four specific points during anaesthesia for this operation when there is maximum stress to the patient.

1. *Endotracheal intubation.* The increase in systemic arterial pressure which accompanies endotracheal intubation and which can be of considerable magnitude, must be minimised to avoid myocardial damage. Attenuation of this response may be achieved by the i.v. administration of β-blockers, or high doses of opioids (e.g. fentanyl 10 μg/kg) prior to intubation. Topical anaesthesia to the larynx prior to intubation is *not* effective.

2. *Cross-clamping of the aorta.* Clamping of the aorta causes a sharp increase in peripheral vascular resistance and afterload. This increases cardiac work, which may result in myocardial ischaemia, arrhythmias and ventricular failure.

3. *Aortic declamping.* Unclamping the aorta causes a sudden decrease in afterload and reperfusion of the lower part of the body. Acid metabolites may enter the circulation causing vasodilatation and metabolic acidosis. Bleeding is a problem throughout the operation, but may be particularly severe at this time as the adequacy of vascular anastomoses is tested. These factors may result in severe hypotension unless circulating volume has been well maintained, and transfusion is continued to maintain an adequate CVP.

4. *The postoperative period*. There is some controversy over the issue of postoperative artificial ventilation in patients who have undergone elective repair of an aortic aneurysm. It is the author's opinion that unless there is severe impairment of pulmonary or myocardial function, such patients do not require elective artificial ventilation in the postoperative period. However, they do require close monitoring of the cardiovascular system, particularly during the first 12–24 h, as vasodilatation occurs in response to increasing body temperature. In addition there may be continued oozing of blood from anastomoses. A satisfactory degree of nursing care is usually available only in a high dependency or intensive care unit.

Emergency repair of abdominal aortic aneurysm

The principles of management are similar to those above. However, the patient is likely to be grossly hypovolaemic and often arterial pressure is maintained only by the tone of the abdominal muscles, causing constriction of the vena cava. All monitoring lines and two i.v. cannulae are inserted under local anaesthesia, while the patient breathes 100% oxygen in the operating theatre. The surgeon then prepares and towels the patient ready for surgery and it is only at this point that anaesthesia is induced. When muscle relaxation occurs, the systemic arterial pressure may decrease precipitously and immediate laparotomy and aortic clamping may be required. Thereafter the procedure is similar to that for elective repair.

The prognosis is poor in this condition for several reasons: there has been no preoperative preparation and the patient may be suffering from concurrent illnesses. He may have undergone a period of severe hypotension, resulting in impairment of renal, cerebral or myocardial function. He may require a massive blood transfusion, which in itself carries significant risks (see p. 405). In addition, postoperative jaundice is common because of haemolysis of damaged red cells in the circulation and of the large retroperitoneal haematoma which usually results from aortic rupture.

Other vascular procedures

Patients suffering from atherosclerotic arterial disease may present with limb or buttock ischaemic pain. Many are heavy smokers and suffer from pulmonary disease, resulting in dyspnoea, productive cough and polycythaemia.

Aortic bifurcation graft

This operation is performed to overcome occlusion in the aorta and iliac arteries and restore flow to the lower limbs. It must be assumed that all patients have widespread arterial disease, even in the presence of a normal e.c.g. Anaesthetic management is similar to that required for surgery of aortic aneurysm. It is normal surgical practice where possible to sideclamp the aorta, maintaining some peripheral flow and to declamp the arteries supplying the legs in sequence; the metabolic changes and hypotension are thus less severe than those seen during aneurysm surgery.

Peripheral arterial surgery

The commonest peripheral arterial grafts inserted are those between axillary and femoral or femoral and popliteal arteries. Because of the prolonged nature of these operations, an IPPV/relaxant anaesthetic technique should be used. Extradural anaesthesia is a useful adjunct, although heparin is often administered i.v. during vascular operations (vide infra), and this may increase the risk of an extradural haematoma if a catheter has been introduced into the extradural space.

Carotid artery surgery

Carotid endarterectomy or subclavian bypass are performed to relieve the symptoms of cerebral ischaemia caused by carotid artery obstruction. The underlying pathology is usually atherosclerosis, which presents typically in elderly hypertensive patients. Cerebral autoregulation is deficient and cerebral blood flow tends to be proportional to systemic arterial pressure.

During surgery the carotid artery is clamped and cerebral perfusion is dependent on collateral circulation. There is a high risk of dislodging atheromatous plaques, with consequent embolisation. Maintenance of perfusion of the brain is achieved by maintenance of a moderately high systemic arterial pressure (up to 170 mmHg systolic), an increased Pa_{O_2}, and a Pa_{CO_2} which is slightly less than normal.

These requirements may be achieved by mild hyperventilation of the lungs using an inspired oxygen concentration of 50% in nitrous oxide (100% inspired oxygen induces cerebral vasoconstriction) and the administration of pancuronium to achieve muscle relaxation. An arterial cannula for pressure monitoring and for sampling for blood gas analysis is mandatory. Under no circumstances must hypotension be allowed to develop. Following surgery, an early assessment of cerebral function is required and residual anaesthetic effects may confuse the diagnosis of intraoperative embolism or ischaemic change. Approx. 30% of patients require control of postoperative hypertension, which may otherwise compromise the graft or cause intracranial haemorrhage. An infusion of trimetaphan, hydralazine or sodium nitroprusside may be required for this purpose.

Heparin

Centres in the U.K. differ in the use of heparin during vascular surgery. In units where it is used systemically, a dose of 100 units/kg is given i.v. after preclotting the graft (where material such as Dacron is used) and at least one circulation time should elapse before arterial clamping begins. Some vascular surgeons rely solely on the local use of heparinised saline. If i.v. heparin has been employed, the anaesthetist may be asked to give protamine (0.5 mg/100 units heparin) before the termination of surgery.

PLASTIC SURGERY

The term 'plastic surgery' is used to describe procedures involving reconstitution of damaged or deformed tissues, the removal of cutaneous tumours and cosmetic alteration of body features. Tissue may be deformed as a result or trauma, burns, infection or congenital abnormality. Division or removal of the abnormality often results in skin cover defects. Major plastic surgery includes the formation and repositioning of free and pedicle grafts and the movement of skin flaps.

There are several important features common to many of the operations. The patient may be grossly deformed as a result of previous trauma or serious disease, and attention must be directed to the patient's psychological state, which is influenced by long periods of confinement and rehabilitation, occasionally chronic pain and concern over disfigurement or loss of limb function. Preoperative drug therapy must be controlled carefully and attention paid to removal of local or generalised infection, the state of nutrition and the haematocrit, all of which are important factors in the outcome of this form of surgery. Cosmetic surgery of the face, tattoo removal, breast augmentation and removal of unwanted adipose tissue are performed usually on healthy patients.

Haemorrhage is a common occurrence during plastic surgery and all but the most minor operations may require blood transfusion. Operations may last many hours, especially those involving vascular reconstruction, and care must be taken to position the patient in such a way that ligament strain and pressure on skin over bony prominences are avoided. The use of lumbar support and soft padding minimises those risks. When surgery has been completed, wound dressing and bandaging may be lengthy procedures. It is common for bandages to be applied round the trunk, and the patient must be lifted carefully during this procedure to avoid injury. Finally, there may be severe postoperative pain, especially from donor skin graft sites.

Head and neck

For surgery in this area tracheal intubation is mandatory using a reinforced tube. It is important to protect the eyes from pressure, the ears from blood and other fluids, and the teeth and anaesthetic tubing from dislodgment. It may be difficult to monitor chest movement and access to the arms may be impossible. An i.v. infusion with extension is essential with a three-way tap accessible for injection of drugs. A foot should be exposed to allow the anaesthetist to monitor colour, capillary filling and arterial pulse. Venous drainage should be adequate with the patient horizontal, although some anaesthetists prefer to position the patient in a 10–15° head-up tilt in an attempt to reduce bleeding from the scalp, which may be profuse.

The anaesthetist must anticipate difficult intubation and have a complete range of equipment available. Tumours or scarring of the neck, deformity of facial bones and cleft palate make endotracheal intubation particularly awkward. Use of muscle relaxants before intubation in such patients may be unwise and the anaesthetist should consider intubating the trachea using local anaesthesia with the patient awake, or inducing general anaesthesia with an inhalational technique. Selection of the method of maintenance will be determined by the condition of the patient, the type and duration of surgery and the experience and preference of the anaesthetist. Hypotensive techniques are employed frequently (see Chapter 35).

Limbs

Local anaesthesia may be advantageous for surgery of upper or lower limbs. However, Bier's block is of limited value since the surgeon often requires cuff deflation to identify bleeding points. The duration of some plastic operations may preclude local techniques, although prolonged neural blockade can be achieved by repeated injection (e.g. through an extradural catheter) or by employing an agent with a prolonged duration of action (e.g. etidocaine or bupivacaine). In order to help the patient endure prolonged immobility on the operating table, sedative drugs or even light general anaesthesia may be required. Specific nerve blocks may be useful. For example, blockade of the femoral and lateral cutaneous nerve of thigh provides analgesia for skin graft donor sites during and after operation.

Trunk

Problems encountered as a result of surgery of the trunk include the adoption of unusual postures and its attendant risks, haemorrhage, prolonged operation and restrictive dressings applied after surgery.

Burns

Hypoxia is the principal cause of rapid death in victims of fire. This may result either from reduction in inspired oxygen concentration in a smoke-filled atmosphere or poisoning by products of combustion. Carbon monoxide has an affinity for haemoglobin over 200 times greater than that of oxygen and even low concentrations cause reduced oxygen carriage in the blood. In addition, there may be direct thermal injury of the airway resulting in ciliary damage, mucosal oedema, surfactant depression and epithelial destruction. These may result in mucosal sloughing and alveolar oedema.

It is not sufficient simply to replace fluid loss in the emergency management of the patient with burns. Account must be taken of disturbances in both ventilation and perfusion and a knowledge of $\dot{V}/\dot{Q}$ mismatch is essential when preparing such patients for emergency surgery. The aim of immediate treatment is to secure the airway and administer 100% oxygen; this may require endotracheal intubation and IPPV until the Pa_{O_2} is adequate. Such patients require humidification of inspired gas, physiotherapy, and bronchial suction. Bronchodilation and PEEP may be necessary.

Burning of flesh produces rapid fluid shifts and formation of tissue oedema, particularly during the first 36 h. The resulting depletion of intravascular volume is greatest in the first few hours and it is essential to commence a fluid replacement regimen as early as possible in order to avoid acute renal failure. An example of a suitable regimen is shown in Table 34.1.

Table 34.1   Fluid regimen for burned patients

1. Estimate/measure weight.
2. Estimate % area of burns using 'rule of nines' for adults (and 'rule of tens' for children)
3. >15% burns (adults) >10% burns (children) — transfusion. Measure:
   haematocrit
   Hb
   electrolytes
   pulse and BP
4. Give fluid replacement (*at least* $\frac{1}{2}$ as plasma) according to *Muir and Barclay*:
   $\dfrac{kg \times \% \; burns}{2}$ ml in each of the six periods from time of burning
   1. 0– 4 h
   2. 4– 8 h
   3. 8–12 h
   4. 12–18 h
   5. 18–24 h
   6. 24–36 h
5. Extensive full thickness burns will require some of the above fluid as whole blood

It should be noted that initially, while there is increased capillary permeability, transfusion of whole blood increases the haematocrit and blood viscosity, thereby impairing perfusion and oxygen supply to the tissues. The hormonal response to burning results in a hypercatabolic state with tachycardia, hyperpnoea and hyperpyrexia.

Once the eschar has formed, there is pure water loss from the body surface with a resultant increase in aldosterone levels. The patient is at risk from water depletion and relative sodium overload. In addition, there is a rapid increase in serum potassium and urea concentrations (caused by release from damaged tissue) and haemolysis, and this is accentuated by acidosis due to infection. In the natural course of recovery there is kalliuresis and anaemia resulting from continuing haemolysis of red cells.

The anaesthetist may be involved with the burns victim at an early stage when hypoxaemia is life-threatening, but it is rare for general anaesthesia to be required before adequate resuscitation has taken place. When fluid balance is restored, hyper-alimentation instituted and 'nonburns' trauma treated, the patient embarks on what may be a prolonged period of surgical treatment requiring multiple administration of general anaesthesia, provision of strong analgesics for changes of dressings, and psychological support.

Anaesthetic problems

Thermal damage to the head and neck of a patient may provide the anaesthetist with a severe test of his ability. In the initial stages, raw and painful tissues may prohibit application of a face mask, while rapid induction incorporating a depolarising relaxant may be inadvisable (vide infra). Later, as soft tissues fibrose and distort, the range of movement in the neck and temporomandibular joints may be grossly restricted rendering laryngoscopic intubation impossible. Thus, the principal problems are difficult intubation and the need for repeated anaesthesia. Tracheostomy may be possible, but is regarded generally as undesirable, mainly because of the risk of infection spreading to damaged skin. Awake intubation may be necessary. Choice of anaesthetic agent is governed by personal preference and the knowledge that repeated administration of certain volatile agents may result in hepatic damage.

Burns dressings

Dressing of a burned area may be very painful and is performed frequently in the early stages, especially in the presence of infection. Several analgesic techniques have been described, which, if to be

successful, are often dependent upon the enthusiasm of the anaesthetist and the nursing staff.

1. *Intravenous administration of strong analgesics.* This should be accompanied by close monitoring for development of respiratory depression. Nausea and vomiting are frequent complications. A combination of an opioid and butyrophenone may be useful.

2. *Entonox.* Nitrous oxide provides good though moderate analgesia. It is administered normally via a face mask and demand valve.

3. *Ketamine.* This is a powerful analgesic in subanaesthetic doses and may be administered i.v. or i.m. It is not safe to assume that the airway is preserved during its administration and it is wise to premedicate with an antisialagogue. Severe dysphoria and hallucinations are not uncommon during recovery and may preclude the use of the drug.

4. *Volatile inhalational anaesthetic agents.* Methoxyflurane and trichloroethylene provide good analgesia, but their physical properties result in prolonged recovery and may interfere with the actions of other drugs. Enflurane may be useful. These agents are administered in air using a draw-over vaporiser.

Suxamethonium

In the presence of muscle damage such as that occurring in burns victims, this drug may cause an increase in plasma potassium concentration in excess of 0.6 mmol/litre. Although the increase is transient, it may result in cardiac arrest. The most dangerous period in this respect is between 3 and 10 weeks following thermal injury. If cardiac arrest does occur, resuscitation is usually effective because the hyperkalaemia is transient.

ANAESTHESIA FOR GYNAECOLOGICAL SURGERY

Either the lithotomy or Trendelenburg position is necessary for most gynaecological procedures, and these positions may have adverse respiratory and cardiovascular effects. In both positions, respiratory excursions are limited by restriction of diaphragmatic movement, a disadvantage exaggerated in the obese, and a potential cause of hypercapnia. Any concomitant reduction in functional residual capacity induced by these positions may result in dependent airway collapse and hypoxaemia, thus reducing further the efficiency of respiratory gas exchange. On completion of surgery, removal of the patient's legs from the lithotomy stirrups, or resumption of the supine position from Trendelenburg, results in pooling of blood in the extremities, thus reducing venous return. The resultant decrease in cardiac output and hypotension may occasionally be clinically significant. It should be apparent that all changes in body position must be accomplished gradually and gently if these untoward effects are to be avoided.

Minor procedures

Dilatation and curettage (D and C), vaginal termination of pregnancy and evacuation of retained products of conception (ERPC) are common minor procedures requiring anaesthesia. All involve dilatation of the cervix, a painful stimulus associated with reflex changes including laryngospasm and bradycardia if a relatively deep plane of anaesthesia has not been achieved.

During D and C, blood loss is not a problem, uterine relaxation is permissible, and mask anaesthesia with N_2O and O_2 supplemented with halothane 1–2% or enflurane 1.5%–3% is satisfactory. Fentanyl 75 μg at induction results in a smoother anaesthetic.

During termination of pregnancy, haemorrhage is the major complication. As vigorous uterine contraction is necessary after expulsion of the conceptus, high inspired concentrations of volatile agents, which cause profound uterine relaxation, are contraindicated. A commonly employed technique involves fentanyl 1 μg/kg followed by a sleep dose of methohexitone, and inhalation of N_2O and O_2. Anaesthesia is maintained with N_2O and O_2 and increments of methohexitone 10–20 mg. Syntocinon 5 units is administered i.v. when the uterus has been cleared and this aids uterine contraction.

Similar anaesthetic considerations apply to evacuation of retained products of conception, which is often necessary after spontaneous abortion. In these patients, however, preoperative blood loss may be significant and, as the procedure is performed as an emergency, there may be considerable gastric residue.

Although the i.v. technique described above is often suitable, hypovolaemia, obesity and the likelihood of aspiration may render a technique employing endotracheal intubation and light anaesthesia with muscle relaxation more appropriate. If intermittent suxamethonium is used, administration of atropine is mandatory before the second dose of suxamethonium.

Laparoscopy

This procedure permits visual inspection of the abdominal cavity using a telescope passed through a small incision in the abdominal wall. For safe insertion of the telescope, preliminary induction of a pneumoperitoneum is necessary. This is accomplished by insufflating either CO_2 or N_2O into the peritoneal cavity through a Verres' needle. The gas is introduced at a rate not exceeding 4 litre/min and adequate abdominal distension is obtained with a total of 3–5 litre.

Most of the problems associated with this procedure are related to the CO_2 pneumoperitoneum. These include:

1. Reduced thoracic compliance from diaphragmatic splinting.
2. Inferior vena caval compression from increased intraperitoneal pressure (especially if intraperitoneal pressure is greater than 50 cmH_2O).
3. Hypercapnia from CO_2 accumulation.

Most of these adverse effects are overcome to some extent by an anaesthetic technique employing endotracheal intubation and mild hyperventilation. It should be noted that gastric dilatation caused by overenthusiastic manual mask ventilation may increase the likelihood of gastric perforation by the laparoscope or trocar, and therefore intubation may best be accomplished using suxamethonium so that mask ventilation can be minimised. Whatever technique is used, careful monitoring of the circulation is essential, together with monitoring of intraperitoneal pressure, which should not be allowed to exceed 30 cmH_2O. Immediate deflation of the pneumoperitoneum is warranted if hypotension occurs as a result of inferior vena caval compression, a problem more likely to occur in hypovolaemic patients (e.g. suspected ruptured ectopic pregnancy).

Other rare complications of laparoscopy include gas embolism (sometimes a problem if N_2O is used as the inflating gas), haemorrhage, mediastinal emphysema, pneumothorax and perforation of an abdominal viscus.

Major procedures

Total abdominal hysterectomy and salpingo-oophorectomy are standard abdominal procedures, and a balanced technique involving muscle paralysis and controlled ventilation is suitable although some authorities employ lumbar extradural block in combination with light general anaesthesia and spontaneous ventilation. During hysterectomy blood loss may be considerable and blood should be cross-matched for these patients, who may be anaemic preoperatively.

Pelvic floor repair and vaginal hysterectomy may also result in considerable bleeding, and lumbar extradural or caudal block plus light general anaesthesia or sedation may improve surgical conditions. Alternatively a balanced technique with controlled ventilation may be employed. Some gynaecologists insist on infiltrating adrenaline locally, and in these cases, the use of halothane should be avoided.

Emergency laparoscopy or laparotomy is often necessary for suspected rupture of a tubal pregnancy. Patients with a suspected tubal pregnancy should be anaesthetised with the utmost caution as catastrophic haemorrhage may occur. Patients may complain only of trivial lower abdominal pain, or be in a state of near exsanguination. Even if volaemic status is judged to be normal a large-gauge i.v. cannula should be inserted prior to induction of anaesthesia and the status of the circulation monitored closely. A 'crash induction' technique with controlled ventilation is appropriate in most patients but those with profound cardiovascular collapse represent a major anaesthetic challenge. These patients may exsanguinate very quickly and resuscitation may be impossible until bleeding has been stemmed surgically (clamping of the internal iliac artery may be necessary). Consequently, it may be necessary to induce anaesthesia in a hypovolaemic patient, and definitive resuscitation performed after surgical haemostasis has been secured. Two large-gauge cannulae are inserted i.v. and colloid given as necessary. As sudden reduction in abdominal muscle tone may result in even more profound haemodynamic compromise,

anaesthesia should be induced in theatre, with the patient towelled and the surgeons gowned. Appropriate monitoring is instituted and after a period of preoxygenation ketamine 0.5–2.0 mg/kg is given i.v. followed by suxamethonium. Anaesthetic agents may be introduced gradually as the patient's circulatory status allows. These otherwise healthy patients should respond quickly to transfusion once the bleeding vessel has been clamped.

RADIOLOGY

It is common for the radiology department to be far removed geographically from the theatre suite, recovery room and intensive care unit, and to be supplied with outdated anaesthetic equipment unwanted in other departments. This, coupled with an unfamiliar environment, poor lighting, or in some instances, near total darkness, may render the anaesthetist's task hazardous.

It is essential to inspect the diagnostic room for the siting of suction, spare laryngoscope blades and batteries, e.t. tubes, spare gas cylinders (only the most modern suites have piped gases), e.c.g. monitor and defibrillator. The anaesthetic machine should be checked by the anaesthetist and only full cylinders used; in a darkened room it may be difficult to spot a rapidly decreasing nitrous oxide pressure. The ventilator should be of a type familiar to the anaesthetist.

Anaesthesia is required for some diagnostic procedures because total immobility may be necessary, and pain may be experienced when certain radio-opaque dyes are injected.

Unusual posturing of the patient may be required either to obtain access to the organ or vessel under investigation, or to obtain satisfactory radiographs, e.g.

1. Translumbar aortography is performed with the patient in the prone position.
2. Bronchography requires a changing posture to permit views of the different pulmonary lobes.
3. Air encephalography is carried out with the patient seated.

Monitoring of vital systems may prove difficult because of inadequate lighting, a moving patient (e.g.

for serial radiography of vasculature of the legs) and restricted access (e.g. during whole body CAT scanning). E.c.g. monitoring is mandatory, and the arterial pressure may be measured by manual or automated sphygmomanometer. Access to a vein should be maintained by an i.v. infusion.

Techniques

Air encephalography. During this procedure, air is injected by lumbar puncture into the c.s.f., and allowed to rise to outline the cerebral ventricles. If the patient is able to sit immobile, mild sedation and local anaesthesia are sufficient for the lumbar puncture. If not, spontaneous breathing using volatile inhalational agents or i.v. neurolept drugs may be considered if intracranial pressure is not raised. A relaxant/IPPV technique is required if intracranial pressure is elevated. An anaesthetised patient is very susceptible to hypotension when placed in the seated position, because of venous pooling. This may be minimised by binding the legs with elastic hosiery, but careful monitoring of arterial pressure and pulse rate is important to ensure that cerebral perfusion is maintained.

Carotid angiography. A relaxant/IPPV technique is used to provide moderate hypocapnia, as a low Pa_{CO_2} tends to constrict normal arteries (in contrast to diseased vessels) and provides radiographs of improved definition. It is important not to decrease Pa_{CO_2} excessively, particularly in patients with a history of cerebral ischaemia.

Abdominal aortography. Translumbar aortography is unpleasant for the patient, but with new, painless dyes, may be performed under local anaesthesia with sedation to help the patient lie still. When general anaesthesia is required, the underlying condition of widespread arterial disease may prove hazardous. Most patients undergoing this investigation are smokers, and are likely to have significant pulmonary pathology.

CAT scanning. Scanning 'slices' of 20 s and, in newer machines, of 4 s, require an absolutely immobile patient. During whole body scanning, apnoea may be required during each 'slice'. General anaesthesia is therefore necessary for young children and unco-operative adults. There may be some distance between the patient and anaesthetic machine with consequent risk of disconnection of circuits.

During exposure the anaesthetist shelters behind lead windows and visual monitors and alarms should therefore be used.

Bronchography. Movement and coughing can mar the results of bronchography and general anaesthesia is often used in children. Spontaneous breathing is usually requested and the patient is required to adopt different postures (see Chapter 28).

ORTHOPAEDIC SURGERY

Orthopaedic surgery is performed principally on the limbs and spine to repair trauma or to correct deformity and dysfunction in diseased tissues. Although the anaesthetic requirements overlap, it is convenient to divide the subject into the following categories.

Trauma

There are two indications for the immediate surgical treatment of fractures. These are:

(a) Concurrent vascular damage which may cause haemorrhage or lead to ischaemia and subsequent development of gangrene.

(b) The risk of infection in a compound wound, which increases as time elapses.

Choice of anaesthesia for emergency orthopaedic surgery is determined by the condition of the patient and nature of the fracture. Local techniques are eminently suitable for operations on or distal to the elbow or knee joints. The skill of the practitioner and the co-operation of the patient are important. Ideally, general anaesthesia should be administered to a patient with an empty stomach and haemodynamic stability. It is important to assess the patient's general condition, and to consider the possibility of hidden blood loss and injury to the head or body cavities. The decision to operate is reached jointly between surgeon and anaesthetist, consideration being given to the surgical problems and the possibility of improvement in the patient's overall condition before surgery.

Disease

Connective tissue disorders, inflammation and the arthritides may cause disruption of joints and muscles. It is not uncommon for these diseases to affect vital organs, and concurrent medical conditions must be sought and treated preoperatively where possible. The nature of many orthopaedic operations demands a relatively fit patient in the immediate postoperative period, e.g. to exercise a joint, to learn to walk with aids or to build up wasted muscles.

Posture

Variations from the supine are required for many orthopaedic operations and there is an increased risk of damaging the patient accidentally.

Skin, muscles and skeleton. Injury to superficial nerves, eyes, pressure areas, hair and genitalia may occur in any anaesthetised patient. Those with backache may suffer severe pain after short periods in a relaxed supine posture. Positioning of limbs or turning the patient increase risks of joint dislocation, stretching nerve plexuses or overstressing the spine.

Lungs and cardiovascular system. The effects of abnormal postures on intra-abdominal pressure and the diaphragm influence the choice of anaesthetic. Spontaneous respiration may be unsuitable in obese patients with a flexed spine because of the resultant reduction in vital capacity. In the lateral position the dependent lung receives a greater proportion of the cardiac output but is not as well ventilated. During IPPV also in the lateral position, the dependent lung tends to be underventilated. (See p. 370.)

Tourniquets

Surgery of the limbs is facilitated by a bloodless field and the use of tourniquets is common. Correctly used, tourniquets are safe, but they are capable of inflicting serious injury. Frequent servicing is mandatory to ensure pressure gauge accuracy and absence of leaks. Application of certain rules improves their clinical safety:

1. Tourniquets are contraindicated in the presence of HbS.
2. Inflation time should never exceed 2 h.
3. Suitable occlusion pressures in the normotensive patient with average sized limbs are:

      arm — systolic arterial pressure + 50 mmHg
      leg — twice the systolic arterial pressure.

Many tourniquets have indicators on the pressure gauge suggesting inflation to 250 mmHg and 500 mmHg for arm and leg respectively. These values are excessive for the normotensive patient.

Nerve and muscle damage due to mechanical disruption by an overinflated cuff may be irreversible.

4. Exsanguination by an Esmarch bandage causes an increase in CVP. Care must be exercised in those at risk from cardiac failure. An adequate bloodless field can often be obtained by simple elevation of the limb for 2–3 min.

5. Tourniquets should be applied only to the upper arm or thigh.

Local anaesthetic techniques

Intravenous regional anaesthesia and specific peripheral nerve blocks are suitable for surgery of the upper limb in the absence of infection. Extradural or subarachnoid blocks are useful for surgery of the hip and lower limb, although careful maintenance of haemodynamic balance is essential, particularly in the elderly patient.

General anaesthetic techniques

1. *I.v. agents for short procedures.* Manipulation of stiff joints and reduction of dislocations may be performed after a single dose of i.v. induction agent. It may be necessary to use a small dose of suxamethonium to provide a brief period of muscle relaxation. If this is required, the trachea should be intubated, and the lungs ventilated with an oxygen/nitrous oxide mixture until adequate spontaneous respiration has resumed.

2. *Spontaneous respiration with inhalational agents.* This technique is suitable for short procedures including meniscectomy, open reduction of fractures under tourniquet or surgery of soft tissues.

3. *Relaxant/IPPV.* For long or complex procedures, e.g. joint replacement, spinal operation, or major bone graft, a technique is preferred employing muscle relaxants and IPPV using nitrous oxide in oxygen, supplemented either by a volatile anaesthetic agent or an opioid analgesic.

A local block combined with a general anaesthetic may result in excellent operating conditions and profound analgesia in the immediate postoperative period.

Special problems associated with orthopaedic surgery

1. Insertion of orthopaedic cement into long bones during prosthetic joint surgery may cause fat or air embolism, resulting in severe hypotension. Close monitoring of the cardiovascular system is mandatory. An oesophageal stethoscope may be used to aid detection of air embolism.

2. It may be necessary to induce anaesthesia while the patient is still in bed and surrounded by traction devices. Not all hospital beds may be tilted into Trendelenburg position. Subsequent movement on to the operating table can be hazardous.

3. Application of dressings or plaster of Paris casts and institution of traction are often required immediately after surgery, and anaesthesia may not be terminated until these have been completed.

SURGERY OF TUMOURS OF THE ENDOCRINE SYSTEM

APUD (amine precursor uptake and decarboxylation) cells are distributed widely throughout the body. Neoplastic change within these cells produces the group of tumours called apudomas. Their presence may be indicated by the inappropriate synthesis and secretion of polypeptides and amines. Apudomas may be orthoendocrine or paraendocrine; the former produce amines and polypeptides associated normally with the constituent cells, while the latter secrete substances usually produced by other organs. There are two orthoendocrine apudomas which may produce significant difficulty for the anaesthetist.

Carcinoid tumour

Carcinoid tumours arise in the enterochromaffin cells of the intestinal tract, are commonly benign and are found most often in the appendix. They may, however, occur anywhere in the gut and, rarely, in the gall bladder or bronchus. Malignant change, occurring in 4%, may give rise to resectable hepatic secondaries. The cells produce the following biologically active compounds:

1. *Serotonin* (5 hydroxytryptamine, 5HT), responsible for abnormal gut motility and diarrhoea and possibly for endocardial fibrosis which may result

in pulmonary and tricuspid stenosis. Serotonin also produces alterations in arterial pressure and hyperglycaemia.

2. *Kallikrein,* an enzyme which acts on circulating plasma kininogen to produce bradykinin. This is a vasodilator which causes flushing and may contribute to bronchospasm, hypotension and oedema.

3. *Prostaglandins,* which produce diarrhoea and facial flushing.

4. *Histamine,* which may produce profound hypotension.

These compounds are normally metabolised in the liver. It is only in circumstances where they escape the portal circulation (hepatic metastases, bronchial primary) that the clinical picture of carcinoid syndrome is seen. Diagnosis is confirmed by the high urinary excretion of 5 hydroxyindoleacetic acid (5 HIAA), a metabolite of 5HT (a level greater than 27 mg/day is diagnostic). Liver scan may show filling defects caused by secondary tumour.

Treatment

The definitive treatment of carcinoid tumours is surgical removal. Patients who present for operation may be taking drugs to control their symptoms (see Table 34.2).

Conduct of anaesthesia

Acute attacks of carcinoid syndrome may be precipitated by fear, hypotension and handling the tumour. The anaesthetist must be aware of the following factors:

1. Hypovolaemia and electrolyte imbalance may occur in patients with diarrhoea.

2. Adequate preoperative sedation with minimal cardiovascular disturbance is essential. Drugs known to release histamine should be avoided. A sedative with antihistamine properties (e.g. promethazine) is suitable.

3. Techniques including extradural block or SAB, which may cause hypotension, should be avoided.

4. The anaesthetist must be prepared for the sudden appearance of bronchospasm, arrhythmias and extreme fluctuations in arterial pressure. Continuous e.c.g. and arterial pressure monitoring are mandatory. Bronchospasm may be particularly resistant to treatment.

Table 34.2 Drugs used in the management of carcinoid syndrome

Compounds produced in carcinoid tumours	Possible pharmacological treatment prior to surgery

5-Hydroxytryptamine (5HT, serotonin)
Bradykinin (following kallikrein activation)
Histamine (esp. gastric carcinoid)
? Prostaglandins
? Neurotensin
? Substance P
? Enteroglucagon
	1. Nicotinamide for associated pellagra
	
	2. Codeine phosphate
	    Diphenoxylate/atropine (Lomotil) } for 5HT induced diarrhoea
	    Loperamide
	
	3. Cyproheptadine } specific 5HT antagonists
	    Methysergide } (NB: methysergide and associated retroperitoneal fibrosis)
	
	4. Phenoxybenzamine
	    or Phenothiazines with α-adrenergic blocking activity } to control flushing
	    (e.g. chlorpromazine)
	
	5. Parachlorophenylalanine — tryptophan hydroxylase inhibitor
	    (NB: high incidence allergic reaction)
	
	6. Antihistamines. H_1 + H_2 receptor blockers — esp. in gastric carcinoid
	
	7. Somatostatin — continuous i.v. infusion — do not stop before surgery

* DO NOT GIVE CATECHOLAMINES *
If vasopressor needed use, e.g. methoxamine

5. Drugs known to release histamine (e.g. curare or morphine) should be avoided. Volatile anaesthetics may prolong recovery time and their use can be hazardous in the presence of valvular lesions.

A suitable technique would include:

Premedication: promethazine, diazepam or droperidol.
Induction: neuroleptanalgesic agents.
Intubation: pancuronium with topical anaesthesia of the vocal cords.
IPPV: using a flow generator capable of overcoming severe bronchospasm.
Monitoring: e.c.g. and direct arterial pressure. Methotrimeprazine 2.5 mg i.v. (or α-blocking drugs) may be used to control hypertensive episodes.
Postoperative: care in a high dependency or intensive therapy unit.

Phaeochromocytoma

In 80% of these apudomas, arising in the phaeochromocytes of the adrenal medulla, adrenaline is the principal hormonal secretion. The remaining 20%, which may appear in the adrenal medulla or any sympathetic ganglion, produce mainly noradrenaline. The symptoms and signs of the disease are shown in Table 34.3 and result from high circulating levels of

Table 34.3 Common symptoms and signs associated with phaeochromocytoma

Symptoms	Clinical signs
Palpitations	Hypertension, paroxysmal or sustained
Headache	Increased basal metabolism and oxygen
Blurred vision	consumption
Fits	Increased blood concentrations of
Pallor	glucose, lactic acid and free fatty acids
Sweating	Haemoconcentration
	Retinopathy
	Renal pathology

these catecholamines. Hypertension is typically paroxysmal but may be continuous.

Diagnosis is confirmed by measurement of plasma catecholamine concentrations or of urinary excretion rates of catecholamines, or of their metabolite 3-methoxy-4-hydroxy-mandelic acid. The tumour(s) may be localised by selective arteriography following α-adrenergic blockade or by CAT scan. Treatment is by surgical removal of all tumour tissue.

The problems facing the anaesthetist are those resulting from high circulating catecholamine concentrations and the perioperative management is determined by two important factors:

1. There is arteriolar constriction with increased systemic arterial pressure *and* venous constriction with a reduced blood volume.

2. Handling the tumour during operation may dramatically raise the catecholamine level in blood, while clamping the venous drainage of the tumour quickly decreases their concentrations. There may therefore be rapid fluctuations in arterial pressure during and immediately after removal of the tumour.

Conduct of anaesthesia

Preoperative drug therapy is employed in order to control hypertension. Phentolamine or phenoxybenzamine is prescribed for several days prior to surgery. These α-adrenergic blockers result in vasodilatation, causing hypotension and reducing the ratio of blood volume to capacitance. An adequate blood volume must be maintained by infusion of fluid under CVP monitoring. Tachycardia may occur, and occasionally necessitates treatment with a β-adrenergic blocker. Treatment with α-methyl-paratyrosine, aimed at interfering with catecholamine synthesis, has also been used.

In anticipation of sudden changes in arterial pressure, monitoring should be instituted before induction of anaesthesia. E.c.g., central venous pressure and direct arterial pressure measurements are *mandatory*.

Premedication should provide sedation alone and agents used for induction and maintenance should be chosen to maintain cardiovascular stability.

Drugs to avoid include:

Atropine	Cyclopropane
Suxamethonium	Diethylether
Gallamine	Trichloroethylene
d-Tubocurarine	Intra/extradural blocking agents

A suitable technique is induction using neuroleptic drugs, followed by normocapnic IPPV using atracurium or vecuronium for muscle relaxation and an opioid for analgesic supplementation. A sodium nitroprusside infusion is probably the most useful method of controlling hypertension peroperatively. β-adrenergic blockade or lignocaine may be required for serious arrhythmias.

Following removal of the tumour, the capacitance volume increases and arterial pressure may decrease if adequate transfusion has not been maintained. With the use of preoperative adrenergic blockade, however, the once common requirement for a postexcision noradrenaline infusion seems to have been rendered unnecessary.

CARDIOVERSION AND ELECTROCONVULSIVE THERAPY

Anaesthesia is provided during cardioversion and electroconvulsive therapy to protect the patient from the unpleasant effects of electric shock. These may include pain and uncontrollable muscle spasm, though the current strengths differ and so, consequently, do the anaesthetic requirements. There are, however, features common to both.

Treatment should be carried out in areas specifically designed for the purpose with a full range of drugs, resuscitation and monitoring equipment available. This must be checked by the anaesthetist prior to every list. Patients should be prepared as for a surgical procedure.

Cardioversion

The technique is successful in converting atrial fibrillation, atrial flutter, supraventricular tachycardia or ventricular tachycardia to sinus rhythm, although maintenance of sinus rhythm depends usually on the subsequent use of antiarrhythmic drugs. Cardioversion is simple, has a low incidence of complications and has little effect on contractility, conductivity or excitability of the myocardium.

Patients may present with a chronic arrhythmia for elective conversion or as an emergency with an arrhythmia which is acutely life-threatening.

Preanaesthetic assessment

Patients may have serious pre-existing cardiovascular pathology including rheumatic disease, arteriosclerotic heart disease, myocardial infarction, congestive cardiac failure or cerebrovascular occlusive disease. Digitalis therapy predisposes to postcardioversion arrhythmias and should be withheld for at least 24 h prior to cardioversion. Accurate knowledge of the medical and drug history, and a thorough clinical examination are essential before selecting the type of anaesthesia. Preanaesthetic sedation, for example with pentobarbitone, reduces circulating endogenous catecholamines. Atropine should be avoided.

Anaesthesia

Insertion of an indwelling cannula and preoxygenation, together with institution of e.c.g. monitoring and measurement of arterial pressure, precede induction of anaesthesia using an i.v. agent. The choice of agent is determined by the cardiovascular stability and recovery period required.

Cardioversion

The attendant physician is responsible for passing a DC shock of from 50 J increasing stepwise to 400 J (duration 2.5 ms) through two paddles positioned on the patient's chest. Electrolyte jelly or saline-soaked gauze is used to prevent burns. The paddles may be sited anterolaterally when the patient is supine or anteroposteriorly with the patient in the lateral position. The shock is synchronised to the e.c.g. to avoid discharge during the initial portion of the T-wave. A shock at this time is liable to result in ventricular fibrillation. If the arrhythmia does not revert to sinus rhythm at the first attempt, further shocks of increasing energy are required and the anaesthetist must ensure continued oxygenation and supply further increments of anaesthetic agent to maintain insensibility.

After successful cardioversion, oxygen therapy is maintained until the patient is fully awake. During the next few hours the patient should be carefully monitored with particular regard to the development of hypotension, cardiac dilatation and pulmonary oedema, and systemic or pulmonary embolism.

Electroconvulsive therapy (e.c.t.)

The term 'e.c.t.' describes the precipitation of a grand mal convulsion by passage of an electric current through the brain. The therapeutic indications have become fewer in recent years as new and more effective drugs have been developed. The principal indication now is severe depression in patients who have failed to respond to tri- or tetracyclic antidepressants. In acute schizophrenia, e.c.t. may produce a transient improvement and there are occasional indications in other psychiatric illnesses.

A course of e.c.t. consists of 2–3 treatments per week over a period of 4–6 weeks. A shock of 30–45 J,

and of 0.5–1.5 s duration is employed, although the range of electrical resistance of the skull (200–500 Ω) results in considerable variation in stimulus to the brain. Only a small proportion of the current traverses the brain.

Passage of the current results in an initial widespread muscular spasm followed in 5–10 s by a typical clonic seizure. Cerebral blood flow is transiently but markedly increased and there are cardiovascular changes similar to those seen during the Valsalva manoeuvre.

Headache and confusion last for 1–2 h, but memory disturbance may persist for several weeks. Skeletal injuries, e.g. dislocated mandible, or clavicular and thoracic vertebral fractures, can occur if muscle relaxants are not employed.

Preanaesthetic assessment

A medical history should be elicited and physical examination performed before a course of treatment is started. The anaesthetist must be aware of the drug history and the patient's particular behavioural problems. While recent myocardial infarction, congestive cardiac failure, raised intracranial pressure and acute respiratory infection are contraindications, the presence of pacemakers, pregnancy or advanced age do not preclude e.c.t.

Anaesthetic techniques

The anaesthetic technique varies. In many centres, methohexitone 0.7–1 mg/kg is used to induce anaesthesia, and inhibition of muscle spasms is achieved by the administration of suxamethonium 0.5 mg/kg. Atropine 300–600 μg may be given i.v. to protect the heart from vagal discharge during the shock, or injected subcutaneously 30–60 min before e.c.t. to reduce secretions, or omitted completely. Thiopentone or other induction agents are favoured in some hospitals. Barbiturates raise seizure threshold; thus the minimum dose required to produce insensibility should be used. Following induction and paralysis, the patient is ventilated with 100% oxygen via a Mapleson C circuit. When the limbs are flaccid, a rubber gag is inserted between the teeth, the electrodes applied to the skull by the psychiatrist, and the current passed. During the seizure, the anaesthetist must ensure that the patient suffers no physical damage.

There is evidence to suggest that artificial ventilation during the fit prolongs the seizure, but cyanosis must be avoided in all circumstances. Ventilation after the fit should be provided to maintain normocapnia in order to avoid prolonging apnoea. When adequate spontaneous respiration has returned, the patient is moved to a recovery area.

FURTHER READING

Brown B R 1980 Anesthesia and the patient with endocrine disease. F A Davis, Philadelphia

Katz J, Benumof J, Kadis L B 1981 Anesthesia and uncommon diseases, 2nd edn. W B Saunders, Philadelphia

Kaufman L (ed) 1982 Anaesthesia review I. Churchill Livingstone, Edinburgh

Kaufman L, Sumner E 1979 Current topics in anaesthesia. Medical problems and the anaesthetist. Arnold, London

Loach A 1983 Anaesthesia for orthopaedic patients. Arnold, London

Muir, I F K, Barclay T L 1974 Burns and their treatment, 2nd edn. Lloyd-Luke, London

35

Hypotensive anaesthesia

Induced hypotension may be defined as the deliberate reduction of systemic arterial pressure in order to reduce bleeding and facilitate surgery. The technique was introduced into anaesthetic practice in the 1940s when few anaesthetic agents were available, spontaneous ventilation the norm, and uncontrolled hypertension common amongst surgical patients. As a result of the changes, both evident and theoretical, produced by this technique, the use of induced hypotension has been controversial since its introduction into clinical practice, but despite this, it has retained a place in modern anaesthesia.

A major source of difficulty in practising hypotensive anaesthesia is the inability to measure oxygen supply to vital organs. Arterial pressure is merely one index of perfusion and existing clinical monitors of the balance between oxygen supply and demand (e.c.g. for myocardium, c.f.m. for brain) are insensitive.

The indications for the use of this technique include:

1. Microsurgery, where small quantities of blood may obscure the operative field.

2. Major cancer surgery; a bloodless operative field facilitates clearance of tumour tissue.

3. When it is desirable to reduce the need for blood transfusion either as a result of its concomitant hazards, or because of patient's objections (Jehovah's Witnesses).

4. To improve the safety of vascular surgery by reducing the risk of haemorrhage and anastomotic disruption.

5. When it is desirable to reduce myocardial oxygen demand in situations when the supply is already compromised, e.g. hypertension in patients with ischaemic heart disease undergoing coronary artery bypass procedures.

In order to reduce systemic arterial pressure, the anaesthetist must interfere with the homeostatic control of the circulation. Arterial pressure is determined by intravascular volume, cardiac output and peripheral resistance. Peripheral resistance is controlled by the calibre of the resistance vessels, capacitance vessels playing a minor role. The intrinsic tone of these vessels may be altered by local metabolites, circulating catecholamines and the activity of the autonomic nerve system. A negative feedback loop exists which enables changes in arterial pressure to be detected by baroreceptors, which modify the level of sympathetic tone within the circulation. The vasomotor centre acts as the integrator of information.

The techniques for interfering with the physiological control of arterial pressure may be classified under three major headings:

1. Intravascular volume may be reduced by haemorrhage. This technique is dangerous and is only of historical interest.

2. Peripheral resistance may be reduced by blocking part of the negative feedback loop.

3. Cardiac output may be reduced.

In general, where a bloodless field is required, it is more appropriate to use a technique which reduces cardiac output. However, blood flow to the surgical field may be reduced by the judicious use of posture, and hypotension by drugs which have little *primary* effect on cardiac output. Where hypotension is utilised for vascular surgery (e.g. intracranial aneurysm), the objective is to reduce the *tension* (and therefore the risk of inadvertent rupture) of the vessel manipulated by the surgeon and indeed reduction in blood flow is of lesser importance unless there is unexpected haemorrhage.

REDUCTION OF PERIPHERAL RESISTANCE

The sympathetic reflex arc may be blocked at six discrete sites (Fig. 35.1).

1. Baroreceptors

A decrease in arterial pressure results normally in an increase in heart rate, mediated by the baroreceptor reflex. The baroreceptors operate over a discrete range of arterial pressure, and their sensitivity to changes in pressure may be reduced by the volatile anaesthetic agents (halothane in particular). Thus, lower levels of arterial pressure may be achieved when halothane is used without a compensatory increase in heart rate.

2. Vasomotor centre

All general anaesthetics depress the central nervous system resulting in a reduction in sympathetic tone and a decrease in arterial pressure.

3. Preganglionic sympathetic nerves

The preganglionic sympathetic nerve fibres (which leave the spinal cord from T1–L2) may be blocked by spinal or extradural analgesia. Blockade of all or part of the sympathetic outflow results in vasodilatation of both resistance and capacitance vessels, the latter promoting venous pooling which enhances the decrease in arterial pressure. The block produced by spinal analgesia is more predictable than that achieved with extradural blockade, and total spinal analgesia has been used to effect a bloodless field. Lesser degrees of blockade may be employed to produce both analgesia and systemic hypotension. Larger volumes of local anaesthetic drugs are required to achieve neural blockade when the extradural route is used and consequently systemic absorption of the local anaesthetic may contribute to the depression of the circulation. During general anaesthesia, both spinal and extradural analgesia produce more profound hypotension than that seen in the conscious patient.

4. Sympathetic ganglia

Transmission through sympathetic ganglia may be blocked by agents which compete with acetylcholine for the postsynaptic receptor sites. A reduction in

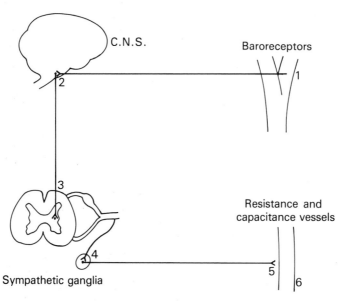

·**Fig. 35.1** Sites of actions of drugs inducing hypotension.

sympathetic tone results in venous pooling and systemic hypotension. All autonomic ganglia are blocked, and this may cause unwanted side effects including cycloplegia. As the arterial pressure decreases, compensatory tachycardia may be troublesome and tachyphylaxis occurs rapidly. Tachyphylaxis may be mediated by pathways through the ganglion which are not cholinergic and therefore not blocked by cholinergic antagonists. Histamine release may be an additional problem, causing profound hypotension and bronchospasm.

The ganglion-blocking drugs in current use include hexamethonium, pentolinium and trimetaphan. The last is administered as an i.v. infusion, since it has a short duration of action. It should be noted that the ganglion-blocked man is exquisitely sensitive to postural changes, which result in pooling of blood in the dilated vascular bed.

5. α-Adrenergic blocking drugs

The chemical transmitters at the postganglionic sympathetic nerve endings may be antagonised by the α-adrenergic blocking drugs. A common problem with the use of these drugs in the young adult is reflex tachycardia. Phentolamine is a short-acting competitive α-antagonist which may be useful during anaesthesia. Phenoxybenzamine produces a more prolonged blockade, and is reserved usually for the management of phaeochromocytoma. Labetalol (a mixed α-and β-antagonist in the ratio 3:7 respectively) has also been used to produce hypotension during anaesthesia, the β-blockade, which predominates, preventing the development of tachycardia.

6. Vessel wall

Several drugs which act as direct vasodilators may be used to induce hypotension. Some have actions which affect predominantly the resistance vessels (e.g. sodium nitroprusside — SNP), whilst others dilate the capacitance vessels (e.g. glyceryl trinitrate — GTN). Although many of these drugs could be used during anaesthesia, the most commonly employed for induced hypotension in general surgery is SNP. In patients with severe coronary artery disease, glyceryl trinitrate has been advocated as an alternative, particularly during coronary artery bypass procedures.

(a) Hydralazine dilates predominantly the resistance vessels, producing a reduction in vascular tone, which persists for up to 45 min when the drug is administered i.v. This drug is employed commonly for treatment of postoperative hypertension.

(b) Sodium nitroprusside (SNP) is a powerful, rapidly acting, smooth muscle relaxant. This property is attributed to the nitroso radicals which combine with the sulphydryl groupings on the cell membrane of the vessel wall. This interaction stabilises the membrane, and prevents the flux of ionised calcium which is necessary to activate the contractile mechanism in the smooth muscle. SNP acts predominantly upon small resistance vessels, the fourth order arterioles. Its evanescent action entails administration as a continous infusion. Once prepared, the solution is extremely unstable and it should be protected from light at all times.

General vasodilatation aids tissue perfusion, which may remain adequate to low levels of arterial pressure. Dilatation of cerebral vessels may cause an increase in intracranial pressure, and SNP should be used with caution in the presence of intracranial hypertension. This problem may be minimised by the slow administration of nitroprusside whilst at the same time reducing intracranial pressure by artificial hyperventilation. Rebound hypertension has been reported, and this has been attributed to the release of renin occurring during the period of hypotension.

Reflex tachycardia is marked, and this tends to maintain cardiac output. The increase in heart rate cannot be prevented completely by β-blockade, and this has led to the suggestion that SNP may have a direct action on the cardiac pacemaker.

Several deaths have been reported following the use of SNP, usually after the administration of excessive quantities. Figure 35.2 shows the possible routes of elimination of SNP from the body. If the rate of breakdown of sodium nitroprusside to cyanide exceeds the rate of removal of cyanide from the plasma, plasma cyanide concentration increases, cellular respiration is impaired and histotoxic hypoxia results. The total dose of SNP should be limited to 1.5 mg/kg body weight to avoid this complication. Recently, it has been suggested that the clinical dosage and potential toxicity of SNP may be reduced

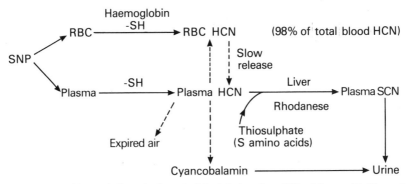

Fig. 35.2 Diagram of nitroprusside metabolism. At the end of the infusion about 98% of the cyanide liberated from the SNP is found in the red cells from which it is slowly released. The half-life of the plasma cyanide is about 30 min.

greatly by the use of a single infusion containing both SNP and trimetaphan.

(c) Glyceryl trinitrate (GTN) acts in a manner similar to SNP, stabilising the membrane and reducing vascular tone, but its action is more pronounced on capacitance vessels. The rate of onset of action is slightly slower than SNP and rebound hypertension is less marked. It may be given continuously as an infusion but it is absorbed onto plastics and polypropylene and should be administered using a glass syringe and pump. Cerebral blood flow is maintained by direct cerebral vasodilatation, but as with SNP, the increase in venous volume leads to an increase in intracranial pressure.

Drugs used to produce a reduction in peripheral resistance are listed in Table 35.1.

REDUCTION IN CARDIAC OUTPUT

Cardiac output is reduced either by a reduction in venous return, as occurs with venous pooling, or by a reduction in myocardial contractility. Thus, in general, when hypotension is produced by arteriolar dilatation as occurs with subarachnoid or extradural anaesthesia, ganglion blocking drugs and SNP (and to a lesser extent GTN), cardiac output is well maintained provided that the patient is not so postured as to produce marked pooling of blood in dependent capacitance vessels. Myocardial depressants, including β-blocking drugs and volatile anaesthetic agents, cause both hypotension and a reduction in cardiac output, leading to an *increase* in right atrial filling pressure.

1. β-Adrenergic blockade

β-adrenergic blockade results in both a decrease in heart rate and a reduction in myocardial contractility. The former action is particularly useful in an induced hypotensive technique as it reduces reflex tachycardia. The majority of β-blockers may be employed, but it is probably wise to use a cardiospecific drug.

Table 35.1 Drugs used for inducing hypotension

Drug	Formulation	Dosage	Duration of action
Trimetaphan	500 mg powder in 500 ml	Slow i.v. infusion of 0.1% solution	1–8 min
Sodium nitroprusside	50 mg in 500 ml in 5% dextrose, protected from light	Slow i.v. infusion of 0.01% solution	$\frac{1}{4}$–5 min
Pentolinium		10–20 mg i.v. 5–10 mg in elderly	5–45 min
Hexamethonium		10–40 mg i.v.	3–20 min
Nitroprusside/ trimetaphan combination	12.5 mg nitroprusside + 125 mg trimetaphan in 500 ml 5% dextose	Slow i.v. infusion	2–10 min
Glyceryl trinitrate	10 mg in 100 ml saline	Slow i.v. infusion of 0.01% solution	$\frac{1}{2}$–5 min

Table 35.2 β-blocking drugs employed by i.v. route in anaesthesia as adjuvants to hypotensive anaesthesia, for attenuation of hypertensive response to endotracheal intubation or in treatment of appropriate arrhythmias (ISA = Intrinsic sympathomimetic activity).

Drug	Intravenous dose (mg)	Plasma half-life (h)	ISA	Cardioselectivity	Membrane stabilising effect
Labetalol (30% α-blocking)	25–30	4	–	–	+
Metoprolol	1–2	3–4	–	+	+
Oxprenolol	1–2	2	+	–	+
Practolol	5–10		+	+	–
Propranolol	1–2	2–3	–	–	+

β-Blocking drugs which have been employed in anaesthesia are shown in Table 35.2.

2. Halothane

Halothane is a powerful direct myocardial depressant, producing a dose related decrease in arterial pressure. During spontaneous ventilation, cardiac output and arterial pressure tend to be maintained by the associated increase in Pa_{CO_2}. However, arterial pressure normally declines during spontaneous respiration and is often marked in the presence of bradycardia. Considerable improvement in arterial pressure is effected by the administration of atropine.

During controlled ventilation with hypocapnia, the use of halothane is associated with a profound reduction in cardiac output (peripheral resistance remaining unchanged, with consequent hypotension) and thus halothane should not be used as the sole agent for hypotensive techniques. In low concentrations, it is a useful adjuvant to other hypotensive techniques.

3. Calcium antagonists

Calcium antagonists have been used to produce hypotension during anaesthesia, but their value needs further assessment.

ADJUVANTS TO INDUCED HYPOTENSION

Posture

The importance of correct positioning must not be forgotten. There is a decrease in systemic pressure in sites elevated above the level of the heart (2 mmHg for every 2.5 cm). In addition, venous pooling occurs in dependent areas, and this may be enhanced by the use of vasodilating agents.

Intermittent positive pressure ventilation

IPPV reduces venous return by increasing mean intrathoracic pressure. The Pa_{CO_2} usually decreases during controlled ventilation, and this results in low levels of circulating endogenous catecholamines.

Good anaesthesia

Increased bleeding at the surgical site is produced by the patient coughing or straining, by an increased intrathoracic pressure (resulting from increased airway resistance e.g. kinked or inappropriately small endotracheal tube), by tachycardia (light anaesthesia) and by hypercapnia resulting from hypoventilation. Thus, induced hypotension must never become a substitute for good anaesthesia, with meticulous attention to oxygenation, carbon dioxide elimination and analgesia. A scheme for management of induced hypotension is shown in Table 35.3.

COMPLICATIONS OF INDUCED HYPOTENSION

A major disadvantage of induced hypotension is that tissue oxygenation may be impaired if arterial pressure is reduced excessively and autoregulation fails. It is therefore important to consider the requirements of the vital organs.

Brain

The brain has high energy requirements and little reserve, so that a reduction in supply of oxygenated blood may have disastrous consequences. Cerebral

Table 35.3 Scheme for inducing hypotension

Assessment	Avoid hypotensive anaesthesia in patients with severe cardiac, respiratory, cardiovascular or renal disease
Premedication	Avoid atropine Objective to produce well-sedated patient Phenothiazine useful
Induction	Thiopentone preferred induction agent Spray larynx with 4% lignocaine Tracheal intubation mandatory
Maintenance	IPPV with at least 50% O_2 in N_2O. Pa_{CO_2} 4 kPa (30 mmHg) dTC relaxant of choice Analgesic drugs to maintain good analgesia Halothane (up to 0.5%) or enflurane as required
Posture	Operation site should be elevated Head should *not* be elevated > 20°
Hypotensive agents	SNP, GTN, trimetaphan or hexamethonium β-blocker if tachycardia results
Monitoring	E.c.g. mandatory Peripheral pulse pick-up Arterial pressure — 1 min reading with Dinamap acceptable Direct arterial pressure recording mandatory if hypotension prolonged or gross — permits measurements of Pa_{O_2}, Pa_{CO_2}, pH
Recovery	O_2 mask, Fi_{O_2} 0.5 E.c.g. HR and arterial pressure Must not be discharged from recovery until arterial pressure restored to preinduction level

blood flow remains constant over a wide range of perfusion pressures (60–130 mmHg). The autoregulatory curve is shifted to the right in hypertensive subjects, and to the left when direct vasodilators (including SNP and GTN) are used.

Autoregulation may be lost completely following an insult to the brain; this includes a period of marked hypotension.

Experimental work suggests than when cerebral blood flow is reduced by 50%, ischaemic signs develop, and damage may be permanent. Patients with pre-existing cerebrovascular disease are less tolerant than normal subjects to this reduction in cerebral blood flow. Some degree of brain protection during hypotensive anaesthesia may be conferred by anaesthetic agents, including thiopentone and Althesin, both of which reduce cerebral metabolism. The level of tolerance varies not only with the patient, but also with the technique chosen. Direct vasodilator agents including SNP and GTN cause potent cerebral vasodilatation, thereby preserving cerebral blood flow to lower levels of arterial pressure.

Monitoring cerebral perfusion during general anaesthesia is difficult and various methods have been employed with limited success. Historically, spontaneous respiration was considered to be a sign of adequate perfusion of vital centres, but this view is no longer held. An approximate index of cerebral perfusion may be obtained by measurement of oxygen extraction by the brain from the oxygen content of jugular venous blood. The cerebral function monitor may be used to demonstrate severe global ischaemia. Despite the limitations of the currently available monitoring techniques, the frequency of reported mishaps remains small, although psychometric testing has shown evidence of temporary cerebral dysfunction following periods of moderate hypotension.

Heart

The myocardium may benefit from a modest reduction in arterial pressure, since myocardial oxygen requirements are also reduced. However, e.c.g. evidence of ischaemia may be detected with increasing frequency when the systolic arterial pressure is diminished below 60 mmHg. The hypertensive subject manifests these changes at higher systolic arterial pressures.

Kidneys

Renal perfusion and glomerular filtration are reduced when the systolic arterial pressure is reduced to levels below 80 mmHg. Oliguria is frequently seen, but is usually only temporary.

Lungs

Physiological dead space increases as arterial pressure decreases and thus meticulous control of ventilation and oxygenation is required. During induced hypotension, the Fl_{O_2} should not be less than 0.5.

Other

Other problems which may result from hypotensive anaesthesia include:

1. Reactionary haemorrhage.
2. Deep venous thrombosis.
3. Retraction anaemia — ischaemia of the brain produced by surgical retraction. This is magnified by hypotensive anaesthesia.

It is difficult to assess the increase in morbidity and mortality associated with induced hypotension. Lindop, using results pooled from several major surveys, suggested that 2.5% of all patients undergoing hypotensive anaesthesia suffer a nonfatal complication, although their causation is uncertain. Various factors increase morbidity and mortality, including poor patient selection and the hypotensive technique employed. Patients with pre-existing hypertension, cerebrovascular disease, hypovolaemia or anaemia are more likely to suffer complications. Hypotension achieved by myocardial depression results in more complications in comparison with other techniques. The complication rate also increases if the mean arterial pressure is reduced below 70 mmHg, the anaesthetist is inexperienced, and there is inadequate monitoring of the patient.

It is mandatory that arterial pressure is measured accurately and frequently, using intra-arterial pressure monitoring when rapid changes in arterial pressure are produced. The e.c.g. must be monitored continuously although it should be remembered that the band width used during anaesthesia is narrower than that of a diagnostic e.c.g. and ischaemic changes may be missed. Hypoxia must be avoided by increasing the Fl_{O_2} during the period of hypotension, and ventilation should be controlled to prevent hypercapnia.

The duration of the period of hypotension must be taken into consideration, and also the importance of fine rapid control of the circulation. It may be essential in some surgical procedures to restore arterial pressure quickly to normal levels so that haemostasis may be achieved, but in other types of surgical practice a gradual recovery may be desirable.

Before embarking upon hypotensive anaesthesia, the anaesthetist must be aware of the potential advantages and disadvantages of the technique. In each instance in which this physiological trespass is used, he must be certain that the increased risk to the patient is justified by the improvement in surgical conditions.

FURTHER READING

Cole P 1979 The safe use of sodium nitroprusside. Anaesthesia 33: 473
Eckenhoff J E (ed) 1979 Controversy in anaesthesiology. W B Saunders, London
Ingram G S 1982 Neurosurgical anaesthesia. In: Kaufman L (ed) Anaesthesia review 1. Churchill Livingstone, London
Lindop M J 1975 Complications and morbidity of controlled hypotension. British Journal of Anaesthesia 47: 799

36

Intercurrent disease and anaesthesia

Many patients presenting for surgery suffer from unrelated disease, for which they may be receiving drug treatment. The course of this disease may be modified by anaesthesia and surgery, while the disease process may also influence the effects of anaesthesia.

The aim of anaesthetic management in such patients is to assess the extent of the medical problem, ensure that the patient's condition is optimised in the time available before surgery (this may vary widely between emergency and elective surgery) and to conduct anaesthesia and postoperative care using drugs and techniques which least affect, or are affected by, the medical condition. To achieve this, all patients undergoing surgery require a full clinical history and examination. A past medical history, including previous anaesthesia, drug and allergy history and examination of previous anaesthetic records (if available) may be particularly important. In addition, special investigations may be necessary depending on the age and fitness of the patient and the nature of the surgery (see Chapter 15).

CARDIOVASCULAR DISEASE

General principles

Anaesthesia for patients with cardiovascular disease involves the application of a number of basic principles.

1. Adequate oxygenation must be maintained throughout.

2. Cardiac output must be maintained at a level commensurate with adequate tissue perfusion.

3. Systemic arterial pressure must be adequate to maintain cerebral and coronary circulation and preserve renal and hepatic function.

4. The balance of myocardial oxygen supply and demand must be preserved, thus minimising the risk of perioperative ischaemia and infarction (Table 36.1).

This demands a knowledge of the physiological mechanisms governing cardiac output, myocardial oxygen availability and consumption, and the adjustments occurring in disease states. An understanding of the effects of i.v. and volatile

Table 36.1 Factors affecting myocardial oxygen supply and consumption

Supply	Consumption	
Coronary Perfusion Pressure α (diastolic pressure — LVEDP)	H.R.	
	Contractility	
Arterial Oxygen Tension		
	Wall tension α	1. LVEDP
Haemoglobin concentration		2. Arterial Pressure
		3. Contractility
Coronary vascular resistance — intraluminal obstruction — external compression α 1. H.R. 2. LVEDP — autoregulation — dependent on myocardial O_2 consumption	External Work α	1. Cardiac Output 2. Arterial Pressure

anaesthetic agents, and muscle relaxants allows a choice to be made of appropriate drugs and techniques. Reversible risk factors (e.g. cardiac failure or hypertension) must be detected and treated preoperatively.

Preoperative assessment

History

Symptoms suggesting cardiovascular disease include dyspnoea, chest pain, palpitations, ankle swelling and intermittent claudication. Severity of symptoms assessed by a history of exercise tolerance is the most useful estimate of severity of cardiovascular disease.

Past medical history and previous medical records usually reveal the nature and severity of disease. The date of a previous myocardial infarct may be important in assessing the risk of perioperative reinfarction. Elective surgery must never be performed within six months of infarction. Angina, increasing in frequency and severity, is associated with an increased risk of perioperative infarction. Previous thromboembolic disease necessitates prophylactic cover, e.g. low-dose heparin, Dextran 70, or intermittent calf compression.

Concurrent drug treatment

Digoxin. The dose should be assessed in the light of age, weight and renal function, and plasma digoxin concentration measured if necessary. Serum potassium concentration should be measured, especially when there is concurrent diuretic therapy, and symptoms of digoxin toxicity, e.g. nausea and vomiting, should be sought. Heart rate and rhythm require assessment. In excessive dosage, especially with concurrent hypokalaemia, ventricular arrhythmias or heart block may occur.

Diuretics. Serum potassium concentration should be checked, and hypokalaemia corrected.

Anticoagulants. Where long-term therapy is indicated, perioperative control must be monitored closely. Warfarin should be stopped 48 h preoperatively, and the prothrombin time monitored daily; it should not be greater than $1\frac{1}{2}$ times control at the time of surgery. (Thrombotest should be greater than 50%.) For emergency surgery, or if undue bleeding occurs, fresh frozen plasma is indicated. Postoperatively, for minor surgery, warfarin may be restarted the following day, while for major surgery, a heparin infusion may be used to maintain anticoagulation (with control by thrombin time estimations) until warfarin therapy is recommenced. This allows reversal of anticoagulation with protamine 1 mg for every 100 unit of heparin if bleeding occurs. Protamine should be administered slowly to avoid hypotension.

β-Adrenergic blockers. In most instances, β-blockade should be maintained throughout the perioperative period. Sudden preoperative cessation may be associated with rebound angina, myocardial infarct, arrhythmia or hypertension postoperatively. Intravenous atropine may be given prior to induction or, if undue bradycardia occurs, intraoperatively. β-Blockers may contribute to and mask the signs of hypoglycaemia.

Calcium antagonists. These drugs block the slow influx of calcium ions which contribute to depolarisation. *Verapamil,* which acts predominantly on the A–V node is used in the management of supraventricular tachyarrhythmias, angina and hypertrophic obstructive cardiomyopathy. Since it increases A–V block, concurrent use with digoxin or β-blockers should be avoided. *Nifedipine,* which acts predominantly on vascular smooth muscle is used in the management of angina, hypertension and as a preload reducer in left ventricular failure. It should be used with caution in patients on β-blocker therapy.

Examination

Preoperative cardiovascular examination should include measurement of heart rate and rhythm, arterial pressure, assessment of peripheral perfusion and detection of signs of cardiac failure. Hypertension and cardiac murmurs are not infrequently a chance finding, and require further assessment before surgery.

Investigations

In addition to routine haematology and biochemical investigations, e.c.g. is important as a baseline before surgery for the diagnosis of arrhythmias, to provide confirmatory evidence of ischaemic heart disease and to assess the severity of cardiac disease, e.g. hypertension, cor pulmonale and valvular heart disease.

Chest X-ray provides information on heart and chamber size, the state of the pulmonary vasculature and evidence of pulmonary oedema and infection.

Ultrasound examination is useful in diagnosing valve lesions, and detection of pericardial effusions.

Cardiac catheterisation and coronary angiography are rarely indicated before routine surgery.

Preoperative treatment

Cardiac failure, arrhythmias, hypertension and angina should be controlled before surgery. Anaemia should be treated, if necessary with blood transfusion, at least 48 h before surgery. Haemoglobin concentration should be greater than 10 g/dl.

Premedication

In ischaemic heart disease and hypertension, premedication should be adequate to allay anxiety. Papaveretum and hyoscine is often satisfactory. In patients with low or fixed cardiac output states, and congestive cardiac failure, premedication should be light, e.g. oral diazepam. In poor-risk patients, preanaesthetic medication should be avoided.

Anaesthesia

In practical terms, this involves maintenance of a normal heart rate, and an arterial pressure adequate to maintain coronary perfusion and oxygenation without increasing cardiac work and thus myocardial oxygen requirements. Excessive myocardial depression should be avoided.

The high risk periods during anaesthesia are:

1. Induction. Most induction agents are cardiovascular depressants, and in patients with low or fixed cardiac output, hypertension or hypovolaemia, hypotension may occur. Etomidate has least cardiovascular effects. Of the numerous neuromuscular-blocking drugs, atracurium and vecuronium produce least (and negligible) cardiovascular effects.

2. Intubation. Tracheal intubation is associated commonly with hypertension.

3. Postoperative period. Rebound hypertension occurs commonly in association with pain and peripheral vasoconstriction. Good analgesia is necessary with careful attention to intravascular volume.

Careful monitoring is essential and always includes heart rate, arterial pressure and e.c.g. The common e.c.g. configuration used for anaesthetic monitoring is standard limb lead II. Whilst this is useful for differentiating arrhythmias, myocardial ischaemia occurs most commonly in the left ventricle and is detected more sensitively with a CM_5 configuration. In high risk patients undergoing major surgery, intra-arterial cannulation, and CVP measurements are indicated. Pulmonary capillary wedge pressure measurement is useful in patients with severe left ventricular failure, shock, or for surgery where major blood loss is anticipated. Monitoring should be instituted before induction, and maintained throughout the immediate postoperative period (if necessary in the intensive care unit).

Hypertension

Untreated hypertension is associated with increased perioperative morbidity and mortality, increased risk of cerebrovascular accident and myocardial infarction. Since arterial pressure increases with age, an acceptable maximum pressure is difficult to define, but elective surgery should rarely be undertaken when the resting diastolic pressure exceeds 110 mmHg. Control of hypertension is achieved using a thiazide diuretic, with the possible addition of a β-blocker and a vasodilator, e.g. hydralazine, or nifedipine in more severe cases.

Where hypertension is a chance preoperative finding, surgery should be delayed until investigation and treatment have been instituted.

Endocrine and renal causes should be excluded (pp. 478 and 482). Complications of hypertension, e.g. myocardial ischaemia, cardiac failure and renal impairment should be sought, and unstable angina and cardiac failure controlled before surgery. Antihypertensive therapy should be continued throughout the perioperative period.

Anaesthesia

Premedication should be generous with, for example, papaveretum and hyoscine. Anaesthetic management should be directed towards avoidance of hypotension and, more particularly, hypertension. Thus close monitoring of arterial pressure and e.c.g. is required from before induction through anaesthesia and the postoperative period. Blood loss should also be monitored carefully, and deficits replaced promptly.

Hypertensive patients are particularly vulnerable to the development of hypotension following induction of anaesthesia or following establishment of subarachnoid or extradural blockade. Etomidate has least cardiovascular effects, but other agents, e.g. thiopentone, are acceptable if carefully administered. Ketamine is contraindicated in anaesthetic dosages. Pancuronium should be avoided in severe hypertension; alcuronium, atracurium and vecuronium are suitable; d-tubocurarine may cause severe but transient hypotension.

Tracheal intubation commonly causes hypertension, tachycardia and arrhythmias. Preoperative administration of a β-blocker is partially effective in obviating this response.

For maintenance of anaesthesia, a nitrous oxide/oxygen/opioid/relaxant technique is appropriate in most instances. Volatile agents (halothane and enflurane) possess marked cardiovascular depressant effects, and require careful administration. However they are suitable for minor procedures with a spontaneous breathing technique.

Intraoperatively, nodal arrhythmias occur commonly, and may produce a decrease in cardiac output. Depending on heart rate, i.v. atropine, β-blocker or decreasing the inspired halothane concentration may be effective in treating arrhythmias. β-Blockers prevent the physiological heart rate response to intraoperative blood loss, while vasodilators prevent vasoconstriction. Thus careful monitoring of blood and fluid loss and CVP is important, and prompt replacement of fluid deficits is necessary to avoid undue hypotension. Local anaesthetic preparations containing catecholamine vasoconstrictors should be avoided.

Postoperative hypertension occurs frequently, partly as result of inadequate analgesia, and partly as a result of peripheral vasoconstriction which occurs during prolonged surgery with associated heat loss and bleeding. Hypertension increases myocardial work and oxygen demand, and in patients with left ventricular hypertrophy or enlargement may cause subendocardial ischaemia or infarction. Good analgesia is essential, and continuous extradural analgesia is safe in treated hypertensive patients if closely monitored.

Postoperative hypertension should be treated promptly and adequate analgesia should be ensured.

In the presence of peripheral vasoconstriction, vasodilators, e.g. i.v. boluses of chlorpromazine 2.5–5 mg, phentolamine 2.5 mg or hydralazine 5–10 mg, are usually effective. All vasodilator therapy requires careful arterial pressure monitoring. β-Blocker therapy is indicated in the presence of tachycardia.

Where the patient has been managed preoperatively with oral β-blockers, a long acting agent, e.g. atenolol or nadolol, should be given before surgery, and oral treatment recommenced on the day following surgery. In certain instances, nasogastric administration or i.v. infusion may be necessary. With propranolol, the i.v. daily dose is approx. one-tenth of the oral dose.

Ischaemic heart disease

Five per cent of patients over 35 yr of age have symptomless ischaemic heart disease. In patients who have had a previous myocardial infarction, anaesthesia and surgery within 3 months of infarction carries a 40% risk of perioperative reinfarction. This rate decreases to 15% at 3–6 months and 5% thereafter. Mortality following postoperative infarction is 50%, considerably greater than after infarction in other circumstances. Elective surgery should be postponed until at least 6 months after infarction.

Unstable angina is associated also with increased risk of perioperative myocardial infarction and should be controlled with β-blockade, nitrates or a calcium antagonist before surgery. There is no evidence that the incidence of postoperative infarction is reduced by using local or regional anaesthetic techniques.

Factors which precipitate further infarction are those which increase myocardial work and thus oxygen requirement, or which decrease coronary blood flow (Table 36.1).

Anaesthesia

Preoperatively, congestive cardiac failure should be treated with diuretics and, if necessary, digoxin. The increase in oxygen consumption resulting from increased contractility is balanced by the beneficial effects on myocardial oxygen supply and demand achieved by decreased left ventricular end-diastolic pressure. Anaemia should be corrected. Premedication should be adequate to allay anxiety.

Anaesthetic management demands the same close monitoring, avoidance of tachycardia and bradycardia, maintenance of normotension or slight hypotension and careful choice of anaesthetic agent which is necessary in the hypertensive patient. β-Blockade should be maintained and this necessitates care in fluid replacement and concurrent drug administration.

Halothane depresses contractility and myocardial oxygen consumption, but coronary blood flow is depressed to a proportionately lesser extent. Thus halothane is tolerated well in small concentrations. However, high concentrations of halothane may produce excessive myocardial depression with a profound decrease in cardiac output, increased LVEDP and myocardial ischaemia. These effects may be potentiated by β-blockade. Normocapnia should be maintained, since hypercapnia may provoke arrhythmias, while hypocapnia causes peripheral and coronary vasoconstriction, and shifts the oxygen dissociation curve to the left.

Postoperatively, monitoring, management of analgesia, and arterial pressure control must be meticulous.

Congestive cardiac failure

Anaesthesia and surgery in patients with cardiac failure carry an increased risk of morbidity and mortality. The cause of the failure should be elucidated, and treatment instituted before surgery.

Left heart failure causes pulmonary congestion and oedema, decreases pulmonary compliance, increasing respiratory work and resulting in hypoxaemia and hypocapnia. Causes include hypertension, aortic valve disease, mitral valve disease, ischaemic heart disease and cardiomyopathy (hypertrophic obstructive cardiomyopathy, HOCM, and congestive cardiomyopathy). It is often precipitated by arrhythmias, e.g. atrial fibrillation in mitral stenosis.

Treatment involves diuretic therapy and, in some instances, digitalisation. In addition, specific therapy is required for the cause of failure, e.g. arrhythmias. The outflow obstruction seen in HOCM responds to β-blockade. If failure is refractory to digoxin and diuretic therapy, venodilatation with glyceryl trinitrate or isosorbide dinitrate decreases preload and may decrease pulmonary congestion.

Right heart failure may be secondary to left heart failure, chronic lung disease (cor pulmonale), idiopathic pulmonary hypertension or pulmonary stenosis. E.c.g. evidence of right atrial and ventricular hypertrophy raises the suspicion of pulmonary hypertension. Hypoxia in such patients causes a marked increase in pulmonary vascular resistance provoking right ventricular failure. Acute right heart failure occurs commonly when patients with chronic obstructive airways disease suffer an acute infective exacerbation with hypoxia. Preoperative treatment of infection is important, and intra- and postoperative maintenance of the airway and avoidance of hypoxia are imperative.

Biventricular failure is also associated with fluid overload and hypoalbuminaemia, e.g. in renal and hepatic disease.

Low subarachnoid and extradural blockade may be useful in certain patients with cardiac failure, the sympathetic block producing venodilatation and reduction in preload.

Shock

Surgery should not be undertaken until adequate resuscitation of the patient has been undertaken. In cases of severe haemorrhage, only initial resuscitation may be possible before surgery, and resuscitation continued until bleeding is controlled. Such patients require adequate oxygenation and ventilation, with blood gas measurements. Monitoring required during resuscitation and anaesthesia includes arterial pressure, heart rate, CVP and urine output, while the core-peripheral temperature gradient provides a useful indication of peripheral perfusion. Active vasodilatation may be considered when full fluid replacement has been undertaken.

Anaesthesia in shock

Minimal doses of induction agent should be employed. Etomidate is associated with least cardiovascular disturbance, but other agents, e.g. thiopentone may be used with care in very low dosage. Ketamine increases myocardial work and may increase oxygen demand excessively in an ischaemic myocardium. A nitrous oxide/oxygen/opioid/relaxant technique, using pancuronium, is usually well tolerated. The effect of a small dose of morphine, administered i.v. prior to induction, often gives an indication of cardiovascular stability. The management of shock is discussed in Chapters 30 and 39.

Arrhythmias (see also Chapter 19, p. 282)

Arrhythmias occurring preoperatively should be treated prior to surgery (which should be postponed if necessary). The most commonly occurring arrhythmia is probably atrial fibrillation, which is caused commonly by ischaemic heart disease, mitral valve disease, or thyrotoxicosis. The ventricular rate should be controlled with digoxin. If the ventricular rate is normal, digoxin should usually be commenced preoperatively to prevent an increase in ventricular rate occurring intraoperatively.

Intraoperative arrhythmias

Approx. 12% of patients undergoing anaesthesia develop arrhythmias but this frequency increases to 30% in patients with cardiovascular disease. Treatment may not be required, depending on the nature of the arrhythmia, and its effect on cardiac output. Single supraventricular or ventricular ectopic beats, and slow supraventricular rhythms do not require treatment unless cardiac output is compromised.

Factors affecting intraoperative arrhythmias include:

1. Spontaneous ventilation. Raised Pa_{CO_2} may cause ventricular extrasystoles.

2. Hypoxia. Initially this causes tachycardia, then bradycardia.

3. Anaesthetic agents. Cyclopropane and halogenated hydrocarbons, e.g. trichloroethylene and halothane, are associated with an increased incidence of ventricular arrhythmias especially if Pa_{CO_2} is raised.

4. Catecholamines. Local anaesthetic preparations containing adrenaline may provoke ventricular arrhythmias especially in patients anaesthetised with halothane in the presence of a raised Pa_{CO_2}. Enflurane is less likely to be associated with adrenaline-induced arrhythmias and isoflurane even less so.

5. Hypokalaemia may be associated with ventricular arrhythmias especially in the presence of digoxin. Hyperkalaemia delays ventricular conduction with eventual cardiac arrest.

6. Reflex arrhythmias tend to occur during light anaesthesia by sympathetic or parasympathetic mediation. They include tachyarrhythmias in response to laryngoscopy and intubation (diminished by β-blockers), ventricular arrhythmias following dental extraction (partially blocked by local anaesthetic infiltration), and oculocardiac reflex (partially blocked by atropine). Reflex arrhythmias in general are prevented by deepening anaesthesia.

Treatment of intraoperative arrhythmias depends on the nature of the arrhythmia. Supraventricular tachycardia may be treated with i.v. verapamil or β-blockers, but concurrent administration of these two drugs should be avoided. Cardioversion may be performed if these drugs are ineffective. If digoxin has been used in an attempt to control atrial flutter or fibrillation, it is advisable to administer lignocaine before cardioversion to prevent ventricular arrhythmias. Ventricular tachycardia responds to i.v. lignocaine 50–100 mg followed by an infusion, but if unsuccessful, mexiletene, procainamide, phenytoin or β-blockers may be tried. Other measures include correction of hypercapnia, hypoxia or hypokalaemia, and reduction of the inspired halothane concentration.

Heart block

The extent of the conduction deficit should be determined preoperatively by e.c.g. monitoring. If the patient has syncopal attacks, or is in cardiac failure, long-term pacing is indicated.

If the patient with heart block presents for surgery without a pacemaker in situ, preoperative insertion of a temporary pacing line is indicated usually in:

1. Complete heart block.
2. Second-degree heart block, notably of Mobitz Type 2 variety.
3. First degree heart block with bifascicular block (right bundle branch block with left anterior or posterior hemiblock).

A decision on whether long-term pacing is indicated or not may be made after the immediate postoperative period by a cardiologist. During anaesthesia, e.c.g. should be monitored continuously, a standby pacemaker should be available and care should be taken to avoid undue blood loss or vasodilatation since heart rate is unable to increase.

Diathermy should be avoided if possible since it may interfere with pacemaker function. Where unavoidable, the diathermy plate should be sited as far away as possible from the pacemaker generator. Temporary generators and demand permanent generators are most often affected. During transurethral prostatectomy, the 'cutting' current may affect the pacemaker while the 'coagulation' current has no effect. With some pacemakers, the reverse may occur. Diathermy should be used in short bursts only. Where first degree heart block only is present, not necessitating external pacing, drugs which slow A-V conduction should be avoided, e.g. β-blockers, digoxin, verapamil.

Sick sinus syndrome

This term covers a number of conduction defects affecting the sino-atrial node, ranging from sinus bradycardia, to sinus arrest. Sino-atrial block may be associated with runs of supraventricular tachycardia (so called tachycardia-bradycardia syndrome). Long-term pacing is indicated if the patient has syncopal episodes. Sinus bradycardia responds usually to atropine while in complete sino-atrial block, atropine accelerates nodal escape rhythm. In the tachycardia-bradycardia group, temporary pacing is indicated to cover anaesthesia and surgery, since treatment of tachycardia with for example, β-blockers, calcium antagonists or digoxin may provoke severe bradycardia.

Valvular heart disease

Aortic stenosis

Isolated aortic stenosis is associated most commonly with calcification often on a congenital bicuspid valve. In rheumatic heart disease, aortic stenosis occurs rarely in the absence of mitral disease, and is combined usually with incompetence. The diagnosis is suggested by the findings of an ejection systolic murmur, low pulse pressure, and clinical and e.c.g. evidence of left ventricular hypertrophy. Aortic systolic murmurs in elderly patients are ascribed frequently to aortic sclerosis, and an assessment of the degree of stenosis present rests on examination of pulse waveform, pulse pressure and e.c.g. evidence of left ventricular hypertrophy. On chest X-ray, heart size is normal until late in disease, while symptoms of angina, effort syncope and left ventricular failure indicate advanced disease.

Perioperative mortality is increased in patients with aortic stenosis; arrhythmias are common and are associated with precipitous decreases in cardiac output. The myocardial oxygen balance is upset by the decrease in coronary perfusion pressure and subendocardial blood flow, and the increase in ventricular afterload. Successful management demands precise maintenance of heart rate, arterial pressure and myocardial contractility. Bradycardia causes a decrease in cardiac output since stroke volume is fixed; tachycardia decreases the time available for coronary filling and therefore both should be avoided. Vasodilatation causes severe hypotension since cardiac output cannot be increased significantly and thus coronary perfusion pressure is reduced.

Most anaesthetic induction agents, and 'first generation' muscle relaxants (d-tubocurarine, pancuronium, alcuronium etc) must be used with extreme caution. The relaxant of choice would be atracurium or vecuronium. Volatile agents (halothane, enflurane) which depress ventricular contractility, may also seriously decrease cardiac output, while halothane predisposes to arrhythmias. Replacement of blood must be prompt. Intensive monitoring is important with intra-arterial pressure and in severe instances, PCWP measurement.

Mitral stenosis

This is usually a manifestation of rheumatic heart disease. Characteristic features may include atrial fibrillation, arterial embolism, pulmonary oedema, pulmonary hypertension and right heart failure. Acute pulmonary oedema may follow the onset of atrial fibrillation.

Patients with mitral stenosis presenting for surgery are frequently receiving digoxin, diuretics and anticoagulants (see p. 217). Preoperative control of atrial fibrillation, treatment of pulmonary oedema and management of anticoagulant therapy is necessary (see Chapter 37, p. 497). During anaesthesia, control of heart rate is important. Tachycardia reduces ventricular filling during diastole and thus cardiac output, while bradycardia also results in a decreased cardiac output since stroke output is limited. As with aortic stenosis, drugs producing vasodilatation may cause severe hypotension.

As a result of pre-existing pulmonary hypertension, patients are particularly vulnerable to hypoxia, including transient episodes. Both hypoxia and acidosis are potent pulmonary vasoconstrictors and may produce immediate right ventricular failure. Thus opioid analgesics should be prescribed cautiously, and airway obstruction avoided.

Aortic incompetence

Acute aortic incompetence resulting, for example, from subacute bacterial endocarditis or Marfan's syndrome rapidly causes left ventricular failure and requires emergency valve replacement.

Chronic aortic incompetence is asymptomatic for many years. Left ventricular dilatation occurs, with eventual left ventricular failure.

Patients with mild to moderate aortic incompetence without left ventricular failure or massive ventricular dilatation tolerate anaesthesia well. A slightly increased heart rate of approx. 100 beat/min is desirable since this reduces left ventricular dilatation. Bradycardia causes ventricular distension and should be avoided. Vasodilator therapy, by decreasing afterload, increases net forward flow, and is useful in severe aortic incompetence, but requires careful monitoring, preferably with PCWP measurement, if severe hypotension is to be avoided.

Mitral incompetence

Acute mitral incompetence commonly results from subacute bacterial endocarditis, or myocardial infarct with papillary muscle dysfunction or ruptured chordae tendineae. Acute pulmonary oedema results, and urgent valve replacement is required.

Chronic mitral incompetence is associated commonly with mitral stenosis. In pure mitral incompetence, left atrial dilatation occurs with a minimal increase in pressure. The degree of regurgitation may be reduced by reducing the size of the left ventricle and the impedance to left ventricular ejection. Thus inotropic agents and vasodilators may be useful. A slight increase in heart rate is desirable except if there is coincident stenosis.

Subacute bacterial endocarditis

This is caused predominantly by the viridans group of streptococci, occasionally by Gram negative organisms or enterococci and also by staphylococci, especially after cardiac surgery or in drug addicts. *Coxiella burnetti* also accounts for a few cases. Patients with rheumatic or congenital heart disease are at risk, the latter including asymptomatic lesions, e.g. bicuspid aortic valve. Infection is caused by transient bacteraemia, frequently after dental extraction or genitourinary investigation or surgery.

Antibiotic cover should be given for all surgical procedures in vulnerable patients. Oral amoxycillin 3 g administered 1 h before dental treatment has been shown to prevent bacteraemia and is a practical prophylaxis for patients having dental surgery, while intramuscular ampicillin 1 g and gentamicin 80 mg 1 h preoperatively provide satisfactory cover for abdominal or genitourinary surgery. Cloxacillin or an alternative antistaphylococcal agent should be included in regimens for cardiac surgery.

Role of local and regional anaesthesia in cardiovascular disease

In appropriate patients with cardiovascular disease, local infiltration, peripheral nerve and plexus blocks provide satisfactory anaesthesia without side effects. However, local anaesthetic preparations containing adrenaline produce tachycardia and should be avoided in patients with severe cardiovascular disease.

Patients undergoing lower abdominal, pelvic or lower limb surgery may be managed satisfactorily with low subarachnoid or extradural anaesthesia. With higher blocks, an increasing sympathetic block produces vasodilatation, reducing preload and afterload on the heart. While controlled vasodilatation may have beneficial effects in ischaemic heart disease, hypertension and cardiac failure, patients anaesthetised with subarachnoid or extradural blockade must be managed very carefully with respect to posture, fluid preloading and replacement to avoid undue hypotension. The sympathetic blockade may produce severe hypotension in patients with untreated hypertension, low cardiac output states, constrictive pericarditis, severe valvular disease or a fixed heart rate resulting from heart block or β-blocker therapy. On the other hand, patients with congestive cardiac failure may benefit from the preload reduction caused by the sympathetic block, and patients with peripheral vascular disease may benefit from peripheral vasodilatation.

High subarachnoid or extradural blockade is contraindicated in patients with cardiovascular disease.

By and large, for anaesthetists with little experience in regional anaesthesia, SAB and extradural blocks should be avoided in patients with severe cardiac disease.

RESPIRATORY DISEASE

Successful anaesthetic management of the patient with respiratory disease is dependent on accurate assessment of the nature and extent of functional impairment, and an appreciation of the effects surgery may have on pulmonary function.

Assessment

History

Of the six cardinal symptoms of respiratory disease (cough, sputum, haemoptysis, dyspnoea, wheeze and chest pain) dyspnoea provides the best indication of functional impairment. Specific questioning is required to elicit the extent to which activity is limited by dyspnoea. Dyspnoea at rest or on minor exertion clearly indicates severe disease. A cough productive of purulent sputum indicates active infection. Chronic copious sputum production may indicate bronchiectasis. A history of heavy smoking or occupational exposure to dust may suggest pulmonary pathology.

A detailed drug history is important. Long-term steroid therapy within three months of the date of surgery necessitates high dose cover for the perioperative period and may cause hypokalaemia. Bronchodilators should be continued over the perioperative period. Patients with cor pulmonale may be receiving digoxin and diuretics.

Examination

A full physical examination is required with emphasis on detecting signs of airways obstruction, increased work of breathing, active infection which can be treated preoperatively, and evidence of right heart failure. Presence of obesity, cyanosis or dyspnoea is noted. In addition, a simple forced expiratory manoeuvre may reveal prolonged expiration.

Investigations

Chest X-ray. The preoperative chest X-ray is a poor indicator of functional impairment but is important for several reasons.

1. As a baseline for assessing postoperative radiographs.

2. To discover any localised disease of lungs and pleura not detected on clinical examination, e.g. neoplasm, collapse, consolidation, effusion.

3. To reveal underlying generalised lung disease in patients presenting with acute pulmonary symptoms, e.g. pulmonary fibrosis, emphysema.

E.c.g. This may indicate right atrial or ventricular hypertrophy (P pulmonale in II; dominant R wave in III, V_{1-3}) while associated ischaemic heart disease is common.

Haematology. Polycythaemia occurs secondary to chronic hypoxia, while anaemia aggravates tissue hypoxia. Leucocytosis may indicate active infection.

Sputum culture is essential in patients with chronic lung disease or suspected acute infection.

Pulmonary function tests (see Appendix XI, p. 562). Peak expiratory flow rate, forced expiratory volume in 1 s ($FEV_{1.0}$), and forced vital capacity (FVC) may be measured easily at the bedside. The $FEV_{1.0}$:FVC ratio is decreased in obstructive lung disease and normal in restrictive disease. In the presence of obstructive disease, the test should be repeated 5–10 min after administration of a bronchodilator aerosol to provide an indication of reversibility.

Fuller investigation involves measurement of FRC, RV and TLC.

Blood gas measurement is indicated where the pulmonary function tests are markedly abnormal, for example, in obstructive disease where the $FEV_{1.0}$ is less than 1.5 litre. A raised Pa_{CO_2} is a good prognostic indication of postoperative pulmonary complications. With a Pa_{CO_2} of 6.7 kPa (50 mmHg) or greater, elective postoperative ventilation may be required for all but minor surgery.

Effects of anaesthesia and surgery

Fitness for anaesthesia and surgery in patients with respiratory disease depends on the type and magnitude of surgery. The effects of anaesthesia alone on respiratory function are generally minor and short-lived, but may tip the balance towards respiratory failure in patients with severe disease. These effects include mucosal irritation by anaesthetic agents, ciliary paralysis, introduction of infection by aspiration or tracheal intubation and respiratory depression by relaxants, opioid analgesics or volatile anaesthetic agents. In addition, anaesthesia is associated with a decrease in FRC, especially in the elderly and in obese patients, which leads to basal airways closure and shunting of blood through underventilated areas of lung. This effect resolves within a few hours after anaesthesia.

Following thoracic and upper abdominal surgery the decrease in FRC is more profound and persists for 5–10 days after surgery with a parallel increase in $(A–a)PO_2$ (see Fig. 21.2). Complications including atelectasis and pneumonia occur in approx. 20% of these patients. Clearly, patients with pre-existing respiratory disease are at much greater risk undergoing upper abdominal rather than limb, head and neck or lower abdominal surgery.

Chronic obstructive airways disease

Chronic bronchitis is characterised by the presence of productive cough for three months in two successive years. Airways obstruction is caused by bronchial oedema and mucus hypersecretion. In the post-operative period, pulmonary atelectasis and pneumonia result if sputum is not cleared. Chronic airways disease may be classified into two groups: the bronchitic group (blue bloaters) and the emphysematous group (pink puffers), although in practice most patients have mixed pathologies. The former group is characterised by hypoxia, hypercapnia and right ventricular failure while patients in the latter group are usually markedly dyspnoeic.

Preoperative management

This should include:

1. Detection and treatment of active infection. Ampicillin, amoxycillin or co-trimoxazole are usually appropriate, the common infecting organisms being *Str. pneumoniae* and *H. influenzae*. Sputum for culture and sensitivities should be obtained to allow appropriate choice of antibiotic. Chest physiotherapy and humidification of inspired gases aid expectoration.

2. Treatment of airway obstruction. Some patients respond to bronchodilator therapy, either β_2 agonist, (e.g. salbutamol), anticholinergic agent, (e.g. ipratropium bromide), or phosphodiesterase inhibitor, (e.g. aminophylline). Existing bronchodilator therapy should be continued perioperatively while in patients not receiving bronchodilators, a trial of oral aminophylline (Phyllocontin) 225 mg bd and salbutamol 200 µg or ipratropium 40 µg (2 puffs) by inhalation may decrease airways obstruction. Steroids may occasionally improve airways obstruction.

3. Chest X-ray examination to exclude spontaneous pneumothorax.

4. Treatment of congestive cardiac failure. Biventricular failure resulting from concurrent ischaemic heart disease and cor pulmonale frequently complicates chronic pulmonary disease. Digoxin and diuretic therapy is indicated.

5. Obese patients. Weight reduction should be encouraged before elective surgery.

Premedication. Opioids should be avoided if severe disease exists. Atropine is useful if copious secretions are present. Diazepam is satisfactory to allay anxiety.

Regional anaesthesia

Regional anaesthesia for operations on head, neck or limbs offers freedom from respiratory side-effects, while avoiding the complications of general anaesthesia. Low subarachnoid or extradural anaesthesia for lower abdominal and pelvic surgery have a similar advantage. Overall, however, the morbidity resulting from general anaesthesia for such operations is low, and it is only, perhaps, in the respiratory cripple that any significant advantage accrues. In these patients, sedation should be kept to a minimum.

In upper abdominal and thoracic surgery, where changes in respiratory function are more profound and prolonged, there is no evidence that extradural anaesthesia is associated with a lower morbidity than general anaesthesia. The advantages accruing from avoidance of volatile anaesthetics, muscle relaxants and opioids are balanced by the effect of extradural blockade on expiratory muscles, decreasing vital capacity. However, the use of extradural analgesia postoperatively may reduce postoperative hypoxaemia by diminishing the decrease in FRC, and result in fewer pulmonary complications.

General anaesthesia

Two approaches may be taken in the presence of severe chronic obstructive disease.

1. The minimal anaesthesia approach involves using minimal sedation, avoiding opioid analgesics and maintaining spontaneous ventilation, usually with a face mask. *Toleration* of endotracheal intubation is improved by spraying the larynx with local anaesthetic solution. Analgesia is provided best by a local or regional technique.

A preoperative Pa_{CO_2} greater than 6.7 kPa (50 mmHg) indicates loss of respiratory centre sensitivity. These patients require controlled oxygen therapy and where general anaesthesia is contemplated, the patient's lungs should be ventilated intra- and possibly postoperatively.

2. With major abdominal and thoracic surgery and in patients with raised Pa_{CO_2}, elective postoperative ventilation may be required, at least until elimination of muscle relaxants and anaesthetic agents has occurred. Care should be taken to achieve optimal ventilation, and to avoid hyperventilation and excessive airways pressure which may cause a precipitous decrease in cardiac output.

Intravenous fluid should be administered with care during the perioperative period. After surgery, salt and water retention occurs, and in combination with overenthusiastic fluid administration, and perhaps a decrease in cardiac output, may result in an increase in lung water which in turn may cause small airway closure, and hypoxaemia.

There is an increased risk of pneumothorax, especially if high inflation pressures are used, and this requires early diagnosis and drainage.

Postoperative care

Elective postoperative controlled ventilation allows adequate oxygenation, analgesia without respiratory depression, clearance of secretions by physiotherapy, tracheal suction and, if necessary, fibreoptic bronchoscopy. Cardiac output and peripheral perfusion may be optimised and fluid overload corrected before restoration of spontaneous ventilation. Unless there is pre-existing pulmonary infection, a period of 24 h elective controlled ventilation is usually adequate. Institution of analgesia by regional (e.g. intercostal, paravertebral, or extradural) blockade often allows earlier return to spontaneous ventilation when the respiratory depressant effects of anaesthetics and relaxants have terminated.

Oxygen. With spontaneous ventilation, controlled oxygen is required using a 24% or 28% Ventimask with frequent checks on arterial blood gases. Hypoxaemia may seriously aggravate existing pulmonary hypertension, precipitating right ventricular failure.

Analgesia. Simple, nonopioid analgesics, and/or local and regional techniques should be used if possible. Fifty per cent nitrous oxide in oxygen (Entonox) is useful for physiotherapy and painful procedures. Opioid analgesics are best administered, where necessary, in small i.v. doses, e.g. morphine 2 mg, under direct supervision.

Physiotherapy, bronchodilators and antibiotics should be continued postoperatively. Doxapram in a single dose of 1.5–2.0 mg/kg i.v. may decrease the frequency of postoperative alveolar collapse and infection.

Restrictive lung disease

This category includes a wide range of conditions affecting lung and chest wall. Lung diseases include sarcoidosis and fibrosing alveolitis, while lesions of chest wall include kyphoscoliosis and ankylosing spondylitis. Pulmonary function tests reveals a decrease in both $FEV_{1.0}$ and FVC with a normal $FEV_{1.0}$/FVC ratio and a decreased FRC and TLC. Small airway closure occurs during tidal ventilation, with resultant shunting and hypoxaemia. Lung or chest wall compliance is decreased; thus work of breathing is increased and the ability to cough and clear secretions impaired. There is an increased risk of postoperative pulmonary infection.

Anaesthesia causes little additional decrease in lung volumes, and is tolerated well provided hypoxaemia is avoided. Postoperatively, however, inadequate basal ventilation and retention of secretions may occur, partly as a result of pain, opioid analgesics and the residual effects of anaesthetic agents. High concentrations of oxygen may be used without risk of respiratory depression. A short period of mechanical ventilation may be necessary in patients with severe disease to allow adequate analgesia and clearing of secretions. High extradural anaesthesia should be avoided in these patients since it causes a further reduction in VC.

Bronchiectasis

The patient should be admitted several days before surgery and regular postural drainage carried out. Appropriate antibiotics, based on sputum culture, should be commenced. Disease localised in one lung should be isolated using a double lumen tube.

Bronchial carcinoma

Patients with bronchial carcinoma frequently suffer from coexisting chronic bronchitis. In addition, there is frequently infection and collapse of the lung distal to the tumour. Patients with bronchial carcinoma may have a myasthenic syndrome (see p. 488), while oat cell tumours may secrete a number of hormones, among the commonest being ACTH, producing Cushing's syndrome, and ADH, producing dilutional hyponatraemia.

Tuberculosis

Tuberculosis should be considered in patients with persistent pulmonary infection, especially if associated with haemoptysis or weight loss. If active disease is present, all anaesthetic equipment should be sterilised after use to avoid cross-infection of other patients.

Bronchial asthma

This common disease, which affects all age groups, is characterised by recurrent generalised airways obstruction, caused by bronchial smooth muscle spasm, mucus plugs and bronchial oedema. Asthma may be classified into two types: *extrinsic,* where an external allergen is demonstrable, and *intrinsic.* Intrinsic asthma tends to occur in adults, is more chronic and continuous and often requires long-term steroid therapy.

Preoperative management

The current state of the patient's disease is assessed by:

1. History: frequency and severity of attacks, factors provoking attacks, drug history.
2. Examination: presence or absence of rhonchi, prolonged expiratory phase, overdistension, evidence of infection.
3. Pulmonary function testing: $FEV_{1.0}/FVC$ before and after inhalation of bronchodilator. Blood gas analysis may be required in severe disease.

Elective surgery should not be undertaken until asthma is well controlled. This involves the use of one or more of a number of drugs: sodium cromoglycate, to control the allergic component; bronchodilators (phosphodiesterase inhibitors, e.g. aminophylline, and β_2 adrenoceptor agonists, e.g. salbutamol) and steroids, systemic or inhaled. Pulmonary infection requires treatment where appropriate. An appropriate bronchodilator drug to commence several days preoperatively is salbutamol by inhaler, 200 μg (2 puffs) 4 times daily, possibly in combination with aminophylline (Phyllocontin) 225 mg bd. Patients with intrinsic asthma sometimes respond well to ipratropium bromide, an anticholinergic agent, by inhaler, 40 μg (2 puffs). A dose of bronchodilator should be given with the premedication 1 h before induction of anaesthesia.

Patients with severe asthma, receiving topical or systemic steroid therapy, or not responding to conventional bronchodilator therapy, require systemic steroid therapy to cover the anaesthetic and postoperative period. Prednisolone 40–100 mg daily may be given preoperatively, hydrocortisone 100 mg i.m. with premedication, and 100 mg 4 times daily for the first postoperative day, the dose reducing thereafter.

Premedication should consist of a sedative agent, e.g. diazepam, with atropine to block vagal reflex-induced bronchospasm. Pethidine and promethazine are also satisfactory.

Anaesthesia

The volatile agents halothane and ether are bronchodilators, and therefore well tolerated. Bronchoconstriction may be triggered by tracheal intubation or by surgical stimuli during light anaesthesia. The larynx and trachea should be sprayed with local anaesthetic and adequate depth of anaesthesia maintained. Drugs which are associated with histamine release (d-tubocurarine and morphine) are best avoided while pancuronium and pethidine or fentanyl are preferable. β-Blocking drugs should also be avoided.

With controlled ventilation, a prolonged expiratory phase is required if there is evidence of severe airways obstruction, while the inspiratory time should be adequate to avoid unduly high inflation pressures. Pneumothorax is a possible complication requiring early detection and prompt drainage. Humidification is necessary if ventilation is prolonged.

If bronchospasm occurs, aminophylline 250–500 mg or salbutamol 125–250 μg should be administered by slow i.v. injection under e.c.g. monitoring. Thereafter an infusion of aminophylline, up to 5 mg/kg 6 hrly or salbutamol, possibly in combination with nebulised salbutamol by positive pressure ventilation (solution of 50–100 μg of 'ventilator solution' per ml of water) should be maintained until improvement occurs. Intravenous hydrocortisone 100–200 mg should be given simultaneously, although it has no immediate effect. Intravenous ketamine has also been used with success when other agents have failed in acute bronchospasm.

GASTRO-INTESTINAL DISEASE

Dysphagia

Patients with dysphagia resulting from oesophageal stricture or achalasia may be severely malnourished and fluid depleted. Fluid and electrolyte depletion should be corrected preoperatively, and anaesthetic drug dosage should be reduced appropriately to avoid hypotension at induction of anaesthesia.

There may be considerable food debris in the oesophagus, and the usual precautions should be taken to avoid regurgitation and aspiration at induction.

Hiatus hernia

There is a risk of regurgitation and inhalation of gastric contents, especially in obese patients. In addition to the usual measures to avoid aspiration, administration of magnesium trisilicate or a histamine H_2-receptor antagonist (cimetidine or ranitidine) preoperatively may decrease the risk of pneumonitis.

Intestinal obstruction

The principal anaesthetic problems in these patients are extreme fluid and electrolyte depletion with consequent risk of cardiovascular collapse on induction of anaesthesia, and the increased risk of vomiting and inhalation of gastric contents. A large nasogastric tube should be used to empty the stomach as effectively as possible before induction. The tube itself should be removed to allow effective cricoid pressure to be applied.

Patients who have severe vomiting and diarrhoea also pose problems in relation to fluid and electrolyte depletion. All such patients undergoing surgery require appropriate fluid and electrolyte replacement preoperatively dependent on blood urea and electrolyte estimation and with CVP monitoring.

In general, subarachnoid and extradural anaesthesia should be avoided where significant fluid depletion is suspected.

LIVER DISEASE

Anaesthesia and surgery may affect liver function adversely even in previously normal patients. In addition, liver dysfunction may have effects on the conduct of anaesthesia, for example on the metabolism of anaesthetic drugs.

Preoperative assessment should be directed towards detection of jaundice, ascites, oedema and signs of hepatic failure (encephalopathy with flapping tremor). Routine preoperative investigation should include a coagulation screen, measurement of haemoglobin concentration, white cell and platelet counts, and concentrations of serum bilirubin, alkaline phosphatase, transaminase, urea, electrolytes and proteins, including albumin and blood sugar. Blood should also be taken for detection of hepatitis B antigen. If positive, appropriate measures must be taken to protect theatre staff from possible contamination.

Particular problems of relevance to the anaesthetist include:

1. *Acid-base and fluid balance.* Many patients are fluid overloaded. Hypoalbuminaemia results in oedema and ascites, and predisposes to pulmonary oedema. Secondary hyperaldosteronism produces sodium retention and hypokalaemia. Diuretic therapy, often including spironolactone, may also affect serum potassium concentration. In hepatic failure, a combined respiratory and metabolic alkalosis may occur, which shifts the oxygen dissociation curve to the left, impairing tissue oxygenation.

2. *Hepatorenal syndrome.* Jaundiced patients are at risk of developing postoperative renal failure. This may be precipitated by hypovolaemia. Prevention involves adequate preoperative hydration, with i.v. infusion for at least 12 h before surgery, and close monitoring of urine output, intra- and postoperatively. Intravenous 20% mannitol, 100 ml, is recommended immediately preoperatively, and is indicated postoperatively if the hourly urine output decreases below 50 ml. Close cardiovascular monitoring is essential.

3. *Bleeding problems.* Production of clotting factors II, VII, IX and X are reduced as a result of decreased vitamin K absorption. Production of factor V and fibrinogen is also reduced. Thrombocytopenia occurs if portal hypertension is present. Vitamin K should be administered and fresh frozen plasma given to cover surgery with regular checks made on coagulation. Infusion of platelet concentrate is indicated to cover surgery in cases of severe thrombocytopenia or if there is overt bleeding in thrombocytopenic patients.

4. *Drug metabolism.* Impairment of liver function slows elimination of many drugs including anaesthetic induction agents, opioid analgesics, benzodiazepines, suxamethonium, local anaesthetic agents and many others. Since the duration of action of many of these is determined initially by redistribution, prolongation of action may not become apparent until a subsequent dose has been given. Altered plasma protein concentrations affect drug binding, and may account for resistance to d-tubocurarine and pancuronium in liver failure.

In addition, a large number of drugs have toxic effects on the liver. Rarely, halothane is associated with postoperative hepatitis when used more than once within a 6-week period. The mechanism appears to be induction of reductive enzymes in the liver, which, in the presence of hypoxia, causes an increase in hepatotoxic, reductive metabolites. A single halothane anaesthetic is safe in patients with liver disease provided cardiac output and hepatic blood flow are not unduly depressed. If postoperative jaundice occurs, other causes should be sought before accepting a diagnosis of halothane hepatitis.

5. *Hepatic failure.* In such patients, all sedative drugs should be administered with extreme care, since they aggravate encephalopathy. All opioids and benzodiazepines are eliminated by the liver. Benzodiazepines in small doses are probably the best sedatives to use, the short-acting midazolam being first choice. Patients with hepatic failure require intensive management, including close metabolic, fluid and electrolyte monitoring. Hypoglycaemia which occurs as a result of depleted liver glycogen stores should be avoided by the administration of dextrose infusion and sodium intake should be restricted. Amino acids, fat emulsions and fructose should be avoided. Mechanical ventilation is often required, and this diminishes the risk of sedative administration.

Conduct of anaesthesia

If liver function is severely impaired, no premedication should be given. Otherwise, a light benzodiazepine premedication is suitable.

The liver is particularly vulnerable to hypotension and hypoxia. During anaesthesia, cardiac output should be maintained as stable as possible. Blood loss should be replaced promptly, and overall fluid balance maintained with CVP monitoring. Drugs which depress cardiac output, including halothane, enflurane, isoflurane and β-blockers should be used with caution to avoid decreasing hepatic blood flow unduly. Cyclopropane directly depresses hepatic blood flow and should be avoided.

Pancuronium is currently the muscle relaxant of choice in view of its cardiovascular stability, but atracurium may prove preferable in view both of its lack of cardiovascular effects and its elimination which is independent of liver and renal function. Opioid analgesic drugs should be administered with caution unless ventilatory support is planned postoperatively. Pethidine may be preferable to morphine, and is best titrated initially against pain in small i.v. doses, e.g. 20 mg, in the immediate postoperative period.

Controlled ventilation to a normal Pa_{CO_2} is important since hypocapnia is associated with decreased hepatic blood flow. Hypoxia should be avoided throughout, with blood gas monitoring if necessary into the postoperative period.

RENAL DISEASE

Renal dysfunction has a number of important implications for anaesthesia, and therefore full assessment is required before even minor surgical procedures are contemplated.

Measurement of blood urea and electrolyte concentrations should be undertaken before all major surgery and in all elderly or potentially unhealthy patients; a raised blood urea demonstrated pre-operatively may be the first indication of renal disease. Severity of renal dysfunction may be assessed further by measurement of serum creatinine and creatinine clearance, urinary:plasma osmolality ratio and urinary urea and electrolyte excretion.

Preanaesthetic assessment of the patient should be directed to a number of specific problems which require correction before embarking on anaesthesia.

1. *Fluid balance.* In both acute and chronic renal failure, fluid overload may occur. In acute failure, the overload develops suddenly and is uncompensated. In chronic failure, overload may be controlled with diuretic therapy or dialysis. Congestive cardiac failure and hypertension may result from overload, and must be treated before induction of anaesthesia. This may require dialysis.

In patients with nephrotic syndrome, hypoalbuminaemia results in oedema and ascites. Circulating blood volume in these patients is often decreased, and care should be taken at induction of anaesthesia to avoid hypotension.

2. *Electrolyte disturbances.* Sodium retention occurs in renal failure, and through increased ADH secretion is associated with water retention, oedema and hypertension. Hyponatraemia is also common in renal disease. It is caused usually by reduced renal tubular ability to conserve sodium, e.g. in pyelonephritis or analgesic nephropathy. Hyponatraemia also occurs in patients with renal failure as a result of vomiting and diarrhoea or diuretic therapy.

Hyperkalaemia typically occurs in renal failure, frequently in association with metabolic acidosis. A raised serum potassium may be controlled in the short-term by infusion of glucose and insulin: 80 ml of 50% dextrose, with 20 unit of soluble insulin may be given for acute control, followed by an infusion of 50% dextrose with insulin as required using a modified sliding scale governed by BM-test blood sugar estimation. In the longer term, correction of the metabolic acidosis with sodium bicarbonate, and administration of an ion-exchange resin, e.g. calcium polystyrene sulphonate in a dose of 15 g tid orally or as a 30 g retention enema, are useful in controlling hyperkalaemia. Administration of calcium chloride antagonises the cardiac effects of potassium. Dialysis is required if these measures are ineffective. Suxamethonium should be avoided in hyperkalaemic patients in view of its effect in releasing potassium from muscle cells. An increase of up to 0.6 mmol/litre may be expected in normal dosage. Hyperkalaemia is associated with delayed myocardial conduction and ultimately cardiac arrest.

Hypokalaemia commonly occurs in patients receiving diuretic therapy. These patients require preoperative measurement of serum potassium, and replacement if necessary. Hypokalaemia is associated with ventricular irritability, notably in patients taking digoxin.

3. *Cardiovascular effects.* Hypertension may occur for a number of reasons. A raised plasma renin concentration occurring as a result of decreased perfusion of the juxtaglomerular apparatus results in hypertension through increased secretion of angiotensin and aldosterone.

Fluid retention also causes hypertension by increasing the circulating blood volume. Conversely hypertension from other causes results in renal impairment. The precise cause of hypertension in these patients should be sought and the hypertension treated. Anaesthesia for hypertensive patients is discussed on page 467.

Both pulmonary and peripheral oedema may occur

from a combination of fluid overload, hypertensive cardiac disease or hypoproteinaemia. Cardiac failure should be treated preoperatively.

Uraemia may cause pericarditis and a haemorrhagic pericardial effusion, which may embarrass cardiac output and require aspiration.

4. *Neurological effects.* Uraemia causes drowsiness and eventually coma. Electrolyte disturbances and rapid fluid shifts, e.g. during dialysis, may also affect conscious level. Sedative drugs including morphine should be used with care in these patients. In addition, a combined motor and sensory peripheral neuropathy may occur in uraemic patients.

5. *Haematology.* Patients with chronic renal failure suffer from normochromic anaemia, which results from marrow depression, partly as a result of erythropoietin deficiency. They also have an increased incidence of gastro-intestinal bleeding and so an iron deficiency component may be present. These patients are well compensated with an increased cardiac output, and excessive preoperative blood transfusion should be avoided.

6. *Other factors.* Patients with chronic renal failure are frequently undernourished. They tend to be vulnerable to infection. Patients who have received renal transplant, and are immunosuppressed are particularly vulnerable to low-grade pathogens, e.g. *Pneumocystis carinii*. Patients undergoing chronic haemodialysis are not infrequently carriers of hepatitis-B antigen, and if so, appropriate precautions should be taken by theatre staff.

7. *Drug treatment.* Many patients with renal disease are receiving diuretics, antihypertensive therapy, including β-blockers, and digoxin.

Anaesthesia

A light premedication with benzodiazepine or opioid analgesic is satisfactory. Minor procedures, e.g. to establish vascular access for dialysis, are carried out most satisfactorily under regional anaesthesia; brachial plexus block for upper limb and combined femoral and sciatic block for lower limb.

The i.v. cannula for induction and fluid infusion should be sited in the contralateral limb from the arteriovenous shunt or fistula (in those patients undergoing dialysis) and care should be taken to protect the shunt during the operation. Careful monitoring of arterial pressure and e.c.g. is required,

and CVP measurement is indicated in patients who are clinically fluid-overloaded. Intravenous fluid administration should be cautious, and in some instances titrated against CVP measurements. Excessive sodium administration should be avoided, and potassium-containing solutions avoided completely in renal failure. Where the patient is anaemic preoperatively, intraoperative blood loss should be replaced promptly.

Drugs excreted primarily via the kidneys should be used with caution in renal failure. In anaesthetic practice, the principal drugs involved are the muscle relaxants, but in addition other drugs including morphine are conjugated in the liver before excretion in the urine. Depending on the activity of the conjugated metabolite, these drugs may have adverse effects following repeated doses. The muscle relaxants gallamine and fazadinium must be avoided, but d-tubocurarine, pancuronium and alcuronium may be used since alternative excretion in the bile occurs. It is prudent, however, to use reduced dosage, and to monitor respiration closely postoperatively in case of recurarisation. Atracurium (elimination of which is independent of kidney and liver function, and which has minimal cardiovascular effects) would appear to be the relaxant of choice.

Methoxyflurane should be avoided in renal impairment, since the concentrating ability of the kidney is reduced by the effect of fluoride ion on the distal tubule. Enflurane, to a much lesser extent, is also metabolised to fluoride ion, and should be used with caution in cases of severe renal impairment.

Postoperative renal failure

This is not infrequently a problem in patients undergoing major surgery involving large blood loss, in surgery following trauma and in septic patients. Jaundiced patients are also at risk of developing acute renal failure — the hepatorenal syndrome. Avoidance of renal failure in these patients involves close monitoring of the cardiovascular state including CVP and urinary output, avoidance of hypotension, adequate fluid and blood replacement and the use of vasodilators to improve peripheral perfusion. Inotropic support may be required to maintain adequate cardiac output.

Stimulation of urinary output by an osmotic diuretic (mannitol 100 ml of 20% solution over 15 min and repeated once if no response occurs), followed by dopamine 2–5 $\mu g/kg/min$ by infusion should be undertaken if no diuresis occurs following correction of fluid depletion and attainment of cardiovascular stability. If severe fluid overload exists, high dose i.v. frusemide should also be given.

Postoperative oliguria may also be the result of postrenal causes. Patients with prostatic enlargement are particularly liable to develop acute retention. Examination to exclude a full bladder, and catheterisation, should always be carried out in the anuric postoperative patient.

MISCELLANEOUS DISORDERS

Carcinoid syndrome

See Chapter 34, page 452.

Myeloma

This neoplastic condition affecting plasma cells has a number of points of significance to the anaesthetist.

1. Widespread skeletal destruction occurs and careful handling of the patient is essential on the operating table. Pathological fractures are common.

2. Hypercalcaemia occurs as a result of bony destruction, and may precipitate renal failure.

3. Anaemia is almost invariable, and preoperative blood transfusion is often necessary.

4. Infection. Patients are liable to infection, including chest infection, especially during cytotoxic therapy.

5. Bleeding disorders. During cytotoxic therapy, thrombocytopenia is common.

6. Increased plasma immunoglobulin concentrations may raise blood viscosity, predisposing to arterial and venous thrombosis. Drug binding may be affected, e.g. resistance to d-tubocurarine may occur.

7. Neurological manifestations include spinal cord and nerve root compression.

Porphyria

The porphyrias are an inherited group of disorders of porphyrin metabolism characterised by increased activity of δ-aminolaevulinic acid synthetase with excessive production of porphyrins or their precursors. In the U.K., *acute intermittent porphyria*

is the most common type. It is characterised by acute attacks which may arise spontaneously or be precipitated by infection, starvation, pregnancy or administration of certain drugs. Inheritance is Mendelian dominant and thus a family history of porphyria requires further investigation. Clinical features include:

1. *Gastro-intestinal:* abdominal pain and tenderness, vomiting, constipation, and occasionally diarrhoea.

2. *Neurological:* a motor and sensory peripheral neuropathy is common. It may involve bulbar and respiratory muscles. Epileptic fits and a psychological disturbance may occur.

3. *Cardiovascular:* Hypertension and tachycardia often occur during the attacks. Hypotension has been reported also.

4. *Fever and leucocytosis* occur in 25–30% of patients.

Drugs which provoke the attack include alcohol, barbiturates, chlordiazepoxide, steroid hormones, chlorpropamide, pentazocine, phenytoin and sulphonamides.

Anaesthesia in such patients is directed to avoiding drugs which may provoke attacks. Induction with ketamine, followed by muscle relaxation with suxamethonium, d-tubocurarine or gallamine, ventilation with nitrous oxide, halothane and oxygen and analgesic supplementation with morphine or pethidine is satisfactory. If fits occur, diazepam is a suitable anticonvulsant, while chlorpromazine, promethazine or promazine are suitable sedatives.

CONNECTIVE TISSUE DISORDERS

Rheumatoid arthritis

Rheumatoid arthritis is a multisystem disease, with a number of implications for anaesthesia which must be considered on preoperative assessment.

1. *Airway problems.* The arthritic process may involve the temporomandibular joints, rendering laryngoscopy and intubation difficult. The cervical spine may be fixed, or subluxed, and thus unstable, especially when the patient is anaesthetised and paralysed. Crico-arytenoid involvement should be suspected if hoarseness or stridor is present.

2. *Respiratory function.* Costochondral involvement causes a restrictive defect with reduced vital capacity.

Pulmonary involvement with interstitial fibrosis produces $\dot{V}/\dot{Q}$ abnormalities, a diffusion defect and thus hypoxaemia.

3. *Cardiovascular system.* Endocardial and myocardial involvement may occur. Coronary arteritis, conduction defects and peripheral arteritis are other features. Immobility caused by arthritis may mask symptoms of cardiorespiratory disease.

4. *Anaemia.* A chronic anaemia, hypo- or normochromic, but refractory to iron occurs. Preoperative transfusion to approx. 10 g/dl is advisable before major surgery. Treatment with salicylates or other nonsteroidal anti-inflammatory drugs may cause gastro-intestinal blood loss.

5. *Renal failure,* or nephrotic syndrome, may occur as a result of amyloidosis.

6. *Steroid therapy.* Many patients are receiving long-term steroid therapy and require augmented steroid cover for the perioperative period (see p. 485). They are more vulnerable to postoperative infection. Thus, routine preoperative investigation should include full blood count, urea and electrolytes, chest X-ray and e.c.g. Other investigations, e.g. pulmonary function tests and cervical spine X-rays, may be required in certain instances.

Conduct of anaesthesia

Particular care should be taken with venepuncture and placing of i.v. infusions because of atrophy of skin and subcutaneous tissues and fragility of veins. Careful positioning of the patient on the operating table is required since these patients may have multiple joint involvement. Padding may be required to prevent pressure sores.

The anaesthetist should be prepared for difficult intubation, and spinal, extradural or regional techniques are useful for many limb or lower abdominal operations.

Other collagen diseases

Scleroderma

Scleroderma (systemic sclerosis) is characterised by many of the above features including restricted mouth opening, lower oesophageal involvement with increased risk of regurgitation, pulmonary involvement, renal failure, steroid therapy and peripheral vascular disease.

Systemic lupus erythematosus

Anaemia, renal and respiratory involvement may be severe. Steroid therapy is usual.

Polyarteritis

There is diffuse vasculitis, with possible coronary involvement, and neuropathy. Pulmonary involvement and steroid therapy are additional problems.

Ankylosing spondylitis

The rigid spine makes intubation difficult, and spinal and extradural anaesthesia may be technically impossible. Costovertebral joint involvement restricts chest expansion.

Marfan's syndrome

This is a disorder of connective tissue of autosomal dominant inheritance, which is characterised by long, thin extremities, high arched palate, lens subluxation and aortic and mitral regurgitation. Regurgitation may be severe, and the valve lesions may be complicated by subacute bacterial endocarditis. Antibiotic cover is therefore necessary for dental and other surgical procedures.

NUTRITIONAL PROBLEMS

Obesity

Obesity poses a number of problems to the anaesthetist and surgeon.

1. *Cardiovascular function.* Obesity is associated with increased blood volume, cardiac work, hypertension and cardiomegaly. Atherosclerosis and coronary artery disease are common. Diabetes may coexist.

2. *Respiratory function.* Vital capacity and functional residual capacity are decreased. Closing volume is increased. As a result, increased shunting occurs through underventilated dependent lung regions with consequent hypoxaemia. These changes, brought about by abdominal splinting of the diaphragm, are accentuated in the supine, Trendelenburg and lithotomy positions. Lung/chest wall compliance is decreased, the work of breathing

increased, and increased oxygen consumption and CO_2 production cause hyperventilation.

3. *Other factors.* Surgery is technically more difficult, with heavy blood loss, and increased incidences of wound infection and wound dehiscence. Hiatus hernia with risk of regurgitation is more common, and maintenance of the airway and tracheal intubation may be more difficult.

Obese patients require careful preoperative respiratory and cardiovascular assessment (see p. 464). The inspired oxygen concentration should be increased to 40%. Fluid balance should be monitored carefully. Elective postoperative ventilation should be considered, especially after abdominal surgery. Pulmonary, thrombo-embolic and wound complications are more common, and appropriate prophylactic measures and/or early recognition and treatment is important.

Pickwickian syndrome

Pickwickian syndrome is characterised by a combination of obesity, episodic somnolence and hypoventilation with cyanosis, polycythaemia, pulmonary hypertension and right ventricular failure. Avoidance of hypoxia is important, and elective postoperative ventilation may be necessary, especially after abdominal surgery

Malnutrition

As a result of persistent anorexia, dysphagia or vomiting, malnourished patients may be severely fluid and electrolyte depleted. Anaemia and hypoproteinaemia are common.

Preoperative correction of fluid and electrolyte deficit is required with CVP monitoring in severe cases. Infusion of albumin may be advisable in certain instances to raise the colloid osmotic pressure. Doses of induction agents should be administered carefully to avoid hypotension, while smaller doses of relaxants are required, pancuronium being the agent of choice.

ENDOCRINE DISEASE

Pituitary disease

The clinical features of pituitary disease depend on the local effects of the lesion and its effect on the secretion of pituitary hormones. Local effects include headache and visual field disturbances. The effects on hormone secretion depend on the cells involved in the pathological process.

Acromegaly

Acromegaly is caused by increased secretion of growth hormone from eosinophil cell tumours of the anterior pituitary. If this occurs before fusion of the epiphyses, gigantism results. Problems for the anaesthetist include:

1. Upper airway obstruction resulting from an enlarged mandible, tongue and epiglottis, thickened pharyngeal mucosa and laryngeal narrowing. Maintenance of a clear airway and intubation may be difficult, and postoperative care of the airway must be meticulous.

2. Cardiac enlargement, hypertension and congestive cardiac failure occur commonly and require preoperative treatment.

3. Growth hormone increases blood sugar. Hyperglycaemia should be controlled perioperatively.

4. Thyroid and adrenal function may be impaired because of decreased release of TSH and ACTH. Thyroxine and steroid replacement may be required.

Treatment involves hypophysectomy which requires steroid cover preoperatively, and steroid, thyroxine and possibly ADH replacement thereafter.

Cushing's disease

Cushing's disease results from basophil adenomas, which secrete ACTH (vide infra).

Hypopituitarism (Simmond's disease)

Causes include infarction following postpartum haemorrhage, chromophobe adenoma, tumours of surrounding tissues, e.g. craniopharyngioma, skull fractures and infection. Clinical features include loss of axillary and pubic hair, amenorrhoea, features of hypothyroidism and adrenal insufficiency, including hypotension, but with a striking pallor in contrast with the pigmentation of Addison's disease (see p. 484).

The fluid and electrolyte disturbance is not as marked as in primary adrenal failure as a result of intact aldosterone production, but may be unmasked by surgery, trauma or infection.

Anaesthesia in these patients requires steroid cover (p. 485) cautious administration of induction agent and volatile anaesthetic agents, and careful cardiovascular monitoring. Pancuronium is probably the relaxant of choice.

Diabetes insipidus

This is caused by disease or damage affecting the hypothalamic-posterior pituitary axis. Commonest causes are pituitary tumours, craniopharyngiomas, basal skull fracture, infection, or as a sequel to pituitary surgery.

Dehydration follows excretion of large volumes of dilute urine. Patients require fluid replacement and treatment with vasopressin (DDAVP — desmopressin 2–4 µg i.m. daily).

Thyroid disease

Goitre

Thyroid swelling may result from iodine deficiency (simple goitre), autoimmune (Hashimoto's) thyroiditis, adenoma, carcinoma and thyrotoxicosis. Nodules of the thyroid gland may be 'hot' (secreting thyroxine) or 'cold'.

The goitre may occasionally cause respiratory obstruction. Retrosternal goitre may in addition cause superior vena caval obstruction. The presence of a goitre should alert the anaesthetist to the possibility of tracheal compression or displacement. A preoperative X-ray of neck and thoracic inlet may be useful, and a selection of small diameter endotracheal tubes should be available. Preoperative assessment of thyroid function is essential.

Thyrotoxicosis

This is characterised by excitability, tremor, tachycardia and arrhythmias (commonly atrial fibrillation), weight loss, heat intolerance and exophthalmos. Diagnosis is confirmed by measurement of total serum thyroxine and T_3 resin uptake.

Elective surgery should not be carried out in hyperthyroid patients. They should first be rendered euthyroid with carbimazole or radioactive iodine.

Urgent surgery and elective subtotal thyroidectomy may, however, be carried out safely in hyperthyroid patients using β-adrenergic blockade alone or in combination with potassium iodide. Emergency surgery carries a significant risk of thyrotoxic crisis. Control in these circumstances is best achieved by i.v. potassium iodide and β-blockers. Where patients are unable to absorb oral medication, i.v. infusion is indicated. (For propranolol, the daily i.v. dose is approx. one-tenth of the oral dose.)

The dosages of sedative drugs for premedication, and of anaesthetic agents should be increased to compensate for faster distribution and elimination. Spinal nerve block reduces the effects of hyperthyroidism, provided solutions containing adrenaline are not used. Larger than normal doses of sedative drugs are required to avoid anxiety when procedures are carried out under regional anaesthesia.

Preparation for thyroidectomy. Previous conventional management involved at least 6–8 weeks administration of carbimazole to render the patient euthyroid, followed by potassium iodide 60 mg tid for 10 days to decrease the vascularity of the gland.

Many anaesthetists now use β-blockers to prepare the hyperthyroid patient for thyroidectomy. Propranolol 160–480 mg daily for 2 weeks preoperatively and a further 7–10 days postoperatively provides adequate control in most patients. However, control with β-blockers depends on maintaining an adequate plasma concentration of the drug. Since β-blockers, in common with other drugs, are cleared faster in thyrotoxic patients, propranolol should be prescribed more frequently (e.g. 4 times daily). Alternatively, a long acting β-blocker, nadolol 160 mg once daily (including the morning of surgery) provides satisfactory control, and avoids the problems of drug absorption immediately postoperatively. A combination of β-blocker and potassium iodide 60 mg tid provides reliable control in even the most severely thyrotoxic patient.

Hypothyroidism

This may result from primary thyroid failure, Hashimoto's thyroiditis, as a consequence of thyroid surgery, or secondary to pituitary failure. The diagnosis is suggested by tiredness, cold tolerance, loss of appetite, dry skin and hair loss. It may be confirmed by the finding of a low serum thyroxine concentration, associated, in primary thyroid failure, with a raised serum TSH.

Basal metabolic rate is decreased. Cardiac output is decreased, with little myocardial reserve and hypothermia is usually present. Treatment is with thyroxine, which should be commenced in a small dose of 0.05–0.1 mg daily. Rapid correction of hypothyroidism may be achieved using i.v. tri-iodothyronine, but is inadvisable in elderly patients and those with ischaemic heart disease, since the suddenly increased myocardial oxygen demand may provoke infarction. E.c.g. monitoring is advisable.

Elective surgery should be avoided in myx-oedematous patients, but where emergency surgery is necessary, close cardiovascular, e.c.g. and blood gas monitoring is essential. Drug distribution and metabolism is slowed and thus all anaesthetic agents must be administered in reduced dosage.

ADRENAL DISEASE

Adrenal cortex

Clinical syndromes are associated with increased and decreased secretion of cortisol and aldosterone.

Hypersecretion of cortisol (Cushing's syndrome)

Most instances are caused by pituitary adenomas secreting ACTH and thus causing bilateral adrenocortical hyperplasia (Cushing's disease). In 20–30% of patients, an adrenocortical adenoma or carcinoma is present. Rarely, an oat-cell carcinoma of bronchus secreting ACTH is the cause. ACTH or corticosteroid therapy presents a similar picture. Clinical features include obesity, hypertension, myopathy, diabetes mellitus and hypokalaemia. Depending on the cause, treatment may involve hypophysectomy or adrenalectomy.

Anaesthetic management of these patients involves preoperative treatment of hypertension and congestive cardiac failure, and correction of hypo-kalaemia. Intraoperative management is directed towards careful monitoring of arterial pressure, and maintenance of cardiovascular stability, with careful choice and administration of anaesthetic agents and muscle relaxants. Etomidate and atracurium or vecuronium would be an appropriate choice of induction agent and relaxant. Postoperative steroid cover is required for hypophysectomy and adrenal-ectomy (vide infra). Fludrocortisone 0.1–0.3 mg daily is required after bilateral adrenalectomy.

Hypersecretion of aldosterone (Conn's syndrome)

Conn's syndrome is caused by an adenoma of the zona glomerulosa of the adrenal cortex and presents with hypertension, hypernatraemia, hypokalaemia and polyuria. Anaesthetic management involves preoperative treatment of hypertension, the administration of spironolactone and potassium replacement, while intra- and postoperative monitoring of arterial pressure is essential.

Adrenocortical hypofunction

Primary adrenocortical insufficiency (Addison's disease) may be caused by an autoimmune process, tuberculosis, amyloid, metastatic carcinoma, following bilateral adrenalectomy or, acutely, from haemorrhage into the glands in association with meningococcal septicaemia. Secondary failure results from hypopituitarism or prolonged corticosteroid therapy. In secondary failure resulting from pituitary insufficiency, aldosterone secretion is maintained and fluid and electrolyte disturbance less marked.

Clinical features include weakness, weight loss, pigmentation, hypotension, vomiting, diarrhoea and dehydration. Hypoglycaemia, hyponatraemia and hyperkalaemia are characteristic biochemical find-ings. The stress of infection, trauma or surgery provokes profound hypotension. Diagnosis is made by measurement of plasma cortisol levels, the response to ACTH stimulation and to insulin-induced hypoglycaemia.

All surgical procedures in these patients must be covered by increased steroid administration (vide infra). Patients with acute adrenal insufficiency require urgent fluid and sodium replacement with arterial pressure and CVP monitoring, dextrose infusion to combat hypoglycaemia and hydro-cortisone 100 mg 6-hourly i.v. Antibiotics are advisable to cover the possibility of infection provoking the crisis. In cases of primary adrenal failure, mineralocorticoid replacement with fludro-cortisone is required. If emergency surgery is required in acute adrenal failure, all precautions necessary for anaesthetising the shocked patient should be taken (p. 394).

Congenital adrenal hyperplasia (Adrenogenital syndrome)

This is associated with overproduction of androgens as a result of deficiency of hydroxylase enzyme required for production of cortisol. Hydrocortisone treatment overcomes adrenal insufficiency and, by suppressing ACTH production, decreases androgen accumulation. Augmented steroid cover is required for surgery in these patients.

Steroid therapy

Replacement therapy in cases of primary adrenocortical failure and hypopituitarism is given as oral hydrocortisone 20 mg in the morning and 10 mg in the evening. Fludrocortisone 0.05–0.1 mg daily is given additionally to replace aldosterone in primary adrenocortical failure. Equivalent dosage of other steroid preparations is shown in Table 36.2. Prednisolone and prednisone have less mineralocorticoid effect, while betamethasone and dexamethasone have none. Requirements increase vastly following infection, trauma and surgery.

Table 36.2   Equivalent doses of glucocorticoids

Betamethasone	3 mg
Cortisone acetate	100 mg
Dexamethasone	3 mg
Hydrocortisone	80 mg
Methylprednisolone	16 mg
Prednisolone	20 mg
Prednisone	20 mg
Triamcinolone	16 mg

Corticosteroids are prescribed also for a wide range of medical conditions including asthma and collagen diseases. Prolonged therapy suppresses adrenocortical function.

Steroid cover for anaesthesia and surgery

Indications for augmented perioperative steroid cover include:

1. Patients with pituitary-adrenal insufficiency, on steroid replacement therapy.

2. Patients undergoing pituitary or adrenal surgery.

3. Patients on steroid therapy for more than 2 weeks prior to surgery.

4. Patients on steroid therapy for more than 1 month in the year prior to surgery.

Topical fluorinated steroid preparations applied widely to the skin may be absorbed sufficiently to produce adrenal suppression.

Preoperative assessment should involve appropriate fluid and electrolyte correction. Evidence of infection should be sought in patients on long-term steroid therapy.

Corticosteroid cover for operation should be given as follows:

1. Minor diagnostic procedures: single dose of hydrocortisone 100 mg i.m. 1 h preoperatively.

2. Intermediate operations (e.g. inguinal herniorrhaphy): hydrocortisone 100 mg i.m. with premedication; 100 mg 6 hrly for 24 h.

3. Major surgery: hydrocortisone 100 mg 6 hrly for 72 h commencing with premedication.

The requirements may need to be increased if infection is present or be continued beyond 3 days if infection or the effects of major trauma persist. Oral administration may be resumed after 24 h.

Where steroids are prescribed for asthma or other medical conditions, the perioperative dosage may require modification according to the activity of the disease.

Adrenal medulla

Phaeochromocytoma

See page 453.

NEUROLOGICAL DISEASE

There are several points of significance.

1. *Medicolegal*. Perioperative alteration in neurological deficit may be attributed to anaesthesia. This may render subarachnoid or extradural anaesthesia inadvisable in certain patients.

2. *Respiratory impairment*. Motor neuropathy from various causes, e.g. motor neurone disease, acute polyneuritis (Guillain-Barré syndrome), disorders of the neuromuscular junction and high spinal cord lesions may produce respiratory inadequacy. These patients are sensitive to anaesthetic agents, opioids and relaxants, and if intraoperative IPPV is undertaken, a period of elective postoperative ventilation may be necessary until full recovery from

the effects of anaesthesia has occurred. If possible, procedures should be carried out under local or regional block. If bulbar muscles are involved, protection of the airway from regurgitation and aspiration may require prolonged intubation or tracheostomy. Surgery should be postponed if a chest infection is present preoperatively.

3. *Altered innervation of muscle, and potassium shifts.* An altered ratio of intracellular to extracellular potassium tends to produce a sensitivity to nondepolarising and resistance to depolarising relaxants. Where there is widespread denervation of muscle in lower motor neurone disease, e.g. in Guillain-Barré syndrome, disorganisation of the motor end-plate occurs, resulting in hypersensitivity to acetylcholine and suxamethonium, with increased permeability of muscle cells to potassium. A similar potassium efflux occurs with direct muscle damage, widespread burns involving muscle, upper motor neurone lesions, spinal cord lesions with paraplegia, and tetanus. In upper motor neurone and spinal cord lesions, the reason for this shift is less clear.

The resulting increase in serum potassium after suxamethonium may be 3 mmol/litre (in comparison with 0.5 mmol/litre in the normal patient) and may occur from 24 h after acute muscle denervation or damage until 6–12 months later. In such patients, suxamethonium is clearly contraindicated.

4. *Autonomic disturbances* may occur as part of a polyneuropathy, e.g. diabetes, Guillain-Barré syndrome and porphyria. Sympathetic stimulation, for example during light anaesthesia, intubation or following administration of pancuronium or catecholamines may produce severe hypertension and arrhythmias. More commonly, blood loss, head-up posture or IPPV may be associated with severe hypotension.

5. *Increased intracranial pressure.* Elective surgery should be postponed where raised intracranial pressure (ICP) is suspected until investigation and treatment have been undertaken. Anaesthetic agents which cause an increase in cerebral blood flow must be avoided. Hypercapnia must also be avoided and controlled ventilation to a Pa_{CO_2} of approx. 4 kPa (30 mmHg) is indicated. This is discussed fully in Chapter 27.

6. *Cerebrovascular disease.* In patients with suspected widespread cerebrovascular disease, the principal aim of anaesthetic management should be to maintain normotension and normocapnia. While hypercapnia increases cerebral blood flow, it may produce 'steal' from ischaemic to well perfused areas of brain. Hypocapnia decreases cerebral blood flow and is also contraindicated.

Epilepsy

In most patients with epilepsy, no identifiable cause can be found. Epilepsy may also be associated with birth injury, hypoglycaemia, hypocalcaemia, drug withdrawal, fever, head injury, cerebrovascular disease and cerebral tumour, the most likely cause depending on the age of onset. Epilepsy developing after the age of 20 yr usually indicates organic brain disease.

Anaesthesia

Patients should be maintained on anticonvulsant therapy throughout the perioperative period. Certain anaesthetic agents, e.g. enflurane and methohexitone, have cerebral excitatory effects and should be avoided. Local anaesthetic agents may cause convulsions at lower than normal concentrations and the safe maximum dose should be reduced.

The anticonvulsants phenobarbitone and phenytoin induce hepatic enzymes and accelerate elimination of drugs metabolised by the liver.

In cases of late onset epilepsy, where increased ICP may be present as a result of tumour, controlled ventilation is advisable to avoid any increase in ICP.

Multiple sclerosis

Deterioration of symptoms tends to occur after surgery, but no particular anaesthetic technique is implicated. It is usually advisable to avoid extradural and subarachnoid anaesthesia, if only for medicolegal reasons, but there is no evidence that these techniques affect the disease adversely and they may be used in certain cases if a full explanation has been given to the patient.

If a larger motor deficit of recent onset is present, there may be increased potassium release from muscle following suxamethonium, which should thus be avoided.

Peripheral neuropathies

These may exhibit axonal 'dying back' degeneration or segmental demyelination. They are classified by anatomical distribution, the commonest being a symmetrical peripheral polyneuropathy. Motor, sensory and autonomic fibres are involved. Causes include (1) metabolic (diabetes, porphyria), (2) nutritional deficiency, (3) toxic (heavy metals, drugs), (4) collagen disease, (5) carcinoma, and (6) infective. Problems for the anaesthetist include the effects of autonomic neuropathy, respiratory and bulbar involvement.

Guillain-Barré syndrome (acute infective polyneuropathy)

The polyneuropathy appears some days after a pyrexial illness. Progression is very variable, ranging from near total paralysis in 24 h to progression over several weeks. Respiratory and bulbar muscles may be affected, and if so endotracheal intubation followed by tracheostomy and IPPV are required. Autonomic neuropathy may result in hypotension following institution of IPPV. This may be minimised by adequate fluid preloading and gradual increases in minute volume. Suxamethonium should be avoided.

Motor neurone disease (Progressive muscular atrophy, amyotrophic lateral sclerosis, progressive bulbar palsy)

Motor neurone disease is characterised by slow onset and progressive deterioration in motor function. Several patterns of motor loss occur with both upper and lower motor neurone loss. Problems for the anaesthetist include sensitivity to all anaesthetic agents and muscle relaxants, respiratory inadequacy and laryngeal incompetence. Local anaesthetic techniques may be useful. Mechanical ventilation should be avoided if possible, since the motor deficit is irreversible.

Hereditary ataxias

Freidrich's ataxia is the most common. Spino-cerebellar, corticospinal and posterior columns are involved, and the course of the disease is slowly progressive. Problems for the anaesthetist include scoliosis, respiratory failure and cardiomyopathy with cardiac failure and arrhythmias.

Spinal cord lesions with paraplegia

Release of potassium from muscle cells by suxamethonium precludes its use within 6 to 12 months of cord injury.

Huntington's chorea

It has been reported that thiopentone may cause prolonged apnoea, while abnormal serum cholinesterase may prolong the action of suxamethonium.

Myasthenia gravis

This is a disease occurring usually in young adults and is characterised by episodes of increased muscle fatiguability, caused by decreased numbers of acetylcholine receptors at the neuromuscular junction. Treatment involves anticholinesterase (pyridostigmine 60 mg qid or neostigmine 15 mg qid) and a vagolytic agent (atropine or propantheline) to block the muscarinic effects. Steroid therapy is useful in certain cases and thymectomy may benefit many patients considerably, especially young women with myasthenia of recent onset.

The chief problems concern adequacy of ventilation, ability to cough and clear secretions, and the increased secretions resulting from anticholinesterase therapy. If there is evidence of respiratory infection, surgery should be postponed. Serum potassium should be normal, since hypokalaemia potentiates myasthenia. Local and regional anaesthesia including low subarachnoid or extradural block may be suitable alternatives to general anaesthesia, although the maximum dose of local anaesthetic agents used should be reduced in view of their neuromuscular blocking action. The minimum possible dose of induction agent should be used and relaxants should be avoided if possible. For major procedures requiring relaxation, the anticholinesterase may be omitted for 4 h preoperatively, and a small dose of, for example, d-tubocurarine 3–5 mg may be given if necessary. Suxamethonium has a variable effect in myasthenia and is best avoided.

Postoperatively, the patient's lungs should be ventilated electively for 24–48 h after major surgery.

Good chest physiotherapy and tracheal suction are required. Steroid cover, where appropriate, is required. If extreme muscle weakness occurs, i.v. atropine 0.6–1.2 mg and neostigmine 1–2 mg may be given. Care must be taken to titrate the doses of anticholinesterase carefully, or a cholinergic crisis, characterised by a depolarising neuromuscular block, with sweating, salivation, and pupillary constriction may occur. Edrophonium may be used to test the end-plate response to acetylcholine.

A myasthenic state may also be associated with carcinoma, thyrotoxicosis, Cushing's syndrome, hypokalaemia and hypocalcaemia. In these patients, nondepolarising relaxants should be avoided, or used in reduced dosage.

Familial periodic paralysis

This is also associated with prolonged paralysis after nondepolarising muscle relaxants.

Progressive muscular dystrophy

Several types of muscular dystrophy exist, of varying patterns of heredity and described according to their anatomical distribution. Muscular weakness occurs, which must be distinguished from myasthenia and lower motor neurone disease. The anaesthetic considerations consist of sensitivity to relaxants, opioids and other sedative and anaesthetic drugs, and liability to respiratory infection. Myocardial involvement may occur.

Dystrophia myotonica

This is a disease of autosomal dominant inheritance characterised by muscle weakness and muscle contraction persisting after the termination of voluntary effort. Other features may include frontal baldness, cataract, sternomastoid wasting, gonadal atrophy and thyroid adenoma. Problems affecting anaesthetic management include:

1. *Respiratory muscle weakness.* Respiratory function should be fully assessed preoperatively. Respiratory depressant drugs, e.g. thiopentone or opioids, should be used with care, while there is sensitivity also to nondepolarising relaxants. Elective postoperative IPPV may be required. Postoperative

care of the airway must be meticulous in view of muscle weakness. Chest infections are common.

2. *Cardiovascular effects.* Arrhythmias are common, particularly during anaesthesia and this may result in cardiac failure. Careful monitoring is essential.

3. *Muscle spasm.* This may be provoked by administration of depolarising muscle relaxants and anticholinesterases. Suxamethonium and neostigmine should thus be avoided. The spasm is not abolished by nondepolarising relaxants.

DIABETES MELLITUS

Diabetic patients frequently present for surgery for peripheral vascular disease, cataract extraction and drainage of abscesses. Surgical stress and infection cause an increase in insulin demands. In addition, diabetes is associated with various complications which affect anaesthetic management.

The aim of perioperative management is to ensure adequate blood sugar control preoperatively and maintain this control, while avoiding hypoglycaemia which may not be detectable readily in the anaesthetised patient. Management is simplified by frequent blood sugar estimations using Dextrostix (Ames) or BM-Test-Glycemie (Boehringer-Mannheim) preferably in conjunction with a reflectance colorimeter.

Precise management depends on the nature of the diabetes and its treatment (insulin dependent or maturity onset), on the magnitude of the surgery contemplated, including the estimated time to resumption of oral intake, and on the time available for control of the diabetes.

Preoperative assessment

Preoperative assessment is aimed at evaluating (a) blood sugar control, (b) the presence of complications of diabetes and (c) the treatment regimen used.

Blood sugar control

This is assessed from the patient by inspecting records of urine testing, and by a blood sugar profile throughout a 24-h period in patients receiving insulin. If possible, blood sugar should be maintained between 6–10 mmol/litre and dosage should be adjusted to achieve this, with the introduction of twice daily short- and medium-acting insulins if necessary.

The author does not favour changing to short-acting insulin on the day before surgery in well controlled diabetes, provided the dose of the medium- or long-acting insulin is not excessive (< 40 unit); all too often this merely results in loss of control. The type of insulin should be noted and it is important to avoid sudden change from bovine to purified porcine insulin since this may produce hypoglycaemia as a result of increased sensitivity to the latter. Table 36.3 describes some of the insulin preparations available.

Oral hypoglycaemic agents are of two types. Sulphonylureas stimulate insulin release from the pancreatic islets. Chlorpropamide has a very prolonged duration of action and unless stopped 48 h before surgery may cause hypoglycaemia intra-operatively. A change to a shorter acting drug, e.g. glibenclamide or glipizide is preferable. Biguanides are used in obese maturity onset diabetics or in combination with sulphonylureas. Phenformin, especially, and metformin may both cause lactic acidosis, usually, but not necessarily only, in patients with renal or hepatic impairment. This complication carries a high mortality, and these drugs should be discontinued before surgery.

Complications

1. *Cardiovascular disorders.* Widespread athero-sclerosis and small vessel disease are common. Ischaemia is often associated with infection. Coronary artery disease also occurs more commonly in diabetics.

2. *Renal disease.* Microvascular damage produces glomerulosclerosis with proteinuria and eventually chronic renal failure.

3. *Eye.* Cataracts and exudative or proliferative retinopathy may be present. Vitreous haemorrhage and retinal detachment may follow.

4. *Infection.* Diabetics are liable to infection, which in turn increases insulin requirements and may provoke ketoacidosis. Abscesses, infected gangrene, urinary tract infections and pulmonary tuberculosis are more common in diabetics. Surgical drainage of an abscess is followed by a sudden decrease in insulin requirements.

5. *Neuropathy.* A chronic, predominantly sensory, peripheral neuropathy is common, especially in elderly patients. The loss of sensation coupled with peripheral vascular disease may result in ulceration

Table 36.3 Commonly used insulin preparations

	Source	Purity	Duration of action	Comments
Short acting				
Soluble	Bovine	—	5–7 h	3 times daily dosage required
Nuso	Bovine	—	4–6 h	Neutral
Actrapid MC	Porcine	Highly purified	5–7 h	Neutral
Neusulin	Bovine	Purified	5–7 h	Neutral
Intermediate				
Isophane	Bovine	—	18—20 h	Twice daily dosage. Add soluble to improve control. Purified analogues: Neuphane, Insulatard
Semilente (IZS Amorphous)	Bovine	—	12–16 h	Twice daily dosage Purified analogue: Semitard MC
Mixed				
Rapitard MC	Bov. & porc.	Purified	18–24 h	Twice daily dosage. Neutral (porc.) and Crystalline (bov.)
Mixtard	Porcine	Purified	18–20 h	Twice daily dosage. Neutral 30% + Insulatard 70%
Initard	Porcine	Purified	18–20 h	Twice daily dosage. Neutral 50% + Insulatard 70% These preparations give control equivalent to soluble + isophane
Long acting				
IZS Lente (Mixed)	Bovine	—	20–24 h	Once daily dosage. IZS Amorphous 30% + Crystalline 70% Purified analogues: Neulente, Lentard, Monotard
IZS Ultralente (Crystalline)	Bovine	—	24–36 h	Once daily Purified analogue: Ultratard

after trivial trauma. Careful positioning of patients on the operating table is important. Mononeuropathy, acute peripheral neuropathy and diabetic amyotrophy (motor) are associated with poor control. Nerve block should be avoided in patients with these acute neuropathies since the neuropathy may be attributed to or exacerbated by local anaesthetic solutions.

6. *Autonomic neuropathy.* This may cause disturbances of bowel and bladder function, vasomotor instability e.g. postural hypotension, and impaired sympathetic response to hypoglycaemia. Patients should be well hydrated before anaesthesia, and cardiovascular parameters monitored carefully. IPPV and subarachnoid or extradural blockade may produce severe hypotension, and require careful management.

7. *Diabetic ketoacidosis.* Diabetic ketoacidosis results from inadequate insulin dosage or increased insulin requirements, precipitated often by the stress of surgery, sepsis or trauma. Patients with ketoacidosis undergoing emergency surgery require rehydration, correction of sodium and, later, potassium depletion, and soluble insulin by infusion at an initial rate of 6–8 unit/h. Progress is monitored by frequent estimations of blood sugar, urea and electrolytes and arterial pH and blood gases. Correction of the acidosis with sodium bicarbonate is rarely required but a small dose of 50 mmol should be given if arterial pH is less than 7.1. Potassium depletion is present *ab initio*, but hyperkalaemia is present initially as a result of acidosis. Potassium replacement should not commence until the serum potassium concentration has begun to decrease as a result of correction of acidosis. Change of i.v. fluids to

5% dextrose should be made when blood sugar has decreased to approx. 15 mmol/litre. When rehydration has been initiated (1.5–2.0 litre in first 2 h) and some correction of acidosis and hyperglycaemia has been achieved, anaesthesia and surgery may be carried out, continuing diabetic management intra- and postoperatively.

Nonketotic hyperosmolar coma is associated with severe dehydration, and hyperglycaemia, but no acidosis. It occurs frequently in elderly patients or in those who have had an excessive glucose load (e.g. badly controlled i.v. feeding), steroid therapy, or diuretic therapy. Correction with hypotonic saline should be carried out slowly to avoid osmotic fluid shifts which result in cerebral oedema.

Concurrent drug therapy in diabetics

Diuretics including thiazides, frusemide and the hypotensive agent diazoxide tend to increase blood sugar. Adrenergic agents, e.g. salbutamol, and corticosteroids also result in carbohydrate intolerance.

Hypotensive drugs, e.g. ganglion blockers and β-adrenergic blockers, tend to potentiate hypoglycaemia, and may mask the sympathetic response to hypoglycaemia.

Certain drugs, including phenylbutazone, may displace sulphonylureas from protein-binding sites and potentiate the hypoglycaemic effect.

Subarachnoid and extradural anaesthesia block the hyperglycaemic response to surgery, thus avoiding the necessity for increasing insulin dosage. However, when the effects of the spinal block decline the

Table 36.4 Maturity onset diabetics — perioperative management

Preoperative	During operation	Postoperative

Poor control:
  change to insulin (Table 36.5)
	Minor surgery:
	  if blood glucose > 10 mmol/litre
	  no specific treatment
	  Recheck blood sugar postop.
		Minor surgery:
		  recommence hypoglycaemic agent
		  with 1st meal

Good control: chlorpropamide —
  ideally change to glibenclamide
  or glipizide 1 week preop. No
  chlorpropamide within 48 h of surgery
  No glibenclamide or glipizide
  on morning of operation
	Major surgery:
	  treat as insulin-dependent diabetic
	  (Table 36.5)
		Major surgery:
		  treat as insulin-dependent diabetic
		  (Table 36.5). When oral intake restarted
		  tid soluble insulin 8–12 unit
		  before each meal. Restart oral therapy
		  when daily requirement less than
		  20 units

Biguanides — discontinue		

Table 36.5 Insulin dependent diabetics — perioperative management

Preoperative	During operation	Postoperative
Stabilisation for 2–3 days. Most patients b.d. soluble + isophane. If large dose isophane, change to short acting only on day before operation	Start infusion of 10% dextrose 500 ml 4-hrly with soluble insulin 10 units and 10 mmol KCl at 8 a.m.	Continue 4–5 hrly infusions until oral intake established. If delayed, change to decreased volumes of 20—50% dextrose by central line. 2–4 hrly dextrostix. Insulin by independent infusion. When oral intake re-established tid soluble insulin
No subcutaneous insulin on day of operation	Preop. and subsequent blood sugars:	
	5–10 mmol/litre — infusion as above. <5 mmol/litre — insulin 5 unit/500 ml 10% dextrose 10–20 mmol/litre — insulin 15 unit/500 ml 10% dextrose >20 mmol/litre — insulin 20 unit/500 ml 10% dextrose 4–5 hrly.	
	Adjust K^+ dosage depending on plasma K^+ concentrations	
	K^+ <3.0 — add KCl 20 mmol K^+ >5.0 — omit KCl	

hyperglycaemic response occurs. By avoiding general anaesthesia, hypoglycaemia may be recognised readily.

Perioperative diabetic control for elective surgery

Tables 36.4 and 36.5 describe a scheme of management for patients on oral hypoglycaemic or insulin therapy undergoing major or minor surgery.

The combination of a glucose solution with insulin is designed to avoid the problem of inadvertent discontinuation or acceleration of either glucose or insulin which may occur if they are administered separately. The scheme described may need to be modified for certain patients, and different concentrations of glucose and insulin may be used. Management depends on preoperative measurement of blood glucose with repeat measurements 2-hrly thereafter.

FURTHER READING

Aitkenhead A R, Grant I S 1983 Intercurrent disease and medication. In: Henderson J J, Nimmo W S (eds) Practical regional anaesthesia. Blackwell Scientific Publications, Edinburgh

Alberti K G M M, Thomas B J B 1979 The management of diabetes during surgery. British Journal of Anaesthesia 51: 693

Bevan D R 1979 Renal function in anaesthesia and surgery. Academic Press, London

Bevan D R 1979 Shy-Drager syndrome. A review and a description of anaesthetic management. Anaesthesia 34: 866

Bevan D R 1978 Symposium on clinical assessment. British Journal of Anaesthesia 50: 1

Diamond A W, Piggot R W, Townsend P L G 1975 Immediate care of burns. Anaesthesia 30: 791

Fisher A, Waterhouse T D, Adams A P 1975 Obesity: Its relation to anaesthesia. Anaesthesia 30: 633

Jones R M, Healy T E J 1980 Anaesthesia and demyelinating disease. Anaesthesia 35: 879

Katz J, Benumof J, Kadis L B 1981 Anesthesia and uncommon diseases. W B Saunders, Philadelphia

Lown B 1967 Electrical reversion of cardiac arrhythmias. British Heart Journal 29: 469

Mason R A, Steane P A 1976 Carcinoid syndrome: its relevance to the anaesthetist. Anaesthesia 31: 228

Muir I F K, Barclay J L 1962–1974 Burns and their treatment. Lloyd-Luke, London

Nunn J F 1981 Anaesthesia and the patient with respiratory disease. In: Gray T C, Nunn J F, Utting J E (eds) General anaesthesia. Butterworths, London

Philbin D M 1979 Anaesthetic management of the patient with cardiovascular disease. International Anesthesiology Clinics 17, 1. Little, Brown, Boston

Prys-Roberts C 1980 Hypertension, ischaemic heart disease and anesthesia. International Anesthesiology Clinics 18, 4. Little, Brown, Boston

Strunin L 1977 The liver and anaesthesia. W B Saunders, London

Stamenkovic L, Spierdijk M D 1976 Anaesthesia in patients with phaechromocytoma. Anaesthesia 31: 941

Stoelting R K, Dierdorf S R 1983 Anaesthesia and coexisting disease. Churchill Livingstone, Edinburgh

Vickers M D 1982 Medicine for anaesthetists, 2nd edn. Blackwell Scientific Publications, London

Welbourn R B, Joffe S N 1977 The apudomas. Recent advances in surgery, 9. Churchill Livingstone, Edinburgh

37

Haematology

Surgery and anaesthesia make heavy demands on departments of haematology and blood transfusion. Consultation between the anaesthetist and haematologist should be frequent both in the operating theatre and intensive care unit if the provision of, for example, appropriate blood products and the correct investigation of the bleeding patient are to proceed smoothly and expeditiously.

ANAEMIA

Anaemia is present when the red cell mass (the erythron) is reduced below that which is normal for the patient's age and sex. There are many causes and these are classified conventionally as:

1. *Blood loss* which may be acute or chronic.

2. *Failure of erythropoiesis* resulting from, for example, inadequate supplies to the bone marrow of nutrients: iron, vitamin B_{12}, folate, certain hormones, protein. Erythropoiesis may be impaired also by bone marrow infiltration in leukaemia or other malignant disease. Most chronic disorders produce what is termed a secondary or symptomatic anaemia. This is seen in inflammation, infection and malignant disease (even when the marrow is not infiltrated). Secondary anaemias are seen commonly in rheumatoid arthritis, renal failure and chronic sepsis.

3. *Shortened red cell lifespan* — the haemolytic anaemias. These are subdivided into those conditions which are inherited and congenital; examples are hereditary spherocytosis, sickle cell anaemia and certain red cell enzyme defects; and those which are acquired sometime after birth e.g. autoimmune haemolytic anaemia, paroxysmal nocturnal haemoglobinuria and drug induced haemolysis.

It is obvious that alternative classifications are possible, and also true that many forms of anaemia may be allocated to more than one category. Thus, chronic blood loss produces negative iron balance with eventual failure of erythropoiesis from iron deficiency. Pernicious anaemia is an erythropoietic failure resulting from lack of correct digestion of vitamin B_{12}, but red cell precursors and mature red cells in this disease have a shortened lifespan.

Anaemia is demonstrated by the measurement of the amount of haemoglobin in a known volume of blood. Haemoglobin is reported as gram per decilitre (g/dl) and it remains one of the few laboratory measures not reported as gram per litre of blood. Anaemia is said to be present in an adult male if the haemoglobin is less than 13.5 g/dl and in an adult female if less than 11.5 g/dl. In the first year of life the haemoglobin decreases from 18–20 g/dl at birth to 9.5 g/dl at one month to attain levels at 12 months close to those of female adults. In pregnancy, haemoglobin levels should not decrease below 11.5 g/dl if iron and folate are taken as prescribed.

Modern electronic blood counting equipment provides accurate red cell indices in addition to haemoglobin estimation and provides guidance on the type of anaemia before resort to further investigation.

With the notable exception of acute blood loss, reduction in red cell mass is accompanied by an increase in plasma volume thus preserving blood volume. The mechanism for this is not clear but it is one of the compensatory mechanisms adopted during anaemia of any duration. Of equal importance is a shift of the oxygen dissociation curve to the right through increased synthesis of 2,3-diphosphoglycerate (2,3-DPG) in the red cell via the Embden-Meyerhof pathway of anaerobic glycolysis and the Rapaport-Luebering shunt. Increases in

2,3-DPG render the haemoglobin molecule less avid for oxygen at given partial pressures and improve tissue oxygenation. Two remaining compensatory mechanisms in anaemia are an increase in cardiac stroke volume and an increase in heart rate.

In acute blood loss, red cells and plasma are lost together such that in the first few hours, haemoglobin and haematocrit measurements change little and cannot be used to estimate blood loss. Surgeons have always attributed much importance to the haematocrit but in continued acute bleeding the haemoglobin and haematocrit move in parallel as haemodilution takes place, being complete by 24–48 h if transfusion is not carried out.

HAEMOGLOBINOPATHIES AND THALASSAEMIAS

The haemoglobinopathies and thalassaemias are a complex and diverse series of inherited abnormalities of globin chain synthesis. The thalassaemias are characterised by absent or reduced production of the affected globin chain whilst the other chains which make up the haemoglobin molecule are normal. In the haemoglobinopathies the affected chain, usually the β or α chain, has an amino acid substitution which, if it affects the structure or function of the haemoglobin molecule as a whole, may produce clinical effects.

Beta thalassaemia

Beta thalassaemia, in which β globin chain synthesis is impaired, is classified into three clinical grades.

1. *Beta thalassaemia trait (thalassaemia minor)* is the heterozygous state and produces little clinical effect. There may be slight anaemia and the condition may be mistaken for iron deficiency. In pregnancy the haemoglobin level may decrease below the normal range.

2. *Thalassaemia intermedia,* as the name implies, is associated with more marked anaemia than thalassaemia trait and generally is caused by homozygosity of a less severe β-thalassaemia gene. Occasionally, patients may require transfusion.

3. *Thalassaemia major (Cooley's anaemia)* is the homozygous inheritance of a severe β-thalassaemia gene. No β-chains are produced thus preventing the synthesis of adult haemoglobin. Without blood transfusion, the condition is generally fatal in the early years of childhood and even with regular transfusion support, patients may not live beyond their early twenties as a result of iron overload. Long-term iron chelation therapy may prevent transfusional iron overload.

Alpha thalassaemia

Alpha thalassaemia is a genetically variegate disorder which ranges in severity from fetal death in utero in the homozygous form to a mild hypochromic disorder in the heterozygous form. Patients with 3 of the 4 α-chain genes deleted suffer HbH disease of intermediate severity, and some require transfusion with red cells.

Haemoglobinopathies

More than 100 haemoglobin variants have been described but only 1 has significant global clinical impact — haemoglobin S. Ten per cent of patients of African extraction carry the S gene. It is also seen in Italy, Greece, Arabia and the Indian subcontinent. Haemoglobin S has valine substituted for glutamine in position 6 of the β-globin chain and this confers notable physical differences on the haemoglobin molecule with profound clinical consequences in homozygotes. Haemoglobin S becomes insoluble at oxygen tensions in the venous range (5–5.5 kPa) and crystallises, imposing the sickle-cell shape on the red cell. The sickled red cell is rigid and does not pass easily through capillaries, leading to occlusion, tissue infarction and pain which is characteristic of clinical episodes known as crises. Red cell survival is greatly reduced and homozygous patients invariably have anaemia (6–10 g/dl) and jaundice. Heterozygotes are almost asymptomatic and their red cells sickle only when oxygen tensions are unphysiologically low (2 kPa). Sickle haemoglobin may be demonstrated rapidly in patients' blood using a commercial kit, e.g. Sickledex. The presence or absence of HbS should be established before anaesthesia in all patients of affected ethnic groups. It may be necessary to pretransfuse electively homozygotes with HbA or consider exchange transfusion to raise percentages of HbA compared with HbS. Clearly it is essential to maintain good oxygenation of the homozygous patient pre-, intra- and postoperatively and consideration should be given to oxygen therapy for 24 h after anaesthesia. Postoperative infarctive episodes may occur even with the most meticulous attention to detail. Sickling is enhanced by low blood pH, high red cell 2,3-DPG, stasis, dehydration and increased plasma osmolality.

HAEMOSTASIS AND FIBRINOLYSIS

The haemostatic mechanism

There are three principal components: platelets, coagulation and what may be termed limiting mechanisms including fibrinolysis. These may be altered individually or collectively in disease to produce haemostatic failure. Investigation of the bleeding patient should include all three components.

Platelets

Primary haemostasis depends solely on the presence of adequate functional platelet numbers (Fig. 37.1). The normal whole-blood platelet count is 150–400 × 10^9/litre. The lower limit of 'normal' depends upon the method used for their quantitation but a platelet count below 100 × 10^9/litre is considered thrombocytopenia. The risk of haemostatic failure increases as the platelet count decreases and when levels below 30 × 10^9/litre are reached spontaneous bleeding may occur. Bleeding is precipitated if there is local pathology, for example peptic ulcer or if there is a surgical wound. Thrombocytopenic bleeding occurs less at a particular platelet count if the low platelet numbers result from peripheral destruction with a functional bone marrow (e.g. autoimmune thrombocytopenia) than if platelet production is impaired, for example in bone marrow disorders (e.g. leukaemia or myeloma).

For adequate primary haemostasis the platelets should also function normally. In comparison to the rare inherited platelet functional disorders, drug-induced platelet metabolic damage occurs more commonly. Nonsteroidal anti-inflammatory drugs (NSAIDs) impair prostaglandin synthetic pathways by inhibition of the enzyme cyclo-oxygenase. Aspirin (acetylsalicylic acid) is the prime example and its effect on measured in vitro function of platelets lasts up to 14 days. Other therapeutic agents affecting platelet function include sulphinpyrazone, dipy-

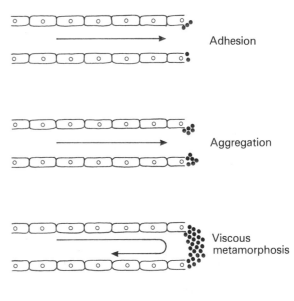

Adhesion

Aggregation

Viscous metamorphosis

Reinforcement with fibrin

Clot retraction

Fig. 37.1   Formation of a platelet plug.

ridamole and dextran. Drug-induced platelet dysfunction may cause bleeding in the face of adequate platelet numbers and patients should be encouraged to discontinue the drug, preferably 2 weeks before major surgery, particularly with respect to the NSAIDs. Uraemia is accompanied by acquired platelet dysfunction which may be corrected by dialysis. Platelets in the myeloproliferative disorders including certain leukaemias may function poorly.

Stored whole blood for transfusion contains few viable platelets; after storage for only 3 days, platelet recovery in vivo is only 20%. Thus, in massive transfusion (more than 10 unit), platelet numbers decline progressively but rarely decrease below 50 × 10^9/litre even when twice the patient's blood volume has been transfused.

Platelet function in vivo is best measured by the bleeding time carried out by haematology staff according to strict methodology. This should not be undertaken unless platelet numbers have been shown to be normal, or bleeding is out of proportion to platelet numbers and coagulation is demonstrably normal. Careful examination of the patient reveals clues to thrombocytopenia: petechial purpura particularly below the knee, blood-filled blisters in the mouth and fundal haemorrhages. In the patient in theatre, oozing at the operation and venepuncture sites acts as an indicator. The strategy of platelet transfusion is described below.

Table 37.1 International nomenclature of clotting factors

Factor	Synonym
I	Fibrinogen
II	Prothrombin
III	Tissue thromboplastin
IV	Calcium ions
V	Labile factor
VI	Unassigned
VII	Stable factor
VIII	Antihaemophilic factor (AHF)
IX	Christmas factor
X	Stuart-Prower factor
XI	Plasma thromboplastin antecedent (PTA)
XII	Contact factor
XIII	Fibrin stabilising factor

Coagulation

The second phase of haemostasis involves the coagulation proteins (Table 37.1) which stabilise the haemostatic plug provided by the platelets. Central to this is the production of thrombin (Fig. 37.2) from prothrombin by the action of activated factor X. Thrombin cleaves fibrinogen to form fibrin. Two pathways lead to the conversion of prothrombin and are composed of linked proteolytic enzymes which act first as substrates and then as activated enzymes. The first pathway is intrinsic (all components circulate in plasma). Its first component is the contact factor XII which requires an exposed subendothelial surface for its activation. A series of reactions follows involving coagulation factors and cofactors which culminate in the prothrombin–thrombin reaction. Extrinsic coagulation joins the cascade at the pivotal factor X requiring tissue juices for its inception. Activated by thrombin, factor XIII stabilises the fibrin polymer by cross-linkages between amino acids in adjacent fibrin strands.

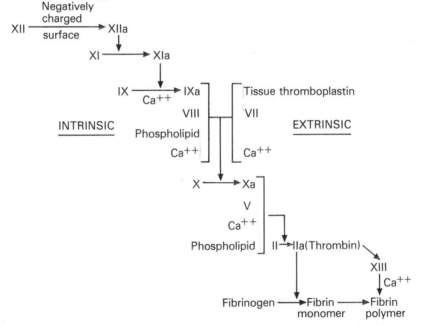

Fig. 37.2 Intrinsic and extrinsic coagulation pathways; 'a' indicates activation of the factor concerned. Phospholipid is provided by platelets and plasma.

Limiting factors

The third set of reactions serves to inhibit the unbridled extension of thrombus and vessel occlusion. Firstly, as the vessel relaxes, returning blood flow dilutes activated clotting proteins and mechanically discourages extension of the plug. Vascular endothelial cells secrete prostacyclin, a powerful inhibitor of platelet aggregation. Circulating inhibitors neutralize clotting intermediates, the most important being antithrombin III.

Lastly, and of great importance, is the fibrinolytic system (Fig. 37.3). Plasmin (the active enzyme of fibrinolysis) cleaves fibrin and fibrinogen and is derived from an inactive precursor, plasminogen. Activator of plasminogen is released from damaged endothelial cells and activated factor XII also converts plasminogen. Thus fibrinolysis has similar triggers to coagulation. The resulting fibrin fragments (fibrin degradation products, FDP) are both anticoagulant and interfere with fibrin polymerisation. The interaction of and balance of coagulation and fibrinolysis is essential in maintaining vessel integrity and patency following injury.

DISSEMINATED INTRAVASCULAR COAGULATION (DIC)

This is also referred to as *consumption coagulopathy* which suggests the pathogenesis. Essentially, the process represents the inappropriate triggering of the coagulation cascade in flowing blood by particular disease processes. There is considerable variation in severity ranging from the coagulopathy being the predominant clinical manifestation (with haemostatic

failure) to merely a laboratory sign of the underlying disease with no clinical haemostatic lesion. Some possible causes are listed in Table 37.2.

Table 37.2 Clinical associations of disseminated intravascular coagulation

Immediate cause	
Release of tissue thromboplastin	Eclampsia
	Placental abruption
	Fetal death in utero
	Amniotic fluid embolism
	Disseminated malignancy including acute leukaemia
	Head injury
	Burns
Infection	Malaria,
	Bacteria, especially Gram negative
	Viruses
Miscellaneous	Incompatible blood transfusion
	Extracorporeal circulation
	Antigen-antibody complexes
	Fat embolism
	Pulmonary embolism
	Shock

The principal laboratory findings are produced by the consumption of platelets during intravascular coagulation with reduction of fibrinogen and elevation of FDP in the serum as secondary (physiological) fibrinolysis breaks down thrombus. Thrombocytopenia, hypofibrinogenaemia and elevation of serum FDP are thus the hallmarks of DIC. Scrutiny of the blood film may reveal red cell distortion or fragmentation if there is associated microangiopathy.

As the majority of clotting tests rely on the fibrinogen-fibrin reaction as the end-point, the prothrombin time, partial thromboplastin time and

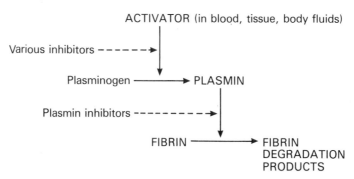

Fig. 37.3 The fibrinolytic system.

thrombin time are prolonged as a result also of the anticoagulant effect of FDP and consumption of other coagulation factors (II, V, VIII). DIC which is associated with endotoxaemia and endothelial damage tends to have more profound thrombocytopenia. There is some suggestion too that in severe DIC there is, in addition, an induced platelet functional defect. DIC is inevitable in some degree where there is tissue damage (particularly the brain), hypotension, shock and poor organ perfusion.

Variants of the syndrome (with similar laboratory findings) may occur with localised extravascular consumption, e.g. placental abruption and localised intravascular consumption (e.g. thrombotic thrombocytopenic purpura). Occasionally primary pathological fibrinolysis (PF) occurs without the microthrombosis seen in DIC, e.g. in neoplasia. Laboratory tests are not dissimilar to DIC but platelet counts tend to be higher. Differentiation of the commoner DIC from the less common PF rests on a careful clinical assessment and informed interpretation of additional laboratory tests which may require haematological advice.

The management of DIC depends on clinical rather than laboratory severity. Whatever the degree of DIC, the first principal is an attempt to alleviate the underlying cause. In septicaemia, the infection should be treated vigorously along conventional lines. In hypovolaemic shock with DIC, adequate blood volume expansion is required and in placental abruption the uterus requires emptying. After successful treatment, most patients with DIC settle spontaneously and only in those with significant and continuing coagulation failure is there a need to repair the haemostatic mechanism with blood products. The approach to the particular patient depends on clinical circumstances and laboratory results but measures may include the administration of fresh frozen plasma (FFP), cryoprecipitate (fibrinogen, factor VIII and fibrinectin), platelets and heparin (rarely). Advice should be sought from the haematologist.

THE BLEEDING PATIENT

The anaesthetist and surgeon are confronted not infrequently with a patient who is known to have a pre-existing haemostatic defect and the haematologist is asked if the patient is either fit for surgery or can be rendered operable.

Inherited coagulation abnormalities

These comprise classical haemophilia (haemophilia A) arising from coagulation factor VIII deficiency, Christmas disease (haemophilia B) from deficiency of factor IX (and clinically identical to classical haemophilia) and von Willebrand's disease from absence of part of the factor VIII molecule. Other inherited coagulation factor deficiencies occur but are rare.

The bleeding manifestations in the haemophilias are related directly to the degree of deficiency. The patient with severe classical haemophilia, with coagulation factor VIII levels of less than 1% (0.01 i.u./ml) of average normal, bleeds spontaneously particularly into joints. In those with higher levels (1 to 3% of average normal) spontaneous bleeding is less common. In those moderately affected (3–16%), spontaneous bleeding is uncommon. The least affected group (16–40%) may remain undiagnosed until late in life. However, any haemophiliac patient of whatever grade of severity bleeds excessively if challenged by trauma or by surgery and an occasional patient is diagnosed initially under those circumstances.

For surgery to proceed safely, the appropriate factor has to be raised to and maintained at a haemostatic level. How this is achieved depends on the type of surgery envisaged, the native factor level in the plasma, the half-life of the factor concerned after infusion, the type of factor concentrate available and the number of days to healing (which in turn depends on the procedure which has been performed). With the availability of factor VIII and IX concentrates, surgery of any kind may now be contemplated safely. Six per cent of severe haemophiliacs develop antibodies to factor VIII, making management much more difficult. Surgery of any type, however minor, should be carried out only in designated haemophilia centres which have the staff, technical facilities and experience to supervise the haemostatic management of such patients. In the emergency situation, recourse should be made to telephonic communication with the haematologist at the nearest designated centre.

The anticoagulated patient

A more commonly encountered problem is that of the orally anticoagulated patient who presents as an emergency requiring surgical intervention within a short time. Although major surgery may be carried out in the fully orally anticoagulated patient, surgeons are generally reluctant to proceed without at least partial reversal of the coumarin lesion.

The oral anticoagulant drug of choice in the United Kingdom is warfarin sodium, and maintenance doses range from 3 to 10 mg daily. This prolongs the prothrombin time to 2 to 4 times normal (the therapeutic range). Phytomenadione (vitamin K_1) may be used (orally, i.m., or i.v.) to treat the warfarinised patient to reverse the warfarin lesion. Its effect is equally rapid by each route. It should be noted that if an excess is given, it renders the patient refractory to further warfarinisation for up to several weeks. The dose of vitamin K_1 in warfarin-induced haemorrhage or overdosage is 2.5 to 20 mg but in the therapeutically anticoagulated patient about to undergo surgery, doses as small as 0.5 to 1.0 mg may be sufficient. Reversal takes up to 12 h to be adequate and the affected vitamin K-dependent clotting factors II, VII, IX and X return to the plasma in order of their half lives. If the planned surgical intervention cannot wait for the 12 h required, the vitamin K-dependent factors require replacement using blood products. The most widely available material is FFP. The material from 3 donations (approx. 540 ml) should be administered and the effect on prothrombin time measured. Meanwhile phytomenadione is given. FFP takes up to 20 min to thaw, so foresight is required. Further FFP may be given (group O and group A is available) if the desired effect is not obtained. Resort to freeze-dried preparations containing vitamin K-dependent factors is rarely necessary and is not recommended presently because of the dangers of triggering DIC.

In patients who are receiving permanent anticoagulation therapy, e.g. for atrial fibrillation or prosthetic cardiac valves, it is prudent to give prophylactic s.c. heparin during the period when warfarin is suspended in an attempt to prevent thrombo–embolic sequelae. The suggested dose is 5000 units of calcium heparin 8 to 12 h s.c. until warfarinisation is re-established. These sub-pharmacologic doses of heparin do not induce bleeding during surgery. The use of heparin assay ensures that desirable levels of plasma heparin are attained.

Liver disease

Hepatocellular disease (cirrhosis or acute liver failure) results in diminished synthesis of vitamin K-dependent clotting factors (II, VII, IX and X) and fibrinogen, producing a laboratory lesion similar to that resulting from oral anticoagulants. In addition, these patients may be thrombocytopenic and clear FDP from the plasma at a reduced rate. Recourse to vitamin K, FFP and platelet support may be required.

HEPARIN

Heparin is a potent, naturally occurring anticoagulant which commercially is isolated from animal intestinal mucous membranes. Bearing a strong negative charge, it interferes with the thrombin–fibrinogen reaction and potentiates the physiological antagonist of activated clotting factors, antithrombin III. It is given i.v. preferably continuously, at a dose of 24–48 000 unit in 24 h (for deep vein thrombosis). Its action is immediate and if given by bolus, it has a half-life of only 40 to 80 min. It has now gained wide acceptance in some but not all forms of major surgery as a successful means of preventing post operative deep vein thrombosis. For this indication, the dose by the s.c. route is 5000 units 8 or 12 hrly given for 7 to 10 days.

If a patient who is therapeutically heparinised requires emergency surgery, cessation of the infusion may suffice because of the short half-life of the drug. The laboratory test of choice used to monitor adequacy of full heparinisation is the partial thromboplastin time with kaolin (PTTK) which should be 1.5 to 4 times prolonged compared to the control time. This desired ratio may differ between laboratories. Prior to emergency surgery in the heparinised patient, recourse to the PTTK may indicate that there is little risk of bleeding if the test is prolonged less than 1.5:1. Reversal of heparin in an emergency may be achieved using protamine sulphate given by slow i.v. injection at a dose of 1 mg per 100 units of heparin. Not more than 50 mg of protamine sulphate should be given as, in addition to side effects of flushing, bradycardia and hypotension, it is itself an anticoagulant.

PLATELET THERAPY

Unlike red cells, platelets have an inconveniently short shelf-life. Whereas red cells in citrate-phosphate dextrose with adenine have a safe storage life of 28 days, platelets in the same anticoagulant are only satisfactory when given to the recipient within 2 days of donation. This places obvious constraints on the supply of viable platelets to hospitals by transfusion centres. Improved survival of platelets following donation may follow the introduction of new materials for blood bag manufacture. Platelets are supplied usually as concentrates, that is platelet rich plasma (PRP) (produced by low g spun freshly donated blood) spun down again and much of the supernatant plasma removed.

The indications for platelet transfusion remain controversial. In patients with, e.g. acute leukaemia, who (because both of bone marrow disease and cytotoxic chemotherapy) are producing no endogenous platelets, the debate centres on the need for prophylactic versus therapeutic platelet transfusions. Because of rapid development of platelet antibodies, leukaemia centres are tending to limit prophylaxis to particular situations when the risk of haemorrhage is high, e.g. during serious infective episodes, and opting to treat other haemorrhagic episodes vigorously as they occur. Seventy per cent of patients develop platelet-destroying alloantibodies after repeated transfusions.

In surgical practice, as a general rule, significant bleeding should not occur if platelet numbers are greater than 100×10^9/litre. Below 30×10^9/litre, bleeding may be anticipated. Between 30 and 100×10^9/litre operative and postoperative oozing depends on the nature of the surgical procedure and the aetiology of the thrombocytopenia.

In autoimmune thrombocytopenia (e.g. idiopathic thrombocytopenic purpura and Felty's syndrome) patients who have failed medical treatment may be referred for splenectomy with very low platelet counts. They do not require platelet transfusion for two reasons. Firstly, therapeutic platelets would be of short survival, being cleared by the same immune mechanism which is causing the patient's thrombocytopenia. Secondly, following the tying of the splenic pedicle, platelet counts may increase rapidly ensuring adequate intra- and postoperative haemostasis. However the local regional transfusion centre should be notified of the elective splenectomy in order that platelets might be furnished at relatively short notice if required.

If surgery is to be covered with platelet transfusions, the standard dose is 4 unit per square metre of body surface, a unit being the platelets from a single donation. Currently, platelets are not cross-matched but where possible, ABO and Rhesus compatible platelets should be chosen. This dose may need to be given twice on the day of surgery and half of the first dose at least 60 min preoperatively. One further dose on the first postoperative day may be required but the need for further platelets should be assessed on the patient's progress and demonstration of normal coagulation proteins if haemostasis is not total. Countable platelets should increase in the patient's blood after a transfusion for there to be any chance of success.

In DIC of any cause, platelet transfusions are rarely needed but should be given if platelet consumption has been documented as severe, and haemorrhage is a clinical problem. In the massively transfused patient with haemostatic failure, platelets may be required if thrombocytopenia is unusually low (less than 50×10^9/litre) and the coagulation mechanism is not judged to be at fault on laboratory testing.

BLOOD TRANSFUSION

The ABO blood groups first described in 1901 by Landsteiner and the Rhesus system described by Landsteiner and Weiner in 1940 together form the important blood group systems for those practising blood transfusion primarily at the bedside. However, there are many other clinically important blood group systems which are the more immediate concern of the blood transfusion laboratory staff. Problems relating to these groups are normally resolved by the laboratory before blood products are issued as compatible for use in the patient.

ABO groups

In the United Kingdom, 47% of persons are group O, 42% group A, 8% group B and 3% group AB. Patients, and thus donors, have these percentage distributions (Table 37.3). Proportions vary elsewhere in the world mainly from increased gene frequency of B. ABO blood group substances may be

Table 37.3 Distribution of ABO blood groups in the United Kingdom their red cell antigens and antibodies

	%	RBC antigen	Serum	
O	47	—	Anti-A Anti-B	'Universal donor'
A	42	A	Anti-B	
B	8	B	Anti-A	
AB	3	A + B	—	'Universal recipient'

Rhesus D positive 85%
Rhesus D negative 15%

found also on leucocytes and platelets and 77% of persons secrete ABO blood group substances in body fluids. ABO antibodies are said to be naturally occurring, that is they are a constant feature of the system in all persons and do not arise as a result of exposure to A or B blood group substances at some time during life. Although A and B blood group substances appear in RBC early in fetal development, the corresponding antibodies appear only after birth at 3–6 months of age and are present in greatest strength at the age of 10 yr. After the early months of life, Anti-A and anti-B are present invariably in the serum when the red cells lack the corresponding antigen. Table 37.3 shows the old rationale, now outmoded, for the designation of group O persons as Universal Donors, because they lack group A and B substances in their red cells, and persons of group AB as Universal Recipients as their serum does not contain either anti-A or anti-B. ABO antibodies are predominantly IgM and thus do not cross the placenta. An occasional person, usually group O, may have 'immune' anti-A (or less commonly anti-B), an IgG molecule capable of crossing the placenta and active at 37°C. Such persons are called 'dangerous' donors and are screened at transfusion centres. If pregnant with a group A (or B) fetus, ABO materno-fetal incompatibility may ensue with haemolytic disease of the newborn.

Whenever possible blood transfusion laboratories try to provide blood of the same ABO group as the recipient. If a patient of group AB requires an emergency transfusion of more than a few units, further AB units may be unavailable and A blood is used, being likely to be more plentiful than B. If ABO compatible blood is unavailable for a group B patient, group O is used with suitable preceding cross matching tests.

ABO incompatible transfusion accidents are the most serious of the transfusion incompatibilities and have significant morbidity and mortality. Properly conducted routine cross-matching techniques detect such incompatibilities in vitro and they occur only where there has been an error of patient identification or sample identification. Most accidents of this type result from clerical errors.

Rhesus groups

Shortly after the discovery of the Rhesus groups it was recognised that some haemolytic transfusion reactions and haemolytic disease of the newborn (erythroblastosis fetalis) resulted from incompatibilities in this system. In bedside blood transfusion practice, the Rhesus D antigen is the most important of the Rhesus antigens and units of blood or blood products labelled Rhesus positive are D positive although they may also be positive for C and E antigens. Units labelled Rhesus negative lack all three antigens C, D and E and thus have the Rhesus phenotype cde/cde. The Rhesus factors are inherited in a 'packet', one from each parent, each 'packet' containing one of each pair of alleles C or c, D or d and E or e. The commonest genes are CDe (gene frequency 0.41) and cde (0.39) followed by cDE (0.14). The other genes are much less common.

Antibodies of clinical significance occur in the Rhesus system and these rarely occur naturally, i.e. they are formed as the result of exposure to Rhesus antigens which the patient does not naturally possess. The commonest circumstance is the bearing of a Rhesus positive fetus by a Rhesus negative woman. The most common antibody is anti-D and at least two pregnancies are required. Such antibodies are detected readily in cross-matching techniques but, if undetected, may result in an immediate transfusion reaction, or at best, impaired survival of the transfused cells.

Other blood groups

The known number of blood group antigens is increasing constantly usually because of the discovery first of the corresponding antibody. Many are of little clinical significance. Ability to react at 37°C and specificity characterise those antibodies in recipient serum which necessitate the provision of red cells lacking the corresponding antigen. Of greatest importance are, in order of frequency, Kell, Duffy, Kidd, Ss and Lewis. Of all clinically significant alloantibodies, 83% are in the Rhesus system (Table 37.4).

Table 37.4 Percentage frequency of clinically important 37°C alloantibodies detected in recipients

Anti-D	61
Anti-C (± D)	11
Anti-E	7
Anti-Kell	6
Anti-C	4
Anti-Duffy	2.2
Anti-Kidd	0.9
Anti-e	0.5
Anti-Ss	0.04
Others (Lewis included)	7

Storage and preservation of blood

Until recently, blood for transfusion was collected into ACD (acid citrate dextrose solution containing trisodium citrate, citric acid and dextrose) which acted both as an anticoagulant and red cell preservative. This was superseded in some parts of the world in the 1970s by CPD (citrate phosphate dextrose) in which the addition of sodium dihydrogen phosphate raised the pH of the solution and improved red cell survival in vivo. The duration of storage considered suitable with an anticoagulant is such that on the last day of storage, 70% of red cells are recoverable in the circulation at 24 h after transfusion and subsequently have a normal survival pattern. In this context red cell survival is related to cellular levels of ATP. The addition of adenine to CPD assists maintenance of ATP levels and this preferred anticoagulant-preservative known as CPD-A enables the shelf life of stored blood to be increased to 28 days or even 35 days compared with 21 days for ACD and standard CPD. Storage of red cells for transfusion should be at 2 to 6°C in a blood bank refrigerator. Resort to other domestic-type refrigerators is hazardous because of the risk of inadequate thermostatic control leading to the possibility of freezing of blood and lysis of red cells on warming in the event of equipment failure. Ministry of Health-type insulated boxes maintain precooled red cells for transfusion at a satisfactory temperature, when used with ice inserts, for up to 24 h.

At appropriate storage temperatures, bacterial replication in blood is inhibited and red cell glycolysis is slowed with some preservation of 2,3-DPG levels.

Red cell survival in vitro is thus preserved. The prime function of the erythrocyte is delivery of oxygen to the tissues and this is dependent on red cell levels of 2,3-DPG. In ACD, red cells lose 40% and 90% of 2,3-DPG at 1 and 2 weeks respectively with a resulting shift to the left of the oxygen dissociation curve. In CPD, 2,3-DPG is better maintained (20% loss at 2 weeks) but slightly less so in CPD-A. Whatever the storage medium, however, levels of 2,3-DPG return to normal in 6–24 h after transfusion.

Blood grouping and cross-matching tests

Elective grouping is now being undertaken more commonly using automated apparatus suited to large batches. This process may take up to half a day. In the emergency situation, if the patient's group is not known it can be ascertained rapidly, using a tile, in 5–10 min after receipt of the samples.

There is incomplete agreement as to what constitutes the ideal cross-matching test system to ensure compatibility between donor red cells and patient's serum. Essential components include a test at room temperature to detect the important ABO incompatibilities between donor and patient and two or more tests at 37°C to detect Rhesus and other allo-antibodies in the patient's serum which would result in transfusion reaction and reduced red cell survival. The clinically important antibodies are shown in Table 37.4. The introduction of low ionic strength saline (LISS) to replace ordinary saline as a red cell suspension medium has resulted in incubation times being greatly reduced and an acceptable 30 min cross-match is now a reality.

Trends towards the elective screening of all patients' sera for irregular antibodies simultaneously with automated grouping may soon obviate the need for any cross-matching technique. This would ensure that once a patient had been shown to be free of alloantibodies to blood group antigens, blood of appropriate ABO and Rhesus group would simply be selected and given without matching (and the resultant time delays).

Red cell concentrates ('packed cells', plasma-reduced cells)

In the U.K. regional transfusion centres issue a large minority of red cells to hospitals as red cell concentrates. This is achieved by the removal of 150–200 ml of citrated plasma from the final donated volume of 490 ml (420 ml blood plus 70 ml of CPD anticoagulant). The fresh plasma thus harvested is used as raw material for blood product manufacture, particularly factor VIII concentrate and plasma protein fraction. Red cell concentrates produced in modern plastic closed sterile blood-bag systems have the same shelf life as whole blood. Cryoprecipitate manufacture from freshly donated units results in a unit of whole blood with the normal amount of plasma and labelled 'cryoprecipitate poor'. Many hospital blood bank laboratories now provide the first two units of blood being matched for surgery as red cell concentrates which are more viscous than whole blood.

Future developments include the provision of red cells from transfusion centres suspended in preservative solutions which contain little plasma, and may include the development of artificial blood in the form of oxygen-carrying plasma volume expander solutions.

Transfusion reactions

In addition to the haemolytic transfusion reactions referred to above there are other types of reaction which may interfere with the completion of transfusion of blood or blood products. About 2% of all transfusions are followed by some form of reaction and three-quarters of these are febrile reactions. These latter result from antibodies to white cells in the HLA system. Such reactions may be accompanied by rigors, hypotension, dyspnoea, occasionally cyanosis, nausea and vomiting. It is worth remembering that the symptoms and signs of any form of transfusion reaction may be obscured or abolished by general anaesthesia. Fever following platelet transfusion in patients with platelet alloantibodies is less common but platelet preparations are always contaminated by white cells. Prevention of reactions to white cells includes the transfusion of buffy coat-poor blood, washing of red cells or the use of white cell filters at the bedside.

Milder anaphylactic reactions are associated frequently with urticaria (weals or hives) and very occasionally with flushing, dyspnoea and hypotension and are thought to result from reaction between IgA in the transfused blood and anti-IgA in the recipient.

Less commonly, other antibodies in an atopic subject may be implicated.

Nonimmunological reactions to stored blood include induced hypothermia from transfusion of large volumes of cold blood and citrate toxicity in similar circumstances. Other consequences are air embolism, transfusion of particulate matter from transfusion equipment and reactions to cellular debris in blood, for example 'postperfusion' lung. Some complications of blood transfusion are listed in Table 37.5.

Table 37.5   Complications of blood transfusion

Transmission of disease, e.g. viral hepatitis, syphilis, malaria,
  AIDS
Bacterial contamination
Pyrogenic reactions
Incompatibility reactions
Haemolytic reactions
Allergic reactions
Citrate toxicity
Hypothermia
Hyperkalaemia
Metabolic acidosis
Circulatory overload
Air embolism
Microaggregate embolism

Plasma volume expanders

In acute hypovolaemia plasma volume expanders are frequently used whilst blood is being prepared. Transfusion is commenced with electrolyte solutions but continued with volume expanders.

There are two nonhuman-source materials in use:

Gelatins

In these bovine gelatin is partly degraded to produce a molecular weight of approx. 35 000. The product Haemaccel has a pH, colloid osmotic pressure and viscosity similar to that of plasma and a half-life of at least 4 h. It is eliminated from the body by 12 days (80% cleared in 48 h). It should not be allowed to mix with citrated blood. It has a shelf-life at ambient temperatures of 8 yr. Occasionally, too rapid infusion may result in the release of vasoactive substances causing rash, hypotension and tachycardia treated best by antihistamines and/or hydrocortisone and discontinuing the infusion. It does not interfere with blood grouping or cross-matching. Renal function is not impaired by gelatins which are excreted unchanged in the urine thereby exerting an osmotic diuretic effect. Not more than 1 litre of gelatin solution should be transfused before whole blood is available (or in extreme circumstances 1.5 litre).

Dextrans

Dextran 70 injection B.P. (6% dextran) is most frequently employed in 5% dextrose or in 0.9% saline. The average molecular weight of the material is 70 000. They should not be administered to patients with renal impairment, severe congestive heart failure and thrombocytopenia. The dextrans are believed to interfere with the haemostatic mechanism if transfused in large quantity and in the laboratory cause difficulty with grouping and cross matching tests by promotion of rouleaux. No acutely haemorrhagic patient should receive more than 1.5 litre and, as unpredictable anaphylactic reactions may occur with erythema, bronchospasm, urticaria and hypotension, the patient should be observed carefully during the first few minutes of the infusion. If such a reaction occurs, the infusion should be stopped immediately and resuscitation measures instituted.

Human plasma protein fraction (PPF)

This is prepared both by the DHSS Blood Products Laboratory from donor plasma and by the pharmaceutical industry. It contains 4.5 g/dl protein, principally as albumin in saline. It is heat treated, and present evidence suggests that this inactivates hepatitis-producing agents. It has a 3-yr shelf-life (away from light). It is singularly free from adverse effects.

Unfortunately the DHSS material is in short supply and has to be supplemented from commercial sources. This may be remedied in the next few years.

The relative prices of these volume expanders (March 1983) for 400 ml to hospital pharmacies are Haemaccel £3.40, Dextran 70 in saline £3.35 and commercial PPF £27.37.

FURTHER READING

Jamieson G A, Greenwatt T J (eds) 1978 Progress in clinical and biological research, vol 19. Alan R Liss, New York
Bloom A L, Thomas D P 1981 Haemostasis and thrombosis. Churchill Livingstone, Edinburgh & London
Hardisty R M, Weatherall D J (eds) 1982 Blood and its disorders, 2nd edn. Blackwell Scientific Publications, Edinburgh
Harris J W, Kellermeyer R W 1972 The red cell, 2nd edn. Harvard University Press, Cambridge, Mass.

Hoffbrand A V, Pettit J E 1980 Essential haematology, 1st edn. Blackwell Scientific Publications, Edinburgh
Mollison P L 1982 Blood transfusion in clinical medicine, 7th edn. Blackwell Scientific Publications, Edinburgh
Retz L D, Swisher S M N (eds) 1981 Clinical practice of blood transfusion. Churchill Livingstone, London
Serjeant G R 1974 The clinical features of sickle cell disease. Clinical studies, vol 4. North Holland, Amsterdam
Weatherall D J, Clegg J B 1981 Thalassaemia syndromes, 3rd edn. Blackwell Scientific Publications, Edinburgh

38

Cardiopulmonary resuscitation

Cardiopulmonary resuscitation (CPR) is required when the supply of oxygen to the brain is insufficient to maintain function. Since oxygen delivery is dependent upon: (1) cardiac output, (2) haemoglobin concentration, and (3) saturation of haemoglobin with oxygen which is dependent largely on respiratory function, it follows that CPR is required most commonly for low cardiac output states, respiratory failure or a combination of the two.

Cerebral hypoxia

The brain is more sensitive to hypoxia than any other organ, including the heart. It has limited facility for anaerobic metabolism and cannot store oxygen. The cerebral cortex is damaged permanently by ischaemia of more than 3–4 min duration. Thus, although a patient may survive an episode of circulatory arrest, permanent impairment of cerebral function may result if cerebral oxygen delivery is not restored within 3–4 min of the initial cessation of blood flow.

The commonest cause of brain damage following cardiac arrest is delay in starting resuscitation. Therefore, when circulatory arrest has occurred, it is essential to commence CPR as rapidly as possible.

THE SIGNS OF CARDIAC ARREST

These are shown in Figure 38.1. During surgery it may be difficult to distinguish between profound hypotension and circulatory arrest. If neither surgeon nor anaesthetist can feel a pulse, external cardiac massage must be commenced.

THE MANAGEMENT OF CARDIAC ARREST

The aim of resuscitation is to restore oxygen delivery to the body tissues, in particular the brain, as soon as possible. Until a spontaneous circulation is restored, circulation must be maintained by external cardiac massage and oxygenation by artificial ventilation.

External cardiac massage (ECM)

ECM is the only manoeuvre that will circulate blood once circulatory arrest has occurred and it must be commenced immediately. The only exception is cardiac arrest resulting from hypoxia or asphyxia when ventilation takes priority.

The reasons for this are that:

1. The lungs normally contain sufficient oxygen to prevent serious desaturation of blood for at least 30 s, or longer if the patient's lungs were preoxygenated.

2. The brain is more tolerant to hypoxaemia than ischaemia.

3. External cardiac massage is normally easier to commence than artificial ventilation.

4. If commenced immediately before the heart becomes deoxygenated, cardiac massage may itself restart the heart.

Mechanism of blood flow

'Old' CPR. Classically the heart was thought to behave as a simple pump during external cardiac massage. During the compression phase, it is squeezed between the sternum and the vertebral column, the valves act normally and blood is ejected into the aorta and the pulmonary artery. Between

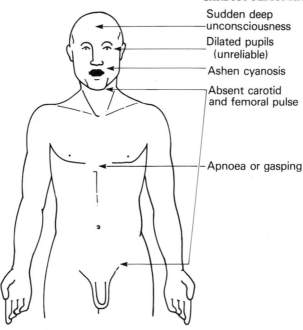

Sudden deep
unconsciousness

Dilated pupils
(unreliable)

Ashen cyanosis

Absent carotid
and femoral pulse

Apnoea or gasping

Fig. 38.1 The signs of cardiac arrest. Sudden loss of consciousness and absence of major pulses are sufficient to justify diagnosis.

compressions the heart refills with blood and oxygenation occurs in the lungs. With 'Old' CPR the lungs are ventilated once every five cardiac compressions.

'New' CPR. When external cardiac compression and ventilation are timed to coincide, cyclical increases occur in intrathoracic pressure. It has been shown that this results in improved forward flow in comparison with 'old' CPR. However, the effect on cerebral oxygen delivery is uncertain and improved survival has not been demonstrated.

Recommended technique for external cardiac massage

This is shown in Figure 38.2. Cardiac compressions should be performed continuously and not

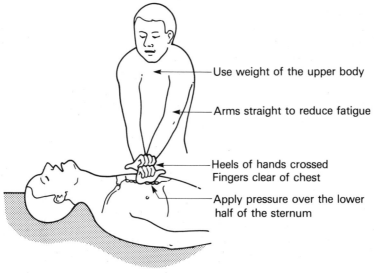

Use weight of the upper body

Arms straight to reduce fatigue

Heels of hands crossed
Fingers clear of chest

Apply pressure over the lower
half of the sternum

Fig. 38.2 External cardiac massage.

interrupted during lung inflations. Ideally the patient should lie on a hard surface but cardiac massage must not be delayed until such a surface is found.

With two operators, the sternum should be compressed 60 times per min and 1 ventilation given every 5 cardiac compressions. For a single operator, two successive inflations interposed every 15 compressions is less tiring.

The time of commencing resuscitation should be noted — this is important for medicolegal and prognostic purposes.

If cardiopulmonary arrest occurs in the operating theatre, the surgeon should be informed, the table tilted head-down, all anaesthetic agents discontinued and the patient's lungs ventilated with 100% oxygen. If the abdomen is open, external cardiac compression is preferable to massage through the diaphragm.

The airway and artificial ventilation

The simplest technique of artificial ventilation is by expired air resuscitation using the mouth-to-mouth or mouth-to-nose methods. This option is always available, requires no special equipment and can be commenced immediately. Expired air contains 16%–18% oxygen and in a patient with normal lungs produces a Pa_{O_2} of approx. 10 kPa, at which level haemoglobin is 89% saturated.

Nonetheless, 100% oxygen should be given as soon as possible, but operator expired-air resuscitation should never be delayed whilst equipment for administering oxygen is found.

Technique of operator expired air resuscitation

The operator clears the airway by extending the patient's neck. If necessary the angles of the jaw are pulled forward. These manoeuvres prevent the tongue from falling back against the posterior pharyngeal wall.

The patient's nose is pinched closed, the operator takes a deep breath, and applying his lips closely over the patient's lips so as to obtain an airtight seal, exhales slowly but forcefully, feeling his expired air enter the patient's chest and watching it expand (Fig. 38.3). The operator then removes his lips and allows the patient to exhale passively. The aesthetics of this technique may be improved if the operator places a handkerchief over the patient's face.

If mouth-to-mouth ventilation proves difficult, mouth-to-nose ventilation should be performed. The operator closes the patient's mouth whilst inflating the lungs via the nose and then the patient's mouth is opened to permit passive expiration to occur.

Other problems which may arise include failure to maintain a patent airway, failure to keep an airtight seal and gastric distension and regurgitation. Suction apparatus should be at hand to remove vomitus.

Adjuncts to expired air resuscitation (e.g. the Brooke, Safar and oesophageal obturator airways) have no place in the anaesthetist's armamentarium. If a patient's airway cannot be maintained, the patient's trachea should be intubated.

Bag and mask ventilation

In an emergency, a self-inflating bag may be used. These units save operator fatigue and can deliver either room air — which has a higher $F_{I_{O_2}}$ than expired air — or room air with added oxygen. A Guedel or nasopharyngeal airway is a useful aid to

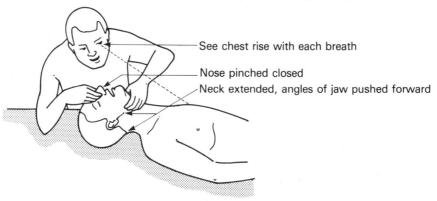

See chest rise with each breath

Nose pinched closed

Neck extended, angles of jaw pushed forward

Fig. 38.3 Operator expired air resuscitation.

lung inflation and may also help maintain patency of the airway in the spontaneously breathing patient. A transparent face mask allows early detection of vomit. In the operating theatre, a face mask in combination with a standard anaesthetic circuit is used.

Endotracheal intubation

This renders resuscitation easier and more efficient and is always desirable. However, it is not essential as a first step unless the airway cannot be maintained by other means, e.g. in the presence of facial trauma or if regurgitation has occurred. However, a cuffed tube placed correctly protects the lungs, guarantees an airway and permits the use of 100% oxygen more easily.

Acute upper airway obstruction

If upper respiratory tract obstruction cannot be obviated by intubation and the situation is desperate the options are:

1. Laryngotomy — the cricothyroid membrane is incised transversely (Fig. 38.4) and the resulting airway maintained with any available piece of tubing, e.g. a 6.0 mm plain endotracheal tube.

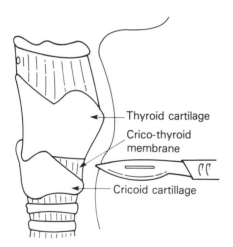

Thyroid cartilage
Crico-thyroid membrane
Cricoid cartillage

Fig. 38.4 The site for laryngotomy. The soft area between the thyroid cartilage and the cricoid is easily palpated and is relatively avascular.

2. Tracheostomy — this can be very difficult as an emergency in the patient without an endotracheal tube in situ.

The re-establishment of a spontaneous circulation of oxygenated blood

With the brain protected by an artificial circulation, measures to recommence adequate spontaneous cardiac contractions must be instituted at once. Therefore without interrupting external cardiac compression or artificial ventilation the following should be instituted:

Intravenous infusion. Intravenous access is necessary not only to give drugs but also to correct a relative hypovolaemia which always occurs in acute circulatory failure; an infusion of 10% of the blood volume offsets this, as does elevation of the legs. In cardiac arrest resulting from haemorrhage, massive transfusion is necessary. If blood is not available, crystalloid or colloid may be lifesaving. Adrenaline 1 mg i.v. should be administered (1 ml of 1:1000 or 10 ml of 1:10 000). This dose is repeated every 2–5 min until spontaneous heart action is restored. Adrenaline may help restart the heart regardless of the cause of the arrest. By its α effect, it increases perfusion pressure and thus myocardial and cerebral blood flow. The β effect is less important during cardiac massage but helps maintain cardiac output once spontaneous heart action is restored. Adrenaline also facilitates defibrillation. Other sympathomimetic amines probably have no advantage over adrenaline, although they are often used empirically.

Sodium bicarbonate should be given in a dose of 1 mmol/kg followed by half this dose every 5–10 min until spontaneous circulation returns (8.4% sodium bicarbonate contains 1 mmol/ml). Sodium bicarbonate corrects the metabolic acidosis resulting from circulatory arrest and from the relative hypoperfusion of cardiac massage. This acidosis depresses the myocardium, renders it more susceptible to ventricular fibrillation, and decreases the effectiveness of sympathomimetic amines. However, it is easy to infuse excess bicarbonate, resulting in an unfavourable alkalotic, hyperosmolar and hypernatraemic state. If possible, arterial blood gas analysis should be used as a guide to therapy and sodium bicarbonate administered according to the following formula:

mmol of sodium bicarbonate required = base deficit × wt (kg) × 0.3.

E.c.g. monitoring should be instituted as soon as possible. If at this stage a major pulse is still absent, the likely patterns are: ventricular fibrillation (or ventricular tachycardia with no cardiac output); asystole (possibly with a few abnormal complexes).

Management of ventricular fibrillation/ventricular tachycardia. An immediate DC countershock of 200 J produces simultaneous depolarisation of all myocardial fibres following which the SA node should assume the initiation of contractions provided the myocardium is well oxygenated and not acidotic. The negative paddle should be applied to the right of the upper half of the sternum and the positive one just below the left nipple, and good electrical contact ensured by the use of electrode jelly. All attendants must stand clear of the patient and the bed prior to discharge.

Failure to defibrillate. If the initial shock is unsuccessful, defibrillation should be repeated with higher energy levels — 300 J followed by 400 J. If ventricular fibrillation persists after adequate doses of adrenaline and sodium bicarbonate, lignocaine 1 mg/kg should be given i.v. to decrease myocardial irritability. Arterial blood gas and electrolyte status (particularly serum K^+) should be assessed and appropriate corrections made.

The witnessed arrest. Immediate DC countershock is indicated in sudden witnessed monitored ventricular fibrillation which may occur in the operating theatre. It is also worth instituting within the first 30 s of a witnessed but unmonitored arrest unless the cause is obviously hypoxia, asphyxia or haemorrhage. Otherwise resuscitation should commence by oxygenating the tissues using cardiac massage and artificial ventilation. It is futile and time-wasting to attempt to defibrillate an anoxic heart.

Management of asystole. Asystole commonly follows hypoxia or exsanguination. It has a worse prognosis than ventricular fibrillation. The aim of treatment is to restore some electrical activity to the heart — for example ventricular fibrillation — which may then be defibrillated. A repeat dose of adrenaline should be given and subsequently other sympathomimetic amines used, e.g. isoprenaline. In asystole secondary to exsanguination, α-adrenergic agents which increase perfusion pressure and thus coronary blood flow may be beneficial, e.g. noradrenaline, phenylephrine. Calcium chloride (5–10 mmol i.v.) is often administered in the presence of asystole. The gluconate salt is unsuitable since the calcium ion is less readily available. Calcium ions have a positive inotropic effect and increase myocardial excitability and contractility. Calcium does, however, promote myocardial ischaemia by producing coronary vasoconstriction. Calcium is the physiological antagonist of potassium and is thus contraindicated in cardiac arrest resulting from hypokalaemia. Calcium potentiates digoxin toxicity and forms a precipitate if mixed with sodium bicarbonate. Probably the best indications for calcium in resuscitation are acute hyperkalaemia, hypocalcaemia or massive transfusion of bank blood.

Table 38.1 Intravenous doses of some drugs used in CPR

Adrenaline	1 mg (1 ml of 1:1000 or 10 ml of 1:10 000) every 2–5 min
Calcium chloride	5–10 mmol every 2–5 min
Sodium bicarbonate	1 mmol/kg then 0.5 mmol/kg every 5–10 min (8.4% solution contains 1 mmol/ml)
Lignocaine	1 mg/kg then 1–4 mg/min by infusion
Dopamine	2–10 μg/kg/min (200 mg in 500 ml at 5–26 standard drop/min)
Isoprenaline	2–20 μg/min (2 mg in 500 ml at 7–75 standard drop/min)
Phenylephrine	2·5 mg every 10–15 min
Noradrenaline	0.1–0.2 mg every 5–10 min
Practolol	5–10 mg repeated to max, 25 mg
Atropine	0.6 mg
Digoxin	0.5 mg i.v. stat then 0.25 mg i.v. 6-hrly until digitalised
Ouabain (for rapid digitalisation)	0.25 mg–0.5 mg i.v. stat then 0.1 mg/h until digitalised

Note
1. Adrenaline, lignocaine and atropine are rapidly effective intratracheally if diluted to 10 ml volume.
2. Suggested dilutions of dopamine and isoprenaline are for emergency use using standard giving sets (15 drop/ml). For longer term, use more concentrated solution and microdrop giving set (60 drop/ml)

Pacing. If asystole persists despite repeated doses of myocardial stimulants, the use of internal pacing should be attempted. A bipolar electrode is passed transvenously into the right ventricle via the antecubital, internal jugular or subclavian route.

Until heart action is restored, cardiac massage and artificial ventilation must be continued with the minimum of interruption.

The return of spontaneous heart action. Restoration of spontaneous cardiac action is signalled by the return of peripheral pulses and circulation. Spontaneous respiration and the return of consciousness usually follow. It is useful to mark the

Table 38.2 Management of important arrhythmias during CPR

Arrhythmia	Significance	Treatment
Ventricular fibrillation	No cardiac output	DC shock 200 J Lignocaine if recurrent (see text)
Ventricular tachycardia	Cardiac output ↓ or absent, may precipitate VF	If cardiac output reasonable, lignocaine. If pulseless, DC shock 200 J
Ventricular ectopics	May herald VF/VT if frequent, multi-focal or R-on-T	Suppress with lignocaine
Complete heart block	May cause profound hypotension or herald asystole	Isoprenaline infusion until transvenous pacemaker in situ
2° Heart block Mobitz type II	May progress to complete block	Transvenous pacemaker
Atrial fibrillation Atrial flutter	Cardiac output ↓ from 1. Loss of atrial contraction 2. Fast ventricular rate	1. Synchronised DC shock 50 J if patient deteriorating 2. Digitalisation 3. Practolol
Supraventricular tachycardia	As atrial fibrillation	1. Carotid sinus massage 2. Synchronised DC shock 50 J if patient deteriorating 3. Digitalisation 4. Practolol
Asystole	No cardiac output	Adrenaline Calcium chloride Pacing (see text)

position of the femoral pulse during resuscitation. Should it disappear at any time, cardiac massage and artificial ventilation must be resumed at once.

Doses of drugs used in CPR are shown in Table 38.1

Aftercare

Once a spontaneous circulation has been restored the time should be noted and recorded in the case sheet with notes on the cause of the arrest and the presence of any complications, e.g. inhalation of vomit. Sometimes recovery is rapid and complete, particularly if resuscitation is prompt and the period of arrest brief. However, some degree of organ failure often persists and requires treatment.

Cardiovascular problems. Cardiac output may remain unsatisfactory as a result of cardiogenic shock and it may be so poor that unconsciousness persists (vide infra). A low cardiac output may result from:

1. Poor myocardial contractility, for example after myocardial infarction or pulmonary embolus. Dopamine 2–10 μg/kg/min by infusion is the treatment of choice. In this dose range it has little if any vasoconstricting effect and causes a preferential increase in renal blood flow. The optimal preload for the failing heart should be ensured by the cautious administration of colloid (Haemaccel or plasma protein fraction) as guided by the CVP. A normal CVP does not rule out the possible development of pulmonary oedema.

2. Hypovolaemia — this requires further transfusion, guided by CVP measurement.

3. Arrhythmias — these require treatment if:

(a) cardiac output is compromised,

(b) they are electrically unstable and therefore predispose to a further episode of circulatory arrest.

Emergency management is summarised in Table 38.2. All arrhythmias are potentiated by disturbances in blood gas or potassium homeostasis.

Respiratory problems. Lung dysfunction is produced by resuscitation for reasons including inhalation of vomit, lung contusion, fractured ribs and pneumothorax. Pulmonary oedema may occur in the presence of heart failure and following head injury, drowning or smoke inhalation. Oxygen therapy for 24 h should follow any episode of circulatory arrest. If overt respiratory failure supervenes, more intensive therapy will be required, including possibly a period of artificial ventilation.

Neurological problems. Efficient cardiac massage and ventilation provide sufficient oxygen delivery to protect the brain from damage though not to prevent depression of function. Therefore, if resuscitation commences immediately circulatory arrest occurs and is continued until restoration of an adequate spontaneous cardiac output, the patient should regain consciousness fairly quickly. Recovery tends to be delayed after prolonged arrest or when general anaesthesia is involved.

Patients may fail to recover consciousness for the following reasons:

1. A low cardiac output (vide supra).

2. Brain damage — which may be present if resuscitation was delayed or if the circulatory arrest was precipitated by hypoxia.

Management of brain damage

The aim of treatment is to provide optimal conditions for recovery of cerebral cells and prevention of secondary neuronal damage.

Basic measures

Care of the unconscious patient. Airway obstruction occurs readily in the unconscious patient and leads to hypoxia and hypercapnia which aggravate cerebral damage. In addition, cough and swallowing reflexes are depressed. Continued endotracheal intubation protects the lungs, secures the airway and renders it easy to institute mechanical ventilation if respiration becomes inadequate. With the airway secure, epileptiform fits may be treated safely with anticonvulsants. In general, if the patient can tolerate the endotracheal tube, it should be left in situ. The spontaneously breathing unconscious patient should be nursed in the lateral position to assist drainage of secretions.

Cardiovascular and pulmonary function should be supported as required and the depth of coma assessed regularly.

Specialised treatment

1. *Hyperventilation.* Mild passive hyperventilation to a Pa_{CO_2} of 4 kPa helps to minimise increases in intracranial pressure secondary to cerebral oedema, although there is no evidence that cerebral damage following cardiac arrest is reduced by hyperventilation if the patient is able to achieve adequate gas exchange when breathing spontaneously. Control of ventilation may be achieved with the aid of muscle relaxants or cerebral depressants. A head-up tilt assists cerebral venous drainage.

2. *Osmotherapy.* Increasing the plasma osmolality decreases cerebral oedema, and mannitol 0.3–0.5 g/kg 2 hrly is often used. Mannitol increases the circulating blood volume and may be dangerous in the presence of pulmonary oedema or a high CVP. In this situation, frusemide or bumetanide may be more appropriate.

3. *Steroids.* There is no evidence that steroids are beneficial following cardiac arrest.

4. *Barbiturates and c.n.s. depressants.* Thiopentone and diazepam are often used in conventional doses to provide sedation, facilitate control of ventilation and suppress seizures. Both these drugs must be used with care following circulatory arrest. In particular, large loading doses of barbiturates are contraindicated, since they produce profound cardiovascular depression. Evidence that they protect the brain is controversial.

Prevention of cardiac arrest

The commonest causes of cardiac arrest during surgery are hypoxia and haemorrhage. Hypoxia may occur with alarming rapidity during periods of apnoea or respiratory obstruction, particularly in obstetric patients and young children. In the latter, bradycardia is an important premonitory sign.

Steady haemorrhage may pass unnoticed until the patient suddenly deteriorates. Other causes include overdose with hypotensive or local anaesthetic agents, infiltrated adrenaline and the use of i.v. induction agents in the presence of hypovolaemia. Vagal reflexes may be involved in surgery on the eye, rectum, carotid sheath and upper respiratory tract.

Generally the outcome following abrupt cardiac arrest is good provided treatment is prompt and effective.

Initiating and terminating CPR

In the first instance, all patients should be resuscitated. If it becomes apparent, once resuscitation has commenced, that CPR would be inappropriate (e.g. because the patient is in the terminal stages of an incurable disease) then it should cease.

Future cerebral function cannot be predicted accurately during CPR and suspicion of brain damage is no justification for terminating resuscitation.

When in doubt, CPR should be continued until there is no doubt that the patient will fail to recover. Good recovery has taken place following 1–2 h of continuous CPR.

FURTHER READING

Goldberger E 1982 Treatment of cardiac emergencies, 3rd edn. C V Mosby, St Louis

Grenvik A, Safar P (eds) 1981 Brain failure and resuscitation. Clinics in critical care medicine. Churchill Livingstone, London

Safar P 1981 Cardiopulmonary cerebral resuscitation. Asmund S Laerdal, Stavanger

Schwartz A J 1981 Current concepts in cardiopulmonary resuscitation. In: A S A annual refresher course lectures. American Society of Anaesthetists

Standards and guidelines for cardiopulmonary resuscitation (CPR) and emergency cardiac care (ECC). 1980 Journal of the American Medical Association 244: 453

39

The intensive therapy unit

The intensive therapy unit (ITU) is the hospital facility within which the highest level of continuous patient care and treatment is provided. The nature of patient care carried out in the ITU has led to the development of specialised layouts which differ markedly from hospital to hospital. A considerably greater area should be allocated to each bed than in ordinary wards because several nurses are required to treat each patient simultaneously and bulky items of equipment often need to be accommodated. Each bed area is supplied with oxygen and piped suction (two outlets per bed), medical compressed air and sometimes nitrous oxide (or Entonox). At least 12 electric power sockets are required and these should be connected to the emergency standby generator. Sufficient local storage space is required to make the nurse self-sufficient for common procedures, e.g. drug administration and tracheal aspiration. Each bed area should be equipped with a self-inflating resuscitation bag to enable the staff to maintain artificial ventilation in case the ventilator fails. In addition, this equipment is used commonly to hyperinflate the lungs during physiotherapy.

Charts

Since considerable information is gathered on the patient undergoing intensive care, comprehensive charts are required for its display. The charts should be easily accessible to the nursing staff who complete them and to the medical staff who utilise them, and they should be placed away from the patient's view. They should provide a record of changes in physiological variables so that significant alterations are recognised easily, of drugs administered to the patient, and of intake and output of fluid. It is desirable that a complete record of what has happened to the patient is collected on a single, necessarily somewhat complex, chart. Medical orders, which inevitably include discretionary elements, should be charted separately. Many units record the results of laboratory tests on a separate chart because of the different time base for these investigations.

While computerised systems have been available for many years to undertake all these data handling functions their cost-benefit ratio in general ITUs has been high and recent applications of microprocessor technology have been aimed at more limited and specific tasks.

WHO SHOULD BE ADMITTED?

Patients admitted to the unit should be those whose lives are in imminent danger but in whom the immediate risk may be averted by active and often invasive therapeutic efforts. A wide range of pathological conditions may lead to such a state, but all involve failure of the respiratory and/or circulatory systems. In addition to these systems may be added dysfunction of one or more of: renal, gastro-intestinal, hepatic, haematological and neurological systems. Involvement of one of these latter systems alone is rarely a reason for admission to the ITU.

Patients admitted to the ITU require active and aggressive therapy for either (a) appropriate treatment of a diagnosed condition, or (b) life-support while a definitive diagnosis is made. Admission should not be sought for patients whose basic condition is essentially untreatable, e.g. the patient whose lungs are almost completely destroyed following chronic bronchitis and emphysema and whose problems cannot be cured by artificial ventilation. It should be appreciated that it is easier to institute heroic therapeutic efforts than to withdraw them once it is clear that restoration of a patient's ability to lead an independent existence is impossible. It should be noted also that it is unethical and almost certainly unlawful to treat a patient against his or her volition.

STAFFING CONSIDERATIONS

The ITU consultant

In the ITU difficult therapeutic and ethical policy decisions may be required at any time. It is essential that they are taken by one whose previous experience is such as to allow a reasonable assessment of the likely outcome, and whose therapeutic expertise is likely to give the patient the optimal chance of recovery. The ITU consultant, if not physically present in the unit, must always be available by telephone and should not be involved in any activity which precludes his or her attendance within half an hour. For effective intensive care, the consultant's basic specialty is relatively unimportant.

The roles of the ITU resident

Communications

Although medical involvement with therapy in the ITU is greater than anywhere else in the hospital except the operating theatre, it should be appreciated that the majority of patient care activities are carried out by nursing staff. The route by which complex instructions and information are transmitted between medical and nursing staff is of vital importance. A system in which a relatively junior clinician serves as a 'final common pathway' for all instructions works well in practice provided the doctor involved is present within the unit at all times so that the nurses may obtain clarification of instructions, report status changes, and receive immediate help in emergencies. Nurses shoulder a greater degree of clinical responsibility if their confidence is sustained by a continuous medical presence and this has important consequences in maintaining therapeutic momentum. Considerable therapeutic difficulties, plus a great deal of frustration, are engendered by a system in which the nurses have to contact one or more doctors outside the unit every time there is an unexpected alteration in a patient's condition.

It causes less confusion if the nursing staff take orders only from the unit staff and not directly from visiting clinicians, however eminent, and even if they are nominally in charge of the patient. This is to ensure that the nurses who execute orders are able to confer with the person who wrote them in case of difficulties. In addition, many patients may be under the care of several clinical teams (e.g. multiple injured patients may be treated by a selection from the orthopaedic or accident team, general surgeons, neurosurgeons or neurologists, dental or plastic surgeons and urologists), so that it is essential that one individual is available to draw attention to and when necessary harmonise what are often conflicting therapeutic regimens. The ITU resident, because of his continuous presence in the unit, should be better informed about the patient's recent diagnostic results, physiological status and therapeutic responses than the visiting clinician and should attempt to utilise his current knowledge to guide treatment along rational lines.

The department which provides the unit staff differs from hospital to hospital; units serving primarily a single specialty (e.g. cardiac surgery or neurosurgery units) are staffed usually by the specialty involved, whereas many central ITUs which serve the hospital as a whole are staffed by the anaesthetic department which is well used to providing round-the-clock emergency services.

Therapeutic functions

As the man on the spot, the resident is the first doctor called in by the nursing staff. It is necessary for him to decide rapidly whether the problem is one with which he can cope, or if more experienced help should be consulted or summoned. For patients already under the care of experienced ITU nurses, the number of occasions when immediate emergency action is required should be relatively small (e.g. unforeseen circulatory collapse, accidental extubation) and resuscitative measures are more likely to be required for patients being admitted to the unit. In these latter circumstances, the ITU should be forewarned about likely admissions (e.g. by the ambulance service or accident department, operating theatre or wards) and the resident should utilise the delay for discussion with the ITU consultant.

It follows, therefore, that most calls to the Unit are the result of a patient behaving in an unexpected manner rather than following a catastrophe. Intubation and obtunded consciousness make direct communication with many patients extremely difficult so that, to assess their problems, reliance is placed on clinical observation and interpretation of patterns of change in the patient's physiological status. The resident should remember that the majority of intensive therapy nurses (and especially the sisters and charge nurses) have an enormous amount of bedside experience with critically ill patients, and considerable reliance may be placed on their observations.

In the following sections a set of systematic guidelines is described to help the resident in his assessment of the patient's condition. Since unusual problems occur commonly during intensive therapy, the flow-charts and the suggested actions are obviously not comprehensive. In addition the proposed order of evaluation of the different physiological variables may prove useful as a checklist on routine rounds.

Initially, the resident should assess the situation by looking at the patient and asking himself questions such as: What changes have occurred since I last saw the patient? Is he or she alert or inert — co-operative or confused — comfortable or distressed — pale or flushed — pink or cyanosed? etc. Simple observations such as these may offer the resident a more reliable indication of the patient's problem than a lengthy examination of the charts!

RESPIRATORY FAILURE

Who should be ventilated?

Patients who are unable to maintain adequate levels of oxygenation or develop hypercapnia may be candidates for artificial ventilation, provided that the pulmonary pathology is potentially reversible. Such ventilatory failure may be actual, in which case arterial blood gas values are abnormal, or anticipated, when blood gas values may be normal.

Hypoxia

The commonest indication for ventilating a patient's lungs artificially in the ITU is an inability to maintain a satisfactory Pa_{O_2}. There are many pathological conditions which produce hypoxaemia but all have the same basic pathophysiological problem — that of an area or areas of lung which have a greater pulmonary blood flow (in litre/min) than alveolar ventilation (in litre/min). Blood flow through areas of lung from which ventilation is completely absent is said to be 'shunted', and hypoxia caused by this mechanism shows little improvement when the inspired oxygen concentration (Fi_{O_2}) is increased. Some clinical conditions which are associated frequently with hypoxia and their common responses to therapy are listed in Table 39.1. Central cyanosis (seen best in the lips) always shows that significant hypoxaemia is present but, if moderate anaemia (Hb

Table 39.1 Some causes of hypoxaemia and usual responses to therapy

Clinical condition	Response to therapy		
	O₂ by mask	IPPV	Need for PEEP
1. Pulmonary oedema			
(a) cardiac	Fair	Good	Uncommon
(b) permeability	Poor	Fair	Often needed
2. Asthma (bronchodilators may make worse)	Good	Good but technically very difficult	Uncommon
3. Chronic bronchitis	Fair (Ventimask)	Good	Uncommon
4. Emphysema	Good (Ventimask)	Good	Rare, beware pneumothorax
5. Pneumonia			
(a) lobar	Poor	Poor	Often disappointing
(b) broncho-	Fair	Good	Useful
6. Pulmonary contusion	Fair	Fair	Often needed, beware pneumothorax
7. Right to left intra-cardiac shunts	Poor	Disastrous	Never
8. Retained secretions	Poor	Good, access for suction important	Helpful
9. 'Exhaustion'	Not accepted	Good	Uncommon

< 10g/dl) is present, as in many patients receiving treatment in the ITU, severe hypoxaemia (Pa_{O_2} less than 6 kPa) may occur without obvious cyanosis.

The initial treatment of hypoxia is to give oxygen by face mask. 6 litre/min should be administered into a Hudson-type mask, and an inspired concentration of approx. 40–50% may be expected. Ventimasks, and other devices which deliver a relatively fixed and low inspired oxygen concentration (24–40%) should be reserved for use in patients with chronic lung conditions in which hypoxic drive may be maintaining ventilation. The effect of this therapy should be assessed by arterial blood gas analysis after 30 min or so. If Pa_{O_2} remains below 7 kPa, the oxygen flow rate should be increased to 10 litre/min and blood gases resampled after a further 20 min. In addition, measures to combat infection, pulmonary oedema or bronchospasm should be introduced, analgesia given if appropriate and chest physiotherapy commenced. Artificial ventilation is required if Pa_{O_2} does not remain above 7–8 kPa.

Patients who are unable to maintain adequate oxygenation often have pulmonary problems in association with other pathology. A persisting inability to cough effectively because of pain and/or weakness leads to retention of secretions and progressive pulmonary collapse. The prophylactic use of IPPV has become common in patients who normally produce significant quantities of secretions and whose ability to cough has been impaired by injury or operation to the chest and/or upper abdomen. Those patients in whom pain rather than weakness is the major defect may often be managed if first class pain relief is provided (e.g. by opioid injection into the thoracic extradural space) together with skilful physiotherapy.

Because of the lower intensity of nursing care provided currently on most general wards, it is often necessary to admit such a patient to the ITU to obtain the medical and nursing supervision necessary to manage the extradural safely, together with regular physiotherapy. Many surgeons regularly 'book' patients into the ITU following major operations of a type which are associated with ventilatory problems, e.g. thoraco-abdominal gastrectomy or oesophagectomy, vascular surgery on the major arteries in the abdomen.

Hypercapnia

Carbon dioxide clearance is related directly to alveolar ventilation. Causes of inadequate ventilation are listed in Table 39.2 together with the likely

Table 39.2 Some causes of inadequate spontaneous ventilation

Site of dysfunction	Common causes	Probable duration of inadequacy
A. Patients usually unable to increase ventilation		
1. Respiratory centre	Brain injury (coning)	Permanent
	Pharmacological depression (e.g. opioids, barbiturates)	Hours (depends on drug[s])
2. Upper motor neurone	High spinal damage	Permanent
3. Lower motor neurone	Poliomyelitis	Weeks, but may be permanent
	Polyneuritis	Months
	Tetanus	Weeks
4. Neuromuscular junction	Myasthenia gravis	Weeks or months
	Neuromuscular blockers	Minutes or hours
5. Respiratory muscles	Myopathies, dystrophies	Permanent
B. Patients who attempt to increase ventilation		
6. Chest wall		
(a) deformity	Kyphoscoliosis	Permanent
	Burn eschars	Until incised
(b) damage	Rib fractures	Days or weeks
7. Lungs — reduced compliance	Pulmonary fibrosis	Permanent
	ARDS	Days or weeks
8. Airways — increased resistance	Upper airway obstruction: croup, epiglottitis	Until relieved
	Lower airway obstruction: asthma	Days
	bronchitis and emphysema	Permanent

duration of the disability since it may be inappropriate to commence IPPV in clinical situations where ventilatory insufficiency cannot be reversed by therapy. Patients whose dysfunction is described by the lower part of Table 39.2 are likely to make vigorous compensatory efforts, while those in whom the dysfunction can be described broadly as 'neurological' are usually unable to help themselves significantly. Artificial ventilation is required if Pa_{CO_2} exceeds 7 kPa in patients who habitually maintain a Pa_{CO_2} in the normal range (4.7–5.3 kPa), or if Pa_{CO_2} increases by more than 2 kPa above the patient's usual level.

Exhaustion

Exhaustion is indicated by a laboured pattern of rapid, shallow breathing which is accompanied often by deterioration in the level of consciousness. This situation may occur in a wide range of clinical conditions, including cardiac failure and severe septicaemia when the institution of artificial ventilation may be followed by an improvement in oxygenation, a reduction in pulse rate and reversal of a trend towards metabolic acidosis. When it occurs in conjunction with myocardial failure, a disproportionate amount of the limited cardiac output is used to maintain ventilation, and institution of artificial ventilation may allow adequate perfusion of vital organs to be resumed. Artificial ventilation is probably required if the respiratory rate remains at or above 45 breath/min for more than 1 h.

Settling the patient on the ventilator

Tracheal intubation

To enable IPPV to be carried out effectively, a cuffed tube must be placed in the trachea via either the mouth or nose, or directly through a tracheostomy. In the emergency situation, an oro- or nasotracheal tube is usually inserted into an unconscious patient. When the patient is initially conscious, anaesthesia should be induced carefully with an i.v. induction agent, and muscular relaxation produced with either suxamethonium or a nondepolarising relaxant. If the patient is

unconscious, a muscle relaxant alone may be necessary (but not obligatory) to facilitate the passage of the tube. Since many patients may be hypoxic, it is essential that 100% oxygen is administered for a few minutes before commencing. The tube should be inserted by the route which is associated with least delay once muscle relaxation has been induced.

Cricoid pressure should be applied to minimise the risk of aspirating gastric contents. Both the oral and nasal tube should be cut short so that the top of the cuff lies not more than 3 cm below the vocal cords. The incompressible plastic connector should lie between the incisor teeth if an oral tube is utilised and in the external nares if a nasal tube is used. After insertion, the head should be placed in a neutral or slightly flexed position (on one pillow) and a chest X-ray taken to ensure that the tip of the tube lies at least 5 cm above the carina.

Endobronchial intubation is the commonest significant complication of artificial ventilation since the tube may migrate down the trachea as the patient is moved for normal nursing procedures. This complication is common when Magill shaped tubes are used but is less likely if an Oxford tube (which has a right-angled bend located in the pharynx) is employed. Intubation of the right main bronchus cannot be detected reliably by observation of chest movements or by auscultation of the chest because of the exaggerated transmission of breath sounds during IPPV although absent or asynchronous chest movement may occur when pulmonary collapse has occurred. Endobronchial intubation is one of the causes of a sudden decrease in compliance, and restlessness and coughing occur if the end of the tube irritates the carina. If this is suspected, the tube should be withdrawn gradually by up to 5 cm while lung compliance and chest expansion are observed carefully. The position of the tube should always be confirmed with a chest radiograph.

Tracheostomy is mandatory only when the upper airway or larynx is obstructed and intubation is not possible (e.g. occasional cases of epiglottitis or laryngeal trauma). The operation is employed more commonly as a planned procedure to make management easier and more comfortable in patients who require ventilation for periods of more than 3 weeks, e.g. tetanus, poliomyelitis and some chest injuries. In such instances it is best performed as a formal operation under general anaesthesia after the airway has been secured using an endotracheal tube.

Setting up the ventilator

There are two main types of ventilator in common use; those which deliver a preset tidal volume (approximately) and those which develop a set pressure during each inspiration. In most units, volume preset machines predominate, and subsequent comments and instructions refer to this general type of ventilator. Since the provision and layout of controls vary considerably between machines, it is essential that the resident is familiar with the ventilator in use in his own unit.

The ventilator should be adjusted to deliver a tidal volume of 12–15 ml/kg body weight (approx. 1000 ml for a 70 kg man) and a minute volume of 8–10 litre/min. The inspired oxygen concentration should be increased until the patient looks pink. If controllable, the inspiratory time should be approx. half the expiratory time. After approx. 10 min, inspired oxygen concentration and arterial blood gases should be measured.

Arterial oxygenation during IPPV

Arterial oxygenation is controlled by manipulating the inspired oxygen concentration and by varying the end-expiratory pressure. Table 39.3 describes measures which may be employed to maintain arterial oxygenation within the desired limits ($Sa_{O_2} > 90\%$ and $Pa_{O_2} < 11$ kPa). More than 50–60% oxygen should not be given for more than a few hours because of the risk of oxygen-induced pulmonary damage.

The application of *positive end-expiratory pressure (PEEP)* or the use of a respiratory pattern in which the expiratory time exceeds the expiratory time (reversed I/E ratio), are methods of increasing FRC, and improving arterial oxygenation. Both methods have inherent dangers in that

1. They raise the mean intrathoracic pressure and hence tend to impair pulmonary blood flow and reduce cardiac output.

Table 39.3 Control of arterial oxygenation. To use this table:
1. Measure the inspired oxygen concentration ($F_{I_{O_2}}$) and arterial blood gases.
2. Adjust $F_{I_{O_2}}$ and/or positive and expiratory pressure (PEEP) depending on results as suggested in Table. Where there is more than one action or step proposed, proceed in the order described. In general, the greater the deviation from adequacy, the larger the steps required.
3. Repeat measurements after 20–30 min and readjust if necessary.

		Arterial oxygenation			
Pa_{O_2}		<8	8	11	>11 (kPa)
Sa_{O_2}		<90	90	96	>96 (%)
	25%				
		Increase $F_{I_{O_2}}$ in steps of 10 to 15%	No change required		Reduce $F_{I_{O_2}}$ to 25% in steps of 5 to 10%
	50%				
		1. Increase PEEP to + 8 cmH$_2$O*	1. Reduce $F_{I_{O_2}}$ to 50% in steps of 5%		Reduce $F_{I_{O_2}}$ to 50% in one step
		2. Increase $F_{I_{O_2}}$ to 60%	2. Minimise PEEP in steps of 4 cmH$_2$O		
Inspired Oxygen ($F_{I_{O_2}}$) Concentration [%]	60%				
		1. Increase PEEP to 16 cmH$_2$O in steps of 4 cmH$_2$O*	Reduce $F_{I_{O_2}}$ to 60% in steps of 10%		Reduce $F_{I_{O_2}}$ to 60% in steps of 20%
		2. Increase $F_{I_{O_2}}$ to 100% in steps of 20%	(PEEP i.s.q.)		
	100%				
		Oxygenation inadequate	adequate		overadequate

* Before and after adding or increasing PEEP, measure P_{O_2} on samples of mixed (or central) venous blood to monitor effect of PEEP on cardiac output and oxygen flux (see text).

2. They increase peak inspiratory pressure and make rupture of alveoli more likely (vide infra).

After the application of PEEP, therefore, the effect on the circulation should be monitored by observing trends in arterial pressure and by measuring changes in the oxygen tension in mixed (or central) venous blood. The supply of oxygen available to the body (the oxygen flux) is the product of cardiac output and arterial oxygen content. PEEP often increases arterial oxygen tension but may depress cardiac output so that oxygen flux is reduced. If this happens, and providing that total body oxygen consumption remains unchanged, less oxygen is returned to the heart and the concentration in the mixed (or central) venous blood decreases. If venous oxygen saturation does decrease after the application of (or increase in the level of) PEEP, then (a) the PEEP should be reduced by 4 cmH$_2$O, (b) the inspired oxygen concentration should be increased by 10% and (c) measurements on arterial and venous blood repeated after 20 min.

Carbon dioxide control

At least initially, it is desirable to minimise the changes in Pa_{CO_2} (especially if elevated,) since a rapid decrease may lead to a marked reduction in cardiac output and arterial pressure. In patients with a normal or low Pa_{CO_2} before IPPV, the minute volume should be adjusted to produce a Pa_{CO_2} of 4–4.5 kPa, a level at which spontaneous ventilatory efforts should be minimal. If the pre-IPPV Pa_{CO_2} is high, the Pa_{CO_2} should not be reduced by more than 1 kPa/h and, if chronically raised (e.g. in chronic bronchitis) to not less than 5.5–6 kPa.

If the Pa_{CO_2} is below 4 kPa minute volume should be reduced by lowering respiratory rate. Because Pa_{CO_2} increases relatively slowly, at least 1 h may elapse before its value is checked.

Management of the ventilated patient

The aims of IPPV are to keep the patient oxygenated with an inspired oxygen concentration of less than 50% and to maintain the Pa_{CO_2} at a satisfactory level. Most patients find the process of receiving artificial ventilation uncomfortable, principally because of irritation from the oral or nasal endotracheal tube.

This is accentuated by movement, particularly of the head. If hypoxic or hypercapnic, the respiratory centre stimulates ventilatory efforts which are not synchronised with those of the ventilator. In pulmonary conditions which increase lung 'stiffness', e.g. ARDS, patients tend to breathe rapidly even when blood gases are normal or the respiratory centre is depressed with large doses of opioids.

A scheme for the assessment of the ventilated patient is shown in Table 39.4.

'Fighting the ventilator'

In managing patients who 'fight the ventilator', the initial step is to determine and, if necessary, correct hypoxaemia or hypercapnia (see Table 39.4). Once these are ruled out, two possible approaches to the problem are possible. The first applies if it is difficult to oxygenate the patient adequately in which case it is likely that the efficiency of the lungs may be impaired further if 'fighting' continues. In this situation, it is necessary to inhibit spontaneous respiratory efforts by administering central respiratory depressants as a continuous infusion (e.g. morphine up to 20 mg/h, pethidine up to 100 mg/h, phenoperidine up to 5 mg/h) limiting the dose if circulatory depression develops. If 'fighting' continues, as it does occasionally, muscular paralysis should be induced. Neuromuscular blockers should be added to the central depressants as a last resort preferably in a continuous infusion (e.g. alcuronium 5–15 mg/h or pancuronium 2–6 mg/h). These techniques should be continued only as long as maintenance of oxygenation continues to be difficult.

If improvement occurs, the second approach to 'fighting' should be utilised, the basis of which is an acceptance of the fact that the spontaneous ventilatory efforts need not harm the patient — although they may disturb the nurses! In this situation weaning may be commenced, or, if pulmonary function is less effective, intermittent mandatory ventilation (IMV) may be employed.

IMV is a pattern of ventilation in which spontaneous ventilatory efforts are interspersed between mandatory breaths delivered by the ventilator. It may be 'dialled in' on more sophisticated ventilators, but can also be applied by using a lightly loaded bypass valve with simpler machines in which it is possible to lengthen the

Table 39.4   Check-list for the artificially ventilated patient

Finding	Some possible causes	Commonly associated features	Suggested action
1. Cyanosis			
YES	Disconnection	Bradycardia, hypotension	Immediate manual ventilation
	Oxygen failure	if terminal	with 100% oxygen
	Cardiac arrest	E.c.g. change, pallor	External cardiac massage
NO ↓			
2. Chest expansion			
ABSENT	Disconnection	Airway pressure down	Reconnect
	Ventilator failure		Manual ventilation
	Total airway obstruction	Airway pressure up	Reintubate
	Tracheal tube in oesophagus	+ gastric distension	
PRESENT ↓			
3. Airway pressure			
DOWN	Leak from system	Tidal and minute volumes down	Manual ventilation unless source of leak obvious
	Improved lung compliance	Tidal and minute volumes up	Check Pa_{CO_2}
	1. Partial airway obstruction		
	(i) Tube kinked	Suction catheter will not pass beyond pharynx or teeth	Reposition tube
	(ii) Tube gripped in teeth		Insert oral airway
	(iii) Tube in right main bronchus	Unequal and/or asynchronous chest movements	Let cuff down, withdraw tube 2.5 cm, chest X-ray
	(iv) Cuff herniation	Expiratory wheeze, overinflated chest, sometimes surgical emphysema in neck	Let cuff down, reinflate until air leak just disappears. Change tube if no improvement
	(v) Inspissated secretions or blood	Cold humidifier	Put 5 ml saline down tube before suction, ?change tube, ?bronchoscope
	2. Bronchospasm	Expiratory ± inspiratory rhonchi, overinflated chest	Bronchodilators
	3. Intrathoracic catastrophes		
	(i) Pneumothorax	Hypotension, tachycardia, surgical emphysema in neck, recent attempts at CVP lines!	Pleural drain if side obvious, chest X-ray if not
UP	(ii) Pulmonary oedema	E.c.g. changes, fine crepitations, copious frothy secretions	Increase FI_{O_2}, diuretics, treat arrhythmias
	(iii) Tamponade	Recent cardiac surgery/trauma; urine flow & BP down, HR & CVP up; reduced loss from chest drains	Unblock drains, reopen chest
	4. Restlessness		
	(i) Hypercapnia	Sweating, vascular pressures up; pyrexia, i.v. nutrition	Check for leaks, increase minute volume
	(ii) Hypoxia	Cyanosis may not be present; falling level of consciousness	Increase FI_{O_2}, ?PEEP
	(iii) Coughing	Characteristic movements	?Tube near carina, review sedation
	(iv) Discomfort or pain	Sweating, grimacing, vascular pressures up	Review analgesia/sedation
	(v) Stimulation of pulmonary stretch receptors	Continuous drive to hyperventilate	Review sedation if oxygenation poor, ?IMV, ?wean

expiratory period to between 8 and 15 s. Since the total minute volume (and hence the Pa_{CO_2}) is effectively under the patient's control during IMV, it is important that muscle relaxants should have been discontinued for some hours and that only moderate doses of respiratory depressants (e.g. opioid analgesics) are being administered.

Reassurance, analgesia and sedation

All but a few patients require some sedation or analgesia while receiving IPPV through an endotracheal tube. If conscious, however, requirements may be minimised by explaining exactly what is happening and stressing that the unpleasant procedures are a temporary measure to tide the patient over the current crisis. Such explanations should be brief, since attention span is short in the sick, and should be repeated frequently, since memory is impaired.

Analgesics should be given if the patient has injuries or wounds which would normally merit these drugs, or complains of the tracheal tube (vide supra).

Sedatives. Diazepam and lorazepam are used commonly as sedative supplements to analgesics, with the aim of reducing distress and awareness during IPPV. While these drugs render management of some patients easier and promote amnesia, they may (a) accentuate disorientation and induce restlessness, (b) produce hypotension in hypovolaemic patients and, (c) if given in large doses, induce a fluctuating level of consciousness as active metabolites are reabsorbed following metabolism and excretion of the parent drug in the liver.

Hypnotics. In units where it is available, nitrous oxide (30–60%) in oxygen has been given to postsurgical patients who require artificial ventilation for relatively short periods of time (e.g. overnight ventilation after cardiac or emergency surgery). This agent should not be given continuously for longer than 18 h because of the risk of bone-marrow depression. Nitrous oxide is useful particularly for patients who are shortly to resume spontaneous ventilation because it is a good analgesic which does not depress respiration and possesses a mild hypnotic effect which disappears within a few minutes of discontinuation. Nitrous oxide may produce hypotension in patients with severely impaired myocardial contractility.

In recent years there has been a tendency to induce light anaesthesia in ventilated patients by infusing continuously the induction agents Althesin or etomidate combined with small doses of opioids. The advantages of this technique are that nursing is made particularly easy since the patient hardly moves but there is a growing conviction that prolonged anaesthesia (up to 2–3 weeks in some instances) and the extremely large total doses of the anaesthetics may have a deleterious effect on hepatic, adrenal and/or renal function so that overall survival may be jeopardised.

Chlormethiazole by continuous infusion may be a useful hypnotic agent in confused patients with hepatic problems in whom opioids are relatively contraindicated. Haloperidol may calm the otherwise almost uncontrollable hyperactivity and confusion observed sometimes (particularly at night) in patients with chronic obstructive airways disease.

Complications

Pulmonary barotrauma. Rupture of alveoli may occur in any patient receiving artificial ventilation but this complication is likely particularly when high mean airway pressures are required because of poor lung compliance or because PEEP has been applied (or both). Air is forced into the substance of the lung and then either into the pleural cavity, when a pneumothorax occurs, and/or up through the hilum and into the mediastinum. Pneumothoraces are particularly likely if there has been previous trauma to the lung, as in chest injuries, and tension almost inevitably develops if IPPV is continued. Drainage of the pleural cavity is mandatory in any patient who develops a pneumothorax while receiving IPPV.

Mediastinal emphysema is diagnosed usually on X-ray, but may appear as surgical emphysema in the neck. Since there is no specific treatment for mediastinal emphysema, its significance is chiefly as a warning that a leak has occurred and that a pneumothorax may develop, though a chest drain is not yet required. Airway pressures should be reduced either by reducing PEEP (and raising FI_{O_2}) or by lowering tidal volume to 10 ml/kg body weight or, perhaps, by switching to a high frequency ventilator if one is available.

It should be noted, however, that surgical emphysema appears first at a site close to the leak so that in a traumatised patient who presents initially with emphysema in the neck, particular attention should be paid to the cervical structures (larynx, pharynx, oesophagus etc) before assuming that the air has tracked up from the thorax.

Weaning from IPPV

Artificial ventilation should be prolonged only if there are specific reasons. It should be routine to consider weaning with each patient each day.

Patients who are otherwise stable should be weaned as soon as (a) pulmonary function seems likely to be adequate during spontaneous ventilation and (b) muscular strength and coordination seem able to maintain an adequate minute volume and cough. Since pulmonary efficiency is usually slightly worse at least initially after discontinuing IPPV and because it is difficult to give an inspired oxygen concentration of more than about 60% through a face mask, patients whose lung function is usually normal should be able to achieve a Pa_{O_2} of more than 10 kPa with an inspired oxygen concentration of 40% or less. If the lungs are permanently damaged (e.g. in chronic lung disease), less effective oxygenation may have to be accepted both during and particularly after IPPV.

The indications for weaning, tracheal extubation and recommencing IPPV are shown in Table 39.5. It is probably safer to wean patients from IPPV and to extubate the trachea early in the day rather than in the late afternoon or evening since less medical and nursing supervision tends to be available at night.

In general, the shorter the period of ventilation, the simpler the weaning procedure; weaning over a period of several days may be necessary after prolonged IPPV, particularly for neuromuscular disorders. In such patients, spontaneous ventilation may be introduced for 5 min each hour, and then gradually increased (by 5–10 min per hour each day) as the patient's strength and confidence improve.

Adult respiratory distress syndome (ARDS) (shock lung)

Almost total pulmonary failure may occur after a wide range of critical conditions including hypovolaemic and septic shock, multiple injuries particularly involving lung contusion and/or long bone fractures, pancreatitis, and as the end-result of severe and often combined viral and bacterial pneumonias. The type that follows shock is characterised by the appearance of tachypnoea,

Table 39.5 Guidelines for weaning, tracheal extubation and recommencing IPPV

1. *When can weaning be commenced?*

   If, when on IPPV (or IMV):
   >   (A) HR <100 in adults — can safely be greater in chilren
   > *and* (B) $Pa_{O_2} >10$ kPa $Fl_{O_2} <40\%$ and zero PEEP
   > *and* (C) $Pa_{CO_2} <6$ kPa with minute volume <10 litre/min (or $V_D/V_T <50\%$)
   > *and* (D) Spontaneous tidal volume >7 ml/kg
   > If answers to A + B + C are YES but D is NO, start or continue IMV

2. *When can the patient be extubated?*

   If patient co-operative and able to cough: extubate
   If unconscious and tolerating tube, leave intubated
   If unco-operative or intolerant of tube, extubate *if* IPPV not required (see below)

3. *When does IPPV need to be restarted?*

   (Assess patient after 5–10 min of spontaneous ventilation then at half-hourly intervals)

   Restart IPPV if:
   >   (a) *Respiratory rate* climbs steadily for 3 successive half hours
   > or   (b) It exceeds 45 beat/min
   > or   (c) *Heart rate* climbs steadily for 3 successive half hours
   > or   (d) It exceeds 130 beat/min
   > or   (e) *Hypoxia* develops ($Pa_{O_2} <8$ kPa — except some chronic respiratory failure patients)
   > or   (f) *Hypercapnia* develops ($Pa_{CO_2} >1.5$ kPa above pre-IPPV level)
   > or   (g) *Level of consciousness* deteriorates

   If one of these conditions does apply, consider *why* spontaneous ventilation cannot be maintained. The appearance of bronchospasm and/or pulmonary oedema are important factors which may be missed.

tachycardia and sometimes pulmonary oedema over a few hours some 6 to 30 h after the insult. The patient is profoundly hypoxic even when receiving maximal amounts of oxygen by face mask. A chest radiograph shows multiple fluffy opacities throughout the lung fields.

The basic defect, which is still poorly understood, appears to be an increase in the permeability of the pulmonary capillaries which permits fluid to flood into the pulmonary interstitial space and alveoli. Insertion of a pulmonary artery catheter confirms that pulmonary oedema is occurring at a low (< 20 cmH$_2$O) pulmonary wedge pressure, and distinguishes the condition from left ventricular failure. In the worst cases, a plasma-like fluid pours from the lungs and there may be a measurable decrease in plasma protein concentration.

IPPV, usually with high levels of both $F_{I_{O_2}}$ and PEEP, is required and even these measures may be insufficient to maintain adequate oxygenation. A high minute volume (15–20 litre/min) is often needed to prevent hypercapnia and, since lung compliance is greatly reduced, very high airway pressures may be generated (N.B. beware pneumothoraces). Fluid overload should be avoided to keep the intravascular pressures to a minimum. The pulmonary artery catheter is valuable in monitoring this aspect of therapy. Crystalloid input must be kept to an absolute minimum (that required to replace losses) and the circulating volume maintained with infusions of colloids, particularly blood or salt-poor albumin. Frusemide should be given initially to produce a brisk diuresis, and urine flow maintained with a low dose of dopamine.

It is possible that large doses of corticosteroids may reduce the severity of the pulmonary insult if given before, or very early in, the development of the condition. Since ARDS has a mortality rate of over 50%, this possible benefit cannot be ignored and so methylprednisolone (30 mg/kg body weight) should be given i.v. as soon as the condition is suspected. Two further but smaller doses (15 mg/kg) should be given at 12 h intervals.

Resolution of the condition is variable. In fortunate patients, oxygenation and lung compliance improve over the subsequent few days, but some remain severely hypoxic for many weeks before making a slow recovery which is often heralded by a spontaneous diuresis and characterised by irrepressible tachypnoea. Other patients die from the effects of infection, multisystem failure or hypoxia following barotrauma.

CARDIOVASCULAR FAILURE (CVF)

While actual or expected ventilatory failure is the commonest reason for admission to most general ITUs, admission as a result of failure of the cardiovascular system is also frequent. When associated with pulmonary problems, the effects of cardiovascular insufficiency may be exacerbated because of reduced oxygenation of blood.

Cardiovascular failure may be acute or chronic. When it develops rapidly (e.g. heart failure after myocardial infarction or peripheral circulatory failure after haemorrhage), it is termed 'shock' and, unless the condition is corrected rapidly, admission to the ITU is necessary. Chronic cardiovascular failure is one of the main *raisons-d'etre* of many departments of medicine (especially cardiology) and surgery (especially cardiac and vascular surgery) but patients who are receiving treatment for one of the varieties of chronic CVF should be placed on a 'short list' for ITU admission if they present with unrelated complaints or complications.

Cardiovascular monitoring

Electrocardiogram (e.c.g.)

Patients are often admitted to ITU because their cardiovascular status is unpredictable and potentially unstable, rendering essential continuous availability of information. All patients in the ITU should be monitored with an e.c.g. which displays both the electrical signal and heart rate. The e.c.g. monitoring system in CCUs is often more complex and may include circuits to recognise, count and display frequency histograms of various arrhythmias.

Arterial pressure

This may be measured intermittently by conventional or automated sphygmomanometer, or continuously by direct intra-arterial recording from the radial, brachial, dorsalis pedis or femoral artery. Percutaneous arterial cannulation is used widely to monitor arterial pressure (Figs 39.1 and 39.2) and

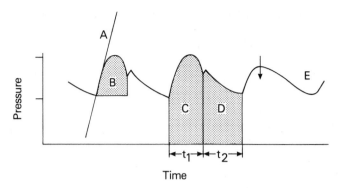

Fig. 39.1 Information to be gained from the arterial pressure signal.
A — Rate of pressure increase α contractility
B — Area under pulse pressure α stroke volume
C — Systolic pressure × time (t_1) α myocardial oxygen consumption
D — Diastolic pressure × time (t_2) α myocardial oxygen supply
E — Loss of waveform detail α catheter occlusion — flush it!)

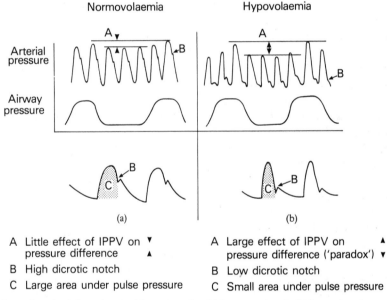

A Little effect of IPPV on ▼
  pressure difference ▲

B High dicrotic notch

C Large area under pulse pressure

A Large effect of IPPV on ▲
  pressure difference ('paradox') ▼

B Low dicrotic notch

C Small area under pulse pressure

Fig. 39.2 Information to be gained from the arterial pressure signal (a) normovolaemia (b) hypovolaemia

provide ready access to arterial blood. Enormous technical efforts are being made to design noninvasive systems which will make invasive procedures less necessary but, at present, their accuracy and dependability are inadequate.

Central venous pressure (CVP)

CVP may be measured from a catheter introduced into the superior vena cava or right atrium and connected to either a water or electronic manometer.

If the latter is used, care must be taken to calibrate in the more conventional 'cmH$_2$O' rather than 'mmHg'. On occasions it may be desirable to measure the pressure in the pulmonary artery using a flow-directed catheter (see Chapter 18), and the type with which cardiac output may be estimated using the thermodilution method has many advantages. The information gained from measurement of wedge pressure permits distinction between pulmonary oedema from a high left atrial pressure and that caused by increased permeability of the pulmonary capillaries. This may be helpful particularly in patients with multiple injuries and pulmonary problems, in those with severe septicaemia and in those with actual or incipient left ventricular failure.

Cardiovascular assessment

A scheme to aid the ITU resident in his or her assessment of the cardiovascular status is shown in Tables 39.6 and 39.7. Further information which may be obtained from the arterial pressure waveform is indicated in Fig. 39.1 and 39.2. A wide range of therapeutic agents is available to modify the behaviour of the cardiovascular system. Some of those used commonly in the ITU are listed in Table 39.8, classified under their major effects.

Shock or acute cardiovascular failure

In shock, there is an acute failure of the circulatory system to supply adequate nutrients to the tissues and to remove metabolites. Under these circumstances cell death eventually takes place following abnormal cell metabolism and impairment of vital membrane functions. This sequence of events may follow severe haemorrhage (from a traumatic or surgical cause) and may also occur after the loss of fluid from the gastro-intestinal tract. Cardiogenic shock is a variant in which the heart is unable to maintain a sufficiently high output and this occurs acutely most commonly after severe myocardial infarction. Septic shock may complicate overwhelming infections of many types but the most frequently encountered in ITU result from Gram-negative infections.

Pathophysiology

In the early stages of circulatory insufficiency, the sympathetic nervous system is activated so that constriction of veins and arteries occurs thereby maintaining perfusion of vital organs (brain, heart and kidneys). These compensatory mechanisms provide a short period during which aggressive treatment may prevent further development of the more severe and irreversible features of shock. If effective treatment is not commenced, however, poor tissue perfusion leads to hypoxia and anaerobic metabolism. The resultant acidosis causes relaxation of precapillary sphincters despite maximal sympathetic activity, though the post-capillary sphincters remain constricted. Fluid becomes sequestered in tissues and the process is exacerbated as capillary permeability increases. The progressive loss of intravascular volume eventually causes hypoperfusion of the previously protected vital organs and respiratory and renal failure develop, followed later by hepatic, cardiac and eventually neurological failure.

Bacteraemic shock

Gram-negative, bacteraemic or endotoxic shock are names which have been given to a clinical state which may appear following localised or systemic bacterial infections. The commonest sources for infection are the gastro-intestinal tract, particularly after laparotomy, and the urogenital tract, particularly after instrumentation. Infections of the respiratory and biliary tracts may also be implicated. Micro-organisms isolated from patients with this condition are usually Gram-negative gut bacteria, e.g. *E. coli*, *Klebsiella*, or *Proteus* although in a small but significant minority, Gram-positive organisms, e.g. *Staphylococcus aureus* or *Pneumococcus* may be found.

Bacteraemic shock is extremely rare outside hospital and occurs usually as a complication of existing clinical problems. Its occurrence (and mortality) are related to the severity of the underlying condition and it is commonest at the extremes of life, in patients in whom resistance to infection is low and following splenectomy (when pneumococcal infection is common).

In early bacteraemic shock, the patient characteristically appears warm and well-perfused, with a normal (sometimes elevated) cardiac output but a low arterial pressure because of reduced peripheral resistance ('warm phase'). If shock persists, a hypodynamic cardiovascular state develops in which cardiac output and blood volume decrease, systemic and pulmonary resistances increase ('cold phase'), and the chances of recovery decrease sharply. In the 'warm' phase, the increased temperature and cardiovascular activity are accompanied by a marked increase in metabolic requirements although, paradoxically, oxygen extraction by the tissues is reduced so that the arteriovenous oxygen content difference is also reduced. Among the factors postulated to contribute to the impaired oxygen utilisation is the opening of arteriovenous capillary 'shunts' in the tissues and the uncoupling of the

Table 39.6 Cardiovascular checklist. Check the primary variables, (systemic arterial pressure [SAP], heart rate [HR], e.c.g. and urine flow) first. Look at 1) absolute values, 2) trends (up, down, variable), 3) relationships with one another — particularly SAP & HR

Use secondary variables (CVP/neck veins, central to peripheral temperature difference, pulmonary artery pressure [PAP] & pulmonary wedge pressure [PWP]) to distinguish between various possibilities.

SAP & HR relationship	Common causes	Confirmatory findings	Suggested action
HR up, SAP up	Sympathetic activation with pain, arousal etc.	Restlessness, CVP up, PAP up	Review sedation and analgesia
HR down, SAP down	1. Heart block	E.c.g. change	Isoprenaline, pacemaker
	2. Severe hypoxia	Cyanosis	Reconnect ventilator or oxygen. Manual IPPV
	3. Response to sedative or analgesic drugs.	Recent drug administration	Reduce subsequent doses of drug
HR down, SAP up	Rising intracranial pressure	Deteriorating level of consciousness, enlarging pupils	Hyperventilate, diuretics, mannitol
HR up, SAP down	1. Shock		
	(a) hypovolaemic	CVP & urine flow down, limbs poorly perfused	Infuse colloid
	(b) septicaemic (early)	CVP & urine flow down, limbs well perfused	Infuse colloid, release pus, give antibiotics & steroids
	2. Tamponade after heart surgery	CVP up, urine flow & lung compliance down	Unblock drains, reopen chest
	3. Pneumothorax	Restlessness, lung compliance down	Chest drain
	4. Tachyarrhythmias	E.c.g. change, CVP up	Antiarrhythmics
	5. Pulmonary embolus	Chest pain, cyanosis, CVP up, ?E.c.g. changes	O_2, ?pulmonary angiography
	6. Allergic reaction	?Rash, recent drug or blood administration	Antihistamines, infuse colloid, ?steroids

Table 39.7 Cardiovascular indicators. It is often not possible to measure certain cardiovascular variables directly, so that it is necessary to use other variables to indicate indirectly what changes are occurring. Changes which are normally undesirable are indicated in the table above. Desirable changes are accompanied normally by alterations in the 'indicator observations' in the opposite direction.

Undesirable change	Indicator observations
1. Cardiac output *down*	Urine flow *down* Central to peripheral temperature difference *up*
2. Blood volume *down*	CVP and PWP *down* Inspiratory to expiratory difference in systolic arterial pressure ('paradox') *up* (see Fig. 39.2) Dicrotic notch *lower* on arterial pressure waveform (see Fig. 39.1) *Large* BP fall in response to IPPV, sedatives or analgesics
3. Right ventricular function *deteriorating*	CVP *up* PAP *down* Peripheral oedema *increasing*
4. Left ventricular function *deteriorating*	PWP or Left atrial pressure *up* SAP *down* Pulmonary oedema *increasing* Oxygenation *deteriorating*
5. Peripheral vascular resistance *increasing*	Central to peripheral temperature difference *up* *Steeper* pressure decay during diastole
6. Myocardial oxygen demand *up*	HR *up* SAP *up* Product of HR × SAP *up*
7. Myocardial oxygen supply *down*	HR *up* Diastolic arterial pressure *down*

Table 39.8 A summary of cardiovascular drugs and initial doses

A. Inotropes

These stimulate the myocardium and increase cardiac output. Often used to raise SAP and increase urine flow

(a) Sympathomimetics
(1) DOPAMINE	i.v. inf. (2–5 μg/kg/min for renal effect, 10–20 μg/kg/min for max. pressor effect)
(2) DOBUTAMINE	i.v. inf. (Up to 15 μg/kg/min)
(3) NORADRENALINE	i.v. inf. (5–10 μg/min)

(N.B. much larger doses of these drugs are required if the patient has received β-blocking drugs)
(4) PRENALTEROL	slow i.v. (2–5 mg in 5 min) or inf. (500 μg/min)
	Used to reverse β-blockade.

(b) Nonsympathomimetics
(1) DIGOXIN	slow i.v. (0.5–1.0 mg in 5 min) (beware hypokalaemia)
(2) CALCIUM	i.v. bolus (10 ml of 10 % Ca gluconate)

B. Chronotropes

These increase the heart rate but a pacemaker is required in heart block
(1) ATROPINE	i.v. bolus (0.2–0.6 mg)
(2) ISOPRENALINE	i.v. inf. (0.5–10 μg/min)

C. Antiarrhythmics

(a) For VENTRICULAR arrhythmias

Before treatment, check that the CVP catheter is not stimulating the heart. All these drugs depress cardiac contractility and tend to reduce SAP
(1) LIGNOCAINE	i.v. bolus (100 mg) + inf. (1–4 mg/min)
(2) DISOPYRAMIDE	slow i.v. (up to 2 mg/kg) + inf. (400 μg/kg/h)
(3) PRACTOLOL	slow i.v. (up to 5 mg)
(4) MEXILETINE	slow i.v. (200 mg in 10 min) + inf. (250 mg in 1 h)

(b) For SUPRAVENTRICULAR tachyarrhythmias
(1) DIGOXIN	slow i.v. (0.5–1.0 mg in 5 min)
(2) AMIODARONE	slow i.v. [via CVP] (150 mg in 30 min and repeat)
(3) VERAPAMIL	slow i.v. (5 mg) + inf. (5–10 mg/h)

D. Antihypertensives

(a) Vasodilators

These lower peripheral vascular resistance and reduce afterload
(1) HYDRALAZINE	slow i.v. (20–40 mg and repeat)
(2) DIAZOXIDE	i.v. bolus (300 mg)
(3) NITROPRUSSIDE	i.v. inf (0.5–5 μg/kg/min)
(4) GLYCERYL TRINITRATE	i.v. inf. (10–150 μg/min)
(5) ISOSORBIDE DINITRATE	i.v. inf (2—10 mg/h)
(6) PHENOXYBENZAMINE	i.v. bolus (20–100 mg)
(7) PHENTOLAMINE	i.v. inf (0.2–2 mg/min)

(b) β-adrenergic blockers

These reduce myocardial contractility and may increase afterload
(1) ATENOLOL	slow i.v. (150 μg/kg over 20 min)
(2) METOPROLOL	slow i.v. (5 mg in 5 min)
(3) OXPRENOLOL	slow i.v. (5 mg in 10 min)
(4) LABETALOL	i.v. bolus (20–50 mg) + inf. (2 mg/min)

normal processes that link energy production and oxygenation. In the 'cold' phase, the pathophysiological picture more closely resembles that seen in hypovolaemic shock.

Treatment

In shock of all kinds, the primary aim of treatment is to restore and maintain an adequate flow of well oxygenated blood. Thus, the initial step in management of the shocked patient is to ensure that arterial blood is well saturated (>95%). To restore the circulating volume, fluid, over two-thirds of which should be in the form of colloid solutions should be given rapidly through a large i.v. cannula. Whole blood is preferred if blood has been lost, although substitutes (e.g. Haemaccel) may be used in septic shock or while awaiting the definitive replacement fluid. Inotropic support and vasodilators (see Table 39.8) may assist in restoration of the circulation, and renal function should be encouraged with diuretics (e.g. frusemide) or low dose dopamine.

In bacteraemic shock, blood should be obtained for culture before antibiotics are commenced, but in this serious condition, large doses of broad spectrum antibiotics are appropriate (cefuroxime + gentamicin + metronidazole). It is essential that every appropriate diagnostic technique including laparotomy be utilised in the search for the source of infection. Collections of pus must be evacuated despite a critical condition, otherwise bacteraemia recurs and progressive multiorgan failure ensues.

DEATH IN THE ITU

The mortality rate of patients in ITU is very high. This is inevitable in view of the pathological processes which necessitate artificial assistance for one or more vital systems. In order to maintain the morale and sense of purpose of the unit staff, it is essential that the need for therapy be the main criterion for admission to the unit rather than the imminence of death.

Often, however, the patient deteriorates despite maximal therapeutic support. This becomes apparent when the patient fails to improve sufficiently to become independent of the measures employed to support ventilation and/or perfusion. The prognosis deteriorates markedly the longer IPPV is required and the more systems require support. The maintenance of a physiologically satisfactory status quo by means of artificial support does *not* augur well and the appropriate message must be transmitted to the patient's relatives. It must be stressed repeatedly that improvement is required to give significant hope of survival, because the patient must not only be able to overcome the effects of the initial near-lethal insult, but also be able to resist the infective episodes which often complicate the recovery period. Failure to improve is usually followed by a slow deterioration in the efficiency of previously unaffected organs, and by a poor response to supportive measures.

Such multiorgan failure may very occasionally be reversed by correcting deficiencies in corticosteroids, phosphate, magnesium or trace elements, and rarely improvement follows withdrawal of all drug therapy. It is extremely difficult to decide for how long therapeutic efforts should be continued in the face of widespread unresponsiveness.

In terms of predicting which patients are unlikely to survive, those who are comatose and unresponsive following severe brain damage are easier to distinguish. The signs of 'brain death' are well

Table 39.9 Recognition of 'brain death'. Brain death may be assumed if (a) the answer to ALL of the 10 questions is 'NO', and (b) if the assessment is repeated, with the same results, after at least four hours. If the answer to any of the questions is 'YES' or 'DON'T KNOW', active treatment must be continued

1. Is there any doubt regarding the cause of coma and brain damage (e.g. trauma, cerebrovascular accident, drowning)?

2. Has the patient received (or taken) any drugs which could either have depressed the central nervous system (e.g. alcohol, sedatives, hypnotics, analgesics), or impaired his or her muscular capabilities (e.g. muscle relaxants)?

3. Are there any metabolic or endocrine disturbances which might affect neural function (e.g. blood glucose changes, uraemia, hepatic dysfunction)?

4. Is the patient's temperature less than 35°C? (Midbrain failure is often followed by a rapid fall in temperature, but hypothermia itself may induce coma. If the temperature is below 35°C, active warming must be started and further cooling minimised with 'space blankets'.)

5. Do the pupils react to light?

6. Are there corneal reflexes?

7. Do the eyes move during or after caloric testing?

8. Are there motor responses in the cranial nerve distribution in response to painful stimulation of the face, trunk or limbs?

9. Does the patient gag, cough or otherwise move following the passage of a suction catheter into the nose, mouth or bronchial tree?

10. Does the patient show any respiratory activity at all when the arterial carbon dioxide level exceeds 7 kPa (checked on an arterial sample)?

Reference: Pallis C 1983 *The ABC of Brain Stem Death*. BMA Publications described (Pallis 1983), and a scheme of assessment is shown in Table 39.9. Formal assessment should be carried out twice by two senior clinicians, at least one of whom must be a consultant.

FURTHER READING

Ledingham I McA, Hanning C D (eds) 1983 Recent advances in critical care medicine 2. Churchill Livingstone, London

Shoemaker W C, Thompson W L (eds) 1980 Critical care: state of the art, vols 1 & 2. The Society of Critical Care Medicine, California

Tinker J, Rapin M (eds) 1983 Care of the critically ill patient. Springer-Verlag, Berlin

40

Relief of chronic pain

Most pain is mild, transitory and of little consequence. Sometimes it may warn of a curable condition, but on occasions it may not be possible to discover the cause, or the cause may be untreatable, and the pain may persist. It is this type of pain that becomes chronic or intractable, and is the stock-in-trade of pain relief clinics.

Patients with chronic pain may be allocated broadly to two groups: (a) those with a normal expectation of life and who are often difficult to treat and (b) those with a short expectation of life (usually resulting from neoplastic disease) and who are normally easier to treat.

Patients seen in a pain relief clinic present usually with one of the following categories of pain.

Neurological

1. Postherpetic neuralgia
2. Trigeminal neuralgia
3. Nerve entrapment syndromes, including back pain and scar pain
4. Disseminated sclerosis
5. Central pain syndromes: 'stroke' pain, thalamic pain syndrome, and phantom limb pain
6. Pain from neuroma formation — stump pain

Vascular

1. Migraine
2. Claudication
3. Raynaud's disease

Orthopaedic

1. Back pain and sciatica
2. Arthritis

3. A variety of vague pains associated usually with the cervical or lumbar spine and often defying conventional diagnosis

Neoplastic

1. Arising from primary tumour
2. Induced by metastases
3. Resulting from treatment, e.g. necrosis following radiotherapy

Unknown or undiagnosable cause

Atypical facial pain

Psychogenic pain

This is defined usually as pain occurring without the presence of an obvious physical cause. However, central pain may also have no obvious cause, which leads to confusion. The distinction is even more intangible as it is argued by some that psychogenic pain results from the existence of some minor disorder, undetectable by normal means, or is produced by some past injury. It is also said that once experienced, pain leaves within the nervous system a memory which is suppressed by inhibitory mechanisms. It is only when these inhibitory mechanisms are removed, usually by psychological factors, that pain becomes apparent.

Szasz has pointed out that 'the notions of physical and mental pain are meaningless. The "common-sense" view that regards this matter as if there were two types of pain — one organic and another psychogenic — is misleading and responsible for numerous pseudoproblems in the borderland between medicine and psychology'.

However, it is important to delineate the relative importance of psychological and physical mechanisms in a patient's pain experience as this influences treatment. Sometimes, distinctive qualities are noted in the pain of patients with psychiatric illness (e.g. in the form of hallucinations) but clinically such cases are not common.

ASSESSMENT OF PATIENTS WITH CHRONIC PAIN

A full history should be obtained and a full clinical examination undertaken (not just of the painful area). Radiological or other investigations may be indicated.

The patient's description of the pain is important. Some pains are described so similarly by different individuals as to be diagnostic, e.g. the pain of trigeminal neuralgia. The patient's choice of words and the vividness of his description provides a pointer to diagnosis (e.g. the burning pain of causalgia) and also reflects the patient's emotional state and his ethnic and cultural background.

Many pain analysis questionnaires exist, but that suggested by Bond is easy to remember and covers all the essential points.

Before treatment of a patient with chronic pain is attempted, it is important that a firm diagnosis is reached and that the patient's pain cannot be relieved by treatment of the cause. This may involve consultation with many other disciplines. In some patients, however, in spite of extensive and lengthy investigations, no diagnosis can be made and these patients have to be accepted and treated symptomatically in the way that seems most appropriate to their pain.

Some attempt should be made to assess the patient's personality and psychological status. In many pain relief clinics held by anaesthetists, this is undertaken in a somewhat amateur fashion, but nevertheless is extremely helpful.

Two formal measurements of personality are available: the Minnesota Multiphasic Personality Inventory (MMPI) and the Eysenck Personality Inventory (EPI). Those personality traits which are important in evaluating the patient with chronic pain include proneness to anxiety and/or depression, and the existence of hysterical, hypochondriacal or obsessional traits. Most patients suffering from chronic pain exhibit some degree of anxiety, or more usually, depression. These may present as an obvious neurosis, in which case the patient should be referred for full psychiatric assessment.

METHODS OF MANAGEMENT OF CHRONIC PAIN

Simple measures

For centuries, rest has been used to relieve pain and suffering and this is still an important measure. This may involve resting the whole patient or just the painful part. Splinting and immobilisation often relieve pain arising from joints or pathological fractures, without the need for potent analgesic drugs.

The relief of anxiety occasioned by pain may produce considerable diminution in intensity of pain. Anxiety may often be relieved more effectively by simple and careful explanation than by anxiolytic drugs.

The injection of tender areas in myofascial syndromes with mixtures of local anaesthetic and steroids is often effective, as may be the use of cold pain-relieving sprays, heat or percussion.

Drugs

For reasons of finance and availability of facilities, the majority of patients with chronic pain are treated with drugs prescribed usually by the general practitioner.

Analgesic drugs

There are many analgesic drugs which may be used (Table 40.1). Prescribing an analgesic regimen for a patient with chronic pain requires the following considerations:

What potency of drug does the patient require? Not all patients need potent opioid analgesics and although the risk of dependence is usually overstated, these drugs should be avoided if possible in patients with a normal expectation of life. However, in general, pain severity (mild, moderate and severe) matches analgesic requirements: low (aspirin); medium (codeine); high (morphine).

Table 40.1 Analgesic drugs in common use

1. *Low potency: antipyretic analgesics*
Salicylates	Aspirin
Aniline derivatives	Paracetamol
Anthranillic acid derivatives	Mefenamic acid
Indole derivatives	Indomethacin
Pyrazolone derivatives	Phenylbutazone

2. *Medium potency*
   Medium duration
Morphine derivatives	Codeine
	Dihydrocodeine
Methadone derivatives	Dextropropoxyphene
Benzmorphinan derivatives	Pentazocine

3. *High potency: opioid analgesics*
   Long acting
   Slow-release morphine
   Buprenorphine
   Oxycodone
   Medium duration
   Morphine
   Diamorphine
   Phenazocine
   Levorphanol
   Methadone
   Short acting
   Dextromoramide

Dose of drug and frequency of administration. The object of treating chronic pain is to provide complete pain relief. The correct dose of an analgesic drug is that dose which relieves the pain for an acceptable period of time without unacceptable side effects. The drug should be administered frequently enough to ensure that the patient remains pain-free.

Route of administration. Ideally, drugs are given orally and injections should be avoided if at all possible. Some drugs (e.g. buprenorphine, phenazocine) may be given sublingually and others (e.g. morphine, diamorphine, oxycodone) by suppository.

Potential duration of treatment. This is usually evident from the aetiology of the pain and influences the choice of drug.

Specific types of pain. Some types of pain or disease make certain groups of drug particularly appropriate. Analgesic drugs either interfere with the production of peripheral pain-producing substances including prostaglandins and kinins (e.g. aspirin and nonopioid analgesics) or act on central mechanisms at endorphin receptors, often including perceptual mechanisms and emotional response to pain (e.g opioid analgesics). Studies of osseous metastases have demonstrated that prostaglandin E_2 (PGE_2) is implicated in the mediation of pain, and prostaglandin inhibitors alone or combined with opioid analgesics provide better pain relief than opioid analgesics alone.

Having established adequate pain relief, the patient should be reassessed at intervals as it is often possible to reduce analgesic drug dosage slowly without pain reappearing. Reappearance of pain on a previously satisfactory drug regimen requires reassessment of the patient before therapy is modified.

Other drugs used in the management of patients with chronic pain

Psychotropic drugs. Analgesic activity appears to be present in most of the tricyclic antidepressant drugs, but is most noticeable in those agents (e.g. amitriptyline, clomipramine) which enhance 5-hydroxytryptamine (5HT) activity by preventing reuptake into presynaptic stores. Pain relief may take up to two weeks to appear. The antidepressant effect is useful in many patients.

Some of the phenothiazines also appear to have analgesic activity, particularly when used in combination with a tricyclic antidepressant. Currently there is interest in enhancement of these effects with transmitter precursors including L-tryptophan.

Anticonvulsants. These drugs have membrane stabilising properties and the principal use is for the treatment of epilepsy. Carbamazepine was the first drug to be used for trigeminal neuralgia and has proved particularly successful. However, anticonvulsants are also useful in other conditions with a 'shooting' component to the pain, e.g. postherpetic neuralgia.

Steroids. Steroids may be useful in several ways.

1. They interfere with the synthesis of prostaglandins

2. They may reduce oedema in neoplastic tissue (either primary tumour or metastasis), so relieving pain by reducing pressure on adjacent pain-sensitive structures.

3. They are very effective by the extradural or intrathecal route in treatment of low back pain and sciatica. The mechanism of action is not clear, but may be a result of reduction of oedema in nerve roots and adjacent structures.

Cytotoxic drugs. Cytotoxic drugs may reduce the size of tumour tissue and relieve pressure on adjacent structures.

Nerve blocks

Blockade of a peripheral pain pathway reduces or obviates the need for potent analgesic drugs and unwanted effects of these agents. Nerve blocks are appropriate for pain confined to an area with a discrete nerve supply.

Blockade of nerves may be carried out at various sites (Fig. 40.1) either temporarily with local anaesthetic for diagnostic or prognostic purposes or permanently or semipermanently for therapeutic purposes (with neurolytic solutions, radiofrequency or cryotherapeutic lesions).

The practice of nerve blocking techniques has been improved greatly by the use of the image intensifier and nerve stimulator.

Before undertaking a permanent nerve block the consequent effects should be assessed by an initial local anaesthetic block. This confirms the presumptive effect of the block (which does not always conform to anticipated effects) and permits the patient to experience effects including anaesthesia, which may result.

Not infrequently the duration of pain relief afforded by local anaesthetic blocks outlasts the duration of action of the local anaesthetic. The reasons for this are not clear.

The following are some of the more common useful blocks.

Somatic nerve blocks

Spinal nerves may be blocked paravertebrally from the cervical to the sacral region, although the precise technique varies with the region. In all instances, the use of an image intensifier is advisable to ensure accurate placement of needles.

It is unusual to require block of more than a limited number of nerves in order to ascertain which are responsible for transmitting the patient's pain. It is important that the block is discrete, i.e. not involving adjacent nerves, and so provides an unequivocal response, especially when a subsequent permanent block is contemplated.

If permanent block of a single nerve is contemplated, this is carried out most conveniently with a radiofrequency lesion (if necessary in the dorsal root ganglion).

Trigeminal nerve and its branches

Blockade of the peripheral branches of the trigeminal nerve is often helpful in the management of facial pain.

Diagnostic blocks are performed with local anaesthetic followed by neurolytic drugs (alcohol, phenol) or, increasingly, the production of a radiofrequency lesion. The standard approaches are described in textbooks of local anaesthesia. Additional help is obtained from an image intensifier.

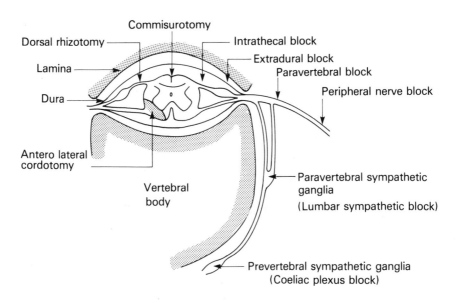

Fig. 40.1   Potential sites for interrupting pain pathways.

These blocks may be helpful for the pain of trigeminal neuralgia and that of head and neck malignancy, although blockade of the peripheral branches of the trigeminal nerve is often insufficient and trigeminal rhizotomy may be required (vide infra).

Extradural blocks

Extradural blocks may be performed at any level of the spinal cord from cervical to caudal. Blocks may be either therapeutic or diagnostic for distinguishing between low back pain of organic or psychogenic origin.

In patients with a limited life expectancy, the block may be repeated with a neurolytic solution (usually phenol), but comparatively large doses are required and the block is less precise than the intrathecal, which is usually preferred.

Mention has been made earlier of the use of extradural steroids, usually methylprednisolone, for the treatment of low back pain and sciatica. This indication probably accounts for the largest number of extradural blocks carried out in pain clinics. Useful pain relief is achieved in at least 60% of patients although the block may need repeating.

The pain of spinal nerve compression from spinal metastases may also respond dramatically to extradural steroids, presumably as a result of reduction of oedema and hence reduction in compression of nerve roots.

Intrathecal blocks

One of the most important historical developments in the management of pain of malignant origin was the introduction in 1931 of intrathecal neurolysis with alcohol by Dogliotti. This was refined subsequently by Maher in 1953 who used a hyperbaric solution of phenol in glycerine (in place of hypobaric alcohol).

The technique is ideally suited to those patients with pain confined to a few dermatomes, and although simple, requires meticulous attention to detail. Following full explanation of the technique and description of possible side-effects, lumbar puncture is performed under local anaesthesia with the patient lying on the painful side on an adjustable table.

A 22 G spinal needle (the finest through which it is possible to inject the viscous phenol in glycerine solution) is inserted with the bevel pointing downwards to just penetrate the dura. The patient is then rotated approx. 45° backwards so that the dorsal roots are most dependent (Fig. 40.2) and phenol in glycerine injected in small increments. Between each increment, the patient is questioned for the presence of sensations.

Usually the patient experiences a sensation of

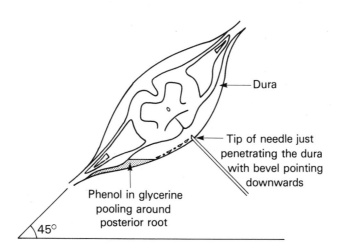

Fig. 40.2 Intrathecal phenol block.

warmth or paraesthesia in the area supplied by the roots bathed in phenol. If this coincides with the area in which the patient experiences pain, then the positioning is correct; if not, the table is tipped in order to move the solution in either a cephalad or caudad direction by gravity.

Further increments (maximum 1.0 ml) are injected until analgesia exists in the painful area. Occasionally patients do not experience paraesthesia and the only indication of the effect of the phenol is the development of anaesthesia, which must be sought in case it does not conform to the correct area.

Side-effects are confined usually to loss of sensation, which is frequently inevitable, but this may be accompanied by paraesthesiae, usually lasting only a few days. Motor block is rare, but if it occurs is probably the result of incorrect positioning.

A more common complication with blocks of sacral roots is disturbance of sphincter action. Unless there are pre-existing sphincter problems this is rare provided the block is unilateral. The resulting urinary retention requires catheterisation, but bladder function usually returns to normal within 2–3 weeks. Spinal headache is surprisingly rare.

The mean duration of analgesia is 3–4 months, but there is considerable variation. However, the technique is easily repeated if necessary.

Autonomic blocks

1. *Stellate ganglion block.* Stellate ganglion block is helpful in managing pain of vascular origin in the upper limb. Repeated blocks with local anaesthetic may be effective, but in view of the adjacent structures and the risks of intravascular or intrathecal injection, neurolytic blockade should be undertaken only by the expert.

2. *Coeliac plexus block.* Pain resulting from intra-abdominal malignancy (especially neoplasms of pancreas and stomach) is ablated readily by blocking the coeliac plexus with alcohol. The use of an image intensifier makes the positioning of needles more precise. The surface landmarks are shown in Fig. 40.3. A 12.5 cm needle is inserted below the 12th rib at a point level with the spinous process of L1. Depending on whether or not the angle of the 12th rib is wide or narrow, the point of insertion of the needle varies in distance (5–10 cm) from the midline, but the further from the midline the easier it is to direct the point of the needle medially in front of the vertebral body of L1.

The needle is inserted at an angle of approx. 45° to the skin and directed medially and slightly cephalad towards the spine of T12 so as just to pass in front of the upper part of the body of L1. The needles usually require insertion to a depth of approx. 10 cm and are inserted bilaterally for a complete block. Twenty five ml of 50% alcohol are injected through each needle. This injection is painful and should be preceded by local anaesthetic; alternatively the patient should be sedated.

The only significant complication of this technique is hypotension. This is occasionally profound and may be prolonged. It may be ameliorated by the use

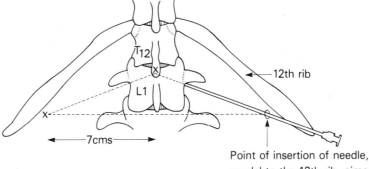

Point of insertion of needle,
caudal to the 12th rib, aimed
at the tip of the spine of T12
and inclined at 45° to the skin
to pass just anterior to the
body of L1

Fig. 40.3   Coeliac plexus block.

of elastic stockings and if necessary an abdominal binder.

3. *Lumbar sympathetic block*. Lumbar sympathetic block with phenol solution (chemical sympathectomy) may be useful for the relief of pain resulting from vascular insufficiency of the lower limbs. However, improvement in blood flow tends to be in the superficial tissues. Claudication may not be improved, and may even be worsened as a result of shunting of blood away from muscles.

The pain of claudication may be relieved by lumbar plexus block using a strength of neurolytic solution which blocks mainly small C fibres.

Radiofrequency lesions

Radiofrequency current may be used to produce lesions within the nervous system. This is a relatively recent technique which has proved very useful.

The radiofrequency electrode comprises an insulated needle with a small exposed tip. A high frequency alternating current flows from the electrode tip to the tissues, producing ionic agitation and a frictional heating effect in tissue adjacent to the tip of the probe. The magnitude of this heating effect is monitored by a thermistor in the tip of the electrode.

Damage to nerve fibres sufficient to block conduction occurs at temperatures above 45°C although in practice most lesions are made with a probe tip temperature of 60°–80°C. The size of the lesion is determined by the size of the exposed electrode tip and the duration and magnitude of heating. The lesion produced comprises all areas heated to 45°C or higher.

Since the lesion is small (average size 10 mm × 7 mm) most radiofrequency lesion generators are equipped with a nerve stimulator to aid accurate placement of the probe. Radiofrequency lesions may be made in almost any peripheral nerve or within the central nervous system (percutaneous cervical cordotomy, mid-brain tractotomy, thalamotomy, etc.)

An example of the use of radiofrequency lesions is the treatment of trigeminal neuralgia.

Trigeminal neuralgia is managed normally with one of the anticonvulsant drugs, e.g. carbamazepine. However, in a proportion of patients the pain is not controlled or the patient finds the side-effects of the drugs intolerable. These patients are treated by radiofrequency trigeminal rhizotomy. Under local or general anaesthesia an electrode is passed through the foramen ovale under image intensifier control so that the tip is amongst the trigeminal rootlets behind the ganglion (Fig. 40.4).

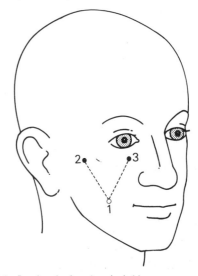

Fig. 40.4   Landmarks for trigeminal rhizotomy.
1 — Point of electrode insertion 2.5–3 cm lateral to labial commissure.
2 — A point 3 cm anterior to the external auditory meatus.
3 — A point below the medial border of the pupil with the patient looking straight ahead.

If anaesthetised, the patient is allowed to awaken and gentle electrical stimulation of the rootlets produces paraesthesia in the division in which the electrode lies. If this does not coincide with the distribution of the patient's pain, the patient is reanaesthetised if necessary, and the electrode manipulated until stimulation coincides with the area of pain.

Incremental radiofrequency lesions are made, monitoring the degree of sensory loss after each lesion. Results of this technique are excellent, affording patients good pain relief with minimal sensory loss.

Cryotherapy

Lesions may also be produced in the nervous system by cold. The cryoprobe consists of an insulated needle, but of larger gauge than the radiofrequency electrode. Cooling is effected by the Joule-Thompson effect using nitrous oxide as the refrigerant. The probe also carries a nerve stimulator for accurate localisation of the nerve.

Nerve destruction is produced by the disruptive effect of the formation of ice crystals within the cells and is enhanced by the application of more than one freeze-thaw cycle. The probe tip may reach a temperature as low as $-80°C$.

Blocking of peripheral nerves by cryotherapy appears to be completely reversible and this may offer advantages in certain situations. The technique has been used not only in chronic pain patients, but also for postoperative pain relief, e.g. at thoracotomy by cryotherapy of intercostal nerves.

Electrical nerve stimulation

It has been known for centuries that an electrical current (from electric catfish, rays, eels, etc.) can relieve pain. More recently, the use of electrical stimulation techniques has been based on the gate control theory of pain which is still accepted as valid, although it has undergone several revisions and has been criticised (see Chapter 5).

The simplest method of applying electrical stimulation to the nervous system is transcutaneous nerve stimulation (TNS). A small battery-powered stimulator is used to apply an electrical stimulus to the skin via flexible carbon electrodes.

The stimulator supplies a square wave or spike pulse with variable voltage, pulse width and frequency. Stimulation is applied at an intensity which the patient finds comfortable, with the electrodes positioned over the painful area, on either side of it, or over nerves supplying the area. The initial response is often good, but judgement of the efficacy of the technique should be delayed for a month or two as the placebo response rate is high. Adverse effects are minimal and are confined usually to allergic responses to the electrodes, gels or tapes, although electrical burns occur occasionally.

Electrical stimulation applied to the dorsal columns is also effective in relieving pain. Electrodes may be implanted either surgically over the dorsal columns or positioned in the extradural space via a Tuohy needle. Stimulation is applied and many patients obtain worthwhile pain relief. However, long-term results have been disappointing, possibly as a result of poor patient selection.

Stimulation by implanted electrodes of the periaqueductal and paraventricular grey matter of the brain, and also of various regions of the thalamus have been successful in abolishing pain, but these techniques are still experimental.

Acupuncture

For four thousand years the Chinese have known that the insertion of needles at certain points of the body may produce analgesia. Understandably this has been treated with some scepticism by Western physicians. However, there now seems little doubt that acupuncture or 'needle effect' has a useful part to play in the management of pain.

The mechanism of action of acupuncture analgesia is gradually becoming understood. It has been known for some time that naloxone reverses the effects of acupuncture and that injection of naloxone into the periaqueductal grey matter of animals also reduces the effect. Increases in c.s.f. endorphin levels have also been demonstrated. Furthermore, lesions of the anterolateral tracts have been demonstrated to prevent the occurrence of acupuncture analgesia. It appears, therefore, that acupuncture analgesia is mediated via Aβ Aδ and C fibres which, via the anterolateral tracts, relay to the periaqueductal grey matter and nucleus raphe magnus. It is possible that descending inhibitory pathways are then activated. There is also a correlation between acupuncture points and trigger points in myofascial syndromes.

Acupuncture points are described usually by the Chinese nomenclature, which provides a useful shorthand. They appear to be areas of low skin electrical resistance (in comparison with surrounding skin) and may be detected by a variety of point detectors which assess electrical resistance.

Modern acupuncture needles are of stainless steel and approx. 30 G. The points for treatment are selected and the needles (which should be sterile) inserted to depths varying from a few millimetres to several centimetres, according to the point.

For acupuncture analgesia to be effective it seems that patients must experience a sensation known as Te-Ch'i. It is described variously as a numbing, tingling or heavy sensation spreading from the acupuncture site. The needle should be manipulated until this sensation is elicited.

Stimulation of the points comprises mere insertion of the needles, manual stimulation by rotation between thumb and finger, electrical stimulation which may last 20 min or more, or a combination of these manoeuvres. Patients usually appreciate some change in level of pain, either during or shortly after treatment. This may last for a variable length of time, but it is customary to give a course of treatments. Acupuncture is now generally accepted as having a useful place in the pain relief clinic.

Pituitary alcohol injection

It has been known for many years that hormonal manipulations influence the course of malignant disease and associated pain.

Oophorectomy, adrenalectomy and hypophysectomy are all used in attempts to induce regression of hormone-dependent tumours, but have the disadvantage of being major operative procedures in patients whose general condition may be poor.

Chemical hypophysectomy is a technique designed to ablate the pituitary with minimal upset to the patient, and is achieved by injecting absolute alcohol into the gland. This is a remarkably simple and safe method of treating the pain of malignant disease and also, unlike other methods of pain control, carries the potential for regression of the tumours.

Cordotomy and other neurosurgical procedures

At first sight it would appear that the interruption of pathways in the central nervous system is an attractive way of relieving pain, since the lesion produced should not recover normal function and pain relief should be permanent.

In practice this is not so since pain eventually returns, although it is not clear if this is induced by regeneration or by development of alternative pathways. However, neurosurgical procedures are useful for some patients with a limited expectation of life.

In general, the closer to the periphery the surgical section of the pain pathway, the more certain is the subsequent pain relief; the more central the section, the more uncertain is pain relief as a result of multiple pain pathways. Section of peripheral nerve is followed rapidly by axonal regeneration, and dorsal root section also has a failure rate for reasons which are not understood fully.

Anterolateral cordotomy is probably the most widely used surgical procedure for the relief of pain. The anterolateral tracts of the cord are sectioned midway between root levels, and anaesthesia for pain and temperature are obtained on the contralateral side of the body, from three to four dermatomes below the level of section.

This technique has been refined in the form of a percutaneous technique at C1–2 level. A spinal needle is introduced under local anaesthesia into the neck approx. 1 cm below and posterior to the mastoid process. Under radiographic control it is aimed at the space between the first and second cervical vertebrae so that its tip pierces the dura just anterior to the dentate ligament. This is identified by injecting Myodil emulsion, and if the position is correct, a fine electrode, insulated except at the tip, is introduced through the needle into the spinal cord. The position of the electrode is checked by stimulation, when the patient should experience paraesthesia in the painful region on the opposite side of the body. If this occurs, incremental lesions are produced using radio-frequency current.

The patient will have anaesthesia to pain and temperature on the contralateral side in a zone dependent on the size and placement of the lesion.

Percutaneous cervical cordotomy with radio-frequency current is a procedure which may be undertaken in patients who are a relatively poor risk, since unlike surgical cordotomy, it does not entail a major surgical procedure.

Radiotherapy

Pain is often a feature of malignant disease, and where radiotherapy is given in the expectation of curing the patient's disease, relief of pain is incidental. However, even when there is no prospect of curing the patient, palliative radiotherapy may be valuable for controlling pain.

Reduction in tumour bulk often relieves pain by relief of pressure on adjacent nerves and other structures. This applies also to metastases, particularly those in bone. A similar effect may be achieved by the use of cytotoxic drugs and hormones.

Psychiatric aspects of pain relief

It is important that a pain relief clinic should have the help and advice of a skilled psychiatrist who is interested in the problems of patients with pain. The need for a psychiatrist illustrates the many facets of chronic pain and emphasises that the division between organic and psychogenic pain is largely false. His functions are threefold. Firstly, to diagnose and treat those patients presenting with frank psychiatric syndromes. Secondly, to offer advice and guidance on the use of psychotropic drugs, psychotherapy, hypnosis and other specialised techniques. Thirdly,

he will recognise personality disorders and patterns of behaviour which are maladaptive, and advise on treatment.

He is also of great help in the support of those patients in whom treatment appears impossible, but for whom the pain clinic may at least play a useful supportive role, preventing their endless search for further consultation and treatments.

FURTHER READING

Bond M R 1979 Pain. Its nature and treatment. Churchill Livingstone, London

Bond M R 1978 Psychological and psychiatric aspects of pain. Anaesthesia 33: 355

Budd K 1978 Psychotropic drugs in the treatment of chronic pain. Anaesthesia 33: 531

Budd K 1982 Pain. Update postgraduate series. Update Publications, London

Lipton S 1979 Relief of pain in clinical practice. Blackwell Scientific Publications, Edinburgh

Swerdlow M 1978 Relief of intractable pain. Excerpta Medica, Amsterdam

Szasz T S 1957 Pain and pleasure. Basic Books, New York

Trimble M R 1981 Neuropsychiatry. John Wiley & Sons, New York

Wood K M 1978 The use of phenol as a neurolytic agent. A review. Pain 5: 205

41

The operating theatre environment

The process whereby a patient is brought to the operating theatre, has an operation, and is returned safely to the surgical ward is complex. The environment in which this process is carried out may affect the outcome either to the benefit or to the detriment of the patient.

IDEAL ENVIRONMENT

A successful working environment should permit the achievement of certain objectives. The medical and nursing staff involved should be able to work together effectively. Patients and staff should be safe from hazards, e.g. infection, and mechanical or electrical dangers. The environment should permit a balance of economy and optimum utilisation of the facilities available. It is obvious that as surgical operations increase in complexity so also must the supporting activities of preoperative care, anaesthesia, monitoring and postoperative care. In the current economic climate, resources are likely to become scarcer despite demands for increasingly sophisticated facilities and equipment.

The objects of this chapter are to consider briefly several parts of the environment which excite current interest, and to speculate on possible innovations.

RECOVERY ROOM

The postoperative recovery room may be defined as a special-care facility adjacent to the operating theatre, offering close surveillance and care for patients, usually for a period of 1–4 h after surgery (or, in the absence of a separate facility, for up to 24 h). The period immediately following surgery is one of increased danger to the patient for many reasons which have been described in earlier chapters. During this period, the patient may develop respiratory complications which may be classified into three categories:

1. *Airway obstruction.* This occurs commonly with loss of consciousness. It may also be caused by aspiration of gastric contents following loss of protective reflexes.

2. *Hypoventilation.* Respiration may be inadequate because of drugs given to the patient in the operating theatre, for example muscle relaxants the effects of which are incompletely antagonised or opioid analgesics producing central respiratory depression.

3. *Hypoxaemia* may also be present because of ventilation-perfusion alterations in the patient's lungs associated with surgery and postoperative pain.

Cardiovascular instability may also be present during this period for a variety of reasons.

The patient's preoperative state is obviously important as is the magnitude of the surgery performed. The effects on the heart and circulation of some anaesthetic drugs may extend into the postoperative phase. Changes in blood volume may occur resulting from continued blood loss from wounds, or other fluid losses. A combination of pain and hypoxia increases the demand on a diseased heart perhaps to the point at which it may no longer maintain an adequate cardiac output. Pain and restlessness also occur in the immediate postoperative period.

It was only after the Second World War that attention was focused on the problems encountered during the early postoperative period. A study carried out at that time revealed that over 60% of anaesthetically related deaths were caused by poor monitoring of patients leading to unrecognised respiratory obstruction and death, and could therefore be classified as preventable. It would seem reasonable from the above discussion to assume that measures would have been taken to ensure the patient's safety throughout this time of recognised risk. Apparently, such an assumption may not be made even today according to the report of the Association of Anaesthetists of Great Britain and Ireland on morbidity and mortality (Lunn and Mushin, 1982). Lack of recovery room facilities was still a contributory factor in patients' deaths in a number of instances.

The value of a recovery room lies in the opportunity to detect complications at an early stage and to institute prompt treatment which may avert disaster.

Design of the recovery room

The size of the recovery room facility obviously depends on the number and type of operations being performed in the surgical suite. The DHSS, in the Hospital Building Note (1967) issued approximate guidelines for an average facility and recommends 1.5 spaces per theatre, each of 100 sq ft.

It would appear reasonable to place the unit close to both the operating suite and the intensive care unit so that patients are close to staff skilled in dealing with the problems outlined above.

Emphasis on recovery room nursing as a specialist service has emerged only in the last decade, and training of nurses remains discretionary rather than mandatory. Recent E.E.C. regulations offer a slight improvement in that all student nurses must spend one week in the recovery room.

Airway maintenance continues to be the most important task of the recovery room nurse, but nowadays this may include also care of those patients who benefit from short-term mechanical ventilation in the postoperative period.

Monitoring of patients and recording of vital signs enable the nurse to detect and prevent potentially life-threatening situations.

The recovery room offers distinct advantages over the ward for effective treatment of postoperative pain. Such therapy as i.v. titration of opioid analgesics or continuous extradural analgesia may be applied safely because of the higher nurse to patient ratio. It is obvious that a ratio of one fully trained recovery room nurse per patient would be ideal. Lower staffing ratios may be attractive financially in the short term but may prove to be a false economy in the light of recent court awards for damages sustained by patients under circumstances of poor postoperative supervision.

A recovery room should be equipped both to monitor the patient and to treat any complication which may arise. Each bedspace should have the monitoring capability for arterial pressure and e.c.g. and should have individual oxygen and suction outlets. There are several designs of bedhead unit which incorporate individual monitors and storage and shelf space for commonly used pieces of equipment, for example, airways, resuscitation bellows, i.v. fluids, and oxygen masks. In addition a trolley should be available which should contain the main items for resuscitation, e.g. laryngoscopes, endotracheal tubes, drugs and i.v. infusion apparatus, and defibrillator. It is also necessary to have a ventilator available for any patient who may require or benefit from short-term ventilatory support postoperatively. The trolley or bed on which the patient lies must be capable of tipping head-down.

A major improvement in postoperative care will be the expansion of these facilities to provide more prolonged care (up to 24 h) for those patients undergoing routine but major surgery, or those patients in whom optimum control of postoperative pain is vitally important and for whom special techniques, e.g. extradural anaesthesia, have been provided. In these groups may be included patients undergoing major vascular or thoracic surgery, those with morbid obesity having procedures such as gastroplasty, or those with poor respiratory function. The alternative at present may be either to send the patients back to the ward or to admit them to the intensive care unit where they may be exposed to the risk of nosocomial infection.

In a sense two major surgical specialities, cardiac and neurosurgical, have already utilised this approach and the terms recovery and intensive care are synonymous when applied to their patients.

HEALTH HAZARD IN THE OPERATING THEATRE ENVIRONMENT

The anaesthetic literature of the past 50 yr has suggested that personnel working in the operating room environment are at an increased risk of disease and ill health.

These reports have included complaints of a fairly minor nature, e.g. headache and fatigue, and also a variety of serious medical conditions which include a higher incidence of certain types of cancer, a higher frequency of spontaneous abortion amongst exposed female workers, and an increased risk of congenital abnormality in the offspring of exposed mothers. Pollution of the operating room by waste anaesthetic gases has been singled out as the culprit for most of these problems. The concentrations involved are in the order of 10 parts per million (ppm) of halothane and 600 ppm of nitrous oxide. However, the epidemiological studies which have been published have been criticised severely on methodological grounds. Most of the studies published have been retrospective in nature and have relied on the return of completed questionnaires from both the group under investigation and a control group. The quality of the data and validity of the inferences which may be drawn depend for example on high response rates to questionnaires for both study and control groups, an accurate memory for the events under investigation, and the absence of unforeseen differences between control and study group. The data gathered from such studies has tended to be contradictory.

Mortality

An earlier study revealed an apparent increased incidence of death from lymphoid and reticulo-endothelial tumours in anaesthetists than in the general population over the period 1947–66. However, when the same authors reviewed the mortality data for the years 1966–71, they found that anaesthetists had a lower incidence of these diseases than the general population. In fact it would seem that anaesthetists probably have lower death rates than physicians as a whole and are less likely to develop cancer than the average person.

Reproduction

The available data suggest that females exposed to the operating room environment have a higher incidence of spontaneous abortion than control females not exposed. However, there is no convincing data that this is causally related to contamination of the theatre environment and there may be other factors involved, e.g. stress.

Malformation

There does not appear to be any good data to support the view that offspring of operating room workers are at greater risk of having congenital abnormalities.

Laboratory studies

In animal studies, the effects of anaesthetic agents on fertility, reproduction, carcinogenesis and terato-genesis have been well investigated. Fertility was not affected by exposure to either trace concentrations of anaesthetic agents or to repeated exposure to surgical anaesthetic concentrations. It is possible however to demonstrate increased rate of spontaneous abortion following prolonged exposure to anaesthetic concentrations of anaesthetic gases and, in one experiment, to concentrations of nitrous oxide of 15 000 ppm. Abnormalities of the skeleton were found also in those animals exposed to surgical concentrations of anaesthetic agent. No currently used anaesthetic agent has been found to be carcinogenic in animal experiments even at levels which produce surgical anaesthesia. The balance of evidence is that these experiments do not provide convincing evidence that trace concentrations of anaesthetic gases are associated with a health hazard.

Stress and other factors

It is possible that other factors may be important in explaining the higher incidence of abortion in operating room staff. It is accepted that emotional and psychosomatic factors enter into the pathogenesis of spontaneous abortion. In this context the stress which the anaesthetist may feel during the performance of her work, in addition to fatigue, anxiety and irregular routine, may have a more important role to play than that of trace concentrations of anaesthetic agents.

Performance

Trace concentrations of anaesthetic agents have been implicated in another area of great concern to the anaesthetist in that it has been suggested that professional performance may be impaired. While it is obviously impractical to conduct experiments on the anaesthetist in the operating theatre, it is also difficult to develop a suitable laboratory study to measure performance. Motor aspects of performance have been tested by audiovisual reaction time tests which require a subject to respond to combinations of changes in a presented auditory signal, usually a fast or slow metronome beat, and a visual signal, usually an e.c.g. trace on the upper or lower part of the oscilloscope screen. This test is affected particularly by changes in the subject's state of vigilance. Memory and intelligence functions of performance may be measured by using the Wechsler Adult Intelligence scale. The initial study carried out using these methods revealed significant decrements in performance when subjects breathed concentrations of both nitrous oxide 500 ppm and halothane 15 ppm or nitrous oxide 500 ppm alone. However, these studies have been repeated in several laboratories in different countries and have failed to confirm these findings. Indeed more recent work suggests that concentrations of the order of 8–12% nitrous oxide are required before decrement in performance can be demonstrated.

It is possible that the anaesthetist may be at greater risk than other members of the operating room staff. His proximity to the expiratory valve and to the mask as this is applied to and removed from the patient may cause him to be exposed to much higher concentrations of waste gases. He is also in the operating room at the point of maximum exposure for the greatest amount of time and therefore would be at risk of any hazards related to chronic exposure.

Notwithstanding the lack of definite evidence linking pollution by waste anaesthetic gases to specific health hazards, the consensus of medical opinion appears to be to place the burden of proof on those who would argue their lack of harmful effects. In the meantime, scavenging of waste anaesthetic gases from the operating room has been recommended.

In this context, scavenging entails the collection of waste gases at the relief valve of the anaesthetic apparatus and its disposal outside the building. The regulations laid down in the U.S.A. to control pollution permit a maximum level of 25 ppm of nitrous oxide and 2 ppm of halothane in the environment of medical workers.

Air conditioning

The ventilation system of an operating room serves to prevent airborne bacterial contamination of wounds, to provide comfort for personnel, and to prevent arcing of electrostatic charges by maintaining high levels of humidity. Precise flow patterns of air in the operating room depend on a variety of factors. These include the positions of the ventilation ducts both for intake and output, the shape of the room, its temperature, the presence of people and pieces of equipment in the room and the effects of door opening. The precise flow patterns of gas within the room also affects the concentration of waste anaesthetic gases at various locations in the room. This variation in concentration of waste gases has important implications when attempts are made to measure pollution in the operating room. Attempts can be made by the use of smoke to detect flow patterns in the room in order to predict the sites of highest contamination.

It is obvious that an air conditioning system which permitted recirculation of air would be ineffective in reducing levels of anaesthetic contamination.

Methods of scavenging (see Chapter 16)

Before discussing specific methods for scavenging, it is worth mentioning that escape of anaesthetic gases may be minimised if a good seal between mask and patient is maintained, if the flow of gases is commenced only after anaesthesia is induced and if fresh gas flows are switched off when the patient is disconnected from the circuit.

Most scavenging systems comprise modification of the normal expiratory valve, usually of a type designed by Penlon or Enderby. Expired gases are removed from the valve by a length of attached tubing for disposal. One of the earliest concepts was simply to divert gas through a canister of activated charcoal, as in the Cardiff Aldasorber, which was capable of removing halogenated agents by the process of adsorption. This method was not effective for elimination of nitrous oxide. The short length of scavenging hose used in this system did not increase significantly the resistance to expiration. However, as alternative methods of waste disposal were investigated with longer pieces of hosing, it became necessary to add a suction source to the scavenging system to avoid any increase in resistance to expiration (a system of *active scavenging*). It is obviously important that such a system should not permit the direct application of negative pressure to the patient circuit. The simplest and most efficient method of scavenging is to dump the waste gas into the exhaust duct of a nonrecirculating air-conditioning system. Such a system should be designed into an operating room to ensure that there are conveniently sited exhaust grills. Failure to do so usually results in long lengths of tubing being laid along the floor and this carries the risk of accidental occlusion and respiratory obstruction.

Another solution has been to convey waste gases to the outside of the building directly by individual lengths of large diameter hosing which do not produce excessive back pressure in the breathing system. Each operating room however requires a separate system to prevent cross-contamination. This is commonly called a *passive scavenging system*.

The efficacy of whichever system is employed should be measured regularly as part of an air-monitoring programme. The mass spectrometer is a useful tool in permitting collection and analysis of pollutants and permits identification of the sites of greatest concentration in the room.

THE CHANGING ENVIRONMENT

It is interesting to consider the changes which may take place in the next decade in the anaesthetist's working environment.

Increasing numbers of operations

There appears to be a growing demand for operative surgical treatment of disease. A variety of factors is responsible for this phenomenon. Amongst the more important are increases in the numbers of elderly people in the population, recently conceived surgical operations (e.g. coronary artery bypass grafting for ischaemic heart disease, or extracranial to intracranial arterial anastomotic surgery for cerebrovascular disease), and not least are improvements in anaesthetic management of poor risk patients undergoing major surgery.

It is apparent, however, that the resources available to finance health care are limited and in order to provide additional services the system must be made to work more efficiently.

Computers

It seems likely that computers will feature prominently in the operating suite of the future. In certain institutions in the U.S.A., computer systems are used to facilitate management of large numbers of operating rooms. Their functions include co-ordinating the scheduling of patients for surgery, with the provision of the appropriate medical and nursing staff to carry out the procedure. The computer will also be utilised more as a tool for the rapid access of patient data.

A system already in use, the Hospital Information System (HIS), performs a series of useful tasks in improving efficiency in handling patients. This device stores information, both clinical and laboratory, on every patient and this information can be retrieved from any computer terminal in the hospital. The terminal may be used also to request additional investigations on the patient or to relay instructions on patient management to nursing staff.

The computer may be used to provide rapid access to information on topics of importance to the anaesthetist. For example, it is possible to establish a database containing guides for drug dosages or fluid balance in paediatric patients. Finally, use may be made of the ability of computers to perform rapid calculations in the operating room itself, e.g. to obtain derived haemodynamic variables from measurements of cardiovascular parameters.

FURTHER READING

Dubois R M 1981 Clinical information systems. Current trends and outlook for the '80s. Computers in Hospitals 2: 38

Farman J V 1978 The work of the recovery room. British Journal of Hospital Medicine 19 (6): 606

Laufman H 1981 Controversial issues in the design of surgical suites. In: Laufman H (ed) Hospital special-care facilities. Academic Press, New York

Lunn J N, Mushin W W 1982 Mortality associated with anaesthesia. Nuffield Provincial Hospitals Trust, London

Mishelevich D J 1981 Success factors in the implementation of a comprehensive hospital information system. Computers in Hospitals 2: 26

Smith G, Shirley A W 1978 A review of the effects of trace concentrations of anaesthetics on performance. British Journal of Anaesthesia 50: 701

Smith W D A 1978 Pollution and the anaesthetist. In: Atkinson R S, Langton-Hewer C (eds) Recent advances in anaesthesia and analgesia no 12. Churchill Livingstone, Edinburgh

Spence A A 1980 Uses of anaesthesia; postoperative care. British Medical Journal 281: 367

Vessey M P 1978 Epidemiological studies of the occupational hazards of anaesthesia. A review. Anaesthesia 33: 430

Appendices

APPENDIX I(a)
Abbreviations

Abbreviations in appendices

BP	boiling point	Eq	equivalent (physical chemical term)
mol.wt	molecular weight	SI	Systeme International d'Unites
SVP	saturated vapour pressure		(International system of units)
mmHg	millimetres mercury $\simeq$ 130 pascals (Pa)	TWC	total water content
Flam	Flammability	e.c.f.	extracellular fluid
°C	degrees Celsius	i.c.f.	intracellular fluid
E/T	endotracheal	CHO	carbohydrate
μg	microgram (10^{-6} gram)	N/A	not available
mg	milligram (10^{-3} gram)	Respiratory	
μlitre	microlitre (10^{-6} litre)	physiology	see XI(a)
kg	kilogram (10^{3} gram)	cp	centipoise
mol	mole		
osmol	osmole		
h	hour		
min	minute		
s	second		

SI units (bracketing μg, mg, μlitre, kg)

APPENDIX I(b)
SI System

The Systeme International d'Unites (SI system) has been developed to reduce the large number of units in everyday physical use, to a much smaller number, with standard symbols.

The seven base units are derivatives of the M.K.S. System of physical measurement.

Length	metre	m
Mass	kilogram	kg
Time	second	s
Electric current	amp	A
Thermodynamic temperature	kelvin	K
Amount of substance	mole	mol
Luminous intensity	candela	cd

Any other units are derived units and may be expressed by multiplication or division of base units.

Volume	cubic metre	—	m^3
Force	newton	N	$kg.m.s^{-2} = J.m^{-1}$ (J/m)
Work	joule	J	$kg.m^2s^{-2} = N.m$ (Nm)
Power (rate of work)	watt	W	$kg.m^2.s^{-3} = J.s^{-1}$ (J/s)
Pressure (force/area)	pascal	Pa	$kg.m^{-1}.s^{-2} = N.m^{-2}$ (N/m²)

The solidus (/) has been used in preference to X^{-1}, either of which is specified in the standard.

Nonstandard units such as the litre, day, hour, and minute may be used with SI but are not part of the standard.

Volume

The SI unit of volume is the cubic metre, but for medical purposes the litre (1 dm³) is retained.

Temperature

A temperature difference of 1 kelvin is numerically equivalent to 1 degree Celsius. In everyday use the degree Celsius is retained. The Fahrenheit scale is no longer used medically and is being phased out of use with the general public.

The magnitude of a unit is expressed by the additions of standard prefixes and symbolic prefixes. The magnitude of SI units usually changes by 10^3 per step.

Fraction	SI prefix	Symbol	Multiple	SI prefix	Symbol
10^{-1}	deci	d	10	deca	da
10^{-2}	centi	c	10^2	hecto	h
10^{-3}	milli	m	10^3	kilo	k
10^{-6}	micro	μ	10^6	mega	M
10^{-9}	nano	n	10^9	giga	G
10^{-12}	pico	p	10^{12}	tera	T
10^{-15}	femto	f			
10^{-18}	atto	a			

It can be seen that the SI handling of 'kilogram' is slightly nonstandard in that the name of the base unit already contains a preficacial multiple. Names of decimal multiples and submultiples of the unit of mass are formed by attaching prefixes to the word 'gram'.

Moles

$$\text{Moles} = \frac{\text{Weight in g}}{\text{molecular weight}}$$

$$\text{thus, 1 mole } H_2O = \frac{18 \text{ g}}{18}$$

$$18 \text{ g } H_2O = 1 \text{ mole}$$

For univalent ions, moles and equivalent are numerically similar, but for multivalent ions, the number of equivalents must be divided by the valency to obtain the molar value. Thus 10 mEq Ca^{++} = 5 mmol Ca^{++}.

APPENDIX II
Anaesthetic agents — physical properties

Name	Formula	Mol. wt	BP (°C)	SVP mmHg (at 20°C)	MAC (%)	Flam. in O_2(%)	H_2O Gas	Oil Gas	Blood Gas	Oil H_2O
Chloroform	$CHCl_3$	119	61	160	0.5	0	40	260	10	100
Cyclopropane	$CH_2CH_2CH_2$	42	−33	4800	9.2	2–60	0.20	11.5	0.45	34.4
Enflurane	$CHFCl.CF_2$ O CF_2H	184.5	56	175	1.68	6	0.78	98	1.9	120.1
Ether (diethyl)	C_2H_5 O C_2H_5	74	35	425	1.9	2–82	13	65	12	3.2
Ethyl chloride	C_2H_5Cl	64.5	13	988	2.0	4–67	1.2	—	3.0	—
Fluroxene	CF_3CH_2 O $CH.CH_2$	126	43	286	3.5	4	0.85	48	1.4	90
Halothane	$CF_3CHClBr$	197	50	243	0.8	0	0.8	220	2.5	220
Isoflurane	CF_3CHCl O CF_2H	184.5	49	250	1.15	6	0.62	97	1.4	174
Methoxyflurane	$CHCl_2.CF_2$ O CH_3	165	105	23	0.2	5–28	4.5	950	13	400
Nitrous oxide	N_2O	44	−88	(39 800)	105	0	0.44	1.4	0.47	3.2
Trichloroethylene	$CHCl . CCl_2$	131	87	60	0.17	9–65	1.7	960	9.0	400

Ostwald coefficients of solubilities @ 37°C

APPENDIX III
Chemical pathology — biochemical values

These values are given for example only — each reporting laboratory provides 'normal values' for its own population and method. This is especially true of enzyme assays. Values given are those obtained from Chemical Pathology in Leicester, where these are available. No inference should be made about the molecular weight of a substance by reference to US and SI values

Name	US units	SI units
Adrenaline	100 pg/ml	0.55 nmol/litre
Amino acid nitrogen	4–8 mg%	3–6 mmol/litre
Ammonia	80—110 µg%	47–65 µmol/litre
Amylase	80–180 Somogyi units%	70–300 i.u./litre
Base excess	± 2 mEq/litre	± 2 mmol/litre
Bicarbonate — actual	22–30 mEq/litre	22–30 mmol/litre
standard	21–25 mEq/litre	21–25 mmol/litre
Bilirubin — total	0.3–1.1 mg%	3–18 µmol/litre
Buffer base (pH 7.4, Pa_{CO_2} 5.3) (Hb 15 g/dl)	48 mEq/litre	48 mmol/litre
Calcium — total	8.5–10.5 mg% (4.5–5.7 mEq/litre)	2.25–2.6 mmol/litre
ionised	4–5 mg%	1.0–1.25 mmol/litre
Chloride	95–105 mEq/litre	95–105 mmol/litre
Cholesterol	140–300 mg%	3.6–7.8 mmol/litre
Cholinesterase plasma (pseudo-cholinesterase)	Dibucaine number >80% usually normal	
	Dibucaine number <20% usually homozygote for atypical cholinesterase	
Copper	80–150 µg%	13–24 nmol/litre
Urinary copper	15–50 µg/24 h	0.2–0.8 µmol/24 h
Cortisol — 0900 } RIA tech 2400	9–23 µg/24 h <7.2 µg%	200–650 nmol/litre <200 nmol/litre
neonatal (competitive protein-binding tech.)	30 µg/litre	110–1076 nmol/litre
Creatine phosopho-kinase (CK)	100 i.u./litre — male 60 i.u./litre — female	25–200 i.u./litre 25–200 i.u./litre
Creatinine	0.5–1.4 mg%	45–120 µmol/litre

Name	US units	SI units
Fibrinogen	150–400 mg%	1.5–4.0 g/litre
Folate	3–20 ng/ml	3–20 µg/litre 2.1–27 nmol/litre
Glucose — fasting	55–85 mg%	3.0–4.6 mmol/litre
post prandial	<180 mg%	<10 mmol/litre
Gamma glutamyl transpeptidase	7–25 i.u./litre	10–55 i.u./litre
Hydroxybutyrate dehydrogenase (HBD)		100–240 i.u./litre
Iodine — total	3.5–8.0 µg/litre	273–624 nmol/litre
[131]I uptake	20–50% of administered dose in 24 h	
Iron	80–160 µg%	14–30 µmol/litre
Iron binding capacity	250–400 µg%	45–69 µmol/litre
Lactate	0.6–1.8 mEq/litre	0.6–1.8 mmol/litre
Lactate dehydrogenase	30–90 i.u./litre	100–300 i.u./litre
Lead		<1.8 µmol/litre
Magnesium	1–2 mg% 1.5–2.0 mEq/litre	0.7–1.0 mmol/litre
Methaemoglobin	<3% of total haemoglobin.	
Nitrogen (non-protein) (urea + urate + creatinine + creatine)	18–30 mg%	12.8–21.4 mmol/litre
Noradrenaline	200 pg/ml	1.25 nmol/ml
Osmolality	280–300 mOsmol/kg	280–300 mosmol/kg
Phosphate	2.0–4.5 mg% 3.0–6.0 mg% (children) <8.1 mg%	0.8–1.4 mmol/litre 1.0–1.8 mmol/litre (children) <2.6 mmol/litre (neonatal)
Phosphatase — acid (total) acid (prostatic) alkaline	1–5 KA units% 3–13 KA units%	1–9 i.u./litre 0–3 i.u./litre 17–100 i.u./litre
Potassium	3.4–5.3 mEq/litre	3.4–5.3 mmol/litre
Protein — total albumin globulin	6.0–8.0 g% 3.5–5.0 g 1.5–3.0 g%	60–80 g/litre 35–50 g/litre 15–30 g/litre
Pyruvate	0.4–0.7 mg%	34–80 µmol/litre
Sodium	133–148 mEq/litre	133–148 mmol/litre
Thyroxine (T_4)	4.7–11 µg%	52–140 nmol/litre

Name	US units	SI units	Name	US units	SI units
Transaminase:			Triglycerides (fasting)	71–160 mg%	0.8—1.8 mmol/litre
Aspartate			Triiodothyronine (T$_3$)	90–170 ng%	0.8—2.5 mmol/litre
transaminase			T$_3$ uptake	95–117%	95–117%
— AST	5–40 units/ml	5–30 i.u./litre	Urea	15–48 mg%	2.7–7.0 mmol/litre
Alanine transaminase			Urea nitrogen (BUN)	10–20 mg%	1.6–3.3 mmol/lire
— ALT		2–53 i.u./litre	Urate — men	4–9.5 mg%	240–590 μmol/litre
Transferrin	220–400 mg%	2.2–40.0 g/litre	women	3–7.5 mg%	170–460 μmol/litre

APPENDIX IV(a)
Cardiovascular system

NORMAL VALUES FOR VARIABLES

Blood flows	% of cardiac output	Flow (ml/min) (70 kg man)
Heart	4	200
Brain	14	700
Liver	25	1250
Kidneys	24	1200
Lung	3	150
Muscle	19	950
Skin	5	250
Fat	5	250
Remainder	1	50
Total	100	5000

E.C.G. TIMES

P wave	< 0.10 s
PR interval	0.12–0.20 s
QRS time	0.05–0.08 s
QT time	0.35–0.40 s
T wave	< 0.22 s

PRESSURES (mmHg)

	Range	Mean
Central venous pressure (CVP)		
(Zero reference point right atrium)	0–7	
Right atrium (RA)	1–10	5
Right ventricle (RV)	14–30 / 0–7	25 / 3
Pulmonary artery (PA)	15–30 / 5–12	23 / 9
Pulmonary artery wedge (PAWP)	5–15	10
Left atrium (LA)	8	8
Left ventricular end-diastolic (LVEDP)	4–10	8

DERIVED HAEMODYNAMIC VARIABLES

			Normal value (70 kg)
Cardiac output (CO)	=	$SV \times HR$	5 litre/min
Cardiac index (CI)	=	$\dfrac{CO}{\text{Body surface area}}$	3.2 litre/min/m²
Stroke volume (SV)	=	$\dfrac{CO}{HR} \times 1000$	80 ml
Stroke index (SI)	=	$\dfrac{SV}{\text{Body surface area}}$	50 ml/m²
Systemic vascular resistance (SVR)	=	$\dfrac{\text{Mean arterial pressure} - CVP}{CO} \times \dfrac{80}{1}$	1000–1200 dyne s/cm⁵
Pulmonary vascular resistance (PVR)	=	$\dfrac{\text{Mean pulmonary artery} - \text{left atrial pressure}}{CO}$	60–120 dyne s/cm⁵
Left ventricular stroke work index (LVSWI)	=	$\dfrac{1.36 (\text{Mean arterial} - \text{left atrial pressure})}{100} \times SI$	50–60 g m/m²
Rate pressure product (RPP)	=	Systolic arterial pressure $\times$ heart rate	
Ejection fraction (EF)	=	$\dfrac{\text{End systolic} - \text{end diastolic volumes}}{\text{end diastolic volume}}$	greater than 0.6

APPENDIX IV(b)

VASOACTIVE INFUSIONS

Sympathomimetic drugs

Drug	Dilution into 500 ml Dextrose 5%	Typical dosage range
Adrenaline (low — α, β_{1+2}) (higher — α)	5 mg = 10 μg/ml	Start 0.02–0.05 μg/kg/min Most respond to less than 0.2 μg/kg/min Greater than 0.5 μg/kg/min leads to excess vasoconstriction
Dobutamine (β_1)	250 mg = 500 μg/ml	0.5–20 μg/kg/min
Dopamine (low — δ) (moderate — δ + β_{2+1}) (high — α, β_1)	200 mg = 400 μg/ml OR 800 mg = 1600 μg/ml	0.5–5 μg/kg/min (low) 5–10 μg/kg/min (moderate) >15 μg/kg/min (high)
Isoprenaline (β_{1+2})	4 mg = 8 μg/ml	0.02–0.4 μg/kg/min
Metaraminol (α)	50 mg = 100 μg/ml	0.1–1 μg/kg/min infrequent use as infusion
Noradrenaline (α, β_1)	4 mg = 8 μg/ml	0.05–0.2 μg/kg/min
Phenylephrine (α)	25 mg = 50 μg/ml	0.1–0.5 μg/kg/min
Salbutamol (β_2)	5 mg = 10 μg/ml	0.1–0.5 μg/kg/min

Miscellaneous

Disopyramide (membrane stabilisation)	500 mg into 450 ml Dextrose 5% or Saline 0.9% = 1000 μg/ml	5–7 μg/kg/min after loading dose — see data sheet
Glyceryl trinitrate (VENOUS and arteriolar dilator) N.B. Do not use with PVC giving set	50–100 mg into 500 ml Dextrose 5% or Saline 0.9% = 100–200 μg/ml	10–200 μg/min (0.2–3 μg/kg/min)
Isosorbide dinitrate (VENOUS and arteriolar dilator)	50 mg into 450 ml Dextrose 5% or Saline 0.9% = 100 μg/ml	30–120 μg/min (0.6–2 μg/kg/min)
Lignocaine (membrane stabilisation)	1 g into 500 ml Dextrose 5% or Saline 0.9% = 2 mg/ml = 2000 μg/ml	25–50 μg/kg/min after loading dose — see data sheet

APPENDIX IV(b) *(contd)*

Drug	Dilution	Typical dosage range
Mexiletine (membrane stabilisation)	250 mg into 500 ml Dextrose 5% or Saline 0.9% = 500 μg/ml	500 μg/min after loading dose — see data sheet
Sodium nitroprusside (arteriolar and venous dilator) N.B. Protect from light	50 mg into 500 ml Dextrose 5% = 100 μg/ml	0.5–8 μg/kg/min (for hypertensive crisis) 0.1–1.5 μg/kg/min (during hypotensive anaesthesia)

APPENDIX IV(c)

DRUGS USED AT CARDIAC ARREST

Drug	Dose	Action
Adrenaline 1:1000 (1 mg/ml) 1:10000 (1 mg/10 ml)	100 μg–1 mg i.v. or intracardiac	α- and β- receptor stimulator. May cause ventricular tachycardia or fibrillation
Atropine 0.5–1.2 mg/ml	0.6–1.8 mg	Mainly via vagal nucleus, 'blocks vagus'. Decreases vagal tone and increases heart rate especially when due to sinus bradycardia
Bretylium	5–10 mg/kg	Prolongs action potential. 'Pharmacological defibrillator'. Used in refractory ventricular fibrillation
Calcium chloride 10% (0.68 mmol Ca^{++}/ml) Calcium gluconate 10% (0.225 mmol Ca^{++}/ml) (Physical incompatibility with bicarbonate)	10 ml	Inotropic. May cause ventricular asystole in tonic contraction
Diphenylhydantoin (phenytoin) 50 mg/ml	50–100 mg	Membrane stabilisation. Especially in digitalis induced arrhythmia. Disopyramide or mexiletine may be preferred.
Disopyramide 10 mg/ml	50–150 mg	Membrane stabilisation. ↓ tendency for tachyarrhythmias (inc. digitalis-induced)
Lignocaine 2% 20 mg/ml	100 mg	Membrane stabilisation. ↓ tendency for tachyarrhythmias
Mexiletine 25 mg/ml	100 mg	Membrane stabilisation. ↓ tendency for tachyarrhythmias (inc. digitalis-induced)
Practolol 2 mg/ml	5 mg	β-blocker — for SVT. Do not give VERAPAMIL subsequently
Sodium bicarbonate 8.4% 1 mmol/ml (incompatible with Ca^{++})	50 mmol	Corrects acidosis Allows easier recovery of spontaneous activity
Verapamil 2.5 mg/ml NOT with β-blockers	5–10 mg	Calcium antagonist. Supraventricular tachyarrhythmias such as Wolff-Parkinson-White syndrome

APPENDIX V
Endotracheal and tracheostomy tube size

Age (yr)	ET and tracheostomy tube size int. diam. (mm)	ET length (cm) Oral	Nasal	Age (yr)	ET and tracheostomy tube size int. diam. (mm)	ET length (cm) Oral	Nasal
0–3 month	3.0	10		9	6.0	16	19
	3.0	10–11		10	6.5	17	20
3–6 month	3.5	12	15	11	6.5	17	20
6–12 month	4.0	12	15	12	7.0	18	21
2	4.5	13	16	13	7.0	18	21
3	4.5	13	16	14	7.5	21	24
4	5.0	14	17	15	7.5	21	24
5	5.0	14	17	16	8.0	21	24
6	5.5	15	18	17	9.0	22	25
7	5.5	15	18	18	9.5	22	25
8	6.5	16	19	20	9.5	23	26

Below 8–10 yr, noncuffed tubes should be used.
It is always advisable to have available a tube one size smaller than calculated.

APPENDIX VI(a)
Fluid balance

FLUID COMPOSITION OF BODY COMPARTMENTS

Blood volumes
Infant   90 ml/kg body weight
Child   80 ml/kg body weight
Adult male   70 ml/kg body weight
Adult female   60 ml/kg body weight

Total water content (TWC)
60% ♂ 55% ♀ of body weight (18–40 yr)
55% ♂ 46% ♀ of body weight (>60 yr)

Volume of e.c.f. 35% TWC
Volume of i.c.f. 65% TWC

APPENDIX VI(b)

FLUID, ELECTROLYTE AND NUTRITIONAL REQUIREMENTS

Minimum daily requirements per kg for adults and children and neonates.

	Adults *(per kg)*	*Children and neonates* *(per kg)*		*Adults* *(per kg)*	*Children and neonates* *(per kg)*
Water	30–35 ml	100–150 ml	Mn^{++}	0.6 μmol	1 μmol
Energy	35–40 kcal	90–125 kcal	Zn^{++}	0.3 μmol	0.6 μmol
	(0.15 MJ)	(0.38–0.5 MJ)	Cu^+	0.07 μmol	0.3 μmol
Amino acids			Cl^-	1.3–1.9 mmol	1..8–4.3 mmol
(nitrogen)	90 mg	330–350 mg			
Protein	0.6–0.9 g	1.8 g			
Glucose	2–3 g	12–18 g			
Fat	2 g	4 g			
Na^+	1–1.4 mmol	1–2.5 mmol			
K^+	0.7–0.9 mmol	2 mmol			
Ca^{++}	0.11 mmol	0.5–1 mmol			
Mg^{++}	0.04 mmol	0.15 mmol			
Fe^{++}	1 μmol	2 μmol			

Neonates

1st day — $\frac{1}{4}$ calculated fluid requirement.
2nd day — $\frac{1}{2}$ calculated fluid requirement.
3rd day — $\frac{3}{4}$ calculated fluid requirement.
4th day — normal calculated fluid requirement.
Premature babies have differing requirements.

APPENDIX VI(c)

INTRAOPERATIVE FLUID REQUIREMENTS (This does not apply in first 3 days of life.)

  (1) Initial volume — 1.5 ml/kg/hr for duration of preoperative starvation

+ (2) Maintenance — 1.5 ml/kg/hr

+ (3) Operative insensible loss — e.g. 1–2 litre for abdominal surgery in adult

+ (4) Blood loss — replace with blood when loss exceeds 20% of estimated blood volume in adults

or 10% of estimated blood volume in children

APPENDIX VI(d)

COMPOSITION OF COMMON I.V. FLUIDS

Name	pH	Calculated* osmolality	Na+	K+	Cl–	HCO3–	Misc	CHO g/litre	Protein g/litre	MJ/ litre
Sodium chloride 0.9%	5.0	308	154	0	154	0	0	0	0	0
Dextrose 5%	4.0	280	0	0	0	0	0	50	0	0.84
Dextrose 4% } Saline 0.18% }	4.5	286	31	0	31	0	0	40	0	0.67
Dextrose 5% } Saline 0.45% }	4.5	430	77	0	77	0	0	50	0	0.84
Lactated Ringer's (Hartmanns solution)	6.5	280	131	5	112	29 (as lact)	Mg^{2+} 1 Ca^{2+} 1	0	0	0.038
Sodium bicarbonate 8.4%	8.0	2000	1000	0	0	1000	0	0	0	0
Haemaccel (Hoechst)	7.4	Colloid oncotic pressure ca. 370 mmH2O	145	5.1	145	0	Ca^{2+} 6.25 PO_4^{2+} Trace SO_4^{2+} Trace	0	35	0
Gelofusin (Consol. Chem)	7.4	Colloid oncotic pressure ca. 456 mmH2O	154	0.4	125	0	Ca^{2+} 0.4 Mg^{2+} 0.4	0	40	0
Dextran 70 in NaCl 0.9%	4–7	N/A	154	0	154	0	0	0	0	0
Dextran 70 in Dextrose 5%	3.5–7	N/A	0	0	0	0	0	50	0	0.84

Human plasma protein fraction 7.4　　　275　　　　　150　2　　120　　　—　　　—　　　　　　—　　　40
(HPPF) (PPF) — 4%　(100 ml 20% salt poor also available — ionic content varies with manufacturer)

Whole blood　　　　　usually > 6.5　　Depends upon donor values. K+ increases with storage time

Plasma reduced blood usually > 6.5　　Depends on donor values. K+ is higher than whole blood — but *quantity* of K+ is similar

Packed cells　　　　　usually > 6.5　　Usually low Na+ and K+ load cf. whole blood, due to late separation of plasma from red cells

Accepted safe storage times at 4°C for whole blood depend upon type of preservative and (in the case of packed cells) time of separation

Heparinised blood — only available for special applications

Acid citrate dextrose (ACD) — 21 days

Citrate phosphate dextrose (CPD) — 28 days

Citrate phosphate dextrose adenine (CPD-A₁) — 35 days

* = Calculated value. Assumes total dissociation of ions.

APPENDIX VII
Gas flows in anaesthetic circuits

	Spontaneous ventilation	IPPV
Magill (Mapleson A) (not suitable for children <6 yr)	MV (theoretically V_A) 70 ml/kg/min	MV × 2.5
Bain (Mapleson D) (suitable for children)	150–200 ml/kg/min	70 ml/kg/min for Pa_{CO_2} of 5.3 kPa 100 ml/kg/min for Pa_{CO_2} of 4.3 kPa
Ayre's T piece (Mapleson E)	2 × MV	As for Bain circuit Minimum 3 litre/min

NORMAL VENTILATION VALUES FOR RESTING AWAKE SUBJECTS

Weight	Minute volume (ml)	Tidal volume (ml)	Frequency (breath/min)
Neonate 2 kg	480	14–16	30–45
3 kg	600	17–24	25–40
10 kg	1680	80	21
20 kg	3040	160	19
30 kg	4080	240	17
40 kg	4800	320	15
50 kg	5200	400	13
60 kg	5280	480	11
70 kg	5600	560	10

APPENDIX VIII(a)
Haematology

NORMAL VALUES

Haemoglobin	men	13.5–18.0
	women	11.5–16.5
	10–12 yr	11.5–14.8
	12/12	11.0–13.0
	3/12	9.5–12.5
	full term	13.6–19.6

g/dl

Red blood cell count (RBC)	men	4.5–6.0 × 10^{12}/litre
	women	3.5–5.0 × 10^{12}/litre

White blood cell count (WBC)	4.0–11.0 × 10^9/litre
Neutrophils	40–70%
Lymphocytes	20–45%
Monocytes	2–10%
Eosinophils	1– 6%
Basophils	0– 1%

Platelet count   150–400 × 10^9/litre

Reticulocyte count   0–2% of RBC

Sedimentation rate	men	0–15 mm in 1 h
	women	0–20 mm in 1 h

Plasma viscosity   1.50–1.72 cp

Packed cell volume (PCV)	men	0.4–0.55
Haematocrit (Hct)	women	0.36–0.47

Mean corpuscular volume (MCV)   76–96 fl

Mean corpuscular haemoglobin concentration (MCHC)   31–35 g/dl

Mean corpuscular haemoglobin (MCH)   27–32 pg

fl = femtolitre (10^{-15} litre)
g = gram (10^{-3} kilogram)

cp = centipoise (not an SI unit)
mm = millimetre (10^{-3} metre)

dl = decilitre (10^{-1} litre)
pg = picogram (10^{-15} kilogram) (10^{-12} gram)

h = hour

APPENDIX VIII(b)

NORMAL VALUES FOR COAGULATION TESTS

Activated clotting time – ACT (Haemochron type)	80–135 s
Antithrombin III	>80% normal
Bleeding time (platelet function)	2–9 min
Clotting time (largely replaced by ACT)	3–11 min
Fibrinogen — plasma	1.5–4 g/litre
Fibrin degradation products — FDP	<10 mg/litre (µg/ml)
Kaolin cephalin clotting time — KCCT (same test as PTTK — vide infra)	35–45 s
KCCT/PTTK — Heparin therapy value	2–4 times control
Partial thromboplastin time Kaolin — PTTK (same test as KCCT — vide supra)	35–45 s
Platelet count	150–400 × 10^9/litre
Prothrombin time	12–14 s

Prothrombin ratio — normal	1.0–1.2
— therapeutic	2.0–4.0

Reptilase clotting time. Heparin independent	<Thrombin CT + 4 s vide infra

Thrombin clotting time — TCT. Heparin dependent   c. 15 s

Thrombotest — normal	70–130%
— therapeutic	5–15%

mg = milligram (10^{-6} kilogram) (10^{-3} gram)
µg = microgram (10^{-9} kilogram) (10^{-6} gram)

APPENDIX VIII(c)

ABNORMAL COAGULATION TESTS

Consumption coagulopathy (DIC)
  Early — decreased platelets
        — increased FDP
        — Presence of $\begin{cases} \text{thrombin/antithrombin complexes} \\ \text{fibrinopeptide A} \end{cases}$

  Late — abnormal PTTK
       — abnormal prothrombin time

Dilutional coagulopathy or *Massive blood transfusion*
  Increased prothrombin time — >20 s
  Decreased Thrombotest — <30%

Abnormal liver
  Early — decreased activity of vit. K-dependent tests — PT —
        (PTTK — later)
  Late — massive derangement of some or all coagulation tests

APPENDIX IX(a)
Paediatrics

DOSES OF DRUGS IN PAEDIATRIC ANAESTHESIA

Premedication

Atropine	20 μg/kg
Hyoscine	20 μg/kg
Glycopyrrolate	5 μg/kg
Diazepam	0.2–0.4 mg/kg
Droperidol	0.1–0.2 mg/kg
Trimeprazine	2–4 mg/kg

Intravenous induction

Thiopentone	4–5 mg/kg
Methohexitone	1 mg/kg
Etomidate	0.3 mg/kg
Ketamine	2 mg/kg

Other induction routes

Thiopentone rectal	30 mg/kg
Methohexitone rectal	25 mg/kg
Ketamine intramuscular	10 mg/kg

Neuromuscular blocking drugs

Suxamethonium	1–2 mg/kg
Tubocurarine	0.5–0.6 mg/kg
Pancuronium	0.08–0.1 mg/kg
Alcuronium	0.25–0.3 mg/kg
Atracurium	0.5 mg/kg

Reversal

Neostigmine	50–80 μg/kg
Atropine	20–40 μg/kg

Analgesics

Morphine	0.2 mg/kg
Papaveretum	0.3 mg/kg
Fentanyl	0.5–1.5 μg/kg
Alfentanil	2.5–5 μg/kg

Local analgesics (maximum safe dose)

Lignocaine	5 mg/kg
Bupivacaine	2 mg/kg
Prilocaine	6 mg/kg

APPENDIX IX(b)

FLUID AND ELECTROLYTE REQUIREMENTS IN INFANCY AND CHILDHOOD

Weight	Rate
Up to 10 kg	100 ml/kg/day
10 to 30 kg	1000 ml + 50 × [wt (kg) − 10] ml/kg/day
20 to 30 kg	1500 ml + 25 × [wt (kg) − 20] ml/kg/day

Fluid requirements in the first week of life

Day	Rate
1	0
2, 3	50 ml/kg/day
4, 5	75 ml/kg/day
6	100 ml/kg/day
7	120 ml/kg/day

	Age (yr)									
	1 week	1	2	3	4	5	6	7	8	9	10
Weight (kg)	3.5	10	13	15	17	19	21	23	25	28	32
Insensible water loss (ml/kg/day)	30	27.5	27	26.5	26	25	24	23	22	21	20
Water requirement (ml/kg/day)	120	100	88	83	80	76	73	68	65	61	56
Na^+ requirement (mmol/kg/day)	4	3	2.5	2	2	1.9	1.9	1.9	1.8	1.75	1.7
K^+ requirement (mmol/kg/day)	2.5	2	2	2	2	1.75	1.75	1.5	1.5	1.5	1.5

These are basal requirements. Additional fluid (10–20%) is required during major surgery, in addition to replacement of overt losses. During the postoperative period, fluid requirements are increased in the presence of pyrexia. Fluid and electrolyte balance should be adjusted after measurement of serum electrolyte concentrations and serum osmolality.

APPENDIX X
Renal function tests

Clearance tests

Inulin clearance $\simeq$ glomerular filtration	100–150 ml/min
PAH clearance $\simeq$ renal plasma flow	560–830 ml/min
Creatinine clearance	
$\simeq$ glomerular filtration rate (over-estimates low GFR)	104–125 ml/min

Blood tests

Serum/plasma

Osmolality	280–300 mosmol/kg
Creatinine	45–120 μmol/litre
Urea	2.7–7.0 mmol/litre
Urea nitrogen	1.6–3.3 mmol/litre

Urine tests

Osmolality	300–1200 mosmol/kg
Creatinine	8.85–17.7 mmol/24 h
Sodium	50–200 mmol/24 h

Comparative urinary values

	Sp. gr	Osmolality	U/P urea ratio	U/P osmolality
Normal	1000–1040	300–1200	>20:1	>2.0:1
Prerenal failure	>1022	>400	>20:1	>2.0:1
Renal failure:				
Early	1010	<350	<14:1	<1.7:1
Late			<5:1	<1.1:1

APPENDIX XI(a)
Respiratory function tests

ABBREVIATIONS COMMONLY USED

Primary symbols

C = concentration of gas — blood phase
D = diffusing capacity
F = fractional concentration in the dry gas phase
P = partial pressure — gas
Q = volume of blood
R = respiratory exchange ratio
S = saturation of haemoglobin with oxygen or carbon dioxide
V = volume of gas
$\dot{X}$ = dot above symbol indicates 'per unit time'
$\bar{X}$ = bar above symbol indicates 'mean value'

Example: Pa_{O_2} = partial pressure — arterial — oxygen.

Secondary symbols

Usually typed as subscripts, capital letters indicate gaseous phase; lower case letters indicate liquid phase.

A = alveolar
B = barometric
D = dead space
E = expired
I = inspired
T = tidal
a = arterial
c = capillary (pulmonary capillary)
v = venous

LUNG SPIROMETRY

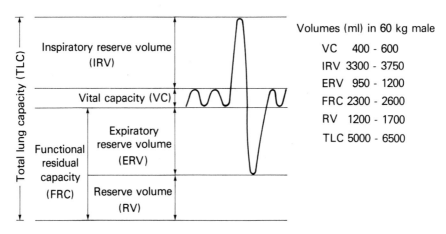

Volumes (ml) in 60 kg male

VC   400 - 600
IRV 3300 - 3750
ERV 950 - 1200
FRC 2300 - 2600
RV 1200 - 1700
TLC 5000 - 6500

Fig. XI(a)   Lung volumes in an average healthy male adult.

APPENDIX XI(b)

PULMONARY FUNCTION TESTS — FEMALES

Age (y)	Height (cm)	$FEV_{1.0}$ (litre)	FVC (litre)	$FEV_{1.0}/FVC$ (%)	PEFR (litre/min)
20	145	2.60	3.13	81.0	377
20	152	2.83	3.45	81.0	403
20	160	3.09	3.83	81.0	433
20	168	3.36	4.20	81.0	459
20	175	3.59	4.53	81.0	489
30	145	2.45	2.98	79.9	366
30	152	2.68	3.30	79.9	392
30	160	2.94	3.68	79.9	422
30	168	3.21	4.05	79.9	448
30	175	3.44	4.38	79.9	478
40	145	2.15	2.68	77.7	345
40	152	2.38	3.00	77.7	371
40	160	2.64	3.38	77.7	401
10	168	2.91	3.75	77.7	427
40	175	3.14	4.08	77.7	457
50	145	1.85	2.38	75.5	324
50	152	2.08	2.70	75.5	350
50	160	2.34	3.08	75.5	380
50	168	2.61	3.45	75.5	406
50	175	2.84	3.78	75.5	436
60	145	1.55	2.08	73.2	303
60	152	1.78	2.40	73.2	329
60	160	2.04	2.78	73.2	359
60	168	2.31	3.15	73.2	385
60	175	2.54	3.48	73.2	415
70	145	1.25	1.78	71.0	282
70	152	1.48	2.10	71.0	308
70	160	1.74	2.48	71.0	338
70	168	2.01	2.85	71.0	364
70	175	2.24	3.18	71.0	394

APPENDIX XI(b) *(contd)*

PULMONARY FUNCTION TESTS — MALES

Age (y)	Height (cm)	$FEV_{1.0}$ (litre)	FVC (litre)	$FEV_{1.0}$/FVC (%)	PEFR (litre/min)
20	160	3.61	4.17	82.5	572
20	168	3.86	4.53	82.5	597
20	175	4.15	4.95	82.5	625
20	183	4.44	5.37	82.5	654
20	191	4.69	5.73	82.5	679
30	160	3.45	4.06	80.6	560
30	168	3.71	4.42	80.6	584
30	175	4.00	4.84	80.6	612
30	183	4.28	5.26	80.6	640
30	191	4.54	5.62	80.6	665
40	160	3.14	3.84	76.9	536
40	168	3.40	4.20	76.9	559
40	175	3.69	4.62	76.9	586
40	183	3.97	5.04	76.9	613
40	191	4.23	5.40	76.9	636
50	160	2.83	3.62	73.1	512
50	168	3.09	3.98	73.1	534
50	175	3.38	4.40	73.1	560
50	183	3.66	4.82	73.1	585
50	191	3.92	5.18	73.1	608
60	160	2.52	3.40	69.4	488
60	168	2.78	3.76	69.4	509
60	175	3.06	4.18	69.4	533
60	183	3.35	4.60	69.4	558
60	191	3.61	4.96	69.4	579
70	160	2.21	3.18	65.7	464
70	168	2.47	3.54	65.7	484
70	175	2.75	3.96	65.7	507
70	183	3.04	4.38	65.7	530
70	191	3.30	4.74	65.7	551

APPENDIX XI(c)

LUNG FUNCTION: ADULT AND NEONATAL VALUES

Examples

	Adult (65 kg)	Neonate (3 kg)		Adult (65 kg)	Neonate (3 kg)
V_D	2.2 ml/kg	2–3 ml/kg			
V_T	7–10 ml/kg	5–7 ml/kg	Respiratory rate	12–18 breath/min	25–40 breath/min
$\dot{V}_E$	85–100 ml/kg/min	100–200 ml/kg/min	Pa_{O_2}	12.6 kPa (95 mmHg)	9 kPa (68 mmHg)
Vital capacity	50–55 ml/kg	33 ml/kg	Pa_{CO_2}	5.3 kPa (40 mmHg)	4.5 kPa (33 mmHg)

Acknowledgements

Many of the figures and diagrams incorporated in the text have been redrawn or modified from original diagrams appearing elsewhere. We therefore gratefully acknowledge permission from authors, publishers and editors in respect of the following:

CHAPTER 1

Fig. 1. 15 *from* Lord Brock 1982 Lung abscess, 2nd edn. Blackwell Scientific Publications, Oxford.

Fig. 1.21 *from* Lee, J.A. & Atkinson, R.C. 1978 Lumbar puncture and spinal anaesthesia. Churchill Livingstone, Edinburgh.

Figs 1.3, 1.4, 1.5, 1.10, 1.11, 1.12, 1.13, 1.14, 1.16, 1.17, 1.18, 1.19 and 1.20 *from* Ellis, H. & Feldman, S. 1977 Anatomy for anaesthetists, 3rd edn. Blackwell Scientific Publications, Oxford.

CHAPTER 3

Fig. 3.14 *from* Smith, J.J. & Kampine, J.P. 1980 Circulatory physiology — the essentials. Williams and Wilkins, Baltimore.

Fig. 3.15 *from* Guyton, A.C. 1967 New England Journal of Medicine 277: 805.

Fig. 3.19 *from* Ledingham, I.McA. & Hanning, C.D. In (Eds) Gray, T.C., Nunn, J.E. & Utting, J.F. 1980 General anaesthesia, 4th edn. Butterworths, London.

Fig. 3.20 *from* Prys-Roberts, C. 1980 The circulation in anaesthesia. Blackwell Scientific Publications, Oxford.

CHAPTER 5

Fig. 5.1 *from* Chapnick, P. 1973 Skin of ourselves. Science, April: 20.

Figs 5.15, 5.17, 5.18, 5.29, 5.30 and 5.41 *from* Bell, G.H., Emslie-Smith, D.M. & Paterson, C.R. 1980 Textbook of physiology, 10th edn. Churchill Livingstone, Edinburgh.

Figs 5.2, 5.3, 5.4, 5.5, 5.6, 5.7 and 5.14 *from* Hendry, B. 1981 Membrane physiology and cell excitation. Helm Croom,

Figs 5.8, 5.9 and 5.10 *from* Maze, M. 1981 Clinical implications of membrane receptor function in anaesthesia. Anesthesiology 55: 160.

Fig. 5.11 *from* Braesrup, C. 1982 Neurotransmitters and CNS disease: anxiety. Lancet 2: 1030.

Fig. 5.13 *from* Spero, L. 1982 Neurotransmitters and CNS disease: epilepsy. Lancet 2: 1319.

Figs 5.19, 5.20, 5.22, 5.23A, 5.25, 5.26, 5.27 and 5.28 *from* Mitchell, G.A. Essentials of neuroanatomy, 3rd edn. Churchill Livingstone, London.

Figs 5.21A and 5.21B *from* Green, J.H. 1976 An introduction to human physiology, 4th edn. Oxford University Press, Oxford.

Figs 5.23B and 5.36 *from* Ganong, W.F. 1979 Review of medical physiology, 9th edn. Lange Medical Publications, California.

Fig. 5.24 *from* Patten, J.P. 1977 Neurological differential diagnosis. Starke, London.

Fig. 5.31 *from* Jessel, T.M. 1982 Neurotransmitters and CNS disease: pain. Lancet 2: 1084.

Fig. 5.32 *from* Lipton, S. 1979 The control of chronic pain. Edward Arnold, London.

Fig. 5.33 *from* Gray, T.C., Nunn, J.F. & Utting, J.E. (Eds) 1980 General anaesthesia, 4th edn. Butterworth, London.

Fig. 5.37 *from* Branthwaite, M. 1980 Anaesthesia for cardiac surgery and allied procedures. Blackwell Scientific Publications, Oxford.

Fig. 5.39 *from* Greenberg, R.P. & Ducker, T.B. 1982 Evoked potentials in the clinical neurosciences. Journal of Neurosurgery 56: 1.

CHAPTER 9

Fig. 9.2 *from* Price, H.L., Kounatt, P.J., Safer, J.N., Conner, E.H. & Price, M.L. 1960 Journal of Clinical Pharmacology & Therapeutics, Vol. I, No. 1: 16.

Table 9.1, 9.2 and 9.4 *from* Dundee, J.W. 1979 Intravenous anaesthetic agents. Edward Arnold, London.

CHAPTER 11

Fig. 11.3 *from* Churchill-Davidson, H.C. 1965 Anesthesiology 26: 224.

CHAPTER 17

Fig. 17.2 *from* Atkinson, R.S., Rushman, G.B. & Lee, J.A. 1982 A synopsis of anaesthesia, 9th edn. John Wright, Bristol.

Fig. 17.3 *from* Lichtiger, M. & Moya, F. (Eds) 1978 Introduction to the practice of anaesthesia, 2nd edn. Harper and Row, Hagerstown, Maryland.

CHAPTER 18

Figs 18.3, 18.4, 18.6 and 18.15 *from* Scurr, C. & Feldman, S. 1982 Anaesthesia, 3rd edn. William Heinemann, London.

CHAPTER 20

Figs 20.2 and 20.6 *from* West, J.B. 1977 Pulmonary pathophysiology — the essentials. Blackwell Scientific Publications, Oxford.

CHAPTER 23

Figs 23.1 and 23.2 *from* Lichtiger, M. & Moya, F. (Eds) 1978 Introduction to the practice of anaesthesia, 2nd edn. Harper and Row, Hagerstown, Maryland.

Figs 23.4 and 23.5 *from* Ellis, H. & Feldman, S. 1977 Anatomy for anaesthetists, 3rd edn. Blackwell Scientific Publications, Oxford.

Fig. 23.6 *from* Moore, D.C. 1979 Regional block, 4th edn. Charles C. Thomas, Springfield, Illinois.

CHAPTER 27
Fig. 27.3 *from* Kitahata, L.M., Galicich, J.H. & Sato, I. 1971 Journal of Neurosurgery 34: 185.

CHAPTER 28
Fig. 28.4 *from* Cameron, E. 1983 Hospital Update, Vol. 9, No. 4: 429.

CHAPTER 31
Figs 31.3 and 31.4 *from* Lichtiger, M. & Moya, F. (Eds) 1978 Introduction to the practice of anaesthesia, 2nd edn. Harper and Row, Hagerstown, Maryland.
Figs 31.1 and 31.2 *from* Cousins, M.J. & Bridenbaugh, P.O. (Eds) 1980 Neural blockade: pain management. J.B. Lippincott Co., Philadelphia.

CHAPTER 35
Fig. 35.2 *from* Cole, P. In Langton Hewer, C. & Atkinson, R.S. 1979 Recent advances in anaesthesia and analgesia, Vol. 13. Churchill Livingstone, London.

CHAPTER 38
Fig. 38.1 *from* Feldman, S. & Ellis, H. 1975 Principles of resuscitation, 2nd edn. Blackwell Scientific Publications, Oxford.
Figs 38.2 and 38.3 *from* Gilston, A. & Resnekov, L. 1971 Cardio-respiratory resuscitation. William Heinemann, London.

APPENDIX XI(b) *from* Cotes, J.E. 1979 Lung function, 4th edn. Blackwell Scientific Publications, Oxford.

Index